HANDBOOK OF CHILD HEALTH ASSESSMENT

WILEY SERIES ON HEALTH PSYCHOLOGY/BEHAVIORAL MEDICINE

Thomas J. Boll, Series Editor

THE PSYCHOLOGIST AS EXPERT WITNESS
by Theodore H. Blau

HEALTH, ILLNESS, AND FAMILIES: A LIFE-SPAN PERSPECTIVE
edited by Dennis C. Turk and Robert D. Kerns

MEASUREMENT STRATEGIES IN HEALTH PSYCHOLOGY
edited by Paul Karoly

HEALTH AND INDUSTRY: A BEHAVIORAL MEDICINE PERSPECTIVE
edited by Michael F. Cataldo and Thomas J. Coates

CHILD HEALTH BEHAVIOR: A BEHAVIORAL PEDIATRICS PERSPECTIVE
edited by Norman A. Krasnegor, Josephine D. Arastch, and Michael F. Cataldo

HANDBOOK OF STRESS, REACTIVITY, AND CARDIOVASCULAR DISEASE
edited by Karen A. Matthews, Stephen M. Weiss, Thomas Detre, Theodore M. Dembroski, Bonita Falkner, Stephen B. Manuck, and Redford B. Williams, Jr.

TYPE A BEHAVIOR PATTERN: RESEARCH, THEORY, AND INTERVENTION
edited by B. Kent Houston and C. R. Snyder

HANDBOOK OF CHILD HEALTH ASSESSMENT: BIOPSYCHOSOCIAL PERSPECTIVES
edited by Paul Karoly

HANDBOOK OF CHILD HEALTH ASSESSMENT

BIOPSYCHOSOCIAL PERSPECTIVES

Edited by

PAUL KAROLY

WILEY

A Wiley-Interscience Publication

JOHN WILEY & SONS

New York / Chichester / Brisbane / Toronto / Singapore

This publication is designed to provide accurate and authoritative information in regard to the subject matter covered. It is sold with the understanding that the publisher is not engaged in rendering legal, accounting, or other professional service. If legal advice or other expert assistance is required, the services of a competent professional person should be sought. *From a Declaration of Principles jointly adopted by a Committee of the American Bar Association and a Committee of Publishers.*

Library of Congress Cataloging in Publication Data:

Handbook of child health assessment.

(Wiley series on health pyschology/behavioral medicine)

Includes bibliographies and indexes.
1. Pediatrics—Psychological aspects. 2. Clinical health psychology. 3. Children—Diseases—Diagnosis—Psychological aspects. 4. Behavioral assessment of children. I. Karoly, Paul. II. Series [DNLM: 1. Child Behavior. 2. Child Development. 3. Child Health Services. WS 105 H2353]

RJ47.5.H37 1988 155.4 88-29482
ISBN 0-471-83628-1

Printed in the United States of America

10 9 8 7 6 5 4 3 2 1

For

my daughter

Hollis Catherine

Contributors

J. Gerald Beales, Ph.D., District Health Promotion Officer, North Derbyshire Health Authority, Scarsdale Hospital, Chesterfield, Great Britain

Steven J. Beck, Ph.D., Associate Professor of Psychology, Department of Psychology, The Ohio State University, Columbus, Ohio

Robert Berg, M.D., Director, Pediatric Clinic, Maricopa County General Hospital, Phoenix, Arizona

Thomas J. Boll, Ph.D., Professor of Psychology, Director, Medical Psychology Program, University of Alabama in Birmingham, University Station, Birmingham, Alabama

Andrew S. Bradlyn, Ph.D., Assistant Professor of Psychology, Department of Clinical Psychology, University of Florida, Gainesville, Florida

Laurie Chassin, Ph.D., Professor of Psychology, Department of Psychology, Arizona State University, Tempe, Arizona

Edward R. Christophersen, Ph.D., Professor of Pediatrics, Chief, Behavioral Sciences Section, College of Health Sciences and Hospital, The University of Kansas Medical Center, Kansas City, Kansas

Anne P. Copeland, Ph.D., Associate Professor of Psychology, Department of Psychology, Boston University, Boston, Massachusetts

Daniel L. Coury, M.D., Assistant Professor of Pediatrics, Department of Pediatrics, Children's Hospital, The Ohio State University, Columbus, Ohio

Erich G. Duchmann, M.A., Graduate Student, Department of Psychology, Louisiana State University, Baton Rouge, Louisiana

Julia L. Eisenstein, M.A., Graduate Student, Department of Psychology, Boston University, Boston, Massachusetts

Pauline D. Elkins, M.A., Graduate Student, Department of Psychology, The University of Alabama, University, Alabama

Debra Fanurik, M.A., Graduate Student, Department of Psychology, The University of Alabama, University, Alabama

Sally Flagler, M.A., Graduate Student, Department of Psychology, The University of Oklahoma, Norman, Oklahoma

Alice G. Friedman, Ph.D., Psychologist, Department of Psychiatry and Behavioral Sciences, The University of Oklahoma, Norman Oklahoma

David S. Gochman, Ph.D., Professor, College of Urban and Public Affairs, Kent School of Social Work, University of Louisville, Louisville, Kentucky

Roger S. Hamada, Predoctoral Intern, Department of Psychiatry, Judge Baker Guidance Center and Children's Hospital, Boston, Massachusetts

James H. Johnson, Ph.D., Associate Professor of Psychology, Department of Clinical Psychology, College of Health Related Professions, University of Florida, Gainesville, Florida

Paul Karoly, Ph.D., Professor of Psychology, Director of Clinical Training, Department of Psychology, Arizona State University, Tempe, Arizona

Mary Klinnert, Ph.D., Pediatric Psychologist, National Jewish Center for Immunology and Respiratory Medicine, Denver, Colorado

Thomas R. Kratochwill, Ph.D., Professor and Director, School Psychology Program, Department of Educational Psychology, University of Wisconsin—Madison, Madison, Wisconsin

William E. MacLean, Jr., Ph.D., Assistant Professor of Psychology, Peabody College, Vanderbilt University, Nashville, Tennessee

Diane Marques, Clinical Fellow in Psychology, Department of Psychiatry, Harvard Medical School, Cambridge, Massachusetts

Judith R. Mathews, M.A., Intern in Behavioral Pediatrics, The University of Kansas Medical Center, Kansas City, Kansas

Hamilton I. McCubbin, Ph.D., Dean, School of Family Resources and Consumer Sciences, University of Wisconsin—Madison, Madison, Wisconsin

Marilyn A. McCubbin, Ph.D., School of Nursing, University of Wisconsin—Madison, Madison, Wisconsin

John McGrew, Graduate Student, Department of Psychology, Indiana University—Bloomington, Bloomington, Indiana

Sandra J. McKenzie, M.A., Graduate Student, Department of Psychology, Louisiana State University, Baton Rouge, Louisiana

David A. Mrazek, M.D., M.R.C. Psych, Director, Pediatric Psychiatry, National Jewish Center for Immunology and Respiratory Medicine, Denver, Colorado

James M. Perrin, M.D., Chief, Ambulatory Care Programs and General Pediatrics, Children's Service, Massachusetts General Hospital, Boston, Massachusetts

James Popejoy, Graduate Student, Department of Psychology, Wichita State University, Wichita, Kansas

Clark C. Presson, Ph.D., Associate Professor of Psychology, Department of Psychology, Arizona State University, Tempe, Arizona

Jeanetta Rains, Graduate Student, Department of Psychology, Wichita State University, Wichita, Kansas

Michael C. Roberts, Ph.D., Associate Professor of Psychology, Department of Psychology, The University of Alabama, University, Alabama

Vivienne Roseby, M.S., Graduate Student, Department of Educational Psychology, University of Wisconsin—Madison, Madison, Wisconsin

Dennis C. Russo, Ph.D., Director, Behavioral Medicine Program, The Children's Hospital, Boston, Massachusetts

Morgan T. Sammons, M.C., Graduate Student, Department of Counselor Education, Arizona State University, Tempe, Arizona

Ronald Seifer, Ph.D., Psychologist, Bradley Hospital, Brown University, East Providence, Rhode Island

William Shaw, Psy.D., Psychologist, Department of Psychiatry and Behavioral Sciences, The University of Oklahoma, Oklahoma City, Oklahoma

Steven J. Sherman, Ph.D., Professor of Psychology, Indiana University, Bloomington, Indiana

Lawrence J. Siegel, Ph.D., Associate Professor, Department of Pediatrics, Child Development Division, The University of Texas Medical Branch, Galveston, Texas

Laura K. Smith, M.A., Graduate Student, Department of Psychology, Ohio State University, Columbus, Ohio

James Snyder, Ph.D., Associate Professor of Psychology, Department of Psychology, Wichita State University, Wichita, Kansas

C. Eugene Walker, Ph.D., Professor and Director of Pediatric Psychology, Department of Psychiatry and Behavioral Sciences, University of Oklahoma College of Medicine, Oklahoma City, Oklahoma

Donald A. Williamson, Ph.D., Associate Professor and Director of the Psychological Services Center, Department of Psychology, Louisiana State University, Baton Rouge, Louisiana

Logan Wright, Ph.D., Professor of Psychology, Department of Psychology, University of Oklahoma, Norman, Oklahoma

Series Preface

This series is addressed to clinicians and scientists who are interested in human behavior relevant to the promotion and maintenance of health and the prevention and treatment of illness. *Health psychology* and *Behavioral medicine* are terms that refer to both the scientific investigation and interdisciplinary integration of behavioral and biomedical knowledge and technology to prevention, diagnosis, treatment, and rehabilitation.

The major and purposely somewhat general areas of both health psychology and behavioral medicine which will receive greatest emphasis in this series are: theoretical issues of bio-psycho-social function, diagnosis, treatment, and maintenance; issues of organizational impact on human performance and an individual's impact on organizational functioning; development and implementation of technology for understanding, enhancing, or remediating human behavior and its impact on health and function; and clinical considerations with children and adults, alone, in groups, or in families that contribute to the scientific and practical/clinical knowledge of those charged with the care of patients.

The series encompasses considerations as intellectually broad as psychology and as numerous as the multitude of areas of evaluation, treatment, prevention, and maintenance that make up the field of medicine. It is the aim of the series to provide a vehicle which will focus attention on both the breadth and the interrelated nature of the sciences and practices making up health psychology and behavioral medicine.

THOMAS J. BOLL

The University of Alabama in Birmingham
Birmingham, Alabama

Preface

To the traditional medical (biological) perspective on health and illness, there has been added, in recent years, a psychosocial accompaniment—the frameworks of *health psychology* and *behavioral medicine*. The three approaches are considerably more in tune than they are dissonant—despite the sometimes strident voices within each calling for the subjugation of the others. For while medicine examines its subjects organically, and health psychology takes an intradisciplinary tack (drawing on the subdomains within general psychology), and while behavioral medicine claims to wed behavioral science to medical science (interdisciplinarily), the differences are often more apparent than real. Advocates of each framework talk to their patients, probe symptom perceptions and historical background (biographical) factors, consider the relevance of current living arrangements and lifestyle pursuits, and, in general, seek to contextualize the presenting problem(s).

In teaching health psychology and behavioral medicine courses to graduate and undergraduate students over the past 10 years, this author has drawn a multidimensional conceptual roadmap that highlights the *what*, *why*, and *how* of the terrain and shows quite clearly that the three "distinct" models converge in both their targets (the *what*) and their purposes (the *why*). All approaches, for example, focus upon: (1) acute illness and its focal problems; (2) chronic illness and its focal problems; and (3) the vulnerabilities (risk factors) of the physically healthy. Similarly, all share three common purposes: (1) intervention and education; (2) prevention; and (3) assessment. While it may seem obvious or even trivial, the key points of demarcation among the various perspectives are strictly procedural—there are important differences in *how* the varied purposes are articulated. Further, these differences are not always sharply defined.

It is not in the best interests of the public (whether healthy or ill) for psychologists, physicians, epidemiologists, sociologists, physical therapists, social workers, nurses, or other "allied health professionals" to utilize the same methods or tools. This is not what *interdisciplinary* study is about. What *is* critical is for each field to appreciate and understand the unique perspective of the other.

I have found it useful, then, further to characterize the terrain by delineating several general dimensions along which investigative procedures differ. These include: (1) levels of analysis; (2) modes of analysis; and (3) the temporal framework. *Levels of analysis* vary from the *micro* to the *macro*, beginning (molecularly) with biochemical and physiological assays and moving to overt motor responses, self-descriptive (trait) accounts, cognitive (information processing) styles, social (interactional) analyses, familial transactions, ecological, sociocultural, and historical accounts. Clearly, biomedical perspectives tend toward the "micro" end, while psychological accounts are middle level. Any content domain (such as pain in acute illness, compliance in chronic illness, or AIDS susceptibility in the physically healthy) can be fruitfully apprehended via any level of analysis; and each has its unique contribution to make in capturing potentially important realities. *Modes of analysis* refer in our multidimensional roadmap to different ways of interpreting the data obtained across levels. Specifically, one can adopt a unitary, static, or content-oriented stance versus a systematic, dynamic, dialectical, relational, or process-oriented stance. For example, we can think of stress as a set of life events happening to a person or as changing interaction between such occurrences and their internal appraisals. Finally, we can examine health and illness in terms of distinct *time-related foci*—in the here and now (contemporaneously), as a pre–post change, cross-sectionally, or truly developmentally.

It has been my didactic objective to show how the behavioral sciences (particularly psychology) and medicine examine their shared targets and pursue their shared purposes along distinct yet compatible procedural pathways. Organized around key analytic targets and multiple levels, my earlier edited text, *Measurement Strategies in Health Psychology* (Karoly, 1985), focused on topics mainly relevant to *adult* illness and health risks from the assessment perspective. Its goals were to review, for behavioral scientists, the current state of the art and to assist medical professionals in appreciating and understanding alternative analytic frameworks. Throughout, it was assumed that intervention and prevention are built upon the bedrock of assessment. Soon after the completion of that book project, it became obvious to me that a companion volume was needed focusing upon the health and illness problems of *children and adolescents*, built around a similar levels-of-analysis framework. The current volume is the end result of the efforts of a large group of health professionals who have addressed the fundamentals of pediatric biopsychosocial assessment. I trust that this book will facilitate the growth of the child assessment enterprise and foster interdisciplinary understanding.

I have many people to thank for their efforts on behalf of this work. First, the contributors must be acknowledged for their willingness to think, write, and revise under time pressure. My colleagues in the department of psychology are acknowledged for creating an intellectual atmosphere conducive to scholarly pursuits. My secretary, LaVaun Habegger, was highly instrumental in the production of a finished manuscript. And finally, my wife, Dr. Linda Ruehlman, provided intellectual and emotional support tirelessly, unselfishly, and affectionately. She loves and hates this book almost as much as I do.

PAUL KAROLY

Tempe, Arizona
March 1988

Contents

PART I

GENERAL CONCEPTS AND ISSUES

1

Child Health Assessment: Toward a Biopsychosocial Frame of Reference

PAUL KAROLY

Since the dawn of civilization, attempts to fix the nature of health and illness have been subject to the peculiar influences of social and historical imperatives. As Ackerknecht (1982) advised:

> A doctor cannot appreciate too early the fact that his profession is a part and product of society, and that it is always closely connected with religion, philosophy, economics, politics, and the whole of human culture. (p. xviii)

However, modern medicine has largely sought to present the face of a highly specific and objective biotechnology, capable of zeroing in upon threats to well-being with apparent mathematical precision. While hardly claiming infallibility, today's medical health professionals can nonetheless draw upon such an impressive arsenal of proven methodologies for diagnosing and treating disease that few

---

The preparation of this chapter was supported in part by grant #PMH 39246-03, establishing the Preventive Intervention Research Center (PIRC) at Arizona State University.

"outsiders" can claim to understand their methods, let alone offer alternative rationales or analytic frameworks. Understandably, the "whole of human culture" has not found a firm place in the typical medical school curriculum.

The study of children's health (pediatrics) has likewise become a domain requiring a wide range of technical skills relevant to the diagnosis, treatment, and prevention of disorders of growth and development. In recent years, the field of pediatrics has, in fact, seen even greater pressures toward specialization, with office-based practitioners and hospital- or clinic-based subspecialists often competing for a role in child and family health care (Haggerty, 1986). So-called developmental disabilities have become an area of special concern for a new breed of physicians—*developmental pediatricians*—for whom an additional 2 years of study is required after the pediatric residency (Msall & Ichord, 1986). Until recently, the liaison between pediatrics and a broader spectrum of professionals knowledgeable about developmental features in adaptation has existed solely via child psychiatry and traditional child clinical psychology (cf. Appendix 2 of this volume).

Fortunately, despite mounting economic pressures and a technological knowledge explosion that strongly justifies a consolidation of didactic efforts, major changes in the nature of illness patterns and the causes of death (morbidity and mortality) have given renewed meaning to the wisdom of the whole person (or whole child) approach to clinical practice.

Decreasing rates of infant mortality, improvements in survival from infectious diseases (such as measles, influenza, and pneumonia), and vast improvements in the care of children with chronic illnesses have all dramatically altered the conceptual as well as the practical bases of pediatrics. Child health professionals must now learn to think in terms of early illness detection, prevention of accidents and addictive disorders, and the maintenance of adaptive functioning in healthy youngsters, as well as in the terms of long-term behavioral compliance for those children with chronic conditions. As Haggerty (1986) has suggested:

> It is clear that pediatric practice will be more concerned in the next two decades with health promotion, care of children with behavior problems and prevention of such problems (especially biopsychosocial disorders). . . . A special role for the pediatrician is to care for children with psychosomatic problems. (p. 14)

The so-called new morbidity has been met with renewed calls for a widening of perspectives—far short of "the whole of human culture," but clearly inter- and multidisciplinary in nature. Words like *psychosomatic* have taken on special vitality, promising to replace the de facto dualism and mechanism of traditional biomedicine with an integrated, multicause–multieffect model of functioning that elevates environmental, psychological, nutritional, and social forces to an equal footing, etiologically and predictively, with biology and genetics. This *biopsychosocial* perspective is an emergent rather than a tangible accomplishment. To embrace a viable guiding framework, workers within all relevant disciplines have to work more closely together or, at the very least, truly understand, respect, and make use of each other's expertise.

Unlike their medical colleagues who work exclusively with adults, child health specialists have rarely had the luxury of approaching their patients in isolation. Pediatrics, as a discipline, has long sought a longitudinal or process view of child patients, appreciating by necessity the role of emotional and cognitive growth, family influences (for better and for worse), academic demands, and peer influences.

The major new development is that the advancement of pediatrics now requires a more formal commitment to the study of (1) how attitudes and behaviors maintain health and prevent disease, (2) various forms of hidden psychiatric morbidity among children and adolescents, (3) the role of stress and other contextual factors in disease onset and/or maintenance, and (4) individual differences in vulnerability and resilience among youngsters in families. In essence, the purpose of this volume is to acquaint both social scientists (psychologists, sociologists, medical anthropologists, and public health specialists) and child health specialists from the world of medicine, dentistry, and nursing with procedures, currently available and under development, for assessing the psychosocial processes, outcomes, and mediators of children's health status.

In order for the biopsychosocial framework to be more than an "everybody has a piece of the action," pseudocollaborative enterprise, creating new job titles in the absence of new insights, the field of child health must come to embrace a *systems* rather than a reductionist–mechanistic worldview. The distinction between a systems-centered and a reductionist perspective in some ways parallels the clash of doctrines in physics between the Newtonian (deterministic) view of the universe and the insights of quantum theory. As a way of knowing (an epistemology) rather than a set of facts, the systems framework takes as axiomatic that adaptive functioning emerges out of the interaction of key ingredients in a bounded context. Open systems (as humans in their environment are said to be) accept, process, and respond to input (information) and operate in the service of maintaining at least one system variable within a specified range (a preferred state). Systems operate through the coordination of components. Further it is assumed that systems operate within systems, and that their functioning is dependent upon their structures (cf. Berrien, 1968; Kuhn, 1974).

> In terms of health and illness, an example of systems thinking could be represented by the belief that specific diseases, which consist of patterns or constellations of symptoms, represent complex interactions of specific environmental, biological, and psychosocial stressors with the organism. (Schwartz, 1984, pp. 154–155)

Hence the beliefs that knowledge is relational (not absolute), that causation is never simply linear (from the body outward or the environment inward), and that one must search for patterned relationships among elements rather than static indicators of an organism's functional status characterize this potentially unifying framework. Physical aspects of a human system interact with cognitive, social, temporal, and contextual parameters in a creative organization the nature of which cannot be revealed to anyone or any group unwilling to consider all components and all potentially available levels of analysis. Good medicine is thus good systems thinking; and the assessments of physical health status, psychosocial adjustment, and social well-being should be seen as facets of a singular enterprise (cf. also Stein & Jessop, 1984).

BIOPSYCHOSOCIAL ASSESSMENT: PROVIDING THE LAST TWO-THIRDS

An examination of the usual process of child health assessment in medical settings at its most basic level—the *units* of analysis employed—and at its most abstract—the guiding *conceptual model*—yields a concern for *signs* and *symptoms* at base and for *biogenesis* as the overarching etiologic (causal) assumption. Contemporary medical diagnosis, in fact, represents a highly refined science and art whereby relatively specific behavioral or clinical manifestations (e.g., physical changes, sensory phenomena, pain, sleep or eating disturbances, cognitive dysfunctions, etc.) are traced to a causative agent or agents from a vast array of possible sources (e.g., toxins, infections, injuries, cancers, metabolic disorders, nutritional deficiencies, allergies, immune system dysfunctions, vascular problems, hereditary disorders, endocrine problems, etc.). Despite the added assessment burden, the present zeitgeist calls for a renewed recognition that even acute but particularly chronic physical symptoms can possess subjective (personal) and social meaning as well as short- and long-term educational, vocational, motivational, interpersonal, and intrapsychic consequences—all of which can influence the display of illness signs and the operation of biomedical mediators.

This volume is, therefore, designed to provide to health practitioners of varied backgrounds an overview of the strategies for multidimensional child health assessment as a necessary foundation for intervention and/or prevention. It can be read by behavioral scientists as a compendium of procedures deriving from psychology and education that may permit them to contribute to the analysis of child health problems. Relatedly, medical professionals can gain greater familiarity with many of the cognitive, emotional, and behavioral pathogens and immunogens not yet included as a systematic part of their formal training experience.

Assessment, in the current context, should not be taken to mean only *diagnosis* in the traditional sense. Rather, in systems terms, it implies diverse levels of evaluation capable of indexing not only problem precipitants, but also personal, social, and familial competencies. Further, it demands that skills and/or deficiencies be evaluated together, in transaction, connected to each other through the goals, values, and regularities contained within the social units, psychological constructions, and the nervous system of the child and adolescent.

GENERAL CONSIDERATIONS

The first part of this book offers a general orientation to the intrinsic but often overlooked multidimensionality of child health and the implications of such a perspective.

In Chapter 2 a physician and a psychologist (Drs. Perrin and MacLean) provide a fundamentals course on the "new survivors"—America's one million-plus chronically ill children whose lives are being prolonged by technical advances, but whose daily adjustment cannot easily be predicted or orchestrated. Both the biomedical and the psychosocial realities of this population are considered, from basic epidemiology and public policy issues to the role of stress, coping, and family functioning.

In Chapter 3, Russo, Hamada, and Marques discuss various models of child assessment in an effort to illustrate the interventive advantages of a multilevel, contextual systems approach. These authors illustrate how a careful analysis of physical status, developmental level, coping strategies, family functioning, the physical care environment, and "generic" assessment factors can assist in clinical decision making and in treatment planning.

LEVELS OF PEDIATRIC ASSESSMENT

Part 2 contains eight chapters that depict the assessment enterprise as varying along a molecular-to-molar continuum, with each unique perspective having a significant part to play in informing clinicians and consumers about children's health, both descriptively and predictively.

Robert Berg, a practicing pediatrician, outlines the pediatric history and physical examination process in Chapter 4. Berg's caring approach to the conduct of a potentially painful and embarrassing task does much to dispel the common image of the physician as a health technician.

The talents and perspectives of contemporary experimentally oriented psychologists are highlighted in the next chapter. Williamson, McKenzie, and Duchmann's account of psychophysiological methods illustrates how a body-centered approach to measurement can serve to illuminate potential mechanisms of disease onset and maintenance and point to noninvasive treatments.

In Chapter 6, Thomas Boll focuses on central nervous system functioning and the assessment of children's neurological status. The nature of brain–behavior relationships can be objectified only in the experimental animal laboratory, where one or the other of these elements can be manipulated, and its effect on the other carefully charted. In the world of neuropsychological testing, *inference* is an essential analytic tool, aided by an appreciation of context and adaptive interdependence.

The separation of mind from body and of both from context is even more difficult in the domain of temperament, the subject of Seifer's Chapter 7. In his account, the author shows how stylistic aspects of behavior (a controversial topic) can be assessed within a systems framework and translated into useful information for the child health assessor. An assumption of goodness of fit helps to unify the usually distinct components of the *biopsychosocial* perspective.

In the next chapter in this section, the intrapsychic level of analysis is penetrated. Eisenstein and Copeland review methods for assessing the cognitive underpinnings of illness adjustment in children. Children's expectations, knowledge base, self-efficacy attributions, and styles of self-environment appraisal emerge as important sources of influence in the stress–illness relationships.

In Chapter 9, Beck and Smith move up the generality ladder to consider such molar concepts as personality and social competence and their roles in illness adaptation and health maintenance. Beck and Smith show how standardized questionnaires, interviews, and role-play analyses can assist the health practitioner in identifying children's strengths and weaknesses and predicting, preventing, or modifying maladaptive health adjustment patterns.

In a detailed review, Kratochwill and Roseby make the often overlooked connection between physical illness and school performance. While health history takers may inquire about school grades or class standing, little is usually done to help disentangle motivational from ability-centered dysfunctions in sick or injured youngsters. Chapter 10 provides a thorough introduction to the unique perspective of school psychologists in health assessment.

In the final chapter of Part 2, Hamilton and Marilyn McCubbin provide an account of family systems assessment concepts and methods and their applicability to the study of child and adolescent health and illness. A number of promising self-report indices of family functioning are reviewed in conjunction with analyses of varied conceptual approaches that link family systems to health and rehabilitative outcomes. McCubbin and McCubbin's chapter should prove valuable in basic as well as clinical applications.

SPECIALIZED FOCI OF ASSESSMENT

Part 3 presents eight chapters dealing with some of the core content dimensions of contemporary pediatric psychology. Outcomes such as medical adjustment and pain, important mechanisms such as stressful life events and children's health concepts, and specific illness categories such as asthma, arthritis, and disorders of eating and elimination are considered, with special emphasis upon assessment issues and methodologies. Many pediatric conditions are omitted (cancer, cardiovascular disease, diabetes, cystic fibrosis, and others)—for even handbooks have limits. Yet the coverage in this section is broad, highlighting (1) factors that are common to the experience of being a child with a health-compromising medical condition, and (2) considerations that are common to the continuing search for psychometric precision in health assessment.

In Chapter 12, Lawrence J. Siegel addresses the assessment of children's adjustment to the effects of hospitalization, dental treatment, surgery, and similar forms of medical intervention. Despite methodological shortcomings in much of the published literature, efforts at multilevel, ecologically sensitive measurement are returning dividends in the form of increasingly reliable assessment tools and broader knowledge of adjustment mediators (including the role of parents and health personnel).

Stressful life events as perceived by children can precipitate, exacerbate, or maintain physical health–related problems. To the degree that this assumption is consistent with the data from careful prospective studies, the tools used to ascertain life event impact will prove invaluable in treatment and preventive efforts. Johnson and Bradlyn provide an excellent overview of both issues and procedures for the evaluation of life change in children and adolescents.

Children's beliefs about illness causality, hospitalization, the workings of the human body, and related forms of emergent health understanding represent still another domain of potent psychological mediation. David Gochman, a major contributor to this literature, articulates what is currently known about children's health and illness constructions and the needs for the future.

Chapters 15 and 16 concern the most common symptom of acute and chronic illness—pain. Despite the centrality of pain and distress in pediatric disease and in routine medical care, assessment efforts generally remain highly circumscribed and minimally attuned to the developmental status of child and adolescent patients. Karoly (in Chapter 15) offers a systems-oriented conceptual model of pain experience and a review of pain assessment practices in pediatrics. The companion chapter, by Morgan Sammons, focuses upon the most common psychosomatic pain complaint of childhood, recurrent abdominal pain, illustrating the current status of pediatric algesimetry and the utility of a multidimensional assessment framework.

Asthma is the topic of Chapter 17 by Mrazek and Klinnert. Both medical assessment procedures and psychological evaluation methods are discussed. The chapter is a brief yet comprehensive analysis of the multidisciplinary approach to one of the most common chronic disorders of childhood.

Enuresis, encopresis, bulimia, anorexia nervosa, and obesity constitute the subject matter of Chapter 18, by Walker and Shaw. The wisdom of an interdisciplinary, systematic approach to problems of eating and elimination is aptly illustrated throughout, and the dangers inherent in considering such problems exclusively psychiatric as opposed to organic are likewise apparent. Pretreatment, process-oriented, and posttreatment assessment parameters are highlighted.

In the last chapter in this section, J. Gerald Beales discusses arthritis and related disorders. Subtitled "The Human Side of Health–Illness Evaluation," Beales's contribution contains a host of sensitive observations on children's struggles to cope with the pain, fear, and embarrassment attendant on physical illness and on parental efforts to manage their own as well as their children's reactions. A unique aspect of Beales's chapter is his analysis of some of the often overlooked dangers of psychosocial assessment stemming from the value-laden assumptions of clinicians and the self-deceptive practices of children and their parents.

SCREENING AND PREVENTION-CENTERED ASSESSMENT

The potential for health-compromising behavior in otherwise healthy children and adolescents has become a central concern among health professionals, educators, legislators, law enforcement personnel, and the public. Risky behaviors from drunk driving to "unsafe" sexual practices (and the potential for exposure to the AIDS virus) are, and probably will continue to be, headline news. Child health assessment must include, therefore, attempts to screen and deter potential threats to health and safety. Part 4 includes four chapters whose focus is the early identification of *preventable* patterns of attitude and action that place our children in harm's way.

Logan Wright, Sally Flagler, and Alice Friedman (Chapter 20) present an analysis of assessment for accident prevention in children. Epidemiologic and demographic facts on diverse forms of injury, diverse models for accident risk assessment, and an appraisal of measurement instruments are included.

Chapter 21 by Mathews and Christophersen focuses upon the prevalent problem of noncompliance (or nonadherence) to medical advice and prescriptive regimens among children. A review of factors underlying child and parent noncooperation is provided as a prerequisite to the authors' consideration of assessment strategies.

The assessment of addictive behaviors is the subject of the next chapter, by Chassin, Presson, Sherman, and McGrew. These authors, who have been involved in longitudinal studies of preadolescent and adolescent smoking patterns, provide a realistic appraisal of the current state of the science in the assessment of risk for such norm-violating behaviors as cigarette smoking, excessive alcohol consumption, and drug taking (so-called substance abuse). Like other chapters, this account illustrates the importance of guiding conceptual models in the design and evaluation of clinical efforts.

The prevention of child abuse and family violence rests upon the ability to assess "risky" patterns of family interaction. Concepts and methods of assessment in this emergent domain are presented by Snyder, Rains, and Popejoy in Chapter 23. The role of participant and independent observation, along with the more traditional interview and self-report methods, is highlighted by the authors. Once again, a multitiered, systems view seems to offer considerable promise.

DIRECTIONS AND ISSUES IN TRAINING

Clearly, multidisciplinary assessment protocols that genuinely integrate the elements of a biopsychosocial worldview will not be produced by narrowly trained specialists. In Appendix 1 of this volume, Michael Roberts, Debra Fanurik, and Pauline Elkins discuss the past, present, and future of training in child health psychology. In Appendix 2, Daniel Coury, a physician and medical educator, reviews the status and direction of behavioral science training in pediatrics. While less concerned with assessment methods per se, these two appendixes provide insights into the broader question of assessor preparation and its limitations.

Child health assessment, in its psychosocial manifestation, is a yet unfinished enterprise whose significant accomplishments are exceeded only by its unmet challenges. It is hoped that this volume will adequately chronicle the former, while illuminating pathways to the latter.

References

Ackerknecht, E. H. (1982). *A short history of medicine*. Baltimore: Johns Hopkins University Press.

Berrien, F. K. (1968). *General and social systems*. New Brunswick, NJ: Rutgers University Press.

Haggerty, R. J. (1986). The changing nature of pediatrics. In N. A. Krasnegor, J. D. Arasteh, & M. F. Cataldo (Eds.), *Child health behavior: A behavioral pediatrics perspective*. New York: John Wiley.

Kuhn, A. (1974). *The logic of social systems*. San Francisco: Jossey-Bass.

Msall, M. E., & Ichord, R. (1986). Developmental pediatric assessment. In D. L. Wodrich & J. E. Joy (Eds.), *Multidisciplinary assessment of children with learning disabilities and mental retardation*. Baltimore: Paul H. Brookes.

Schwartz, G. E. (1984). Psychobiology of health: A new synthesis. In B. L. Hammonds & C. J. Scheirer (Eds.), *Psychology and health. The master lecture series* (Vol. 3). Washington, DC: American Psychological Association.

Stein, R. E. K., & Jessop, D. J. (1984). General issues in the care of children with chronic physical conditions. *Pediatric Clinics of North America, 31*, 189–198.

2

Biomedical and Psychosocial Dimensions of Chronic Illness in Childhood

JAMES M. PERRIN
WILLIAM E. MACLEAN, JR.

CHILDHOOD CHRONIC ILLNESS: AN INTRODUCTION

Epidemiology of Childhood Chronic Illness

Ten to 20 percent of children in America have some chronic health condition (Gortmaker & Sappenfield, 1984). Most chronic conditions are physiologically benign, creating few ongoing problems for the child and interfering little with the child's ability to do the sorts of things other children do. These minor conditions rarely limit the child's development or his or her schooling, although there is some evidence that even minor health conditions may influence the child's psychosocial functioning (Haggerty, Roghmann, & Pless, 1975). About 10 percent of children with chronic illnesses, or 1 to 2 percent of the total childhood population, have

The work for this chapter was supported in part by a grant (82-0836-00) from the William T. Grant Foundation.

physiologically severe conditions that may interfere on a regular or daily basis with their ability to go to school, play with other children, perform household chores, or do other things that children their age expect to do.

The mild (or minor) chronic childhood conditions include such problems as chronic acne, hay fever, mild migraine, or refractive errors. Cystic fibrosis, juvenile-onset diabetes, certain congenital heart diseases, sickle cell anemia, juvenile arthritis, and leukemia are examples of more severe conditions. Only a few chronic health conditions are common in childhood. Three categories occur with some frequency (Pless & Roghmann, 1971). Allergic disorders, mainly hay fever, eczema, and asthma, affect perhaps 10 to 15 percent of the total childhood population. Asthma is the most common severe chronic illness of childhood; however, most of the 3 percent of children with asthma have a mild form of the illness (Williams & McNicol, 1975). These children typically have the onset of asthma around age 5, have one to two episodes of wheezing every year or so for a period of 6 or 7 years, and then stop having asthma. Only about 10 percent of children with asthma have a severe form that causes frequent hospitalizations, necessitates long-term medications, and may interfere significantly with the child's schooling and growth.

Beyond allergic conditions, the two common chronic illness groups in childhood are (1) neurological conditions and developmental handicaps and (2) behavioral disorders. Essentially, all other childhood chronic conditions occur rarely. Juvenile diabetes, the most common endocrinological illness of childhood, occurs in approximately 1 in 1000 children under the age of 16 (Drash & Berlin, 1985). Cystic fibrosis and sickle cell anemia are slightly less common than diabetes. Juvenile arthritis affects approximately 1 in 10,000 children. Other conditions, such as phenylketonuria, are even more rare, and it is not unusual to identify children with syndromes so rare that they have been described in only 5 or 10 children previously. Although on an illness-by-illness basis, most of the chronic illnesses of children are quite rare, when taken together, approximately 2 children out of every 100, or *more than 1,000,000 children in the United States*, have severe chronic illnesses that may significantly impair their daily activities, their school performance, or their psychosocial functioning as they develop (Hobbs, Perrin, & Ireys, 1985).

The incidence and prevalence of chronic illnesses vary relatively little across social class and ethnic groups. Specific conditions are more common in certain social classes or groups of certain racial or ethnic descent. Cystic fibrosis, as an example, is much more common in White children than in Black. Sickle cell anemia is predominantly a disease of Black children in the United States. Spina bifida and other neural tube defects have a curious geographical variation in incidence. Some of this variation may reflect different patterns of nutrition, although not all the variation can be explained in this way (Smithells et al., 1981). Although, in general, social class seems not to influence the incidence or prevalence of chronic illness, children from lower socioeconomic classes have more *severe* chronic illness. Whether poorer children are biologically at greater risk for severe illness or whether their illness is worsened through lack of access to adequate health care is unclear. Despite the advent of Medicaid and other public programs, poor children still have significantly greater problems with access to health services than do children from wealthier families. And poor children with chronic illness are about twice as likely as their able-bodied poor age-mates to lack any form of third-party health insurance, public or private (Butler, Budetti, McManus, Stenmark, & Newacheck, 1985).

The epidemiology of childhood chronic illness is distinctly different from that of adult chronic illness. Adults face a relatively small number of common chronic conditions: diabetes, degenerative osteoarthritis, hypertension, and the like. Diabetes, which is relatively rare in children, becomes much more common with increasing age, such that as many as 50 percent of people over age 70 may have signs of diabetes. The fact that these illnesses occur frequently in adults is evident in the observation that most people with high blood pressure know other people who are similarly affected. By the same token, most physicians and other health professionals who see patients with hypertension are likely to have extensive clinical experience with this condition. They are sensitive to the variations in the disease from person to person and to the idiosyncracies of treatments commonly used. The situation is quite different for the chronic illnesses of childhood. When a child develops diabetes, it is unlikely that his or her family will know other families with children with diabetes. Or if a child is born with a rare orthopedic condition, especially a nonfamilial disorder, it is unlikely that anyone in the same community or city will have a similar condition. And for the child whose condition is so rare that it has occurred only a handful of times before, it is unlikely that any health provider in that child's community will have seen a previous case of the disease. For the moderately rare condition like spina bifida, the typical obstetric and nursery unit may experience only one such child a decade, and the professional staff may be unaware of changes in the care of this condition or the different approaches that potential referral sources may take in treating it. Early identification, appropriate referral, and adequate transfer of information to allow effective monitoring of child health and development are all made difficult by the rarity of each condition. Self-help groups and parent support activities all seem to benefit families facing a chronic stressor, such as a chronic illness in their child. However, the logistics of forming such groups are surely difficult where only one child in the city may have Klippel-Feil syndrome, for example, or methylmalonic aciduria.

The numbers of children with severe chronic illnesses *appear* to be increasing. Where approximately 1 percent of parents in the mid-1960s reported their children as having a severe chronic health condition interfering with usual daily activities, by the early 1980s that number had doubled to 2 percent (Gortmaker, 1985; Newacheck, Budetti, & Halfon, 1986). However, there is little evidence of changing or increasing incidence of the severe chronic illnesses of childhood. Rather, this doubling reflects the real advances of new technologies and improved medical care over the past two decades. Many children who would have died two decades ago now survive well into young adulthood. Children with cystic fibrosis, for example, currently have a life span averaging 22 years. Twenty years ago, the expected span was about 6 years. Similarly, children with the most common form of leukemia, acute lymphoblastic leukemia, had essentially a uniformly fatal disease. In the mid 1980s, conservatively at least 50 percent of children with this disease will have a long-term remission and apparent cure. For some conditions, such as muscular dystrophy or certain malignancies, there has been little improvement in survival; but for most, such as congenital heart diseases or chronic renal disease treated with dialysis or transplant, the change in mortality has been dramatic. Indeed, current estimates are that at least 80 percent of the achievable improvement in mortality has already occurred (Gortmaker, 1985). In other words, in the event that survival of children with chronic illnesses rose to 100 percent, the percentage of children with severe chronic illnesses would rise from approximately 2 percent currently to 2.5 percent. Insofar as the numbers of children born per year have remained fairly constant over the last few years (and are likely to do so over the next couple of decades) and insofar as the incidence of most chronic conditions appears to be stable, the doubling that occurred between 1960 and 1980 is unlikely to occur again between 1980 and 2000.

The New Survivors

Many children with severe chronic illness survive to young adulthood with a major ongoing disability. Children with arthritis may have crippling deformities of their joints; children with sickle cell anemia may be stunted in their growth and experience problems with fertility; and children with diabetes may develop blindness or severe chronic renal disease. For others who may survive to young adulthood in apparently good health, uncertainties lie ahead. Will the person who has survived childhood leukemia develop a second cancer in his or her thirties or forties? Will scarring associated with the surgical repair of congenital heart disease lead to important cardiac rhythm problems or other problems in the functioning of the heart musce in middle age? Although efforts must continue to improve mortality rates for many childhood illnesses, attention now must go to improving the lives of those children who do survive and to supporting the types of services that will permit appropriate monitoring of these people over the years.

CHARACTERISTICS OF ILLNESS AND DISEASE

Severity

The severity of a chronic illness is a complex concept (Hobbs et al., 1985). Although intuitively one would expect it to be easy to distinguish a child with severe arthritis from one with mild arthritis, in fact the gradations in classifications can be quite difficult. Most classification schemes are confounded by the interaction of some biologic predilection to illness and the response to treatment. As an example, the severity of asthma is most often defined by the frequency of attacks of asthma, the number of days of hospitalization, the number of days absent from school, the use of medications, and the presence of pulmonary involvement between attacks. Yet most of these criteria are affected both by the biological severity of the condition and by the adequacy of the response to treatment. A child who complies with an appropriately prescribed regimen of treatment, including medications and avoidance of inciting events or allergens, is likely to miss fewer days of school and to have fewer attacks than a child with the same "biological" severity who does not comply with prescribed treatment.

In addition to clinical severity, one may consider severity in terms of its impact on the child's growth and development, on the family's functioning, on family finances, or on the child's school performance. All of these variables reflect a kind of severity; yet for any childhood disease there may be poor correlation among these different forms of severity. An illness causing significant financial hardship may have little impact on the child's psychological development.

These observations have led to the development of techniques to assess severity in a more comprehensive manner. Some important work has been done by Stein and colleagues (Stein & Jessop, 1982a), who have developed measures of functional status for children with long-term illnesses (Stein & Jessop, 1984) and of the impact of illness on the family (Stein & Riessman, 1980). McCubbin, Patterson, McCubbin, and Wilson (1983) have also developed measures of parents' ability to cope with health-related problems.

Despite the difficulties encountered in defining and measuring severity, the gestalt of severity remains an important clinical variable that warrants assessment. Perhaps the most illustrative example is the relationship between clinical severity and psychological adjustment of children. Several early reports noted that children with long-term illnesses had a greater incidence of significant psychiatric problems than did healthy control groups (Pless & Roghmann, 1971; Rutter, Tizard, & Whitmore, 1970). More recent work has to some degree challenged this increased risk (Drotar & Bush, 1985; Tavormina, Kastner, Slater, & Watt, 1976). However, the weight of the evidence supports the view that chronically ill children continue to be at higher risk for psychological problems than are able-bodied children. Psychological difficulties are presumed to follow from the demands upon the child and family from a chronic illness over and above the complexities of normal development and psychological growth. Among children with chronic illness, who are the ones most likely to have problems in psychological adjustment? Intuitively, one might expect that children with the most severe illnesses have the greatest risk of poor psychological adjustment. Although there is evidence in a few studies for a direct relationship between illness severity and adjustment, most studies suggest that the increased risk affects all children with chronic illness, whatever the level of severity (Bruhn, Hampton, & Chandler, 1971; McAnarney, Pless, Satterwhite, & Friedman, 1974; J. M. Perrin, MacLean, & E. C. Perrin, 1986). Moreover, in several studies, children and young adults with less severe illness had greater problems with psychological adjustment than those with more severe forms (Markova, Lockyer, & Forbes, 1980). Some attribute this finding to the concept of *marginality*; that is, children who are at the border of being healthy and having an illness are less secure in their knowledge of their group membership (healthy or ill) and therefore face greater risk of psychological maladjustment. McAnarney and colleagues (1974), studying children with juvenile arthritis, found that those with more severe disease had fewer problems with psychological adjustment. Furthermore, they found that children with arthritis but no disability often had greater problems with adjustment than those children who had moderate or severe disability. The relationship between severity and adjustment remains complex. It may be that there is a tendency toward greater risk with more severe disease, but it appears that marginality plays a role as well, increasing the risk for those children at the borderline between being ill and being well. The important finding is that systematic assessment for problems of psychological adjustment should *not be limited* to those children with physiologically severe health conditions.

Biomedical Perspectives

The chronic illnesses of childhood are remarkably diverse. Many have major genetic components, reflecting either a chromosome disorder or more subtle genetic defects that may affect the functioning of an enzyme important to a key biologic process. Although conditions that are genetic may run in families, their patterns vary considerably (Hobbs et al., 1985). Conditions that are sex-linked recessives (such as hemophilia or muscular dystrophy) are transmitted by an asymptomatic carrier female through her affected sons. The carrier mother may have brothers or cousins who have been affected by the same condition. On the other hand, some sex-linked recessive conditions represent new mutations, and families may be unaware of the presence of the disease in their children until they have experienced two or three pregnancies. Muscular dystrophy, as an example, typically has few or no symptoms until the child is 4 or 5 years of age. By that time, additional male children may have already been born.

An autosomal recessive pattern is more common, in which, to have the disease, a child must receive a disease-causing gene from each parent. Insofar as most of these genes are fairly rare, mating of two people who carry these genes is uncommon, and it is unlikely that other family members will have the same condition. Thus children with cystic fibrosis may have siblings with the same condition, but they are unlikely to have uncles or aunts with it. For many chronic illnesses, the biologic causation is less clear than for the genetic conditions, likely representing a developmental phenomenon in utero or a combination of environmental factors and genetic predisposition.

Greater understanding of human genetics has been one of the advances of the past decade. New techniques allow the careful elucidation of gene structures and help to pinpoint the precise positions on the gene associated with genetic illnesses. A primary result of these advances has been the increasing ability to diagnose numbers of genetic conditions in utero, allowing, in certain circumstances, pregnancy termination. Newer techniques of gene splicing currently allow the development of large amounts of biologically active substances, such as human insulin, through the insertion of insulin-producing genes into reproducing bacteria. Gene splicing holds some hope for similar efforts in the future to replace missing enzymes in diseased children, carrying the potential to eradicate the disease fully. It is, however, unrealistic to expect that the next decade will eliminate genetic diseases. First, the numbers of such diseases are staggering. Many thousands have been described, and it will likely take years to determine the gene structure of each of these diseases. Furthermore, insofar as many occur unexpectedly (either as mutations in sex-linked–type diseases or as a first affected child in a family with autosomal recessive disease), many children will continue to be born with these chronic illnesses.

New genetic technology may some day allow primary prevention of some diseases. There are, however, other levels of prevention. It may be useful to distinguish primary, secondary, and tertiary prevention (Holtzman & Richmond, 1985). Primary prevention is prevention of the onset of disease or the conception of an affected fetus. Primary prevention might mean that a couple known to be at risk for a genetic disease would choose not to have children or to have their genes altered (in the future) to prevent their having an affected child. Secondary prevention is the use of abortion to prevent the delivery of a child with a genetic condition or similar disability. Technologies now becoming available mainly influence this form of secondary prevention. Tertiary prevention is the prevention of the side effects of disease. The process of tertiary prevention relates to the usual aspects of treatment: to prevent deterioration of body organs, to diminish the impact of the illness on the child's functioning in school and with peers and family, and to diminish the psychological impact of illness on the family and the child.

Although prevention is often thought of in the context of preventing the onset of acquired disease (hypertension, diabetes, anemia) in presumably healthy individuals, there are clear advantages and implications of taking a preventive view in the context of chronic illness as well. Applying a preventive orientation to traditional treatments, involving health and developmental and psychological concerns, carries great promise. As an example, insofar as certain children with long-term illnesses are at greater risk for psychological adjustment problems than are their able-bodied colleagues, a preventive approach in the provision of mental health services seems likely to be of great benefit and of different magnitude and potential from the delivery of treatment services for a disturbed child.

Dimensions of Illness

Although the chronic illnesses of childhood seem quite diverse, with little linking one disease to another, there are underlying themes that may help to categorize illnesses (Pless & J. M. Perrin, 1985). An obvious dimension is the expected course of the disease. Some conditions, such as many childhood malignancies, are uniformly fatal. Other diseases, such as asthma and hemophilia, may be associated with approximately normal life spans. For conditions such as cystic fibrosis, the expected life span has progressively increased over the last several years and may reasonably be expected to continue to do so. There are also illnesses that may resolve in later life. Needless to say, the expectations of child and parents (and educators and health professionals) are highly affected by whether the child will have a normal life span or an early demise.

The age of onset of the condition affects children differently. Those conditions that a child is born with present different tasks for adjustment and adaptation than do conditions that are acquired later in life. Generally, acquired conditions create greater adaptation problems than do congenital conditions (E. C. Perrin & Gerrity, 1984). There are important exceptions to this general rule; for example, children with major sensory deficits, such as blindness, are placed at great disadvantage with respect to the processes by which they explore and understand their world and the objects and people around them. For these conditions, adaptation may be easier when the condition is acquired rather than congenital. Onset of the condition at different ages presents different tasks for a child as a function of developmental stages. A child who develops asthma at age 3 adapts to that illness quite differently from the child who develops a significant respiratory disease at age 15. Similarly, the understanding of illness and the ways in which understanding may improve the child's adaptation differ from age to age. Developmentally, a 5-year-old child with leukemia understands his or her disease, its causation, and treatment in a fashion quite different from that of a 15-year-old with leukemia (Bibace & Walsh, 1980; E. C. Perrin & Gerrity, 1981).

Certain diseases significantly affect cognitive functioning of children, interfering with their ability to learn. Some conditions, such as spina bifida and muscular dystrophy, affect the child's mobility. Certain conditions are visible; others, such as diabetes and epilepsy, are invisible, causing no apparent external indication of the illness for the child.

Commonalities Among Conditions

While the aforementioned illness characteristics help to categorize conditions, no specific typology so far seems satisfactory. More importantly, there is tremendous variation within a disease entity, such that one child with a specific diagnosis may be more affected in any of the realms of functioning or prognosis than another child with the same diagnosis (Stein & Jessop, 1982a, 1982b). As an example, a child with leukemia may have a relatively uncomplicated course, with excellent response to initial medical therapy, entering remission without evidence of ongoing disease and then surviving, apparently cured. Other children with leukemia may face a course characterized by frequent relapses, may have significant cognitive impact from their primary disease or its treatment, and may suffer a fatal outcome. This large amount of within-disease variation makes difficult any attempt to categorize the course of illness outcomes or the nature of the psychosocial problems involved. Indeed, the work of several research groups, especially those led by Pless and Stein, has demonstrated that, despite the tremendous physiological diversity of conditions and the different impact on the human organism, the *fact of chronicity* alone carries implications common to most ill children and their families. These commonalities in many ways distinguish this class of children from most other children in the United States (Hobbs et al., 1985).

Most chronic conditions, for example, are quite costly to treat. Conservatively, the 1 to 2 percent of children with severe chronic illnesses utilize approximately 30 to 40 percent of the child health dollar in America (Butler et al., 1985). This figure does not account for the sizable additional out-of-pocket costs that families face, especially those costs that are not traditionally considered medical, but that may further burden an already financially strapped family. And although most Americans have some form of private health insurance, there are major problems with both access to adequate health coverage and the breadth of health coverage that continue to put many families at great financial risk (Weeks, 1985). This situation can be contrasted with conditions in most other industrialized countries, where the presence of severe chronic illness in the child brings along certain benefits that at least diminish the financial impact of illness on the family's self-sufficiency.

For most Americans, private health insurance is an employment benefit. For many young families, coverage may be limited to the working parent only, leaving the children uncovered. In smaller companies, there may be exclusions that prohibit payment for chronic illness in a covered family member or there may be lengthy waiting periods after someone joins the company. Most private health insurance is designed to meet both acute and catastrophic health problems, being less well designed to meet the severe financial demands of an illness that lasts for months or years.

For children living in poverty, similar problems occur. Despite the presence of Medicaid, many poor children in America are not eligible primarily because of the strong link of Medicaid coverage to Aid to Families with Dependent Children (AFDC) (Starfield, 1982). With the addition of opportunities to cover families not on AFDC and families including both parents, it may be that Medicaid will eventually cover a larger proportion of children in poverty. But until recently, fewer than 50 percent of children in poverty were covered by Medicaid (Butler et al., 1985). Poor children with a severe illness face double jeopardy, insofar as they are twice as likely as other poor children to have no third-party coverage, public or private.

A second common element of chronic illness is that the daily care falls on the family. For the family, the logistical and physical burdens of care can be enormous. A family may have three teenage sons with muscular dystrophy, all of whom are wheelchair bound and all of whom require assistance with toileting, going to school, or getting out of bed. The family of the child with cystic fibrosis may provide an hour or so every day of physical therapy for their child, trying to improve lung function and to help the child breathe better. For example, chest physical therapy may be necessary in the morning prior to school, to allow the child to go to school and participate actively with his or her peers. The burdens of child care exist every day, every week, every month, without respite, and may sorely stretch the limits of a family's stamina.

The organization and delivery of services for children with long-term illnesses are highly fragmented (J. M. Perrin & Ireys, 1984). Typically, families require a wide variety of services, including access to high-quality primary and specialty medical interventions, often in-home nursing care, occupational and physical therapy, counseling around genetic, financial, and psychological issues, and attention to educational problems, especially when a child may be frequently absent from school. Access to these services varies widely from community to community and from disease to disease. One child with a seizure disorder may receive comprehensive services if he lives in one community, but a similar child living in another city or in a rural area may receive only medical monitoring of the medications she is taking. In another community, assistance may be available for a child with hemophilia, but not for one with thalassemia. Medical and surgical services, especially on an inpatient basis, are relatively well reimbursed and, in general, easier to obtain than are many of the other services needed by families.

The fourth common problem is that most chronic conditions entail treatment from a variety of medical, nursing, and other therapists. Where the average child in America receives medical care from a single provider, usually a pediatrician, family practitioner, or nurse, the child with spina bifida may see a neurosurgeon, an orthopedist, a urologist, a pediatrician, an ostomy nurse, a physical therapist, an occupational therapist, and a nutritionist. To expect that all these professionals will have a clear and agreed-upon plan for the child and family is at best unrealistic. Typically, families face conflicting advice from different professionals and the difficult problem of choosing among opinions. Only rarely is help provided to families in sorting out different suggestions, and thus coordination of complex services is a difficult problem for many families.

Specialty services are available primarily in academic health centers, although increasingly they are available as well in the larger multispecialty group practices developing in many parts of the country. Most specialty services are highly centralized and are built around the ability to amass a moderately large population of children with the same or related rare diseases. Doing so also allows better clinical research through larger study samples, and provides a group of clinicians who are experienced with and knowledgeable about the nuances of a given rare disease. For example, a child with diabetes can have blood sugar, diet, and other treatments monitored in the home community. On the other hand, a community practitioner is unlikely to know the most recent information on new therapies for diabetes, the efficacy of such devices as an insulin pump, or unusual complications that should be screened for. This information will be had primarily by the specialists in a central unit. For common conditions, especially asthma and seizure disorders, a community practitioner is likely to have enough experience on an ongoing clinical basis to be aware of new treatments and complications. These children may not need additional specialty services.

For many children, pain and discomfort characterize their disease and its treatment. The degree of pain may be far beyond that understood or experienced by other children with whom they interact on a regular, daily basis. For teenagers especially, some aspects of treatment or its monitoring may be very embarrassing. Testing urine or blood samples in school or the necessity for special diets or special permission to miss athletic events can distinguish the child from his or her able-bodied classmates.

For most conditions, uncertainty is a special problem. When will the child with asthma have another attack? Will the child with leukemia continue to do well or have another relapse? Will this particular hospitalization represent the last, fatal episode for a child, or will he or she survive and then be rid of disease? There is increasing evidence that uncertainty is an especially difficult problem for families. Knowledge of what may happen to a child can be very helpful. That lack of knowledge, or the uncertainty of what lies next, is especially difficult for families.

Finally, as another common element, there is the issue of rarity. It is common for families to feel quite isolated. As noted before, most adult chronic illnesses are common; nearly every affected adult knows someone else with hypertension. For such anomalies as Klippel-Feil or Marden-Walker syndromes, it is unlikely that a family with this condition may ever meet another family with a similar condition. This feeling of isolation tends to diminish the sense of control that many families feel they have over the health and welfare of themselves and their children. The issue of rarity provides still another link among the families with children with chronic illnesses.

Children with chronic illnesses require the same types of health supervision and health maintenance services that are available to able-bodied children in the United States. They require immunizations, advice to parents about normal developmental tasks and progress, screening for other illnesses, and treatment for acute minor illnesses. Yet it appears that children with chronic illnesses are more likely than other children to lack the ordinary rudiments of general health care (Palfrey, Levy, & Gilbert, 1980). Immunization levels are lower, the likelihood that they will be able to identify a general health provider is less, and they will typically have undergone less screening for other diseases than their able-bodied colleagues. To some degree, this pattern of service reflects the tendency to generalize from the disease to the child and his or her needs. All too often, the child is referred to as "an asthmatic" or "a hemophiliac," rather than as " a *child* with asthma" or "a *child* with hemophilia." The focus on the disease rather than the child often limits the expectations for the child and the types of routine services the child may receive.

DEVELOPMENTAL CONSIDERATIONS

Fundamental to the assessment of any child is an understanding of the developmental processes that characterize the childhood period. These processes include the cognitive, sensorimotor, language, social–emotional, and physiological aspects of development. While the developmental tasks are the same for chronically ill and healthy children alike, there is some question whether chronically ill children develop along different pathways. Gliedman and Roth (1980) make the case that the influence of a chronic illness on development is considerable. E. C. Perrin and Gerrity (1984) summarize this point by indicating:

> The manner and extent to which a chronic illness may modify typical developmental processes depend to large degree on details of the illness, such as its severity, its natural history and expected prognosis, the degree of limitation associated with it, the presence or expectation of mental retardation, its genetic background and implications,

necessity for care, and the degree to which the illness is visible and thus known to the wider community. (p. 19)

Perrin and Gerrity also point out that these factors, in combination with individual difference factors, are only a part of the process. Family and environmental influences also have a direct effect on the development of a child with chronic illness.

Developmental processes should be considered in assessing the impact of chronic illness on childhood functioning. Such basic knowledge assists care providers in determining whether a child's response is problematic or typical of a child at that particular developmental level (Bibace & Walsh, 1981). Furthermore, developmental stages, as specified by developmental theories, are more critical elements in assessment than chronological age. Much of the literature on chronic childhood illness makes little mention of developmental level. Where there is consideration of developmental processes, the assessment is limited typically to chronological age. It should be pointed out, however, that there are several instructive exceptions to this generalization. Of particular relevance is the literature that addresses the development of children's understanding of illness.

E. C. Perrin and Gerrity (1981) provided important cross-sectional data on understanding of illness among healthy children. The data were coded according to a Piagetian framework of cognitive development and analyzed across children attending kindergarten through eighth grade. They found that younger children have a very concrete and superficial understanding of illness. For example, preschoolers view illness causation in magical terms or as a result of their transgression of rules. The understanding of illness exhibited by school-aged children is characterized by the emergence of rule-bound thinking. The rules are still very concrete, such as the view that all illness results from germs, but there is a hint of more sophistication than the preoperational thinking described earlier. It is not until the age of 10 or 12 that children begin to understand illness as a complex and multifaceted process. Such formal operational thinking is more evident during early adolescence when children begin to speculate about illness mechanisms in an abstract fashion. Perhaps the most interesting aspect of the data reported by E. C. Perrin and Gerrity was that changes in understanding of illness closely followed conceptual development in other areas (e.g., conservation of mass, weight, and volume). Similar findings had been obtained earlier by Bibace and Walsh (1979, 1980) and Simeonsson, Buckley, and Monson (1979), among others. The basic knowledge derived from such studies is of immense practical importance in fostering empathy with chronically ill children (Bibace & Walsh, 1979), promoting understanding among health providers (E. C. Perrin & J. M. Perrin, 1983), and designing appropriate interventions (Jordan & O'Grady, 1982).

In a recent discussion of the development of children with a chronic illness, E. C. Perrin and Gerrity (1984) described the pervasive influence of a physical illness on each period of a child's development. During infancy, chronic physical illness can have a range of untoward effects. First, the illness may have a primary effect on growth and development by interfering with feeding, exploration of the environment, and social responsiveness. Second, parents and other caregivers may respond differentially either to the infant's level of responsiveness, physical deformity, or irritability, or to their own reactions to parenting a less than perfect child. As a result, attachment may be disrupted, leading to further developmental difficulties. E. C. Perrin and Gerrity speculate further that "frequent and repeated hospitalizations or visits to physicians' offices may interrupt the smooth flow of family development and the transition to parenthood" (p. 21). Furthermore, the need for frequent health care contacts and specialized information may also make it difficult for parents to establish a sense of competence in their interactions with their children.

The influence of physical illness on children ages 18 months through 3 years of age is most evident in the child's attainment of autonomy and self-control. E. C. Perrin and Gerrity indicate that "frequently, chronically ill toddlers manifest increased dependency, difficulty with separation, a tenuous self-image, and poor impulse control" (p. 23). Disruptions during this stage may also have effects on emerging verbal and cognitive abilities. While some of these limits may be a direct consequence of the illness, there are data that suggest that parents may employ overprotective parenting styles that also inhibit the child's opportunity for exploration. Similar effects are apparent among preschoolers in that limits in activity imposed by parents may decrease motor competence and the child's sense of mastery over the environment. A further consideration is the child's social competence. With limited opportunities for peer interaction and social involvement, preschoolers may have decreased self-image and shy away from social situations.

For school-aged children, the presence of a chronic illness can have a major impact upon their social development. They may worry about being different from their peers and attempt to hide the illness from friends and teachers. However, many children are not able to minimize the impact of their illness; and their limited activity in sports, different lunch menus, frequent visits to the doctor, and need for medication during the school day are soon noticed and serve to ostracize them from their peers. E. C. Perrin and Gerrity maintain that approval and acceptance by peers is what every child with a chronic illness would benefit most from. A further consideration is school performance. Given the likelihood that these children will miss large amounts of school and that their chronic illness may have a direct impact on their physical and cognitive functioning, there is little question about the need for careful monitoring of school performance.

Adolescence is a time of particular vulnerability for children with a chronic physical illness. The increased turmoil of this developmental period is widely recognized as a prerequisite for adult functioning. Adolescence is a time of dramatic physical change and striving for independence. Chronic illness can make both of these processes considerably more difficult than for healthy peers. In many cases it is difficult to gain independence from enmeshed family systems that have not fostered independent functioning from the beginning, and to join a peer group that perceives the chronically ill adolescent as "different."

STRESS AND COPING

Stress and Chronic Illness

Over the past 30 years there has been increasing interest in understanding the role of stress in chronic illness (Elliott & Eisdorfer, 1982). Following early work conducted primarily by Holmes, Rahe, and their colleagues, there has been growing recognition that stress is an important construct in understanding a variety of illness-related questions. There are at least three literatures that have emerged with regard to stress and chronic childhood illness: stress and onset of chronic illness, stress and exacerbation of chronic illness, and stress of chronic illness on child and family functioning.

Stress and the Onset of Chronic Illness. The most rigorous of these studies were reported for childhood leukemia (Jacobs & Charles, 1980), diabetes (Stein & Charles, 1971), and juvenile rheumatoid arthritis (Heisel, 1972; Henoch, Batson, & Baum, 1978). In each case, life events such as changes in residence and school, death of a parent, separation and divorce, and family disturbance due to severe physical illness or psychopathology were more prevalent in the lives of chronically ill children prior to the time of the apparent onset of disease as compared with control populations.

What typically remains wanting in reports such as these is direct evidence that the stress did lead to the onset of the chronic illness. However, there is fairly good evidence that family stress is associated with infectious disease. In a study conducted by Meyer and Haggerty (1962), 100 children in 16 families were asked to keep a diary of "upsetting" events and illnesses experienced by family members. It was striking that the number of upsetting events quadrupled from baseline levels in the 2 weeks prior to confirmed streptococcal and upper respiratory infections. While not all infections were preceded by upsetting events, there was a substantial increase in risk following stressful events. Similar results were obtained by Boyce and colleagues (1977). In their sample, the duration and severity of respiratory tract illnesses among young children were directly related to their cumulative life change scores and an index of family routine.

What remains is the observation that for some but not all children psychosocial factors seem related to the onset of disease states. It seems likely that the etiology of disease is multifactorial, determined by historical, organismic, and environmental influences (Plaut & Friedman, 1981). The complex and interrelated physiological responses of the endocrine, immune, and gastrointestinal systems seem to place *some* individuals at considerable risk for disease (Hamburg, Elliott, & Parron, 1982).

Stress and Exacerbation of Chronic Illness. Many diseases, particularly those that affect organ systems, are characterized by periodic manifestations of the disease state followed by a return to a period of equilibrium. This cyclicity is evident in asthma, hemophilia, juvenile rheumatoid arthritis (JRA), and lupus. While there may be many factors that result in exacerbation of chronic disease, we suspect that stress has a quantifiable influence. Indeed, data that support such a conclusion have been reported for hemophilia (Garlinghouse & Sharp, 1968), asthma (Matus, 1981), and juvenile rheumatoid arthritis. For the most part, these reports are based on correlations between illness activity and the frequency of recent stressful life events. Future research should define further the temporal relationship between stressors and exacerbation of the illness so as to ensure that these relationships are not largely due to the stress of the illness. This is an area of immense practical importance. Simply stated, if stress does have a clear contributory role in the exacerbation of chronic childhood illness, then psychosocial interventions could be employed to lessen the occurrence of illness episodes.

Stress of Illness on Child and Family Functioning. The presence of a chronic illness brings on a host of additional demands that frequently exceed the coping resources of children and families. For children, significant disruptions in the normal processes of child development are typical. While children with chronic illness have about twice the risk of children without illness to manifest significant psychological adjustment problems (Pless & Pinkerton, 1975; Rutter et al., 1970), it is far more likely that these children experience decreased functioning across a range of usual childhood activities such as school attendance, participation in after-school activities (clubs, sports, or playing with friends), and performance of household chores (Pless & Pinkerton, 1975).

For families, the impact can be equally devastating (Hobbs et al., 1985; Masters, Cerreto, & Mendlowitz, 1983). Especially given today's spiraling health care costs, the financial burden of a child who requires regular, highly specialized medical services can have profound implications for the quality of family life and lead to even greater levels of ambient stress. This stress can have direct effects upon the mental health of the parents. Many families do not have resources or time to be part of a larger community and this isolation often leads to deficiencies in social support. More commonly, parents differ over child-rearing methods. These difficulties can lead to marital difficulties or further stress tenuous marital relationships.

Parents are also in a position to mediate much of the impact of illness for their children. Their perceptions of what their child may or may not be able to do could greatly affect what the child then believes he or she is capable of accomplishing, regardless of the clinical assessment of the child's health status. The magnitude of this influence is readily apparent in a study conducted by Bergman and Stamm (1967). They found that parental perceptions of the implications of (innocent) heart murmurs diagnosed early in life led to restrictions in the children's activity that endured into the elementary years.

Another area of concern has been the reports of increased adjustment problems among siblings of chronically ill children (Breslau, Weitzman, & Messenger, 1981; Drotar & Bush, 1985; Lavigne & Ryan, 1979). These difficulties may take the form of increased withdrawal and irritability as in the case of cardiology, hematology, and plastic surgery patients described by Lavigne and Ryan (1979) or in the higher perceived social isolation of siblings of children with cancer (Cairns, Clark, Smith, & Lansky, 1979). As of yet there is no explanation of this spillover phenomenon. Investigators point to the increased anxiety among siblings due to the illness, changes at the family level that influence all family members, and differences in interaction patterns between parent and child (Drotar & Bush, 1985). Given this important concomitant of chronic illness, it is clear that siblings should be a focus of assessment.

Coping with Chronic Illness

Any discussion of the stress associated with a chronic illness immediately invokes the concept of coping. Previously, coping was regarded as simply a response to a stressful event. The bulk of the evidence indicates that intervening cognitive factors alter the coping response. Roskies and Lazarus (1980) refer to stress and coping as two faces of the same coin. They point out that "coping is a reaction to stress, but also a shaper of the stress experience" (p. 45). In discussing this point further, we will refer to a model (see Fig. 2.1) described by Moos and Tsu (1977).

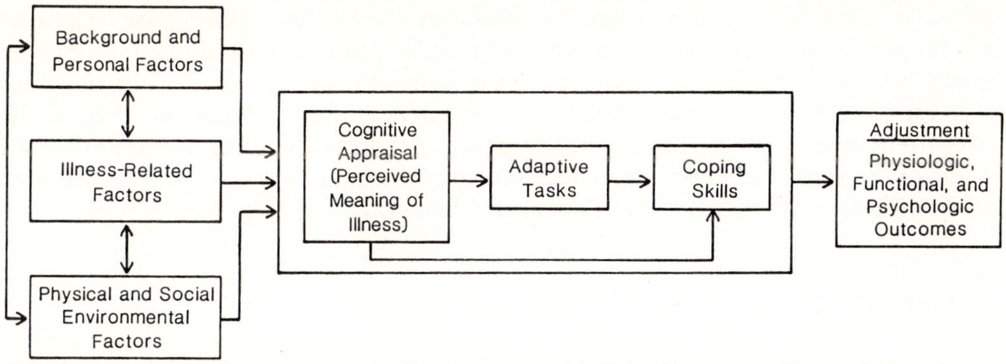

FIGURE 2.1. A model of coping with childhood chronic illness. (From *Coping with Physical Illness* by R. H. Moos, 1977, New York: Plenum Publishing Corp. Reprinted with permission.)

The model has three main components. The first set contains factors that mediate the appraisal of stress. Background factors include age, intelligence, level of cognitive and emotional development, and premorbid psychological adjustment. Illness-related factors include disease characteristics such as age of onset, impact on mobility, severity, visibility, and lethality. Physical and social environmental factors include the school and family.The role of the family is of considerable importance in that it appears likely that the parents mediate much of what children understand about their disease (Drotar & Bush, 1985; Masters et al., 1983). These three types of factors lead then to the first adaptive step, cognitive appraisal of the illness. In other words, how the child perceives illness and its effects will largely determine the methods and problems of adaptation. Adaptive tasks are those demands placed by the illness, as mediated by cognitive appraisal. They include responding to pain or incapacitation and to the health care environment and providers, as well as maintaining emotional balance and family relationships. Coping skills are the techniques applied to the adaptive tasks and are perhaps the least well understood component of the model. With regard to coping with physical illness, Moos and Tsu (1977) describe several major types of coping skills that range from denying or minimizing the seriousness of an illness to learning specific illness-related procedures.

Finally, there is a set of outcomes that stand as an index of how well the coping resources meet the perceived demands. We find it useful to place outcomes into three basic categories: physiological, functional, and psychological. The physiological category typically reflects the activity of the disease, such as frequency of asthma attacks or amount of Factor VIII infused over a period of time. Functional outcomes reflect participation in usual childhood activities, such as school attendance, play, or self-care. Psychological adjustment has received the greatest attention of these outcomes as it has been a focus of inquiry since the 1930s (Hobbs et al., 1985).

The primary objective of research on the psychological adjustment of children with chronic illness has been determining the prevalence of psychopathology among these children relative to comparison groups. Investigators have proceeded from a medical (illness) model where the presence of an abnormal physical condition is presumed to have far-reaching negative effects on the child (Drotar & Bush, 1985).

Taken as a whole, it is now clear that children with chronic illness are at greater risk for psychological disturbance than their healthy peers, but that the relationship is not one to one. That is, most children with chronic illness do not evidence psychopathology. They may, however, experience some disruption of their development due to their illness. Investigators are now directing attention to the study of competence in an effort to elucidate how children cope effectively with chronic illness (Garmezy, 1981; Garmezy, Masten, & Tellegen, 1984).

SUMMARY

Historically, children with long-term illnesses have received relatively little attention, especially in the broader functional, family, and psychosocial aspects of their lives. With changing patterns of child health, and with the real improvement in survival of children with long-term health needs, there is greater interest and opportunity for research into these dimensions of childhood illness. A number of important questions may be raised, as reviewed recently by Starfield (1985): What are the biologic correlates of behavior? How are behavioral phenomena translated into biological representations, including exacerbations of chronic illness? Increasing numbers of studies indicate that stress plays a role in both the initiation and the exacerbation of childhood illnesses. Underlying neuroendocrine, immunologic, and physiologic mechanisms merit careful elucidation. Other questions abound. Why does one child with severe arthritis function well, miss little school, act as a leader in the school environment, being only minimally affected by a severe crippling disease? And yet another child, with clinically minimal disease, difficult to demonstrate on physical examination, is severely debilitated, unable to go to school for more than 2 or 3 days a week, complains of frequent pain, and is often bedridden? What are some of the behavioral aspects that may help to explain the different responses of the human organism to disease or to treatment? Why is it that one child with similar genetic material and similar environmental exposures develops a certain disease while another does not?

Further research is needed in trials of different intervention mechanisms. A number of important studies have examined ways of improving the psychological and biological functioning of children through various behavioral and psychological interventions. Much more needs to be done. The most extensive such study was that of Stein and her colleagues at the Albert Einstein Medical Center through the Pediatric Ambulatory Care Treatment program, which was a controlled trial of a coordination of care experiment for families with children with a variety of long-term illnesses. There is sizable opportunity for experimentation in new interventions, varying from specific psychological treatments to stress management programs to educational interventions to care coordination efforts, and it will be wise to examine outcome broadly in a series of domains in new ventures.

Health psychology is of course not limited to the chronic illnesses of childhood. There is a health psychology of acute illness as well, as with the evidence for ambient stress increasing the likelihood of a number of acute infectious diseases, especially herpes and streptococcal disease. Some of the concepts underlying assessment in the area of childhood chronic illness are applicable as well to the broader field of child health in general.

References

Anderson, K. O., Bradley, L. A., Young, L. D., McDaniel, L. K., & Wise, C. M. (1985). Rheumatoid arthritis: Review of psychological factors related to etiology, effects, and treatment. *Psychological Bulletin, 98*, 358–387.

Bergman, A. R., & Stamm, S. J. (1967). The morbidity of cardiac nondisease in school children. *New England Journal of Medicine, 276*, 1008–1116.

Bibace, R., & Walsh, M. E. (1979). Developmental stages of children's conceptions of illness. In G. Stone, F. Cohen, & N. Adler (Eds.), *Health psychology: A handbook*. San Francisco: Jossey-Bass.

Bibace, R., & Walsh, M. E. (1980). Development of children's concepts of illness. *Pediatrics, 66*, 912–917.

Boyce, W. T., Jensen, E. W., Cassel, J. C., Collier, A. M., Smith, A. H., & Ramey, C. T. (1977). Influence of life events and family routines on childhood respiratory tract illness. *Pediatrics, 60*, 609–615.

Breslau, N., Weitzman, M., & Messenger, K. (1981). Psychological functioning of siblings of disabled children. *Pediatrics, 67*, 344–353.

Bruhn, J. G., Hampton, J. W., & Chandler, B. C. (1971). Clinical marginality and psychological adjustment in hemophilia. *Journal of Psychosomatic Research, 15*, 207–213.

Butler, J., Budetti, P., McManus, M. A., Stenmark, S., & Newacheck, P. W. (1985). Health care expenditures for children with chronic illnesses. In N. Hobbs & J. M. Perrin (Eds.), *Issues in the care of children with chronic illness: A sourcebook on problems, services, and policies*. San Francisco: Jossey-Bass.

Cairns, N., Clark, G. M., Smith, S. D., & Lansky, S. B. (1979). Adaptation of siblings to childhood malignancy. *Journal of Pediatrics, 95*, 484–487.

Drash, A., & Berlin, N. (1985). Juvenile diabetes. In N. Hobbs & J. M. Perrin (Eds.), *Issues in the care of children with chronic illness: A sourcebook on problems, services, and policies*. San Francisco: Jossey-Bass.

Drotar, D., & Bush, M. (1985). Mental health issues and services. In N. Hobbs & J. M. Perrin (Eds.), *Issues in the care of children with chronic illness: A sourcebook on problems, services, and policies*. San Francisco: Jossey-Bass.

Elliott, G. R., & Eisdorfer, C. (Eds.) (1982). *Stress and human health*. New York: Springer.

Garlinghouse, J., & Sharp, L. J. (1968). The hemophilic child's self-concept and family stress in relation to bleeding episodes. *Nursing Research, 17*, 32–37.

Garmezy, N. (1981). Children under stress: Perspectives on antecedents and correlates of vulnerability and resistance to psychopathology. In A. I. Rabin, J. Arnoff, A. M. Barclay, & R. A. Zucker (Eds.), *Further explorations in personality*. New York: Wiley.

Garmezy, N., Masten, A. S., & Tellegen, A. (1984). The study of stress and competence in children: A building block for developmental psychopathology. *Child Development, 55*, 97–111.

Gliedman, J., & Roth, W. (1980). *The unexpected minority: Handicapped children in America*. New York: Harcourt Brace Jovanovich.

Gortmaker, S. L. (1985). Demography of chronic childhood diseases. In N. Hobbs & J. M. Perrin (Eds.), *Issues in the care of children with chronic illness: A sourcebook on problems, services, and policies*. San Francisco: Jossey-Bass.

Gortmaker, S., & Sappenfield, W. (1984). Chronic childhood disorders: Prevalence and impact. *Pediatric Clinics of North America, 31*, 3–18.

Haggerty, R. J., Roghmann, K. J., & Pless, I. B. (1975). *Child health and the community*. New York: Wiley.

Hamburg, D. A., Elliott, G. R., & Parron, D. L. (Eds.) (1982). *Health and behavior: Frontiers of research in the biobehavioral sciences*. Washington: National Academy Press.

Heisel, J. S. (1972). Life changes as etiologic factors in juvenile rheumatoid arthritis. *Journal of Psychosomatic Research, 16*, 411–420.

Henoch, M. J., Batson, J. W., & Baum, J. (1978). Psychosocial factors in juvenile rheumatoid arthritis. *Arthritis & Rheumatism, 21*, 229–233.

Hobbs, N., Perrin, J. M., & Ireys, H. T. (1985). *Chronically ill children and their families*. San Francisco: Jossey-Bass.

Holtzman, N. A., & Richmond, J. (1985). Genetic strategies for preventing chronic illness. In N. Hobbs & J. M. Perrin (Eds.), *Issues in the care of children with chronic illness: A sourcebook on problems, services, and policies.* San Francisco: Jossey-Bass.

Jacobs, T. J., & Charles, E. (1980). Life events and the recurrence of cancer in children. *Psychosomatic Medicine, 42,* 11–24.

Jordan, M. K., & O'Grady, D. J. (1982). Children's health beliefs and concepts: Implications for child health care. In P. Karoly, J. J. Steffen, & D. J. O'Grady (Eds.), *Child health psychology: Concepts and issues.* New York: Pergamon.

Lavigne, J., & Ryan, M. (1979). Psychological adjustment of siblings of children with chronic illness. *Pediatrics, 63,* 616–627.

Markova, I., Lockyer, R., & Forbes, C. (1980). Self-perception of employed and unemployed hemophiliacs. *Psychological Medicine, 10,* 559–565.

Masters, J. C., Cerreto, M. C., & Mendlowitz, D. R. (1983). The role of the family in coping with childhood chronic illness. In T. G. Burish & L. A. Bradley (Eds.), *Coping with chronic disease.* New York: Academic.

Matus, I. (1981). Assessing the nature and clinical significance of psychological contributions to childhood asthma. *American Journal of Orthopsychiatry, 51,* 327–341.

McAnarney, E., Pless, I. B., Satterwhite, B. B., & Friedman, S. B. (1974). Psychological problems of children with chronic juvenile arthritis. *Pediatrics, 53,* 523–528.

McCubbin, H. I., McCubbin, M. A., Patterson, J., Cauble, A. E., Wilson, L., & Warwick, W. (1982). CHIP: Coping health inventory for parents. In H. McCubbin (Ed.), *Family stress, coping and social support.* New York: Springer.

McCubbin, H. I., Patterson, T., McCubbin, M. A., & Wilson, L. R. (1983). Parental coping and family environment. In D. Bagarozzi, A Jurich, & R. Jackson (Eds.), *Marital and family therapy: New perspectives.* New York: Human Sciences Press.

Meyer, R. J., & Haggerty, R. J. (1962). Streptococcal infections in families: Factors altering individual susceptibility. *Pediatrics, 29,* 539–549.

Moos, R. H., & Tsu, V. D. (1977). The crisis of physical illness: An overview. In R. H. Moos (Ed.), *Coping with physical illness.* New York: Plenum.

Newacheck, P. W., Budetti, P. P., & Halfon, N. (1986). Trends in activity-limiting chronic conditions among children. *American Journal of Public Health, 76,* 178–184.

Palfrey, J. S., Levy, J. C., & Gilbert, K. L. (1980). Use of primary care facilities by patients attending specialty clinics. *Pediatrics, 65,* 567–572.

Perrin, E. C., & Gerrity, P. S. (1981). There's a demon in your belly: Children's understanding of illness. *Pediatrics, 67,* 841–849.

Perrin, E. C., & Gerrity, P. S. (1984). Development of children with a chronic illness. *Pediatric Clinics of North America, 31,* 19–32.

Perrin, E. C., & Perrin, J. M. (1983). Clinician's assessment of children's understanding of illness. *American Journal of Diseases of Children, 137,* 874–878.

Perrin, J. M., & Ireys, H. T. (1984). The organization of services for chronically ill children and their families. *Pediatric Clinics of North America, 31,* 235–258.

Perrin, J. M., MacLean, W. E., & Perrin, E. C. (1986). *Health status and psychological adjustment in children with asthma.* Manuscript submitted for publication.

Plaut, S. M., & Friedman, S. B. (1981). Psychosocial factors in infectious disease. In R. Ader (Ed.), *Psychoneuroimmunology.* New York: Academic.

Pless, I. B., & Perrin, J. M. (1985). Issues common to a variety of illnesses. In N. Hobbs & J. M. Perrin (Eds.), *Issues in the care of children with chronic illness: A sourcebook on problems, services, and policies.* San Francisco: Jossey-Bass.

Pless, I. B., & Pinkerton, P. (1975). *Chronic childhood disorder: Promoting patterns of adjustment.* Chicago: Year Book Medical Publishers.

Pless, I. B., & Roghmann, K. J. (1971). Chronic illness and its consequences: Some observations based on three epidemiological surveys. *Journal of Pediatrics, 79,* 351–359.

Roskies, E., & Lazarus, R. S. (1980). Coping theory and the teaching of coping skills. In P. O. Davidson & S. M. Davidson (Eds.), *Behavioral medicine: Changing health and lifestyles.* New York: Brunner/Mazel.

Rutter, M., Tizard, J., & Whitmore, K. (Eds.) (1970). *Education, health, and behavior.* London: Longman.

Simeonsson, R. J., Buckley, L., & Monson, L. (1979). Conceptions of illness causality in hospitalized children. *Journal of Pediatric Psychology, 4,* 77–84.

Smithells, R. W., Sheppard, S., Schorah, C. J., Seller, M. J., Nevin, N. C., Harris, R., Read, A. P., & Fielding, D. W. (1981). Apparent prevention of neural tube defects by periconceptional vitamin supplements. *Archives of Disease in Childhood, 56,* 911.

Starfield, B. (1982). Family income, ill health, and medical care of U.S. children. *Journal of Public Health Policy, 3,* 244–259.

Starfield, B. (1985). The state of research on chronically ill children. In N. Hobbs & J. M. Perrin (Eds.), *Issues in the care of children with chronic illness: A sourcebook on problems, services, and policies.* San Francisco: Jossey-Bass.

Stein, R. E. K., & Jessop, D. J. (1982a). A noncategorical approach to chronic childhood illness. *Public Health Reports, 97,* 354–362.

Stein, R. E. K., & Jessop, D. J. (1982b, May). *What diagnosis does not tell: The case for a non-categorical approach to chronic physical illness.* Paper presented at the Annual Meeting of the Society for Pediatric Research, Washington, D.C.

Stein, R. E. K., & Jessop, D. J. (1984). Relationship between health status and psychological adjustment among children with chronic conditions. *Pediatrics, 73,* 169–174.

Stein, R. E. K., & Riessman, C. (1980). The development of an impact-on-family scale: Preliminary findings. *Medical Care, 18,* 465–472.

Stein, S. P., & Charles, E. (1971). Emotional factors in juvenile diabetes mellitus: A study of early life experiences of adolescent diabetics. *American Journal of Psychiatry, 128,* 56–60.

Tavormina, J. B., Kastner, L. S., Slater, P. M., & Watt, S. L. (1976). Chronically ill children—A psychologically and emotionally deviant population? *Journal of Abnormal Child Psychology, 4,* 99–110.

Weeks, K. (1985). Private health insurance and chronically ill children. In N. Hobbs & J. M. Perrin (Eds.), *Issues in the care of children with chronic illness: A sourcebook on problems, services, and policies.* San Francisco: Jossey-Bass.

Williams, H. E., & McNicol, K. N. (1975). The spectrum of asthma in children. *Pediatric Clinics of North America, 22,* 43–52.

3

Linking Assessment and Treatment in Pediatric Health Psychology

DENNIS C. RUSSO
ROGER S. HAMADA
DIANE MARQUES

The pediatric health psychologist who works with children having frank medical disorders faces emerging and unique challenges and opportunities. One of the most important challenges is determining the place and shape of assessment in the consultation or treatment encounter. The determination will be influenced, to a large extent, by the assessor's conceptual models of health and illness.

Conceptual models in pediatric health psychology are shifting away from unilevel, unifactor, linear constructions, such as the classic biomedical or psychosomatic models (Miller, 1983; Schwartz, 1982). With this shift, the need for multilevel, interactional, systemic assessment becomes paramount. Traditional assessment measures that focus on quantifying the child's pathology or deviation from "normal"

Reprints may be obtained from the senior author, Behavioral Medicine Program, The Children's Hospital, 300 Longwood Avenue, Boston, MA 02115. Equal contribution to the development and writing of this manuscript was made by each of the three authors.

tend not to address adequately the complex and multifaceted presentation of the average child responding to or coping with the extraordinary circumstances of having a physical disorder (Russo & Varni, 1982).

As an integral part of a treatment team, the pediatric health psychologist is predominantly concerned with using assessment not for classifying and categorizing symptomatology, but rather for selecting appropriate targets for intervention. Therefore, the pediatric health psychologist must assess both the modifiability of behaviors or symptoms and the optimal systemic level(s) at which to intervene. This assessment will encompass considerations of the child's underlying medical disorder, the cognitive and emotional state of the child, the child's developmental level, his or her family system, the child's physical and social care environment, and the implicit and explicit expectations that the child and the child's caretakers have regarding the role of the pediatric health psychologist in the particular treatment encounters.

In this chapter, we will argue that treatment-related assessment in pediatric health psychology demands contextual assessment. That is, it should explicitly consider not only certain psychological characteristics of the child but also the multiple and interacting variables of that child's background, family structure, and situational context. In addition, it must attend to the interactions between these variables at the different systemic levels. Although various beginnings have been made at delineating what is "context" and what to assess in contextual assessment, operational guidelines for child health clinicians have yet to be established. Some sense of what comprises contextual assessment may be derived from a comparison of the biopsychosocial model of health and illness that underlies the notion of contextual assessment with more traditional biomedical and psychosomatic models on which "acontextual" approaches to assessment with a pediatric population have been based.

MODELS UNDERLYING ACONTEXTUAL ASSESSMENT

Traditional assessment models have emphasized a unidimensional focus. That is, these models have encouraged the focusing of assessment efforts on a single domain of variables in studying the genesis and maintenance of physical disorders. These domains have generally been restricted to one of three categories: biological, psychodynamic, or environmental. The acontextual models have guided assessors in their choices of both diagnosis and treatment. We shall review these traditional acontextual models as they relate to the evaluation of contemporary pediatric illness and current notions of disease genesis and treatment.

Biomedical Model

The biomedical model has dominated the practice of twentieth century medicine, including the practice of medical assessment. A primary characteristic of this model has been its almost exclusive focus on biological parameters in trying to understand and treat illness to the relative exclusion of psychological and social factors (Miller, 1983). This focus on variables of the biological domain led to the discovery of the etiologies and successful treatment of many infectious disorders.

Assessment within the biomedical model emphasizes measurement and quantification of physical parameters and the detection of any deviations from "normal" for these parameters in a given patient. In this model the primary goal of assessment is diagnosis. The diagnosis of disease should in turn lead directly to the prescription of an effective, etiology-based treatment for the disorder. The biomedical model, with its emphasis on the intraindividual, biological level of assessment, has been successful in treating many diseases and in significantly reducing mortality and morbidity attributable to these diseases. The central role of diagnostic assessment in this model has resulted in an impressive increase in the power and diversity of physical, microbiological, and biochemical diagnostic tests.

Due in large part to the success of the biomedical model, the epidemiology of pediatric illness has been changed so that the model no longer seems to provide an adequate basis for conceptualizing most contemporary physical disorders. Whereas the biomedical model provided a solid framework for the assessment and treatment of acute, infectious diseases, the current pediatric patient population primarily comprises individuals suffering chronic physical disorders. Because cures based on a knowledge of the etiology of these disorders are not readily available, these patients' illnesses must be considered a long-term problem requiring ongoing management. Hence chronic disease has an impact on most aspects of patients' lives, and considerations of the psychosocial aspects of illness are playing an increasingly prominent part in the treatment of the contemporary pediatric medical population.

Psychosomatic Model

A second model of health and illness that has influenced the assessment of children with medical disorders is the psychodynamic model of psychosomatic illness. This model, like the biomedical model, focuses on the intraindividual level of analysis, but it does so by emphasizing intrapsychic rather than biological variables. It is a unilinear model, generalized from the biomedical model of pathology (Miller, 1983). The psychodynamic model of psychosomatic illness posits a causal relationship between specific unresolved unconscious conflicts and specific somatic disorders such as rheumatoid arthritis, bronchial asthma, and peptic ulcer. Alexander (1950) argued that psychosomatic disorders represented symbolic manifestations of specific repressed conflicts. These conflicts were the etiology of the physical illness.

Assessment in this model of illness attempted to uncover the unconscious conflicts underlying illness. Projective techniques are utilized as assessment tools to tap the contents of the unconscious. Psychosomatic illness is assumed to be associated with psychopathology. Little or no attention is paid to proximal causes such as genetic factors, infections, or immunological or traumatic variables. Importantly, assessment based on this model of illness has had little impact on differentially specifying treatment, as individuals diagnosed as having psychosomatic illness would be uniformly treated in psychoanalysis or long-term psychotherapy.

Approaches to assessment based on the psychosomatic model share qualities of acontextual assessment with most methods of traditional psychological assessment. These qualities include a focus on the intraindividual level of analysis and an assumption that the individual characteristics being assessed are stable across situational contexts. Acontextual psychological assessment views variability in behavior across individuals as a function of personality, motivation, and cognitive styles (Messick, 1983).

When the pediatric health psychologist utilizes instruments developed within the traditional psychological assessment framework, that psychologist must be cognizant of the assumptions under which the instruments were developed. In particular, results obtained using norm-referenced or projective instruments must be viewed in the context of what groups comprised the original normative sample.

Behavioral–Operant Model

Behavioral assessment, as traditionally conceived, shares both similarities and differences with the other unidimensional models just reviewed. Traditional behavioral assessment (Mash & Terdal, 1981) is centered on evaluating the functional relationships between a person's environment and his or her behavior. The operant approach's molecular focus on the interactive series of stimulus and consequence events in the child's proximal environment and its insistence on the centrality of such events as the proper locus of inquiry fail to differentiate it from other linear explanatory models (Russo & Tarbell, 1984).

Behavioral–operant models do differ, however, in their supposed locus of functional, controlling variables: the environment. This locus allows obvious advantages in model building, among them a focus on observable events and the ability to test hypotheses by experimental methods. It is noteworthy that experimental outcomes have increasingly demonstrated the need to increase the paradigm's recognition of other variables, such as cognitive and disease factors, which are more temporally distal than the immediate stimulus environment originally considered to be important (Russo, Tarbell, & Follansbee, in press). Recently, the linear, unifactor stimulus–response model that provided the lore for early notions of behavioral assessment has been elaborated upon to posit reciprocal, interactive relationships between multiple levels of stimuli and responses (Evans, 1985; Kanfer, 1985; Russo et al., in press). Such elaboration of traditional models should assist in their integration to explain more adequately contemporary pediatric disease.

CONTEXTUAL MODELS OF ILLNESS

In recent years, unifactor models have evolved into more systemic multicausal, multieffect models. Unifactor models of disease had clinical utility in guiding the discovery of causal mechanisms in infectious diseases. As previously noted, these early models were generalized to study psychopathology with mixed results. However, as infectious diseases were increasingly mastered and medicine largely focused on both preventive care and the management of chronic illness, the inadequacy of unifactor models became apparent (Miller, 1983). Neither biomedical models with exclusive emphasis upon biological factors in disease nor traditional psychosomatic models with exclusive emphasis on psychogenesis of disease were able to explain the interactive role of genetic, developmental, behavioral, cognitive, social, and environmental factors in the mediation of health and disease (Russo et al., in press).

Similarly, recent research on setting events suggests that operant conditioning principles may not always be sufficiently extensive to account for contextual influences beyond immediate organism–environment interactions (Russo et al., in press; Wahler

& Fox, 1981). Although unifactor operant models have led to many successful remediations of maladaptive behavior, a strictly behavioral model also cannot explain the complex interrelationship between biology, behavior, and illness. As the impact of psychosocial factors upon every area of biological functioning including the immune system and smooth muscle functioning previously thought not under voluntary control becomes elucidated (Russo et al., in press), the need for multicausal, multifactor models of both psychological and physical pathology becomes paramount.

Several models suggesting frameworks to understand the complex relationship between etiological, intrapersonal, and environmental factors have been proposed. These models have a common focus on identifying and quantifying both small- and large-scale systemic factors, on studying the effects of interactions, and on considering variables from different domains simultaneously (Schwartz, 1982). These contextual models include the modern psychosomatic models and the biopsychosocial models.

Modern Psychosomatic Models

Modern psychosomatic medicine presents an alternative to the traditional psychodynamic model of psychosomatic illness. Current psychosomatic theory reflects findings on the multicausality of somatic functions and behavior and acknowledges the contribution of biological, psychological, and social factors to the development, course, and outcome of physical disorders. The complex and dynamic interactions of these multilevel factors, modified by feedback effects, are posited to influence changes in health.

The new psychosomatic model (Lipowski, 1977) posits that an individual's constitution is a function of the interaction of genetic factors and early experience, constantly modified by multiple biological and psychosocial variables. Symbolic processes such as perceptions, thoughts, images, and memory influence organismic responding at all levels of functioning, from cellular physiology to behavior.

Three conceptual categories reflecting current psychosomatic theory have been detailed: psychophysiological response specificity; psychosocial stress; and individual susceptibility to disease (Lipowski, 1977). The psychophysiological specificity concept hypothesizes that particular individuals respond to stressful stimulus events and situations with a predictable set of psychological and physiological changes. It follows from this conceptualization that assessment of and intervention either at the level of environment to reduce the probability of stressful events occurring or at the psychophysiological level to modify the predictable response may be beneficial.

Psychosocial stressors are environmental events and social situations that disturb individual homeostasis and stimulate physiological changes. Major life events, particularly if temporally contiguous, have been considered necessary but not sufficient triggers for the onset of physiological illness. Individual susceptibility to disease refers to the notion that inherently vulnerable organ systems in individuals may remain nonproblematic until environmental or psychosocial events trigger stress-related pathology.

Thus the three tenets of new psychosomatic theory suggest the following scenario for the onset of physical disease: A clustering of psychosocial stressors leads to physiological changes in particularly vulnerable organ systems, and particular individuals respond in predictable psychological and physical ways.

Biopsychosocial Model

The biopsychosocial model of health and illness (Engel, 1977, 1982; Schwartz, 1982) represents a systems-based model that argues that assessment and treatment of disease should encompass consideration of the interactions of biological, social, and psychological factors. In addition, the biopsychosocial model assumes that treatments will interact with each other as well as with the person and his or her environment. This model is derived from what Pepper (1942) (cf. Schwartz, 1982) described as contextual and organistic thinking in contrast to categorical, reductionistic, or unicausal thinking. In contextual thinking, the character of natural events is postulated to depend on the context in which they occur as well as on the context of the observer of the events. Organistic thinking is characterized by the contention that the properties of a system as a whole emerge from the functioning of its individual parts, and the system is more than the sum of its parts.

Contextual thinking is exemplified by Fabrega and Van Egeren (1976) in their description of a biopsychosocial paradigm from a systems perspective as consisting of interconnected and hierarchical subsystems. Any changes in one level of a subsystem will thus impact on other levels. Reciprocal relationships are posited to exist among the complex levels of a subsystem, such that psychosocial events that may produce or be associated with concomitant physical changes are communicated through various biochemical changes at the cellular level. Conversely, biochemical or molecular events are posited to be transmitted through the system hierarchy and to result in concomitant psychophysiological, cognitive, and behavioral changes.

As previously stated, biopsychosocial assessment demands a multilevel, interactive approach to evaluating the state of health or illness, to selecting and implementing the necessary interventions, and to monitoring the efficacy of the interventions. However, operationalizing these concepts is a difficult matter. Schwartz (1982) has proposed operationalizing this model through the use of the Patient Evaluation Grid (PEG). The PEG would be used to guide the comprehensive assessment of individuals and to organize clinical data in a manner that acknowledges the interactive, multilevel nature of illness. The PEG provides a multidimensional framework delineating, on one dimension, important categories of biological, personal, and environmental data, and on another, temporal, dimension, the historical, recent, and current status of those categories. The biopsychosocial model with its emphasis on interdisciplinary collaboration and integration of variables at numerous conceptual levels may be closer to the actual practice of contemporary pediatric health psychology than the previously described models of health and illness.

The biopsychosocial model assumes that behavior and psychological events occur not in isolation but in an interacting context that both impacts on and is subsequently influenced by those behaviors and events. In the practice of behavioral pediatrics, one implication of the biopsychosocial model is that "abnormal" or maladaptive behaviors in the chronically ill child are not thought of as stemming from fixed or static internal traits. Instead, the child with chronic disease is best viewed as a "normal" individual who is functioning in the abnormal context occasioned by his or her illness (Russo & Varni, 1982). It is argued that children with chronic illness have been able to cope reasonably well with daily life events prior to their illness, but with the onset of their illness find that their life contexts have been altered in both gross and subtle ways and that they face an unusually large number of disruptive and intrusive stressors. If these children develop maladaptive behaviors, cognitions, or feelings, the symptoms may be attributed to psychosocial stress and to the unusual learning situation afforded by having a chronic illness, rather than to any inherent defect in the child.

The biopsychosocial model, in addition to considering an individual's reaction to illness, considers the course of the illness as being reactive to the individual's behavior and psychological state. For example, the detrimental synergistic effects of inappropriate eating, dieting, exercise patterns, and levels of stress on the course of cardiovascular disease as well as the positive effects of stress management, anxiety reduction, and diet–weight–exercise education in postcoronary patients have been documented (Maccoby, Farquhar, Wood, & Alexander, 1977).

Assessing synergistic relationships between variables at different levels of the subsystems impinging on an individual and choosing a point of entry into the system for treatment are procedures that have not been well operationalized. Assessing a child's symptoms in context simultaneously requires both a narrow focus on the presenting problem and a broader focus on relevant variables at other systemic levels.

Comprehensive medical and psychological treatment requires attending to the disease itself, to the synergistic impact of development, learning, and behavior on the course of the disease, and to the reciprocal impact of the disease on these factors (Russo, Bennett, Harmon & Brown, 1981). Determining the most effective, efficient, and parsimonious intervention from the perspective of this multifactor contextual model is a complicated decision. Based on this biopsychosocial view of illness, the crux of assessment and treatment for the practicing pediatric health psychologist may be framed by two questions: (1) How does one define the problem? (2) At what level does one intervene? The answers to these questions require a consideration of factors above and beyond what may be defined as the presenting problem by the child's caretaking systems. We believe that it is this determination by pediatric health psychologists regarding the appropriate targets and levels for intervention and the intervention of choice that distinguishes their role as health care professionals. Clearly, assessment and treatment are inextricably and symbiotically linked in the accomplishment of this role.

LINKING ASSESSMENT AND TREATMENT

In helping children and families faced with chronic and/or life-threatening conditions, the pediatric psychologist now finds little utility in models as a basis for clinical intervention. On the one hand, recent research has moved away from unifactor models such as personality configurations that predisposed individuals to certain illnesses (Johnson, 1984). On the other hand, behavioral medicine research continues to focus on the treatment of particular ailments in the absence of examination of commonalities of the illness process in distressed individuals (Lazarus, 1985). By addressing symptoms through mechanical or rote interventions, one fails to appreciate the person in the context of his or her physical and emotional reality (Lazarus, 1985). When dealing with children, it is even easier to ignore certain psychological needs and expressions, given the child's relative lack of control or power in the treatment decision.

Multilevel Assessment Factors

The review just presented of the various traditional and contemporary models of disease leaves the pediatric psychologist with little in the way of specific operational guidelines for linking assessment and treatment. Which model will eventually best explain the child with chronic illness is, in many senses, a question best answered as an outcome of practice. For the pediatric psychologist faced with a chronically ill child in obvious distress, the question becomes one of assessing the multiple and specific factors influencing the individual child and family in the process of coping with chronic illness. The remainder of this chapter will focus on describing these areas and suggesting possible strategies for their assessment.

In this section, we shall review six factors central to a contextual assessment of pediatric chronic illness. This assessment framework suggests that complex, often idiosyncratic interactions may exist between several variables and these must be considered for adequate treatment formulation. By identifying strengths and weaknesses at each level in this system, one may then develop multiple hypotheses about the most probable or common causal variables responsible for patient dysfunction. The choice and prioritization of treatment targets are facilitated by identifying common problem themes across factors, determining base rates of problem presentation, identifying treatment options and their probable success, and evaluating the consequences of omitting or delaying treatment on a given problem.

After certain target behaviors are chosen, the treatment must then be justified using ongoing assessment as a part of the treatment process. These guidelines may be recognized as hallmarks of traditional medical diagnosis (Kanfer, 1985), but they are necessary as well in the provision of adequate treatment in pediatric health psychology. This chapter will now examine in detail physical status, developmental level, coping strategy, family functioning, the physical care environment, and generic assessment factors as they relate to a contextual assessment of pediatric chronic illness.

Physical Status. It is imperative that pediatric health psychologists who work with children having frank medical disorders be cognizant of the physical status of their clients (Russo & Varni, 1982). This knowledge is integral to psychologists' responsibilities, defining the extent to which they are capable of helping children and their families. The knowledge is also central to the formulation of intervention programs and to the evaluation of the efficacy of such programs (Russo & Tarbell, 1984). It therefore behooves psychologists working with medically disordered children, in particular those children with chronic illnesses, to acknowledge that psychological intervention should occur only in conjunction with ongoing medical treatment (Cataldo, Russo, Bird, & Varni, 1980). Hence the major responsibility for the patient's care must rest with the physician, with psychologists acting primarily in the role of consultants, albeit consultants who are involved in an ongoing relationship with patients, their families, and their treatment teams (Hovanitz, Gerwell, & Russo, 1984; Schwartz, 1982).

In acknowledging their consultative role, pediatric health psychologists must determine that children presenting with somatic problems receive an adequate medical examination as a prerequisite to psychological intervention. Knowledge about the medical disorder's physiological mechanisms and course will have several implications for psychologists treating children with these disorders. It may be that somatic complaints are not amenable to psychological intervention but are best managed primarily through medical or surgical means. In these cases, a knowledge about patients' physical status will guide psychologists toward selecting appropriate targets for intervention, will help them assist patients in delineating appropriate goals for psychological intervention, and will enable psychologists to predict to some extent at the beginning of treatment the kind, rate, and degree of improvement to be realistically expected (Pelcovits, Silver, & Russo, 1983).

Knowledge of a child's physical status can alert the pediatric health psychologist to potential areas of concern due to general physiological symptoms resulting from any pathophysiologic disorder or from the medical treatment or management of that disorder. Understanding of the pattern of an illness can lead to a recognition of the scope of the illness's effect on the child's daily life and to the stresses a child and his or her family might be expected to encounter. Furthermore, this knowledge can inform the psychologist as to the parameters of a child's physical impairments and possible deterioration in physical status. Finally, information about a child's physical condition can provide some insight into how health care providers might interact with the child (Drotar, Crawford, & Ganofsky, 1984).

A child's disease or its treatment may result in altered physiology or in pharmacological side effects. Children experience pain, nausea, loss of appetite, dizziness, and other symptoms that contribute to subjective distress (Russo et al., 1981). These symptoms, in turn, may motivate maladaptive behavior such as a refusal to eat or a decrease in social and physical activity. Consequences of this maladaptive behavior may include nutritional deficiencies, muscle atrophy, life-threatening weight loss, depression, and psychosocial withdrawal. Physiological alterations and treatment side effects may also lead to nonadherence to medical treatment regimens and medical fears and anxieties.

Psychologists are often asked to intervene with ill children when the consequences of maladaptive behavior become a concern for health care professionals or parents. Formulating an intervention program without an understanding of the patient's medical status and its implications for the child's behavior may compromise the appropriateness and/or the efficacy of an intervention program.

Children with medical illnesses and their families experience anxiety and stress associated with those illnesses. Stress, in turn, often exacerbates symptoms of an illness. An understanding of the pattern of an illness can often inform a psychologist about the nature and extent of the impact an illness has on the lives of children and their families, and about the stresses these individuals may be expected to encounter. For example, the bronchospasms associated with stress and anxiety may exacerbate respiratory distress in both asthmatics and children with cystic fibrosis. This distress may lead to hyperventilation and thus increase the severity of symptoms. Training in coping skills, relaxation, and stress management may be effective in reducing respiratory distress and preventing hyperventilation in both groups. However, the psychologists working with these children will keep in mind how the meanings of respiratory distress may differ for the asthmatics and their families and for those with cystic fibrosis and their families. For some mild asthmatics, while their distress is alarming, the symptoms are fairly readily alleviated, and in many cases, will remit with age. Cystic fibrosis, on the other hand, is a progressively deteriorating, life-threatening disorder with no known cure. As the child approaches the end stages of the disease, frequency of hospitalizations for respiratory distress increases (Spirito, Russo, & Masek, 1984).

Knowing the differing patterns of these diseases that may present with a similar symptom alerts psychologists to the possibility that often issues in addition to the presenting symptom may have a bearing on how they work with these children and their families. Depending on the nature and course of a disease, psychologists may need to help patients and their families cope with physical impairment and deterioration, disruptions in their adjustments to life's routines, impending premature death, and parent's guilt at transmitting a genetically linked disorder to their offspring (Drotar et al., 1984; Koocher & O'Malley, 1981).

An awareness of the typical pattern of a medical illness is also vital to pediatric health psychologists' evaluations of the efficacy of their interventions. For example, biofeedback, relaxation training, and stress management training are frequently used to help children cope with the pain of muscle contraction and migraine headaches (Masek, Russo, & Varni, 1984). When these means are employed, children are often able to decrease the intensity, duration, and frequency of their headaches. A particular subtype of vascular headaches, cluster headaches, typically presents as a series of brief, intense headaches that spontaneously remit, sometimes for months, and then recur without obvious precipitants. Self-control strategies have not proven to be very effective in alleviating this particular kind of headache. However, if one were not aware of the natural course of these headaches, one might erroneously attribute the spontaneous remission of symptoms to the intervention program.

In their work with medically ill children, pediatric health psychologists may have opportunities for psychophysiological and biochemical assessment of their patients that are not readily available to psychologists who work with other patient populations. These assessments can be extremely valuable in providing validation of patients' self-reports, as, for example, in patients who practice relaxation exercises, in providing objective and independent assessment of compliance to medical and psychological treatment, in providing new measures of treatment criteria, and in validating the effects and efficacy of behavioral interventions (Russo, Bird, & Masek, 1980).

Developmental Level. In planning and implementing an individualized intervention program, the pediatric health psychologist will be influenced by his or her assessment of a child's developmental level. Such an assessment will affect decisions about the optimal systemic level at which to intervene and about which intervention techniques will be employed. It is becoming increasingly recognized by psychologists who work with pediatric populations, as well as by child clinical psychologists in general, that intervention programs must be appropriately tailored to a child's level of cognitive, physical, and socioemotional development (Maddux, Roberts, Sledden, & Wright, 1986; Varni, 1983).

Intervention methods applied to pediatric populations have been largely developed for adult patients. Whether the direct application of these methods to children is appropriate is beginning to be explored empirically. Some evidence suggests that there are differences between the responses of adults and children to various interventions (Harris & Ferrari, 1983). However, incorporating assessment of developmental level into treatment decisions involves more than questioning the applicability of adult techniques to children.

Research from developmental psychology strongly suggests that children cannot be considered a homogeneous group with respect to their cognitive, physical, and socioemotional development, but might be more properly viewed as many unique subgroups, each of which shares the homogeneity of a particular developmental stage (Kendall, Lerner, & Craighead, 1984). The implications of this view for the treatment of children with frank medical illness may be illustrated by a consideration of how children's level of cognitive development relates to their conceptualizations of illness.

Research with children who are ill and hospitalized suggests that their concepts of illness fit a cognitive developmental model and parallel general cognitive development. For example, Simeonsson, Buckley, and Monson (1979) used questions designed to test children's notions of the causes of illness in a group of children 4 to 9 years old hospitalized for a variety of medical reasons. Children's responses were assigned to one of three groups, including: (1) global, magical, superstitious, or undifferentiated responses; (2) concrete, specific responses reflecting rule breaking, rule keeping, and specific acts and events; and (3) abstract verbalizations or expressions of a generalizable principle. These researchers found that the children's conceptions of the causes of illness were related to their general cognitive development as reflective in measures of conservation, decentration, and physical causality. These findings are supported by other researchers utilizing similar methods (Campbell, 1975; Myers-Vando, Steward, Folkins, & Hines, 1979).

This research supports the findings of a number of clinically oriented studies that have indicated that young, ill children may conceptualize their illness, hospitalization, and treatment as punishment for misbehavior or breaking rules (for reviews see Nagera, 1978; Weis, 1975). Children's understanding of the causes of their illness and of their treatment will affect how they appraise that illness and treatment and how stressful the experience will be for them. Their understanding may affect the levels of anxiety and dysphoria they experience, as well as their compliance with and adherence to prescribed treatment regimens.

By assessing the cognitive developmental level of a child, which is not reliably predicted by considering chronological age alone, the pediatric health psychologist can minimize or avoid the additional stresses on the sick child due to the child's misconceptions about the illness and its treatment. This task can be accomplished, in part, by being sensitive to the cognitive characteristics of children at specific developmental levels, being alert for misconceptions, and correcting or avoiding such misconceptions by providing information in a manner suited to the child's level of cognitive development. Furthermore, educating the family unit regarding the child's conceptual level may aid the family in helping the child cope with the illness and hospitalization adaptively.

Varni (1983) suggests the following guidelines to facilitate pediatric patient education:

1. Terminology that may have unintended secondary meanings that children may be unable to distinguish should be avoided.
2. Explanations should be very concrete and refer to overt behaviors. Internal

processes should be explained using metaphors appropriate to the child's cognitive level.

3. Use of toys and fantasy play with young children not only provide a vehicle for assessing and clarifying misconceptions and conveying information about medical procedures, but also give the child an opportunity to achieve some sense of mastery over the situation through active participation. Permitting the child to manipulate some of the instruments prior to the actual procedure may help alleviate anxiety.

In addition to being an important consideration in planning patient education, a child's developmental level should be taken into account in the selection of an intervention to alleviate a target problem. The intervention should be appropriate for the child's developing physical, psychological, social, and behavioral characteristics. Kendall and colleagues (1984) underscore the importance of matching interventions to developmental level. They cite the research of Katz, Kellerman, and Siegel (1980), which suggested that older children express anxiety differently than younger children. They noted that younger children's anxiety was manifested as crying and screaming, while the older children evidenced muscle rigidity and expressions of pain. Kendall and colleagues (1984) noted that the focus of anxiety shows age-related shifts, changing from anxiety about specific animals and events in younger children to social anxiety and agoraphobia in early adolescence.

Given these data, the pediatric health psychologist must consider the developmental level of the child in deciding whether to emphasize muscle relaxation in a treatment program for anxiety, whether to focus on in vivo exposure, or whether to include a cognitive component in such interventions. Effectiveness of such cognitively oriented interventions as self-instructional training also relies on an adequate assessment of a child's developmental level.

Knowledge of a child's developmental level will help the pediatric health psychologist in working with the family of a sick or dying child. Parents of a sick child, particularly a child suffering from a chronic illness, may be helped to modify developmentally inaccurate expectations of him or her, and this modification could benefit both child and parents. Chronically ill children whose illness has interfered with a normal developmental course may show uneven attainment of physical, socioemotional, and psychological milestones so that parental expectations may exceed their children's capabilities (Stein & Jessop, 1982). On the other hand, parents may underestimate a chronically ill child's capabilities and therefore fail to encourage the child to express his or her talents fully. The behavior of other people in the child's environment may shape the child's own behavior either toward increasing passivity and dependence or toward developing adaptive coping skills (Russo, 1986).

Considering the developmental level of a child suffering a life-threatening illness will give the pediatric health psychologist some guidelines regarding the child's concerns and conceptions of death (Koocher, 1984). The psychologist, in turn, can guide and support the child's family in coping and helping the child cope optimally with the situation. For example, whereas the parents of a dying young child may react to the impending separation portended by the child's death, the child may be more concerned about whether dying will hurt and about the parents' expressions of distress (Sourkes, 1982). With the psychologist's assistance, parents who understand the child's concerns may be better able to support the child's efforts at coping with the illness, with the often painful and invasive treatment of the illness, and with the terminal stages of illness.

In behavioral approaches to managing disorders associated with pediatric chronic illness, it is often the case that the intervenor's assessment of developmental issues and of his or her ability to control environmental variables translates into using cognitive, physiological, and self-control strategies with adolescents and using operant procedures for younger children (Hovanitz et al., 1984). However, as information accrues regarding the cognitive, socioemotional, and physical development of children with frank medical disorders, and as the use of multilevel, contextual assessment and interventions is explicitly formulated, assessment of developmental level will guide interventions in increasingly sophisticated and subtle ways.

Coping Strategy. Stress researchers and health psychologists have noted that adults demonstrate consistent cognitive strategies for coping with stress (Folkman & Lazarus, 1980; Lazarus, 1966; Leventhal, Nerenz, & Strauss, 1980). Suls and Fletcher (1985) have characterized a number of these strategies as either avoidant or nonavoidant coping strategies. Avoidant strategies are those in which a person "focuses attention away from the source of stress or away from one's psychological/somatic reactions to the stressor" (p. 250). This group incorporates strategies that have been variously termed denial, distraction, repression, and suppression. Nonavoidant strategies, on the other hand, consist of those in which attention is focused toward the source of stress or one's reactions to stress. People characterized as sensitizers or those who are deemed to have accurate reality testing may use nonavoidant coping strategies. In a metaanalysis of the extant experimental research, Suls and Fletcher (1985) argue that choice of coping strategies is associated with how effectively a person is able to cope with stress both in the presence of the stressor and over the long term.

Although most of this research has been carried out with adults, some researchers have begun to examine whether children also demonstrate identifiable and characteristic cognitive strategies for coping with stress (Burnstein & Meichenbaum, 1979; Knight et al., 1979; Siegel, 1981). These studies have generally found that children's styles of coping with medically related stressors, like those of adults, may be broadly classified as avoidant or nonavoidant. Peterson and Toler (1984) have demonstrated how taking children's different cognitive coping strategies into account in designing programs for presurgical preparation may lead to greater postsurgical benefits than if a standard presurgical program is uniformly applied to all children about to undergo surgery.

As evidence continues to mount that a child's reaction to a stressor may be influenced by his or her appraisal of that stressor as much as or more than by the objective characteristics of the stimulus, pediatric health psychologists will want to take individuals' coping strategies into account in planning intervention programs, following the example of Peterson and Toler (1984).

Family Functioning. Assessment of the family functioning of the chronically ill child is essential. There are a number of levels at which a family's organization and behavior both impact on and are influenced by the course of a child's illness. The level the clinician may choose to assess ranges from molecular interactions to more global patterns of behavior, and interventions may also range from specific to more global levels.

On a basic interactional level, the pediatric health psychologist must assess how parental response to the problematic behavior influences its appearance. Because certain medical treatments and care regimens frequently involve necessary restrictions of certain behaviors and activities, chronically ill children often learn sick-role behaviors that later impair their adjustment in more everyday circumstances (Russo & Varni, 1982). If particular sick-role behaviors are being shaped and reinforced by parents, their willingness and capability to reshape more adaptive behaviors must also be assessed. The degree to which the child's symptoms have a function in avoiding or escaping negative or stressful events must be examined, as well as parental limit setting. Often parents of chronically ill children experience difficulty in routine limit setting that may generalize to more serious problems in facilitating compliance with necessary medical regimens in their children. Thus the parents' ideas about the child's illness, parental expectations of normal behavior from the child, and feelings of guilt or responsibility for the presence of the child's illness are types of cognitions that need to be assessed and addressed in the treatment encounter.

On a more global level, it is often useful to assess the function an illness plays in the life of the family. Occasionally families are seen in which an illness such as asthma or epilepsy takes on an unnecessarily restrictive, central role. Given the ample opportunities illness provides for the learning of maladaptive behavior patterns, families may use the symptoms of a child's illness to avoid or escape familial conflicts and stresses, just as the child may learn to do in stressful situations. Using anecdotal observations, Bowen (1976) has extensively documented the "shock wave" pattern in which the appearance of pathology in family members often coincides with a real or functional loss of a significant family member. Occasionally families will appear requesting treatment who have had numerous previous treatment contacts, and an extensive number of specialists and social support personnel in the background. When the most parsimonious interventions fail, more systemic questions such as have been previously detailed are well worth examining.

Finally, the structural life-style of a family may contribute to or exacerbate the course of illness on an instrumental or primary level. High levels of interpersonal conflict, irregular or inadequate nutritional support, poor hygiene, and a host of other factors in the physical environment of the home may be chosen as targets for intervention.

Physical Care Environment. The impact of the health care environment is being increasingly recognized as an important contributing factor not only in reducing mortality but also in speeding recovery (Cataldo, Jacobs, & Rogers, 1982). The actual physical care routines of a hospital, such as the ways in which vital signs are collected, can be critical variables when problems arise. For instance, ICU psychosis appeared as an unexpected and undesirable side effect of the intensive, round-the-clock care in which sensory deprivation and time distortion occur. Care routines that reinforce wellness and facilitate independence create more opportunities for recovery.

Also, staff interactions that foster communication and cooperation lead to clearer behavioral expectations for the sick child. An important point of evaluation is the staff–staff, staff–patient, and staff–parent interaction. Frequently, ward consultations are requested when disagreement exists within a multidisciplinary team, when caretakers perceive a child's behavior with staff as manipulative, or when parents or staff perceive inadequacies on either part. One must assess such "hidden agendas" in order to gauge effectively the resources of the system both to implement changes and to address what is really being requested.

Interactions between the patient and his or her family and the patient's health care providers should be assessed. The care of sick children, particularly chronically ill children, places unique stresses on the relationships between patients and their caregivers. Chronically ill children and their families are often required to negotiate transactions with a number of caregivers in many, often highly specialized, different treatment settings. These treatment settings have distinctive subcultures (Drotar, 1976) with which patients and their families must cope.

In addition, the multiplicity of specialized caregivers, time pressures, the absence of privacy, and structural and organizational problems all work to the detriment of the interactions between families and caregivers, thereby increasing stress in the patient–family system (Drotar, Benjamin, Chuast, Litt, & Vajner, 1981; Tefft & Simeonsson, 1979). Moreover, working with chronically ill children and their families tends to stress the caregivers who must try to remain open and available to their patients while feeling frustrated because of their inability to cure the disease and because this work often requires psychosocial skills that the caregivers may not have received formal training in and that may not be in their repertoires. (Axelrod, 1979; Haggerty, Roghman, & Pless, 1975). Medical treatments may result in unforeseen stresses, and caregivers must struggle with the moral and ethical burden of apparently inflicting added physical and emotional suffering on a child and family when they know that they cannot cure the physical condition. The pediatric health psychologist working with a chronically ill child may well choose, therefore, to target interventions at the level of the health care team as well as at the level of child and family. An assessment of the child's physical status and an understanding of the issues involved will help guide these interventions.

Finally, as in all consultation or liaison contacts, the consultant is confronted with the dilemma of who one's client is—staff, patient, or parents? Consultants must always assess what is in the best interests of the child and who will most benefit from a change in the targeted behavior. Fortunately, most requests for behavior change are in the interests of more effective and therapeutic treatment. Health care team members may encourage a child to take responsibility for aspects of his or her care in an effort to give the child a sense of control of treatment and to combat anxiety-provoking feelings of helplessness or lack of control. It may happen that the degree of responsibility expected is developmentally inappropriate or primarily serves the convenience of caretakers rather than the child's needs. If this is the case, this situation should be brought to the attention of the care team and be resolved with the consultant's assistance.

Generic Assessment Factors. A multilevel, multicausal assessment should attend to the previously delineated systemic levels, to provide information permitting the choice of an appropriate intervention. The principles of assessment delineated in Russo and colleagues (1980) give a contextual approach to assessment.

Issues of reliability and validity remain important assessment concerns affecting quality of treatment (Russo et al., 1980). Objective measures of psychophysiological or biochemical functioning have often been shown to have poor test–retest reliabilities, and medical measures should not be automatically assumed reliable. A social reliability problem presents itself in assessing the influence of behavior on disease or the importance of psychological factors on the course of illness. Frequently, traditional assessments have been used, such as verbal report or psychological tests, rather than observable behaviors. Often, in treating psychophysiological disorders, no overt observable behaviors are available for measurement, self-report of internal response is not assessed for reliability, or measures of targeted psychophysiological response are not obtained outside of the treatment setting. Continued attention to the reliability of assessment measures and the use of multiple assessment techniques then appear necessary to both the determination of treatment and its effectiveness.

Validity of psychological intervention represents a second important issue in the recognition of such treatment as a part of comprehensive medical care (Russo et al., 1980). For physicians to accept the value of psychological treatment, results must address treatment-induced changes in terms that physicians understand. Information that relates treatment outcomes to changes in physical status, such as improved BUN or creatinine values as a result of dietary compliance in the hemodialysis patient or correlations between seizure activity and behavioral treatments, will form the basis for helping us to understand the basic relationships between behavior and disease.

How the thoughts, behaviors, and feelings of our patients influence their physical status and vice versa is what forms the scientific substrate of health psychology. Attention to these issues in both clinical and scientific work not only enhances our understanding of disease–behavior mechanisms but also will strongly influence medical perception of psychological treatment as a primary therapeutic device as well as a supportive treatment. Given that psychological treatment may represent an alternative to pharmacologic or surgical treatment in areas such as migraine (Masek et al., 1984) or fecal incontinence (Parker & Whitehead, 1982), data on physical as well as behavioral or psychosocial outcomes are critical in validating the necessity of such treatment as an alternative to traditional medical management of certain disorders or conditions.

In order for assessment and treatment in pediatric health to meet their maximum potential, specific attention must be paid to communication of both methods and outcomes to collaborating medical professionals. This requires not only the publication of research in medical as well as psychological journals, but additionally the explicit teaching, in every clinical encounter, of the value of psychological intervention, when it should be utilized, and the complexity and multiplicity of resources available to the pediatric health psychologist in the collaborative management of health and disease in children. The training of physicians in how to identify relevant targets for psychological intervention should become a significant part of all treatment encounters. Such efforts should simultaneously result in improved care of the ill child and the increased utilization of pediatric health psychology sevices.

A GUIDE TO CONTEXTUAL CLINICAL ASSESSMENT

When presented with a clinical referral, the pediatric health psychologist is, in essence, faced with a series of decisions related to assessment, clinical intervention, and communication. Such decisions must be based upon a thorough understanding of the psychologist's role in the health care team, the nature of the patient's illness and medical treatment, and the multiplicity of factors delineated earlier in this chapter. Indeed, such a role demands more of the training, energy, and communication skill of the psychologist than any other role in contemporary practice.

As we have progressed through this chapter one fact has emerged clearly: Contextual assessment and treatment that simultaneously address disease, patient and family, and environmental factors must define the role of the pediatric health psychologist. Such assessment and treatment skills are still in their infancy. As Russo and Tarbell (1984) suggest, the dictum *primum no nocere* ("first to do no harm") is an appropriate caveat for psychologists as well as physicians. Clinical practice in pediatric health psychology is still very much at the level of an art rather than a science. This is due to several factors, including the emerging understanding of the relationships between behavior and disease and the lack of rigorous and formal training in health psychology at this early stage of the field (Russo et al., in press).

In clinical practice, the pediatric health psychologist must be acutely aware of the dynamic balance between the practice of medicine and health psychology and the need for continued joint medical and psychological care. While the benefits of such a collaboration are many, the potential for and cost of error on the part of health psychologist, due to overzealous or independent effort, are high. Limits of capability and practice must be a just consideration in the development of any treatment plan.

After such consideration, assessment and treatment require a complex process of examining the patient, the disease, the environment, and the context. Based upon our clinical experience, we would recommend the following issues be considered prior to the implementation of any therapeutic intervention. These should be considered a *minimum*. Each case requires individual consideration, and additional assessment may be necessary.

1. What is the referral problem?
   a. Is the request reasonable?
   b. Does the request take into account multiple factors that may influence psychological treatment?
2. What other areas require intervention (e.g., family issues, stress, behavior problems)?
3. What factors require assessment to provide an adequate formulation?
   a. Medical: physical status, contraindications, drug effects, and so on
   b. Developmental factors
   c. Family function
   d. Stress issues
   e. Care routines, environmental issues
   f. Other factors, as relevant
4. What methods will be used over the course of the assessment and treatment (e.g., interview, history, ratings, behavior recordings, physical data)?
5. What are the goals of treatment?
   a. What is a satisfactory outcome?

   b. Do goals fit with medical care?
6. What are the methods of treatment?
   a. Define specific interventions.
   b. Who will conduct treatment?
   c. How will assessment and treatment be linked?
7. How will communication between health care team members occur?
   a. Who must receive data?
   b. How will joint decisions on treatment course be made?
8. Is the treatment ethical, appropriate, and defendable?
   a. Who is the "patient"?
   b. Does treatment serve the long-term best interests of the child?
9. Under what circumstances should treatment be curtailed or reevaluated?
   a. Specify failure criteria.
   b. Monitor physical parameters as a basis for decision.
10. How will treatment be maintained and generalized?
   a. Plan for parent training or home care.
   b. What will be necessary to assist patient over *course* of chronic disease?
   c. What future problems may arise that should trigger a response by care team?
   d. Who will follow the case to identify these issues?

These guidelines represent some of the questions to be asked prior to any intervention by the health psychologist. It must be stressed that the process of assessment must be based upon the needs of the patient, medical status, and the current context of care, not upon theoretical formulation. In each clinical case the role and contribution of the pediatric health psychologist are defined by the presenting problems and must "fit" within the multiple medical and psychosocial care plans. Unlike traditional psychological formulation, assessment in pediatric health psychology requires both initial and ongoing evaluation to enhance its effectiveness and to protect the patient.

This chapter has attempted to delineate some of the considerations in linking assessment and treatment in the multidisciplinary management of pediatric chronic illness. Like assessment itself, our understanding of such illness and the role of the pediatric health psychologist in comprehensive care will evolve only to the extent that we are cognizant of the multiple and interactive factors that impact upon contemporary disease, the chronically ill child, and current chronic care medicine.

References

Alexander, F. G. (1950). Psychosomatic medicine: Its principles and applications. New York: Norton.

Axelrod, B. H. (1979). The chronic care specialist "but who supports us." In O. J. Sahler (Ed.), *The child and death*. New York: Mosby.

Bowen, M. (1976). Family reaction to death. In P. J. Guerin (Ed.), *Family therapy: Theory and practice*. New York: Gardner.

Burnstein, S., & Meichenbaum, D. (1979). The work of worrying in children undergoing surgery. *Journal of Abnormal Child Psychology, 7*, 127–132.

Campbell, J. D. (1975). Illness is a point of view: The development of children's concepts of illness. *Child Development, 46*, 92–100.

Cataldo, M. F., Jacobs, H. E., & Rogers, M. C. (1982). Behavioral/environmental considerations in pediatric inpatient care. In D. C. Russo & J. W. Varni (Eds.), *Behavioral pediatrics: Research and practice*. New York: Plenum.

Cataldo, M. F., Russo, D. C., Bird, B. L., & Varni, J. W. (1980). Assessment and management of chronic disorders. In J. M. Ferguson & C. B. Taylor (Eds.), *Comprehensive handbook of behavioral medicine: Vol. 3. Extended applications and issues*. New York: Spectrum.

Drotar, D. (1976). Psychological consultation in the pediatric hospital. *Professional Psychology, 8*, 72–80.

Drotar, D., Benjamin, P., Chuast, R., Litt, C., & Vajner, P. (1981). The role of the psychologist in pediatric outpatient and inpatient settings. In S. Tuma (Ed.), *Handbook for the practice of pediatric psychology*. New York: Wiley.

Drotar, D., Crawford, P., & Ganofsky, M. A. (1984). Prevention with chronically ill children. In M. C. Roberts & L. Peterson (Eds.), *Prevention of problems in childhood*. New York: Wiley.

Engel, G. L. (1977). The need for a new medical model: A challenge for biomedicine. *Science, 196*, 129–136.

Engel, G. L. (1982). The biopsychosocial model and medical education. *New England Journal of Medicine, 306*, 802–805.

Evans, I. M. (1985). Building systems models as a strategy for target behavior selection in clinical assessment. *Behavioral Assessment, 7*, 21–32.

Fabrega, H., & Van Egeren, L. (1976). A behavioral framework for the study of human disease. *Annals of Internal Medicine, 84*, 200–208.

Folkman, S., & Lazarus, R. S. (1980). An analysis of coping in a middle-aged community sample. *Journal of Health & Social Behavior, 21*, 219–239.

Haggerty, R., Roghman, K. J., & Pless, I. B. (1975). *Child health and the community*. New York: Wiley.

Harris, S. I., & Ferrari, M. (1983). Developmental factors in child behavior therapy. *Behavior Therapy, 14*, 54–72.

Hovanitz, C. A., Gerwell, E. L., & Russo, D. C. (1984). Behavioral methods in pediatric chronic illness. In B. B. Lahey & A. E. Kazdin (Eds.), *Advances in clinical child psychology* (Vol. 7). New York: Plenum.

Johnson, S. B. (1984). Knowledge, attitudes, and behavior: Correlates of health in childhood diabetes. *Clinical Psychology Review, 4*(5), 503–524.

Kanfer, F. H. (1985). Target selection for clinical change programs. *Behavioral Assessment, 7*, 7–20.

Katz, E. R., Kellerman, J., & Siegel, S. E. (1980). Behavioral distress in children with cancer undergoing medical procedures: Developmental considerations. *Journal of Consulting & Clinical Psychology, 48*, 356–365.

Kendall, P. C., Lerner, R. M., & Craighead, W. E. (1984). Human development and intervention in childhood psychopathology. *Child Development, 55*, 71–82.

Knight, R. B., Atkins, A., Eagle, C., Evans, N., Finkelstein, J., Fukushima, D., Katz, J., & Weiner, H. (1979). Psychological stress, ego defenses and cortisol production in children hospitalized for elective surgery. *Psychosomatic Medicine, 41*, 40–49.

Koocher, G. P. (1984). Promoting coping with illness in childhood. In J. C. Rosen & L. J. Solomon (Eds.), *Prevention in health psychology*. Hanover, NH: University Press of New England.

Koocher, G. P., & O'Malley, J. E. (1981). *The Damocles syndrome: Psychological consequences of surviving childhood cancer*. New York: McGraw-Hill.

Lazarus, R. S. (1966). *Psychological stress and the coping process*. New York: McGraw-Hill.

Lazarus, R. S. (1985). The trivialization of distress. In J. C. Rosen & L. J. Solomon (Eds.), *Prevention in health psychology*. Hanover, NH: University Press of New England.

Leventhal, H., Nerenz, D., & Strauss, A. (1980). Self-regulation and the mechanisms for symptom appraisal. In D. Mechanic (Ed.), *Psychosocial epidemiology*. New York: Neal Watson.

Lipowski, D. (1979). Psychosomatic medicine in the eighties: An overview. *American Journal of Psychology, 134*, 233–244.

Maccoby, N., Farquhar, J. W., Wood, P. D., & Alexander, J. K. (1977). Reducing the risk of cardiovascular disease: Effects of a community-based campaign on knowledge and behavior. *Journal of Community Health, 3,* 100–114.

Maddux, J. E., Roberts, M. L., Sledden, E. A., & Wright, L. (1986). Developmental issues in child health psychology. *American Psychologist, 41,* 25–34.

Masek, B. J., Russo, D. C., & Varni, J. W. (1984). Behavioral approaches to the management of chronic pain in children. *Pediatric Clinics of North America, 21,* 1113–1131.

Mash, E. J., & Terdal, L. G. (1981). Behavioral assessment of childhood disturbance. In E. J. Mash & L. G. Terdal (Eds.), *Behavioral assessment of childhood disorders.* New York: Guilford.

Messick, S. (1983). Assessment of children. In W. Kessen (Ed.), *History, theory, methods* (Vol. 1). In P. H. Mussen (Ed.), *Handbook of child psychology* (4th ed.). New York: Wiley.

Miller, N. E. (1983). Behavioral medicine: Symbiosis between laboratory and clinic. *Annual Review of Psychology, 34,* 1–31.

Myers-Vando, R., Steward, M. S., Folkins, C. H., & Hines, P. (1979). The effects of congenital heart disease on cognitive development, illness causality concepts and vulnerability. *American Journal of Orthopsychiatry, 49,* 617–625.

Nagera, H. (1978). Children's reactions to hospitalization and illness. *Child Psychiatry & Human Development, 9,* 3–19.

Parker, L., & Whitehead, W. (1982). Treatment of urinary and fecal incontinence in children. In D. C. Russo & J. W. Varni (Eds.), *Behavioral pediatrics: Research and practice.* New York: Plenum.

Pelcovits, M. A., Silver, B. V., & Russo, D. C. (1983). Somatic disorders in children. In M. Hersen (Ed.), *Outpatient behavior therapy: A clinical guide.* New York: Grune & Stratton.

Pepper, S. C. (1942). *World hypotheses.* Berkeley, CA: University of California Press.

Peterson, L., & Toler, S. M. (1984, August). *Self-regulated presurigcal preparation for children.* Paper presented at the Annual Meeting of the American Psychological Association, Los Angeles.

Russo, D. C. (1986). Chronicity and normalcy as the psychological basis for research and treatment in chronic disease in children. In N. Krasnegor, J. Aresteh, & M. F. Cataldo (Eds.), *Child health behavior: A behavioral pediatrics perspective.* New York: Wiley.

Russo, D. C., Bennett, A. K., Harmon, W. E., & Brown, D. (1981). Behavioral medicine issues in the management of children with end-stage renal disease. *Behavioral Medicine Update, 3,* 15–19.

Russo, D. C., Bird, B. L., & Masek, B. J. (1980). Assessment issues in behavioral medicine, *Behavioral Assessment, 2,* 1–18.

Russo, D. C., Tarbell, S. E., & Follansbee, D. J. (in press). Learning and the modification of somatic function. In A. Brownstein & P. Harzem (Eds.), *Progress in behavioral studies.* Hillsdale, NJ: Erlbaum.

Russo, D. C., & Varni, J. W. (1982). Behavioral pediatrics. In D. C. Russo & J. W. Varni (Eds.), *Behavioral pediatrics: Research and practice.* New York: Plenum.

Schwartz, G. E. (1982). Testing the biopsychosocial model: The ultimate challenge facing behavioral medicine? *Journal of Consulting & Clinical Psychology, 50,* 1040–1053.

Siegel, L. J. (1981, April). *Naturalistic study of coping strategies in children facing medical procedures.* Paper presented at the meeting of the Southeastern Psychological Association, Atlanta.

Simeonsson, R. J., Buckley, L., & Monson, L. (1979). Conceptions of illness causality in hospitalized children. *Journal of Pediatric Psychology, 4,* 77–84.

Sourkes, B. M. (1982). *The deepening shade.* Pittsburgh: University of Pittsburgh Press.

Spirito, A., Russo, D. C., & Masek, B. J. (1984). Behavioral interventions and stress management training for hospitalized adolescents and young adults with cystic fibrosis. *General Hospital Psychiatry, 6,* 211–218.

Stein, R. E. K., & Jessop, D. J. (1982). A noncategorical approach to chronic childhood illness. *Public Health Reports, 97,* 354–362.

Suls, J., & Fletcher, B. (1985). The relative efficacy of avoidant and nonavoidant coping strategies: A meta-analysis. *Health Psychology, 4,* 249–288.

Tefft, B. M., & Simeonsson, R. J. (1979). Psychology and the creation of health care settings. *Professional Psychology, 10,* 558–570.

Tuma, J. M. (1982). *Handbook for the practice of pediatric psychology.* New York: Wiley.

Varni, J. W. (1983). *Clinical behavioral pediatrics: An interdisciplinary biobehavioral approach*. New York: Pergamon.

Wahler, R., & Fox, J. (1981). Setting events in applied behavior analysis: Toward a conceptual and methodologic expansion. *Journal of Applied Behavior Analysis, 14*, 327–338.

Weis, D. P. (1975). Children's cognitive development—Or how children draw "maps." *Child Welfare, 54*, 567–580.

PART II

LEVELS OF PEDIATRIC ASSESSMENT

4

The Physical Examination of the Child

ROBERT BERG

To many infants, an ear examination is an assault; to many adolescents a probing history is insulting as well as assaultive; but to a physician the pediatric history and physical examination constitute the primary data base. It is commonly stated in medical training that more than 90 percent of the time the correct diagnosis can be deduced from a thorough history and physical examination. In essence, the history and physical examination are the primary tools of the pediatric trade, whereas laboratory evaluations and new "high-tech" diagnostic procedures are often simply confirmatory. The traditional, detailed medical history that is described in this chapter is not appropriate in all circumstances. Data-gathering priorities are different at the first well-baby visit than they are at an emergency room visit for a cardiac arrest. Variations in priorities and depth of history and physical examination will be discussed after the detailed "classic" history and physical examination are described.

The pediatric history and physical examination differ from those of adult medicine in several ways. Frequently the history is obtained from a third person, the parent, rather than the patient. In veterinary medicine the animal is the patient, yet the

The preparation of this chapter was supported in part by grant #PMH 39246-03, establishing the Preventive Intervention Research Center (PIRC) at Arizona State University.

animal owner is the client. In pediatrics the child is the primary patient, yet the parent is the client. The client seeks out services and pays for them. The complexity of these relationships and the potential for distorted data are great. Furthermore, it is not unusual for the family to be the patient or for another person, such as a baby-sitting relative, to be the client.

An important nuance of the pediatric history and physical examination is the consideration of growth and development. Abnormal growth and/or developmental patterns are important clues to pathological states. Furthermore, the child's cognitive and emotional abilities and limitations determine how much the child can contribute to the history and how thoroughly the physician can examine him or her. Knowledge of present growth and development parameters as well as a longitudinal perspective is essential for appropriate interpretation of the pediatric history and physical examination.

The typical medical history begins with the patient's (or parent's) chief complaint. This presenting complaint is the reason the child came to the doctor; the parents are unlikely to be satisfied until the physician adequately explains the cause of the complaint and recommends appropriate treatment (if any is deemed necessary). In order to understand the chief complaint, the physician must put it in the context of the present illness, past medical history, personal demographic data, social history, family medical history, nutritional history, behavioral history, and review of other organ systems.

In eliciting the history of present illness, the physician delves into the what, when, and where of the illness. When was the patient last well? What were the first symptoms? How long did they last? Were they intermittent or continuous? What were the order and date of onset of new symptoms? What evaluations and treatments have been done? What factors seemed to aggravate or alleviate the symptoms? Have there been exposures to infections?

Certain demographic information is important to elicit. The child's age, race, socioeconomic status, ethnic background, educational status, and environmental exposures (e.g., a day-care center) all provide important clues that suggest that certain diagnoses are more or less likely, and that certain treatments are more or less appropriate and/or acceptable. For example, a 2-year-old Black male with severe abdominal pain and anemia may well have sickle cell anemia. A blonde Caucasian infant with frequent respiratory illnesses and chronic diarrhea may well have cystic fibrosis.

Various aspects of the past medical history are often quite significant. Antenatal history includes maternal health, medical supervision of the pregnancy, pregnancy complications, and exposures to teratogenic agents. Medications, illicit drugs, infections (such as rubella or CMV), radiation, alcohol, and various maternal illnesses can have adverse effects on the fetus, resulting in long-term problems for the child. The physician also asks about congenital anomalies, difficult delivery, prematurity, postmaturity, perinatal infection, or perinatal illness, as well as the APGAR score (if available).

Past medical illnesses are also explored, including hospitalizations, surgeries, allergies, accidents, and injuries. Frequent hospitalizations for severe infections may be due to an immunologic disorder. Present medications, including prescriptions and over-the-counter medications, are discussed. These medications may be causing the patient's symptoms or may be masking the true diagnosis by partially treating the problem.

In pediatrics we especially discuss the immunization history and growth and development. Abnormal growth parameters are often clues to pathological states. Growth curves and patterns are even more important than present growth parameters. If the child's head circumference is presently at the fifth percentile, he or she may simply be a small child with a proportionately small head, whose parents are also small. In this case, height, weight, and head circumference would all be near the fifth percentile as well as the parents' height, weight, and head circumference. However, if the child's height, weight, and head circumference were previously progressing at the ninetieth percentile, and height and weight remain at the ninetieth percentile, and the parents' growth parameters are at the ninetieth percentile, the fifth percentile head circumference may indicate significant deceleration of head and brain growth secondary to a serious central nervous system insult (e.g., a serious near-drowning episode or a degenerative neurological disorder). Similar changes in height or weight curves can be important clues to illnesses. Changes in growth curves can often indicate that a pathological process began before the patient or parent noticed any symptoms.

The physician needs at least rudimentary information about the child's developmental status. In infants, motor milestones provide much of that information. For toddlers, physicians inquire about language milestones, social skills, and toilet training. School-age children usually have copious documentation of their cognitive skills, especially if they are dysfunctioning (i.e., school records). Physicians, therefore, usually inquire about the child's academic skills at school as well as his or her social functioning with peers and authorities. Many physicians utilize the Denver Developmental Screening Test or the Denver Parent Developmental Questionnaire on a sequential basis for infants and preschool children in order to follow the child's development more objectively.

Nutritional history is generally assessed more carefully in infants than in adults. The physician inquires about the type of milk (i.e., breast or formula), formula changes, introduction of solid foods, caloric intake, and appetite. This information is crucial with regard to malnutrition, allergies, metabolic disorders, and malabsorptive states. For example, the rare child with hereditary fructose intolerance only develops symptoms after he or she is exposed to fructose (e.g., fruits or table sugar).

Behavioral history includes unusual habits, sleep patterns, peer interactions, family interactions, school behavior, bowel habits, bladder control, and phobias. Frequently, parents are concerned that their child "doesn't mind me" or "is hyperactive." In such cases more detailed information is required about attention span, distractibility, impulsivity, parental discipline, and family functioning as well as evidence of petit mal seizures or partial seizures with complex symptomatology (temporal lobe seizures) or multiple motor and/or vocal tics (e.g., Tourette's syndrome). It is important to separate out the various problems that can masquerade as hyperactivity. For example, children with frequent petit mal seizures often appear inattentive, yet their treatment should be quite different from that of a child with primary attention deficit disorder (i.e., hyperactivity).

Social history includes delineation of the family structure, who lives at home, what sources of family income are, sibling interactions, and parent–child interactions.

Divorces, separations, and frequent family moves are common issues that need further exploration. Social supports, such as extended family, friends, and religious affiliations, are important factors about which the physician should be aware.

Family medical history is often pertinent. Many diseases are hereditary or infectious. Therefore, a history of deaths and illnesses in the family is obtained. If several family members have been hospitalized in psychiatric facilities for bipolar affective disorder (i.e., manic-depressive illness) the physician must consider the possibility that the child has the same disorder (rather than being a hyperactive child).

The *review of systems* is the physician's attempt to leave no stone unturned. The physician specifically asks about symptoms in each body system. For example, review of dermatologic system would include questions about rashes, hives, skin texture, skin color changes, and problems with hair or nails. Questions are asked about each body system: ears, nose, throat, eyes, teeth, chest, cardiovascular, gastrointestinal, genitourinary, musculoskeletal, endocrine, and neurological.

Clearly an exhaustive history as just described would be inefficient and inappropriate if it were utilized at every physician–patient encounter. Certainly, when a 3-year-old child presents with an accidental laceration, the physician would ask a few appropriate questions and simply clean and suture the wound. If the child is coming for the 2-year-old health maintenance visit ("checkup"), the physician will already know much of the history from prior visits and will only pursue appropriate questions for that visit and any intercurrent problems that have arisen since the last visit. If the child arrives at an emergency room or intensive care unit in severe distress with a life-threatening illness, the physician will ask a few pointed questions and provide life-sustaining interventions as quickly as is necessary. Further historical information will be asked when time permits. If the patient is an adolescent with significant psychological problems, the physician may require several visits in order to develop a sense of trust and rapport before exploring many of the areas noted earlier. The classical pediatric history is an essential part of a physician's data base; however, a prudent physician will individualize the depth and breadth of historical exploration in accordance with the presenting problem and social, cultural, psychological, and time constraints of the patient, family, and situation.

The physical examination is usually described as following the history. In fact, the most important aspects of the physical examination precede the history and are concurrent with the history. When the physician first sees the child, he or she quickly but carefully catalogs many observations. Is the child in acute physical distress? Having respiratory difficulty? Alert, lethargic, or unresponsive (comatose)? Does the child have any disfigurements or anomalies? Does he or she appear well or ill? Well-nourished or malnourished? Happy, cooperative, distraught, shy, or hostile? How does the child interact with the parents? The physician must make these observations rapidly. If the child is severely lethargic, unresponsive to the environment, or hyperirritable, he or she may have a life-threatening illness (such as meningitis) requiring immediate diagnostic tests and therapeutic intervention. For many children 8 months to 3 years old, this initial observation may be the last time the physician is able to observe them not crying or throwing a temper tantrum.

Physicians who care for children quickly learn that how they approach them greatly affects the quality of the examination and the entire interaction. Generally, a calm, friendly, unintrusive approach gets the best results. A long, boring history will turn many 2-year-olds into hyperactive tyrants. The complete physical examination to be described may not be appropriate or most efficient in all patients, and the order of examination will vary depending on the patient, the age, and the presenting complaint. Generally, the least threatening aspects of the examination should precede the most threatening. Touching the hand of a 3-year-old will generally be less threatening than looking in the ears through the dreaded otoscope. Parts of the examination that do not require mechanical equipment are generally tolerated best by the toddler. On the other hand, a modest 13-year-old may be made more uncomfortable by a genital or anal inspection. Pediatricians have a myriad of tricks they use to encourage the best (and most fun) physical examination possible. Some pediatricians make animal sounds or make up silly stories or play games or examine mommy's mouth first or let Johnny listen through the stethoscope after the doctor does or simply make noise with keys to distract an infant. For school-age children and adolescents, the quality and comfort of the prior interview set the stage for their level of cooperation and relaxation during the physical examination.

It is important never to tell a child an uncomfortable procedure will be painless. What little (if anything) is gained today will certainly be lost tomorrow. The precedent that responsible adults lie is abhorrent.

The physical examination starts with growth measurements and measurements of the vital signs: heart rate, blood pressure, temperature, and respiratory rate. Generally, these are all done by a nurse before the physician sees the patient. Growth measurements include height and weight for all patients, and head circumference for children less than 3 years old and any children with neurodevelopmental problems. Short stature may reflect familial, genetic potential or may be secondary to endocrinological problems, bone abnormalities, genetic abnormalities (such as Turner syndrome), or inadequate nutrition. Many disease states result in inadequate nutrition because of increased metabolic needs and poor appetite. In general, inadequate nutrition initially affects weight first, then height, and finally head circumference (only if severe enough). Excessively large stature may be a familial variant of normal or secondary to endocrinological problems or genetic problems. We often record the weight and the height and graph the weight for height. Low weight is most often due to inadequate nutrition or appropriate weight for a short person. In the former case, the weight-for-height graph would demonstrate that the weight was low for height, whereas in the latter the weight-to-height graph would be near the fiftieth percentile. Head circumference, or occipitofrontal circumference, is measured from the occiput to the eyebrow and tends to reflect brain size. Severely small head circumference, or microcephaly, is most often due to severe prior neurological insult (e.g., severe birth asphyxia or fetal alcohol syndrome). Borderline microcephaly may be secondary to a neurological problem or simply a variant of normal. Head circumference growth curves for the former usually reveal progressive "falling off the curve" (i.e., lower percentiles over time). The latter tends to remain at the same percentile, and often the normal parent also has a small head. Furthermore, often the height and weight are similarly small (i.e., the head circumference is simply proportional to other growth parameters).

The vital signs are the heart rate, blood pressure, temperature, and respiratory rate. Heart rate varies with age and is best determined in infants by listening to the heart. In older children and adults it is usually derived by palpating the pulse at the wrist. Critically ill children have their pulse rate monitored continuously, usually via painless electrocardiogram leads. Blood pressure should be measured for all children greater than 3 years old and all critically ill children at any age. Blood pressure can be measured by stethoscope and sphygmomanometer cuff, by cuffs attached to machines that use a Doppler method, or by continuous direct intraarterial catheter monitoring. The traditional stethoscope and sphygmomanometer method can be difficult with a squirming infant or toddler and is cumbersome with a critically ill infant or toddler. Therefore, painless mechanical Doppler-derived blood pressures are often used for ill infants and toddlers. Continuous direct intraarterial blood pressure readings are generally the most accurate and are often used with critically ill children. However, the necessary intraarterial catheter placement is painful and invasive. Respiratory rates in infants and toddlers are often erratic and must be counted over at least an entire minute. Rapid respiratory rates are often seen with serious respiratory illnesses, serious infections, and high fevers.

Of the vital signs, probably the least important to most pediatricians is the temperature. If the patient has an acute infectious illness, the level of fever is far less important than the other vital signs and how the child looks. The temperature is somewhat helpful in determining whether the illness is due to an infection. Temperatures can be measured via oral, rectal, axillary, or cutaneous means. The traditional cutaneous method is the hand on the forehead. Unfortunately, even for experienced hands this method is not reliable. Modern technology has developed several methods of determining forehead temperatures more accurately by placing various devices on the forehead. These readings do not reliably reflect internal body temperature, the real temperature that we seek. Rectal thermometers accurately reflect internal temperatures throughout the body, but having a thermometer placed in the rectum is uncomfortable and, on rare occasions, dangerous, if the thermometer should break while it is in the rectum or be poked through the bowel wall. Oral temperatures are frequently used but are unreliable if the patient will not keep the mouth shut or has a rapid respiratory rate resulting in too much cool air entering the nose and mouth. Frequently, axillary temperatures are used in children. The thermometer is placed in the axilla (armpit) between the arm and chest. These readings are safe and more accurate than forehead temperatures, but they are clearly less accurate than rectal temperatures. When it is important to assess body temperature, the oral or rectal method must be used.

The physical examination includes evaluation of the skin, head, eyes, ears, nose, throat, neck, chest, heart and blood vessels, abdomen, genitalia, musculoskeletal system, lymph nodes, anus and rectum, and neurological system. The basic tools of evaluation are visual inspection (looking), manual palpation (feeling), auscultation (listening) via a stethoscope, and percussion (thumping with a finger or reflex hammer).

Skin examination is crucial for strictly dermatologic disorders such as rashes, scabies, lice, malformations, and superficial infections. The color, texture, pattern, and depth of involvement are among the clues to the dermatologic diagnosis. Examination of the skin may also reveal important information about systemic illnesses. Many inflammatory dermatologic conditions are superficial manifestations of inflammatory processes in other organs. Systemic lupus erythematosus, juvenile rheumatoid arthritis, rheumatic fever, Kawasaki disease, and toxic shock syndrome are but a few of the systemic inflammatory conditions that may present primarily with dermatologic manifestations. Numerous infections such as chicken pox, measles, rubella, and forms of overwhelming sepsis often first manifest themselves on the patient's skin. Pallor may indicate anemia, and cyanosis (blue coloration) may indicate inadequate oxygenation. Certain endocrine, genetic, and other diseases have characteristic associated skin findings. Skin is derived embryologically from the neuroectoderm, the same substrate as much of the nervous system. It is, therefore, not surprising that the skin is often a "window" to the brain. Neurocutaneous disorders such as neurofibromatosis, tuberous sclerosis, and Sturge-Weber syndrome are often diagnosed by the cutaneous manifestations. Careful skin examination also reveals important clues regarding the patient's state of hydration and nutrition. The hair and nails, specialized structures of the skin, are also carefully examined visually and manually for evidence of local or systemic disease.

The physician looks at the size and shape of the head and face in order to note any deformations or malformations that may be clues to neurological, teratogenic, genetic, or other disorders. Down's syndrome, fetal alcohol syndrome, myopathies, and storage diseases among literally hundreds of diseases have characteristic craniofacial features. Many bones join together along suture lines to form the mature cranium. The anterior and posterior fontanels (or soft spots) are at the confluence of suture lines and can be distinctly palpated through the first year and the first month, respectively. At the anterior fontanel the brain is initially not covered by bone, so increased intracranial pressure secondary to brain swelling (e.g., with meningitis or Reye's syndrome) or hydrocephalus may be manifested as a bulging fontanel, and decreased intracranial volume (e.g., with significant dehydration) may be manifested as a sunken fontanel.

Examination of the eye includes visual acuity assessment, inspection of the conjunctivae and cornea (coverings of the eye), lens and retinal examination (internal or ophthalmoscopic examination), pupillary examination, and strabismus examination. The physician first looks for gross abnormalities in size, shape, and color of the eyes as well as direction of gaze. Prominent eyes are noted in glaucoma and hyperthyroidism. Inspection of the lids, conjunctivae, and cornea may reveal infectious processes such as an hordeolum (sty) or viral conjunctivitis (pink-eye). Corneal opacities may be seen with metabolic degenerative processes, and lens opacities (cataracts) may be seen with congenital infections (e.g., congenital rubella) or side effects of steroid medication. These opacities may be seen by simply shining a penlight on the cornea and pupils, or by looking through an ophthalmoscope. Ophthalmoscopic examination also involves visualization of the retina, the most easily accessible outpouching of the brain. Various infectious, traumatic, and genetic neurological diseases have characteristic retinal manifestations, such as retinal hemorrhages with shaking injuries in child abuse and the cherry-red spot of Tay-Sachs disease. Strabismus, or misalignment of the visual axis, is a common preventable form of blindness. The corneal light reflex, or reflection of light on both corneas from a penlight several feet away, should be symmetrical. If it is not, the patient has strabismus, which can often be reversed before it causes unilateral blindness. Pupils are examined for shape, size, and reaction to light. Many drugs and pathological states affect pupillary size and reactivity. Visual acuity can be tested by the Standard Snellen chart in school-age children, but more inventive methods, such as coaxing an infant to follow a tongue blade with a boy figure on top, are often needed grossly to assess visual acuity in infants.

Nasal discharge, congestion, bleeding, and malformation are visually sought by either gross visual examination or magnification by looking through an otoscope while slightly nudging the tip of the nose upward. Occasionally, children cleverly sequester foreign bodies such as tissue or parts of toys or food in a nostril, resulting in foul-smelling unilateral nasal discharge that has been shrugged off as a chronic cold or allergies. The nasal mucosa (internal covering) is carefully examined to differentiate an infectious process (a cold) from an allergic process. The former tends to result in an irritated, red mucosa with purulent discharge; the latter tends to result in a pale, blue mucosa with thin discharge.

The ear examination traditionally follows the head, eye, and nose examination in older children and adults. However, the physical and psychological battle that often develops during an ear examination frequently precludes any further physical workup. Therefore, physicians often examine infants' and toddlers' ears last. External ear abnormalities often signal serious internal ear pathology associated with deafness. The ear canal and tympanic membrane are examined through the otoscope. Appearance of the tympanic membrane reflects the presence or absence of fluid or infection in the middle ear. The otoscope is rigid and the ear canal is pliable; therefore, the child must be held very still while being examined in order to avoid painful distortion of the ear canal. Most children 6 months to 2 years old consider being held still a major form of punishment. Unfortunately, earwax often partially occludes the ear canal. Curette removal of the earwax is also uncomfortable. This entire process is generally hated by infants and toddlers, endured by their physicians, and poorly tolerated by their parents. However, ear infections are very common, and they can only be reliably diagnosed through this examination.

Examination of the oral cavity is similarly often deferred to the end of the examination because of discomfort and gagging due to physical restraint and examination with a tongue blade. Painful fissures at the corners of the lips are seen with nutritional deficiencies, especially of the B vitamins. Blisters are seen with cold sores (oral herpes simplex infections). Congenital clefts of the lip (harelip) and palate are sought. Severe clefts present significant cosmetic, nutritional, and speech problems. Subtle clefts of the palate result in frequent ear infections. Unusual mouth odors are noted with severe diabetes and with many poisons. The number and condition of the teeth are important clues to the patient's general health. Delayed tooth development and abnormal teeth are seen with abnormalities in calcium metabolism (such as rickets), generalized malnutrition, and infections (such as congenital syphilis). Dental caries and dental malocclusion are two of the most common maladies of childhood and are carefully noted during the oral examination. The physician examines the gums for nonspecific signs of infection (redness, swelling, and tenderness), as well as specific signs such as Koplik's spots, which are virtually only seen with measles.

The neck is examined for enlarged lymph nodes, a goiter (abnormal large thyroid gland), masses, and normal size and mobility. Large lymph nodes are usually caused by common infections, such as colds or mononucleosis. Less common infections (such as tuberculosis) and some cancers are sometimes the etiology of large lymph nodes. A "stiff neck" may simply be due to musculoskeletal trauma or an infection of structures around the neck. Less commonly, a stiff neck is a manifestation of meningitis.

Simple inspection is the most important part of the chest examination. Respiratory rate, respiratory effort, and respiratory pattern are quite characteristic for acute respiratory infectious illnesses, versus apparent respiratory distress with neurological disorders, versus apparent respiratory distress with metabolic disorders (such as diabetic ketoacidosis or aspirin poisoning). Infants and toddlers frequently cry and hold their breath when the doctor comes close and/or listens with a stethoscope. The initial opportunity to inspect the respiratory rate and pattern is not uncommonly the last opportunity truly to evaluate the youngster's respiratory system. Auscultation (listening) with a stethoscope further aids in separating upper airway diseases (e.g., croup) from lower airway diseases (e.g., asthma) from parenchymal lung disease (e.g. pneumonia).

Inspection and palpation of the chest wall and breast tissue may reveal masses, infectious processes, or musculoskeletal problems. For example, male gynecomastia (breast enlargement) is a normal finding during early stages of puberty, but may be seen at other ages with medications (e.g., digitalis), tumors, drugs (e.g., marijuana), severe liver disease, or testicular dysfunction (e.g., Klinefelter's syndrome).

Inspection, palpation, and auscultation of the heart and blood vessels usually reveal no cardiac disease and adequate tissue perfusion (blood flow). Children may have congenital defects (holes) in their hearts, sometimes resulting in congestive heart failure or cyanosis (inadequate oxygen) or shock (inadequate tissue perfusion). Physicians hear heart murmurs in over half of all children. The vast majority of these heart murmurs are so-called innocent murmurs (i.e., without pathological significance). Occasionally physicians hear murmurs that suggest heart defects prior to the development of congestive heart disease, cyanosis, or shock.

Abdominal palpation is especially helpful in differentiating various causes of abdominal pain, such as appendicitis, urinary tract infection, and hepatitis. Devious distraction, careful observation, and subtle palpation are required for a physician adequately to examine a child with abdominal pain. In children without abdominal symptoms, abdominal cancers (e.g., Wilm's tumor) or metabolic storage diseases (such as Gaucher's disease or mucopolysaccharidosis) may infrequently be discovered. More commonly, an asymptomatic hernia (or outpouching of bowel) is noted in the inguinal area (groin).

Genital examination may reveal disorders of sexual differentiation, precocious puberty, tumors, or infectious processes. Increasingly, physicians are asked to evaluate children for evidence of sexual assault. The physician can note evidence of trauma or sexually transmitted diseases (e.g., gonorrhea),but he or she can rarely be certain of the precise cause of the trauma (e.g., penile penetration vs. deep manual manipulation vs. tampon usage) or the identity of the perpetrator. However, evidence of deep vaginal penetration in a prepubertal child, evidence of bruising, lacerations, and/or sperm in a prepubertal child, and evidence of sexually transmitted diseases certainly are strong indicators of inappropriate sexual activity. Especially for pubertal children such evidence must be correlated with historical information. Appropriate examination of prepubertal children usually requires an external genital examination. For a prepubertal girl, simply spreading her labia majora allows adequate visualization. If there is evidence of discharge or penetration, laboratory specimens are obtained by touching the vulvar or vaginal area with a cotton swab. Occasionally a pelvic examination or internal examination is required. Often general anesthesia is needed for an adequate pelvic examination in prepubertal children.

Pubertal girls with sexual assault or abdominal or gynecological symptoms require a pelvic examination. Sexually transmitted diseases (such as gonorrhea) may present as abdominal pain alone, and the delay in diagnosis can result in sterility. Other gynecological problems (such as ovarian cysts) may also present as abdominal pain alone. There are two major components of a pelvic examination: the speculum examination and the bimanual examination. The speculum is a plastic or metal instrument that is inserted into the vagina and is spread open in order to maintain patency of the vagina for adequate visualization of the cervix and vagina. After obtaining appropriate laboratory specimens the physician removes the speculum and inserts a finger of a gloved hand into the vagina while simultaneously palpating a girl's abdomen with his or her other hand. The uterus, ovaries, and fallopian tubes can thereby be felt between the two hands (ergo, the *bimanual* examination).

Anal examination consists of simply spreading the buttocks of the child and inspecting the anal area for infections, irritations, or malformations. In some circumstances a rectal examination is also indicated. The physician inserts the index finger of a gloved hand through the anus and may detect evidence of internal bleeding, infection, or tumors.

The physician examines the musculoskeletal system (muscles, bones, and joints) mainly by inspection and palpation. The joints, extremities, back, neck, and chest wall are observed for swelling, redness, tenderness, or malformation. The joints are checked for full mobility. Subtle evidence of juvenile rheumatoid arthritis or systemic lupus erythematosis or osteomyelitis (infection of the bone) may only be discovered after a careful musculoskeletal examination. Part of the musculoskeletal examination is careful observation of the child during usual activity (e.g., walking into the office or jumping off the examination table). This is especially important for preschoolers who are often uncooperative during a more structured examination. Physicians are careful to look for scoliosis (curvature of the spine) and kyphosis (humpback deformity) because these conditions often progress rapidly in childhood and adolescence, and because the progression is often avoidable with appropriate early treatment.

Neurological and neurodevelopmental examination can be rather simple or quite extensive. A classical neurological examination includes assessment of general cerebral function, cranial nerves, cerebellar function, motor system, sensory system, deep tendon reflexes, and peripheral nerves. In infants, we also check for protective and primitive reflexes. General cerebral function assessment includes level of consciousness (e.g., comatose, alert, or lethargic), memory, general behavior, intelligence, and communication skills. Most commonly, this is grossly assessed by noting the child's general behavior during the history and physical examination. More detailed evaluation (e.g., psychometric testing and psychological evaluation) is beyond the scope of the typical pediatric physical examination.

Cranial nerve examination includes evaluation of muscles and sensation of the eyes, ears, nose, throat, tongue, and neck. The so-called cranial nerves innervate these structures, and examining the cranial nerves may provide early evidence of many brain tumors. Gait, coordination, and balance are major areas of cerebellar function.

Muscle strength, tone, and unusual muscle movements are noted. Hearing, vision, response to touch and pinprick, and proprioceptive sensation (e.g., awareness of position in space and objects placed in the hand) are components of the sensory examination. Deep tendon reflexes (such as knee jerk and ankle jerk) are complex reflexes requiring afferent (sensory) stimuli, spinal cord reflex, supraspinal modulation, and efferent (motor) response. Asymmetry or other abnormalities of the deep tendon reflexes may provide valuable information.

Much of the appropriate history is tailored to the specific setting, the appropriate physical examination varies depending on various circumstances. An office visit for an acute respiratory illness should not result in the same physical examination as an office visit for a chronic neurological problem (e.g., headaches and seizures associated with worsening in school performance). In the former instance, the neurological examination would be cursory; in the latter, the neurological examination would be detailed. For health maintenance visits (i.e., well-child care) certain aspects of the examination will be stressed at certain ages and ignored at others. For example, careful examination of an infant for congenital hip dislocation is essential, whereas a preadolescent who is walking normally does not require the same hip examination. If the diagnosis of congenital hip dislocation has been missed in infancy, the child is left with a severe permanent hip disability and is unable to walk normally. The neurological examination of an intensive care patient who is comatose after head trauma is obviously quite different from that of a child at a well child visit. A comatose patient cannot participate in evaluation of muscle strength, most aspects of sensation, and most aspects of cognitive functioning. Hospitalized patients need very detailed physical examinations, whereas a child with a laceration of the finger generally needs only a good examination of the finger and extremity. A detailed general physical examination requires only 10 to 15 minutes to be completed. Detailed neurodevelopmental evaluations may require considerably more time.

The pediatric history and physical examination are always a challenge, often a joy, and sometimes a frustration to parent and physician alike. The information obtained is the cornerstone of appropriate medical diagnosis and treatment; the process is the cornerstone of appropriate patient and parent rapport.

5

Psychophysiological Assessment

DONALD A. WILLIAMSON
SANDRA J. McKENZIE
ERICH G. DUCHMANN

The proposition that physiological responses and psychological reactions (e.g., emotions, cognition, or behavior) are highly related can be traced to such philosophers as Galen and Descartes. Over the past 30 years, large strides have been made in the understanding of these relationships. This area of basic scientific research is known as *psychophysiology* (Greenfield & Sternbach, 1972). The earliest research in psychophysiology began with the discovery of the galvanic skin response by Féré (1888) and the electroencephalogram by Caton (1875). From this pioneering work came the development of sophisticated electronic systems for amplifying biological responses using noninvasive electrodes and transducers, thus allowing physiologists, psychologists, and medical researchers to record physiological changes in humans without endangering the subjects. Today it is possible to record heart rate, blood flow, brain waves, muscle activity, and many other responses in an objective, reliable manner with minimal inconvenience. This capability was quickly recognized by early psychophysiologists such as Darrow, Malmo, Davis, and Lacey as a potential means of using objective physiological measures as indices of more subjective psychological phenomena such as emotional states or cognitive processes.

Over the past 40 years, the technology for assessing physiological responses has improved dramatically. Also, principles have been established for interpreting various biological signals as they relate to psychological phenomena.

Psychophysiology has always attracted researchers with clinical or applied interests, as evidenced by the early work by Malmo and Shagass (1949) on stress, and by D. T. Graham (1972) on psychosomatic illness. It was with the evolution of the tripartite conceptualization of behavioral assessment (Lang, 1971) and the development of the area of behavioral medicine that psychophysiology found a firm footing in clinical psychology. In recent years, psychophysiological methods have been used extensively for the assessment of specific disorders, as well as for the assessment of treatment outcome or treatment process, for example, with biofeedback and relaxation (Ray & Raczynski, 1981; Williamson, Waters, & Hawkins, in press). Psychophysiological assessment has been most often applied to adults. In recent years, however, there has been an increasing trend toward using psychophysiological methods with children. This chapter describes the basic methodology associated with this type of assessment and summarizes the clinical research on the psychophysiological assessment of children.

BASIC METHODOLOGY

Equipment

In order to record psychophysiological responses, one must connect the subject to a device that can amplify certain bioelectric signals. This amplifying device is generally called a polygraph or physiograph. The subject is connected to the polygraph using electrodes or certain types of transducers that convert nonbioelective signals into electrical signals that can then be amplified. In many modern laboratories, micro- or minicomputers are used to analyze the amplified signals from the polygraph output so that psychophysiological responses can be converted to digital data. The following subsections describe the varied components of the recording system in more detail.

Polygraph. A polygraph is a device for conditioning (modifying), amplifying, and displaying two or more biological signals simultaneously. Different manufacturers of polygraph equipment configure the conditioning and amplifying components of a recording system in different ways. Generally, a coupler or preamplifer is used to: (1) condition the signal, that is, change its form, and (2) amplify the signal to a level that can be accepted by the power or driver amplifier. The driver amplifier is used to increase the amplitude of the signal so that it can be displayed using an oscillograph pen-writing system. This display involves moving ink writing pens across paper that advances at a constant rate. This type of display allows for a continuous analysis of physiological response changes over a specified time period, for example, heart beats per minute. Because the biological signal often must be amplified more than a million times in order to be displayed, it is necessary to filter unwanted electrical activity from the signal. Most amplification systems allow for filtering both high and low frequencies so that the psychophysiologist can select precise signals to be displayed and recorded.

There are two basic types of preamplifiers: AC and DC. The AC preamplifier is designed to detect or follow rapid changes in a physiological signal. The DC preamplifier, in contrast, reproduces slow-changing responses. The AC preamplifier is used for recording psychophysiological responses such as the electrocardiogram, electromyogram, and electroencephalogram, which change very rapidly. The DC preamplifier is used to record responses such as skin temperature and skin resistance, which change very slowly. In addition to these two basic preamplifiers, there are certain types of couplers or preamplifiers that are designed to convert the physiological signal into a rate measure, for example, heart rate, or into an integrated signal, for example, the electromyogram.

Electrodes and Transducers. Electrodes are used for measuring bioelectric signals from the surface of the skin. The most common type of electrode is a silver–silver chloride disk enclosed in a plastic casing. Electrode gels or pastes are placed over the electrode to enhance the conduction of bioelectric signals. Electrodes are attached to the subject's skin using adhesive collars. The subject's skin should be thoroughly cleaned using alcohol or acetone. It is common to abrade the skin gently with a pad in order to remove oils, dirt, and dead cells on the surface of the skin.

Transducers are devices used to detect a physiological response and to convert the response into an electrical signal that can be processed by the polygraph. Transducers are generally used for recording responses that are not bioelectric, for example, blood flow, blood pressure, and respiration.

Automated Scoring Systems. Most modern psychophysiology laboratories have some type of peripheral equipment that converts analog psychophysiological data into digital data. The most common type of system includes a network of analog-to-digital converters that are connected to a microcomputer. This type of system allows for on-line collection of digital data and eliminates the need for hand scoring of polygraph records.

PSYCHOPHYSIOLOGICAL RESPONSES

Using polygraph equipment, one can record a variety of physiological responses. The following section describes the methodology and equipment required for recording the primary responses that are used for assessing children. Table 5.1 summarizes the basic equipment requirements for recording these responses. For a more detailed description of this methodology, the reader may wish to refer to a basic psychophysiology text such as Greenfield and Sternbach (1972).

Electrocardiogram (EKG) and Heart Rate (HR)

Measurement of the EKG involves recording the electrical activity of the heart. The heart consists of two pumps, one on the left side and one on the right. Each pump is composed of two chambers, the atrium and the ventricle, with the right pump supplying blood to the pulmonary system (to be reoxygenated) and the left pump supplying oxygenated blood to the rest of the body. The blood is distributed throughout the body by a system of arteries (e.g., arterioles, capillaries) and returns to the heart via the veins.

TABLE 5.1. EQUIPMENT REQUIREMENTS FOR RECORDING PSYCHOPHYSIOLOGICAL RESPONSES

Response	Preamplifier	Electrodes–Transducer
1. Electrocardiogram	AC	Silver–silver chloride electrodes
2. Heart rate	Cardiotachograph	Silver–silver chloride electrodes
3. Vasomotor response	DC	Photoplethysmograph
4. Blood pressure	Blood pressure preamp	Sphygmomanometer
5. Electromyogram	AC or integrator	Silver–silver chloride electrodes
6. Skin resistance	DC	Silver–silver chloride electrodes
7. Skin conductance	DC	Silver–silver chloride electrodes
8. Skin potential	AC	Silver–silver chloride electrodes
9. Respiration	DC	Strain gauge or nasal thermistor
10. Electroencephalogram	AC	Silver electrodes
11. Anal sphincter muscle tension	DC	Pressure transducer

The normal EKG signal is composed of several components that correspond to the various pumping actions of the heart. The most notable of these components appears as a pronounced spike in an otherwise fairly straight line. This spike is referred to as the QRS complex (for purposes of component labeling) and is produced by the contraction of the ventricles (i.e., the heartbeat), which can be measured as a large change in voltage potential.

All that is needed to obtain an EKG signal of sufficient quality to measure heart rate is the placement of two active electrodes and one ground electrode on the skin so that they form a triangle around the chest. The most common electrode placement is with the active electrodes on the right arm and left leg and the ground electrode on the right leg. This configuration tends to produce the largest QRS spike, which facilitates the task of interpreting the signal. EKG is generally recorded with an AC amplifier, which gives a stable baseline and makes it easier both to read the chart paper of the polygraph and to perform either computer or cardiotachograph analysis.

Today most researchers use either a cardiotachograph or a computer to analyze the EKG signal. A cardiotachograph is a specialized coupler or preamplifer that measures the time from one QRS complex to the next (i.e., interbeat interval). This information is then represented on the polygraph as a straight line graph moving in a stepwise fashion higher or lower above the baseline as the interbeat interval (i.e., heart rate) increases or decreases. An example of a cardiotachograph record is presented in Figure 5.1

A major distinction between the EKG recording procedure and that of a cardiotachograph is the manner in which cardiac activity is actually measured. The EKG is a representation of each heartbeat, and an analysis of an EKG record yields

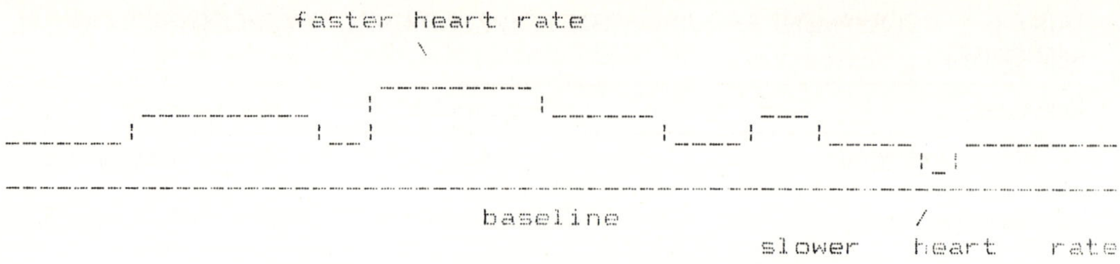

FIGURE 5.1. Illustration of cardiotachograph recording.

heart rate or the number of beats per time period, usually in terms of minutes. A cardiotachograph, however, measures interbeat interval or the time from one QRS complex to the next. Thus cardiac activity could be described as 120 beats per minute or 0.5 seconds depending on the method of measurement being used. It is important to note, however, that the data from these two methods are not linear in relationship (cf. Khachaturian, Kerr, Kruger, & Schachter, 1972). Data originally collected in beats per minute might produce a different distribution when converted to interbeat interval units. This phenomenon of nonlinearity is most problematic when there is a wide range of heart rate scores or interbeat intervals.

Vasomotor Response (VMR)

Vasomotor activity, or the degree of dilation of peripheral blood vessels, is frequently used to assess autonomic activity, with vasoconstriction being related to increased sympathetic activation and vasodilation being related to decreased sympathetic activation.

The most commonly used method of measuring VMR in psychophysiological research is plethysmography. The word *plethysmography* is Greek and can be literally translated as "enlargement" or "fullness." Therefore, following this definition, a true plethysmograph is a device for measuring the change in volume of a given structure such as an arm, leg, finger, or even the entire body.

Although there are a variety of techniques for measuring VMR, the three most frequently used are: (1) photoelectric changes; (2) impedance changes; and (3) volume changes recorded with a strain gauge. Photoplethysmography is by far the most popular technique used by modern psychophysiologists. This method employs a small infrared light source and a photocell to determine the volume of blood in a particular area. There are two basic variations of this method: The light source can either pass through the tissue segment (transmitted), or bounce off the tissue (reflected). The light source produces light in the infrared range, which is scattered (or absorbed) by blood. Therefore, the amount of light that is either transmitted or reflected back to the photocell can be considered to be inversely related to the amount of blood within the region (Brown, 1967; Weinman, 1967).

Only a few sites (e.g., finger, toe, earlobe) are appropriate for use with a transmitting photoplethysmograph, because the light source must be transmitted through the tissue to a photodetector on the other side. With reflecting photoplethysmography, however, the light source and the photodetector are located on the same side of the tissue and can be placed over a vascular bed anywhere on the body.

In psychophysiological research, the two vasomotor measures most commonly used are blood volume and blood volume pulse. Blood volume measures reflect the relatively slow changes in the amount of blood in an arm, leg, finger, or toe and are a direct result of sympathetic nervous system activity (the parasympathetic system is not involved). Blood volume pulse reflects the more rapid changes caused by the pumping action of the heart, and is reflected as the pulse observed in the periphery with each heartbeat.

Measurements of VMR are generally made with a DC amplifier so as to measure blood volume and blood volume pulse accurately. In order to eliminate blood volume, an AC amplifier may be used so that the faster-changing pulses that are associated with the pumping of the heart can be accurately recorded without recording the slow wave changes associated with blood volume.

There are many factors that can influence VMR. One should, therefore, be cautious in interpreting experimental results as well as the actual recordings that are derived from the measurement of vasomotor responding. Daily fluctuations in room temperature, for example, could result in differential results unrelated to the experimental situation. Also, individual differences in skin characteristics make absolute comparisons between subjects impossible. Finally, differences in procedure, for example, placement of the transducers, and the equipment itself can make comparisons only relative. For these reasons, VMR cannot be regarded as an absolute measure. Therefore, comparisons across sessions and across individuals are inappropriate. Only *within-session changes* are considered to be valid. The most common method of expressing VMR is in terms of a percentage of baseline.

Blood Pressure (BP)

Blood pressure is a function of cardiac output, that is, heart rate and stroke volume (amount of blood pumped by the heart) and peripheral resistance (the degree of vasodilation or vasoconstriction in the periphery of the body). In other words, BP = (stroke volume × heart rate) × peripheral resistance.

The two most important characteristics of blood pressure are its maximal and minimal values. The maximal blood pressure, or systole, occurs when the ventricle of the heart contracts. Diastole, or minimal blood pressure, occurs during the relaxation of the left ventricle. Diastolic pressure tends to vary with peripheral resistance while systolic pressure is affected by both peripheral resistance and cardiac output. The average blood pressure of a young, healthy individual is 120 over 80 (systolic over diastolic); however, factors such as age, diet, posture, and weight can influence this reading.

The most common method of measuring blood pressure was introduced by Korotkoff at the beginning of this century. It employs a sphygmomanometer, a device commonly found in a doctor's office consisting of a pressure cuff connected to a tube containing mercury. The cuff is placed on the upper arm and a stethoscope is placed over the brachial artery just below the cuff. The cuff is then inflated with sufficient pressure to cut off all blood flow in that arm. The pressure is slowly released until the first so-called Korotkoff sounds (i.e., thumping sounds) are heard through the stethoscope. The pressure at this level is regarded as the systolic pressure and the cuff pressure is further lowered until the sound can no longer be heard. This level is the diastolic pressure.

In psychophysiological research, automated devices are commonly used to measure blood pressure. These devices are very similar to those used in the manual method, except that the pressure cuff can be inflated from another room and the Korotkoff sounds are recorded by a microphone. In addition, a specialized preamplifier or coupler is used to display the cuff pressure on the polygraph record while the Korotkoff sounds are displayed as marks superimposed on the pressure record as the cuff is deflated. In this way, the systolic and diastolic pressure levels are determined visually rather than aurally.

Although the measurement of blood pressure is a fairly standardized procedure, there are some methodological and experimental problems that exist in recording it. First, blood pressure is not a static measure, but can vary as much as 30 mm Hg in a single recording. There is also a tendency for blood pressure to vary (in repeated measurement) in response to temporary tissue changes caused by the inflation and deflation of the pressure cuff.

Another factor affecting blood pressure measurement is the situation in which it is measured. Some investigators have found higher blood pressure readings when they are taken in a clinical setting than when they are taken during the person's normal day. And finally, individual differences among the experimenters themselves can lead to differences in blood pressure readings.

A new method for measuring blood pressure without a cuff has been developed in recent years. It is called the pulse wave transit time (PWTT) technique, and it involves the measurement of time required for a pulse wave to travel from the heart to some distant location in the body, such as an arm or finger. To determine this variable, psychophysiologists measure the elapsed time between a QRS signal in the EKG recording and the detection of a peripheral pulse as measured by a photoplethysmograph. This procedure is based on the cardiovascular measure of pulse wave velocity. *Pulse wave velocity* refers to the rate of propagation of pressure pulse waves along the arteries, and short-term changes in this measure are considered to be primarily due to changes in blood pressure. It has therefore been suggested (Gribbin, Steptoe, & Sleight, 1976) that pulse wave velocity can be used as an indirect measure of blood pressure (in that it is inversely related to blood pressure).

PWTT is a relatively easy procedure for measuring blood pressure. Also, unlike traditional pressure cuff techniques, PWTT allows for the continuous monitoring of blood pressure, yet does not tend to distract the subject or produce the differential effects that can result from inflation and deflation of a pressure cuff. However, the PWTT technique is not without some problems. Measurement of pulse wave velocity requires the use of pressure transducers, which can be susceptible to movement artifact. Also, research concerning the interpretation of PWTT as a measure of blood pressure has yielded inconsistent findings. Several studies have found PWTT to be most highly correlated with systolic blood pressure and less highly correlated with diastolic blood pressure (Kimper, 1977; Obrist, Light, McCubbin, Hutcheson, & Hoffer, 1979). However, other studies (e.g., Marie, Lo, Jones, & Johnston, 1984; Pollak & Obrist, 1983; Steptoe, Smulyan, & Gribbin, 1976) have found satisfactory correlations between PWTT and both diastolic and systolic blood pressure. There are many methodological considerations in measuring and interpreting PWTT. The interested reader should refer to Pollak and Obrist (1983) and Steptoe, Godaert, Ross, and Schreurs (1983) for a more complete discussion of these issues.

Skin Temperature (ST)

Skin temperature measurement in psychophysiology involves the use of a thermally sensitive transducer called a thermistor, which detects the surface temperature of the skin at some particular area on the body. Like skin resistance, this signal is associated with very slow changes and is best measured using a DC amplifier.

A thermistor is a thermoresistive transducer that changes its resistance in relation to its temperature. This device is very small and very sensitive, and can be placed anywhere on the body that is of interest. The standard procedure, however, is to place the thermistor in a peripheral location, such as on an arm or finger. When it is used in this manner, skin temperature can be conceptualized as an indirect measure of peripheral blood flow, since warm blood in the vascular bed tends to have a warming effect on regional surface skin temperature. It should be noted, however, that skin temperature must be regarded as a slowly changing index of peripheral blood flow changes and is, therefore, an inappropriate measure of blood flow changes to discrete stimuli. The vasomotor response is a much better measure for this purpose.

Because the temperature of the skin is thought to be directly related to peripheral blood flow, skin temperature biofeedback procedures have been designed to teach vasodilation in specific areas of the body. These procedures have been found to be particularly effective in the treatment of migraine headaches and Raynaud's syndrome (Blanchard, Theobald, Williamson, Silver, & Brown, 1978; Jacobson, Manschreck, & Silverberg, 1979; Silver, Blanchard, Williamson, Theobald, & Brown, 1979).

Electromyogram (EMG)

The most common measure of muscle tension is the EMG. The EMG is a direct measure of the electrical activity generated by contraction of skeletal muscles. The most common method for measuring EMG is through the use of three surface electrodes that are placed over a single muscle group. Electrodes should be placed parallel to the fibers of the muscle to be measured. Electrodes are generally placed a few centimeters apart with the ground electrode centered between two active electrodes. As illustrated in the study by Williamson, Epstein, and Lombardo (1980), electrode placement can be a very important variable in measuring EMG. In this study, two methods of electrode placement for frontal EMG were compared. One method used the traditional horizontal placement across the forehead, which measures muscle activity across two muscle groups. The other method used a vertical placement, which measured the muscle activity of only one muscle group. The results showed that both measures were highly correlated, but that the horizontal placement yielded approximately twice the EMG activity of the vertical placement.

The EMG is recorded using the AC preamplifier or coupler. The output of this channel is called raw EMG, which is very difficult to convert to digital data without integration. For this reason, EMG is usually integrated using either an integrator preamplifier on an analog-to-digital converter. The EMG is generally expressed in terms of microvolt-seconds.

Electrodermal Responses

Skin resistance, skin conductance, and skin potential are the three electrodermal responses measured in psychophysiology. Skin resistance and skin conductance are recorded using a DC preamplifier that conducts a small current across the skin. Skin potential is a naturally occurring bioelectric response that is recorded using an AC preamplifier. All of these electrodermal responses are measures of sweat gland activity, which is known to be under control of the sympathetic branch of the autonomic nervous system. Thus electrodermal responses are a good index of sympathetic arousal and have been used extensively in clinical research on emotional and stress reactions.

Skin resistance and skin conductance are recorded using two active electrodes placed on the palmar surface of two fingers. Skin conductance is the reciprocal of skin resistance. The technology for recording skin resistance and that for recording skin conductance are virtually identical. Both measures yield a variety of different wave forms. Baseline or atomic measures are defined as the level of skin resistance or conductance in the absence of stimuli. A skin resistance or conductance response is defined as a response to a stimulus. When a stimulus is presented, skin resistance decreases and skin conductance increases. The latency of the response after the stimulus is presented is usually about 2 to 3 seconds. Spontaneous activity is defined as responses that occur in the absence of stimulation or as responses that are less than a certain amplitude. Skin resistance and skin conductance levels are easily quantified using computer systems. Responses of these measures are much more difficult to automate and require sophisticated computer programs. Skin resistance is quantified in units of kilohms and skin conductance is quantified in units of micromhos (μmhos).

Skin potential is recorded using one active electrode placed on the palmar surface of the hand and one inactive electrode, usually placed on the arm. Skin potential responses have both positive and negative voltage changes, usually recorded in microvolts. Skin potential must be quantified in terms of response amplitude to a stimulus. Because of the complexity of the skin potential wave form, it is not easily recorded using automated computer systems. For this reason, skin resistance and skin conductance are the preferred measures of electrodermal activity in modern psychophysiology.

Respiration

Respiration rate is the most common respiratory measure used in psychophysiological assessment. Measurement of respiration amplitude is much more difficult, in that it requires the recording of expired gases. Respiration rate can be recorded using two methods. The most preferred method is through the use of a strain gauge placed around the subject's chest. A strain gauge measures minute changes in the circumference of the chest as air is inspired and expired. A less frequently used procedure utilizes a temperature thermistor placed below one nostril of the subject. This procedure allows for the measurement of temperature changes as the subject inspires cool external air and expires warm internal air. Both procedures allow for quantification of respiration cycles in terms of cycles per minute. Both procedures require the use of a DC preamplifier. The use of a strain gauge allows for easier automated recording because there is less "drift" of the signal. There are problems with recording of respiration using temperature because of changes in room temperature and heating of the thermistor, which may cause gradual shifts in baseline across the recording session.

Electroencephalogram (EEG)

The EEG is a surface recording of brain waves. It uses an AC preamplifier. Electrode placement for the recording of EEG is very complex. The interested reader should refer to Shagass (1972) for a more complete discussion of these issues. Automated recording of EEG requires the use of filters to isolate specific frequencies of the EEG signal. Table 5.2 summarizes the commonly used frequencies in EEG research.

An average of EEG responses to discrete stimuli is called the evoked potential. The recording of evoked potential requires specialized computer systems that can present a stimulus and record the electrical activity that occurs immediately after the stimulus presentation. These responses are averaged across time (in msec) and trials (presentation of the stimulus).

Sphincter Muscle Tension

The measurement of anal sphincter muscle tension has been developed in recent years for the assessment and treatment of disorders of bowel function (e.g., fecal incontinence). This type of assessment requires the insertion of a specially designed transducer into the rectum (see Engel, 1977, for a more complete description). This transducer simultaneously measures tension of the internal and external sphincter muscles. These measures are recorded using a DC preamplifier. This assessment allows for evaluation of dysfunctional muscular tone and can be used in biofeedback treatment of fecal incontinence.

RELIABILITY AND STABILITY OF PSYCHOPHYSIOLOGICAL MEASURES

Before turning to the clinical applications of psychophysiological measurement, it is important to discuss the reliability of these measurement procedures with both normal and clinical populations. It has been widely assumed that psychophysiological measures are relatively stable over time. This assumption was based upon early psychophysiological research on individual response stereotypy (Lacey, Bateman,

TABLE 5.2. CLASSIFICATION OF EEG ACTIVITY

Category	Frequency	Psychological Correlates
Alpha	8 to 13 Hz	Alert and relaxed
Beta	14 to 30 Hz	Excited
Delta	Less than 4 Hz	Deep sleep
Theta	4 to 7 Hz	Drowsy

& VanLehn, 1953), which suggested that individual autonomic response patterns were relatively stable over time. Several studies prior to 1980 (e.g., Goldstein, 1972) reported good reliability of EMG measurement, although the studies involved only one response and were investigated with outdated equipment.

Researchers have recently begun to investigate these issues utilizing more diverse response systems and more sophisticated measurement procedures and statistical analyses. Most of the studies to date have involved psychophysiological measurement of adults. One study (Giordani, Manuck, & Farmer, 1981), however, demonstrated that task-related heart rate reactivity across two experimental sessions was highly reproducible in boys of elementary school age. The results of this study lend credibility to the assumption that reliability estimates of psychophysiological assessment in adults may be generalized to children.

Arena, Blanchard, Andrasik, Cotch, and Myers (1983) investigated the reliability of psychophysiological measures in a small sample of nonclinical, adult individuals. They measured multiple response systems (i.e., forehead and forearm EMG, HR, SRL, ST, and cephalic VMR), under multiple experimental conditions (i.e., baseline, self-control, mental stressors, and physical stress), on multiple occasions. The findings of this study cast some doubt upon the reliability of psychophysiological measures as commonly used in clinical research and clinical practice. Overall, few psychophysiological responses were highly correlated over time. Specifically, frontalis EMG was stable across experimental conditions and time, heart rate and forearm EMG were reliable across most experimental procedures but not time, skin temperature was only stable over a 1-week period of time, and cephalic VMR and skin resistance were found to be unreliable. However, other current research has indicated some degree of reliability for electrodermal measures (e.g., Baque, 1982) and for cardiovascular measures assessed during experimental cognitive stressors (e.g., Manuck & Garland, 1980; Manuck & Schaeffer, 1978).

A very recent investigation (Williamson, Waters, Bernard, Faulstich, & Blouin, 1985) was designed to reexamine the issues of psychophysiological response reliability and pattern stability in psychophysiological test procedures. The type of statistical analyses used by Williamson and colleagues in the study just cited allowed for the evaluation of both the reliability of multiple psychophysiological responses (pattern) and the reliability of the individual response stereotypy of each subject. With respect to specific experimental procedures, overall reliability for stressful imagery and stressful slide presentations was found to be satisfactory. Reliability of habituation and startle procedures was also found to be satisfactory, although to a lesser degree. An oral intelligence test, however, was found to be unreliable. Heart rate, skin resistance, and skin temperature were found to be the most consistently reliable responses across experimental procedures. However, the degree of reliability for any given psychophysiological response was found to depend upon the experimental test procedure, the method of statistical analysis, and the degree and pattern of individual response stereotypy of the subject tested.

In a follow-up study, Faulstich (1985) found that heart rate, blood pressure, skin temperature, vasomotor response, and skin resistance were very reliable when used in four stress tests: cold pressor, isometric challenge, mental arithmetic, and an oral intelligence test. This study utilized a large sample size and sophisticated multivariate statistical procedures. In combination with the earlier findings of Williamson et al. (1985), it can be concluded that most psychophysiological assessment procedures are stable over time. However, the overall findings suggest that certain measures are more stable than others and that certain experimental tasks may elicit more reliable responses. Therefore, researchers and clinicians using psychophysiological assessment procedures should choose to measure responses that are most stable across the chosen experimental procedures for studies involving repeated measures. Again, it can now only be assumed that these general findings would apply in psychophysiological assessment of children.

CLINICAL APPLICATIONS

Biofeedback

One of the most common uses of psychophysiological measurement is to provide feedback to the individual concerning autonomic or motor activity. Biofeedback involves the presentation of a feedback signal that reflects changes in a physiological response. It entails providing to the individual a visual, auditory, or other type of sensory display of changes in his or her own physiological responses as they are occurring in time. The individual is usually given instructions regarding the "meaning" of the feedback signal and procedures to change the signal in a particular direction as suggested. The direct link in time between the actual physiological response occurring in the body and the sensory display of the same response is the essence of the concept of biofeedback and is thought to be critical in the process of self-regulation (Williamson & Blanchard, 1979a, 1979b, 1979c).

In addition to providing feedback, psychophysiological measurement is often used to document the efficacy of biofeedback training. The degree of change in the targeted psychophysiological response is generally used as a measure of success in biofeedback learning.

Although biofeedback has been provided from many autonomic or motor functions, electromyographic (EMG) and skin temperature biofeedback have been the most commonly selected for use with children (Williamson, McKenzie, & Goreczny, in press). EMG biofeedback training is used to increase the contraction of inadequately functioning muscles and decrease activity in overactive muscles. The raw EMG signal provides limited information and is difficult to interpret as feedback. Therefore, integrative techniques that store and sum the raw EMG are more often used. In children, EMG biofeedback has been used to increase peak expiratory flow rates in asthmatics (Kotses, Glaus, Crawford, Edwards, & Scherr, 1976) and to increase academic performance in hyperactive boys (Denkowski, Denkowski, & Omizo, 1983).

Skin temperature has been used frequently as a model of biofeedback for children. The most significant use of skin temperature biofeedback with children has been in the treatment of childhood migraine (Labbé & Williamson, 1983, 1984). Although degree of improvement of headache activity and degree of temperature increase were not tested, children given skin temperature biofeedback were able to raise their skin temperature 0.5°C. Skin temperature changes during feedback and self-control following feedback were significantly different from baseline and self-control preceding feedback (Labbé & Williamson, 1984). These data suggested that children learned to control skin temperature during biofeedback training, though there was a question whether the children learned self-control of skin temperature in the absence of biofeedback. From these initial studies, it is clear that more basic research using psychophysiological assessment as a measure of biofeedback learning is needed in order to understand better the mechanisms underlying the improvement observed when biofeedback is used as a treatment for childhood migraine.

More generally, it appears that children can learn to control psychophysiological responses using biofeedback (Williamson, in press). There is a need for more systematic research concerning basic issues involved in this learning, for example, the significance of age of the child, type of feedback, and so forth.

Cardiovascular Reactivity

Psychophysiological assessment has been utilized to examine an individual's physiological responses to challenge stressors (both mental and physical) in the laboratory. This type of investigation is particularly important in children who may be at high risk for cardiovascular disease. These children may be identified by relatively high levels of blood pressure at a given age or may be normotensive with a history of parental hypertension. It has been suggested that persons who show a large autonomic response on cardiovascular measures (i.e., heart rate or blood pressure) may be more likely to develop some type of cardiovascular disease, such as hypertension (Sternbach, 1966). This phenomenon was referred to earlier as individual response stereotypy (Lacey et al., 1953).

Several studies have been conducted to investigate cardiovascular reactivity in children. The studies have focused on both normal and clinical populations, and most have involved heart rate and blood pressure responses to experimental tasks in order to investigate reactivity. A study conducted in the early 1960s (Lacey & Lacey, 1962) showed some stability of unique cardiovascular responses among younger subjects who were exposed on two occasions separated by time. However, the subjects varied in age from 7 to 17 years, and the experimental stressor was purely physical in nature (which may have evoked thermal adjustment as well as cardiovascular reactivity).

A later study was conducted to measure heart rate and blood pressure responses to a mental arithmetic task in adolescent "labile" hypertensives, normotensive adolescents with hypertensive parents, and normotensive control subjects with no family history of hypertension (Falkner, Onesti, Angelakos, Fernandes, & Langman, 1979). All subjects were matched for age to control for age-related effects on blood pressure. The results of this study showed greater heart rate and blood pressure responses in both hypertensive adolescents and the normotensive adolescents with hypertensive parents than in the normotensive control subjects. In a related study, Hastrup, Light, and Obrist (1982) examined the response to an experimental stressor in college students with and without a history of parental hypertension. In this study, however, both a mental stressor (i.e., reaction time task) and a physical stressor (i.e., cold pressor) were used. Sons of hypertensive parents showed higher heart rate and systolic blood pressure responses than did sons of normotensive parents during both rest and stress, with the greatest difference occurring during the stressful reaction time task. Both studies (i.e., Falkner et al., 1979; Hastrup et al., 1982) provide support for a familial component of heart rate reactivity in response to stress. In addition, these findings suggest that cardiovascular responses to stress may aid in predicting future risk of hypertension.

In order to determine whether the early individual differences in experimentally induced heart rate reactivity are stable across time, Giordani and colleagues (1981) presented 8-year-old boys with a mental stressor (concept-forming task emphasizing both speed and accuracy) on two occasions separated by 1 week. Previous investigations (Manuck & Garland, 1980; Manuck & Schaeffer, 1978) had shown that adults demonstrated stable differences in heart rate reactivity to the same experimental task (i.e., concept formation) when retested 1 week later. Results of the childhood study (Giordani et al., 1981) showed that task-related heart rate reactivity was highly reproducible. They were able to demonstrate differences between groups of heart rate reactors and nonreactors across the experimental sessions and the stability of relative differences between baseline measures and task measures of heart rate. In other words, those children who responded to the experimental stressor with an increase in heart rate during the first session responded with the same relative increase during the second session. It is important to note that increases in heart rate were not directly related to task performance.

Although heart rate reactivity has been shown to be stable in both children and adults, there are insufficient data to conclude that cardiovascular reactivity is a stable characteristic from childhood through adulthood. Longitudinal studies must be conducted before stability greater than 1 week can be assumed.

Seizures

Seizures may be defined as involuntary alterations in or loss of control of motor, sensory, or autonomic functions of the body. Seizures may involve brief lapses in consciousness or prolonged interruptions of consciousness with associated convulsions. Much of our understanding of seizure activity depends upon detailed knowledge of the electroencephalographic features of the seizures. For this reason, psychophysiological recording of brain wave activity is usually employed in the assessment of seizures. It is important to note, however, that there is no electroencephalographic (EEG) pattern that absolutely defines seizures, and that similar records may be seen in differing types of seizure disorders (Fois, 1963). As a result, it is often desirable to measure other autonomic or motor functions in conjunction with EEG in order to observe temporal sequences or correlations between different physiological or behavioral events. It may also prove beneficial to record EEGs under different experimental settings. For example, examination of brain activity during sleep may indicate specific abnormalities that were not apparent under resting conditions. It may also be necessary to obtain more than one record in order to demonstrate the presence of abnormalities; serial EEGs also provide a measure of consistency of the abnormal brain activity (Gaustaut & Braughton, 1972).

In addition to diagnosis, psychophysiological assessment of brain wave abnormalities has aided in the development of nonpharmacological treatment methods. Early animal studies by Sterman and his colleagues showed that the occurrence of EEG in cats of 12 to 16 cycles per second could be modified by reinforcement (Roth, Sterman, & Clemente, 1967; Wyrwicka & Sterman, 1968). This EEG activity (12 to 16 Hz) was termed sensorimotor rhythm, or SMR (Brazier, 1963), because it tends to occur over the sensorimotor area of the cortex. With training and reinforcement, this rhythm was found to increase as a percentage of EEG in trained animals and was associated with an inhibition of a previously learned motor response and cessation of all movement. This type of training was also shown to delay the effects of a powerful convulsant in the experimental cats (Sterman, LoPresti, & Fairchild, 1969).

Seizure resistance exhibited by SMR-trained cats led to studies employing biofeedback training techniques in human seizure patients, both child and adult (Sterman & Friar, 1972; Sterman, Macdonald, & Stone, 1974). One striking characteristic of psychophysiological measures of brain activity in seizure patients is the absence of a rhythm of 12 to 14 Hz and the presence of a rhythm of 4 to 7 Hz (Olton & Noonberg, 1980). Biofeedback has been used to correct these abnormalities. The EEG is recorded from the scalp, and the person is given feedback about the presence of both activity of 12 to 14 Hz and activity of 4 to 7 Hz. Biofeedback is used to increase the amount of 12 to 14 Hz activity and to decrease the amount of 4 to 7 Hz activity. All of the studies employing this type of biofeedback have utilized continuous psychophysiological measurement of brain wave activity. These clinical studies have shown that EEG biofeedback can lead to substantial seizure reduction in children and adults (Kuhlman & Kaplan, 1979). Thus psychophysiological assessment has been utilized to diagnose seizure patients and to reduce the frequency of seizures through biofeedback procedures.

Asthma

Asthma is a respiratory disorder characterized by involuntary constriction of the bronchial passages. Common symptoms include coughing, shortness of breath, wheezing, labored breathing, and anxiety accompanying a feeling of suffocation (King, 1980; Melamed, 1980; Melamed & Johnson, 1981). Asthma affects 2 to 4 percent of the pediatric population and accounts for 25 percent of all school absences due to chronic illness (Melamed, 1980; Melamed & Johnson, 1981).

Although many asthma attacks are caused by allergic stimuli, several studies have shown that attacks can be precipitated by mere suggestion (Godfrey & Silverman, 1973; Luparello, Lyons, Bleecker, & McFadden, 1968; Phillip, Wilde, & Day, 1972; Strupp et al., 1974). Because of this apparent psychological component in asthma, researchers in psychology have attempted to find ways to help alleviate the symptoms of this disorder.

The assessment of treatment outcome in asthma is generally based on changes in pulmonary functioning. The most frequently used assessment of pulmonary functioning is the peak expiratory flow rate (PEFR) or the measure of the maximum rate of airflow from the lungs during forced expiration. This technique is very reliable and very easy to perform and has been used by numerous researchers to determine pulmonary functioning in asthmatics. For example, Miklich, Rewey, Weiss, and Kolton (1973) used peak expiratory flow rates as an indicator of psychophysiological responses to stress in asthmatic children, while other studies (Davis, Saunders, Creer, & Chai, 1973; Kotses et al., 1975) have examined the effects of EMG biofeedback and relaxation training on the PEFR in children with asthma.

It is a widely held notion among psychologists that anxiety can play a major role in the onset of an asthma attack. Therefore, many researchers have turned to psychophysiological assessment methods to measure autonomic arousal in asthmatic patients. Studies by Hahn (1966, 1967), for example, have shown that asthmatic boys tend to have higher resting heart rates and finger temperatures than do normal boys. In biofeedback relaxation training, psychophysiological arousal is measured and is then visually or aurally displayed so that the subject can see the direct effects of his or her attempts to relax. This relaxation method has been employed effectively in several treatment outcome studies with asthmatic children (Davis et al., 1973; Feldman, 1976; Kotses et al., 1976).

Bulimia

Bulimia is a disorder commonly found in female adolescents and young adults, and it has gained much recognition in recent years. It is characterized by recurrent episodes of bingeing and purging (by means of self-induced vomiting or the use of laxatives or diuretics) in an attempt to control weight. It has traditionally been conceptualized as a variant of anorexia nervosa, but evidence now suggests that bulimia should be regarded as a distinct clinical entity (Fairburn & Cooper, 1982). The latest edition of the *Diagnostic and Statistical Manual of Mental Disorders* (DSM-III) does, in fact, list bulimia as a separate diagnostic category.

An anxiety model of bulimia, such as the one proposed by Rosen and Leitenberg (1982), is frequently used to describe the etiology of this disorder. Williamson, Kelley, Davis, Ruggiero, and Veitia (1985) have proposed a model that incorporates the anxiety model with aspects of a model proposed by Slade (1982). Slade suggests that the motivation of binge eating is the deprivation of energy due to repeated purging of food before it can be absorbed in the stomach and intestines.

Williamson and colleagues' model of bulimia is illustrated in Figure 5.2. This model holds that the central problem of bulimia is a sequence of events such as that enclosed within the broken lines in the figure. Frequent purging of food is thought to cause a state of biological deprivation, subjective feelings of hunger, preoccupation with food, and strong urges to eat. These conditions cause anxiety because of the bulimic's fear of becoming obese. Purging serves to reduce this anxiety, but also deprives the bulimic of energy, producing a state of biological deprivation and continuing the binge–purge cycle. In addition, the model suggests that other psychopathology, such as depression, distorted body image, interpersonal problems, obsessive–compulsive habits, substance abuse, and stress, can interact with the core of the problem of the binge–purge cycle to cause the eating disorder and other psychopathology to worsen over time.

In one study (Williamson et al., 1985), the anxiety component of bulimia was tested by measuring autonomic responses to the feared stimulus of food. Bulimics were allowed to adapt for 15 minutes and were then given a standard meal to consume. Although the bulimic group did show physiological signs of anxiety, only EMG activity was found to be significantly greater than that for obese and normal subjects. Further analyses, however, did find most severe bulimics (in terms of bingeing and purging frequency) to be significantly more anxious than obese and normal subjects as evidenced by increased EMG and heart rate activity.

Recent research from our laboratory shows that bulimics evidence significant sympathetic arousal when faced with having to eat certain "forbidden foods." These psychophysiological data suggest that bulimics may experience strong anticipatory anxiety in response to eating high-calorie foods, which leads to either food avoidance or binge eating followed by purging, as predicted by the anxiety model. This usage of psychophysiological assessment is of importance because it is one of the few

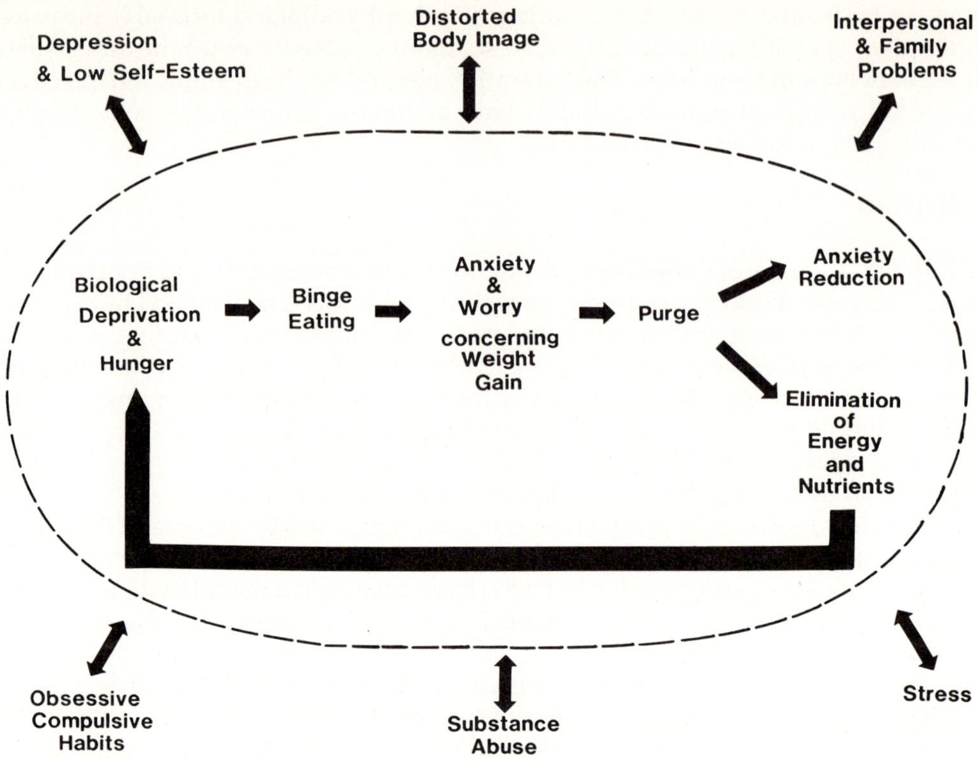

FIGURE 5.2. Anxiety model of bulimia.

uses of psychophysiological methods to measure anxiety in children or adolescents. This application clearly needs to be developed further considering the problems of assessing anxiety in children.

CONCLUSIONS

Psychophysiological assessment with children is a very new and underdeveloped area of research. Many of the basic principles developed in the laboratory with adults should apply to child populations. However, there is a need for basic research concerning the techniques that might best be used with children. For example, common stressors used with adults are mental arithmetic, oral intelligence tests, and cold pressor. It is unclear whether these tasks can be directly transferred to child populations.

Clinical applications of psychophysiology with children have lagged far behind those with adults. Psychophysiological techniques for assessing stress, anxiety, and pathophysiological conditions have been widely used with adults but are only beginning with children. Also, biofeedback treatment approaches have been extensively studied with adults but have only recently been initiated with children.

These observations suggest that psychophysiological methods have great promise as a part of child assessment but have, as of now, gone undeveloped. Given the recent surge of interest in behavioral pediatrics and related areas, it is only a matter of time before this area is more widely investigated. Until then, we must conclude that psychophysiological assessment with children holds much promise and awaits the efforts of basic and applied researchers to tap its potential fully.

References

Arena, J. G., Blanchard, E. B., Andrasik, F., Cotch, P. A., & Myers, P. E. (1983). Reliability of psychophysiological assessment. *Behavioral Research & Therapy, 21,* 447–460.

Baque, E. (1982). Reliability of electrodermal measures: A compilation. *Biological Psychology, 14,* 219–220.

Blanchard, E. B., Theobald, D. E., Williamson, D. A., Silver, B. V., & Brown, D. A. (1978). Temperature biofeedback in the treatment of migraine headaches: A controlled evaluation. *Archives of General Psychiatry, 35,* 581–588.

Brazier, M. A. B. (1963). The problem of periodicity in the electroencephalogram: Studies in the cat. *Electroencephalography & Clinical Neurophysiology, 15,* 287–298.

Brown, C. C. (1967). The technique of plethysmography. In C. C. Brown (Ed.), *Methods in psychophysiology.* Baltimore: Williams & Wilkins.

Caton, R. (1875). The electric currents of the brain. *British Medical Journal, 2,* 278.

Davis, M. H., Saunders, D. R., Creer, T. L., & Chai, H. (1973). Relaxation training facilitated by biofeedback apparatus as a supplemental treatment in bronchial asthma. *Journal of Psychosomatic Research, 17,* 121–128.

Denkowski, K. M., Denkowski, G. C., & Omizo, M. M. (1983). The effects of EMG-assisted relaxation training on the academic performance, locus of control, and self-esteem of hyperactive boys. *Biofeedback & Self-Regulation, 8,* 363–375.

Engel, B. T. (1977). Cardiac arrhythmias. In R. B. Williams & W. D. Gentry (Eds.), *Behavioral approaches to medical treatment.* Cambridge, MA: Ballinger.

Fairburn, C. G., & Cooper, P. J. (1982). Self-induced vomiting and bulimia nervosa: An undetected problem. *British Medical Journal, 284,* 1153–1155.

Falkner, B., Onesti, G., Angelakos, E. T., Fernandes, M., & Langman, C. (1979). Cardiovascular response to mental stress in normal adolescents with hypertensive parents. *Hypertension, 1,* 23–30.

Faulstich, M. E. (1985). *The reliability of psychophysiological assessment: A comparative analysis of mental and physical stressors.* Unpublished doctoral dissertation, Louisiana State University, Baton Rouge.

Feldman, G. M. (1976). The effect of biofeedback training on respiratory resistance of asthmatic children. *Psychosomatic Medicine, 38,* 27–34.

Féré, C. (1888). Note sur les modifications de la tension électrique dans le corps humain. *Comptes rendes des Séances de la societé de Biologie, 5,* 28–33.

Fois, A. (1963). *Clinical electroencephalography in epilepsy and related conditions in children.* Springfield, IL: Charles C. Thomas.

Gaustaut, H., & Braughton, R. (1972). *Epileptic seizures: Clinical and electrographic features, diagnosis, and treatment.* Springfield, IL: Charles C. Thomas.

Giordani, B., Manuck, S. B., & Farmer, J. K. (1981). Stability of behaviorally induced heart-rate changes in children after one week. *Child Development, 52,* 533–537.

Godfrey, S., & Silverman, M. (1973). Demonstration by placebo response in asthma by means of exercise testing. *Journal of Psychosomatic Research, 17,* 293–297.

Goldstein, I. B. (1972). Electromyography: A measure of skeletal muscle response. In N. S. Garfield & R. A. Sternbach (Eds.), *Handbook of psychophysiology.* New York: Holt, Rinehart, & Winston.

Graham, D. T. (1972). Psychosomatic medicine. In N. S. Greenfield & R. A. Sternbach (Eds.), *Handbook of psychophysiology.* New York: Holt, Rinehart, & Winston.

Greenfield, N. S., & Sternbach, R. A. (1972). *Handbook of psychophysiology.* New York: Holt, Rinehart, & Winston.

Gribbin, B., Steptoe, A., & Sleight, P. (1976). Pulse wave velocity as a measure of blood pressure change. *Psychophysiology, 13,* 86–90.

Hahn, W. W. (1966). Autonomic responses of asthmatic children. *Psychosomatic Medicine, 28*, 323–329.

Hahn, W. W., & Clark, J. A. (1967). Psychophysiological reactivity of asthmatic children. *Psychosomatic Medicine, 29*, 526–534.

Hastrup, J. L., Light, K. C., & Obrist, P. A. (1982). Parental hypertension and cardiovascular response to stress in healthy young adults. *Psychophysiology, 19*(6), 615–622.

Jacobson, A. M., Manschreck, T. C., & Silverberg, E. (1979). Behavioral treatment for Raynaud's disease: A comparative study with long-term follow-up. *American Journal of Psychiatry, 136*, 844–846.

Khachaturian, Z. S., Kerr, J., Kruger, R., & Schachter, J. (1972). A methodological note: Comparison between period and rate data in studies of cardiac function. *Psychophysiology, 9*, 539–545.

Kimper, T. (1977). *Biofeedback of blood pressure information in normotensive subjects using pulse wave transit time measurements*. Unpublished doctoral dissertation, Pennsylvania State University, State College.

King, N. J. (1980). The behavioral management of asthma and asthma-related problems in children: A critical review of the literature. *Journal of Behavioral Medicine, 3*, 169–189.

Kotses, H., Glaus, K. D., Crawford, P. L., Edwards, J. E., & Scherr, M. S. (1976). Operant reduction of frontalis EMG activity in the treatment of asthma in children. *Journal of Psychosomatic Research, 20*, 453–459.

Kuhlman, W. N., & Kaplan, B. J. (1979). Clinical applications of EEG feedback training. In R. J. Gatchel & K. P. Price (Eds.), *Clinical applications of biofeedback: Appraisal and status*. New York: Pergamon.

Labbé, E. E., & Williamson, D. A. (1983). Temperature biofeedback in the treatment of children with migraine headaches. *Journal of Pediatric Psychology, 8*, 317–326.

Labbé, E. E., & Williamson, D. A. (1984). Treatment of childhood migraine using autogenic feedback training. *Journal of Consulting & Clinical Psychology, 52*, 968–976.

Lacey, J. I., Bateman, D. E., & VanLehn, R. (1953). Autonomic response specificity: An experimental study. *Psychosomatic Medicine, 15*, 8–21.

Lacey, J. I., & Lacey, B. C. (1962). The law of initial value in the longitudinal study of autonomic constitution: Reproducibility of autonomic responses and response patterns over a four-year interval. *Annals of the New York Academy of Sciences, 98*, 1257–1290.

Lang, P. (1971). The application of psychophysiological methods to the study of psychotherapy and behavior modification. In A. E. Bergin & S. L. Garfield (Eds.), *Handbook of psychotherapy and behavior change: An empirical analysis*. New York: Wiley.

Luparello, T. J., Lyons, H. A., Bleecker, E. R., & McFadden, E. R. (1968). Influence of suggestion on airway reactivity in asthmatic subjects. *Psychosomatic Medicine, 30*, 819–825.

Malmo, R. B., & Shagass, C. (1949). Physiological studies of reaction to stress in anxiety states and early schizophrenia. *Psychosomatic Medicine, 11*, 9–24.

Manuck, S. B., & Garland, F. N. (1980). Stability of individual differences in cardiovascular reactivity: A thirteen-month follow-up. *Physiology & Behavior, 24*, 621–624.

Manuck, S. B., & Schaeffer, D. C. (1978). Stability of individual differences in cardiovascular reactivity. *Physiology & Behavior, 21*, 675–678.

Marie, G. V., Lo, C. R., Jones, J. V., & Johnson, D. W. (1984). The relationship between arterial blood pressure and pulse transit time during dynamic and static exercise. *Psychophysiology, 21*, 521–522.

Melamed, B. G. (1980). Behavioral psychology in pediatrics. In S. Rachman (Ed.), *Contributions to medical psychology* (Vol. 2). Oxford: Pergamon.

Melamed, B. G., & Johnson, S. B. (1981). Chronic illness: Asthma and juvenile diabetes. In E. J. Mash & L. G. Terdal (Eds.), *Behavioral assessment of childhood disorders*. New York: Guilford.

Miklich, D. R., Rewey, H. H., Weiss, J. H., & Kolton, S. (1973). A preliminary investigation of psychophysiological responses to stress among different subgroups of asthmatic children. *Journal of Psychosomatic Research, 17*, 1–8.

Obrist, P. A., Light, K. C., McCubbin, J. A., Hutcheson, J. S., & Hoffer, J. L. (1979). Pulse transit time: Relationship to blood pressure and myocardial performance. *Psychophysiology, 16*, 292–301.

Olton, D. S., & Noonberg, A. R. (1980). *Biofeedback: Clinical applications in behavior medicine*. Englewood Cliffs, NJ: Prentice-Hall.

Phillip, R. L., Wilde, G. J. S., & Day, J. H. (1972). Suggestion and relaxation in asthmatics. *Journal of Psychosomatic Research, 16*, 193–204.

Pollak, M. H., & Obrist, P. A. (1983). Aortic-radial pulse transit time and ECGQ-wave to radial pulse wave interval as indices of beat-by-beat blood pressure change. *Psychophysiology, 20*(1), 21–28.

Ray, W. J., & Raczynski, J. M. (1981). Psychophysiological assessment. In M. Hersen & A. S. Bellack (Eds.), *Behavioral assessment: A practical handbook*. New York: Pergamon.

Rosen, J. C., & Leitenberg, H. (1982). Bulimia nervosa: Treatment with exposure and response prevention. *Behavior Therapy, 13,* 117–124.

Roth, S. R., Sterman, M. B., & Clemente, C. D. (1967). Comparison of EEG correlates of reinforcement, internal inhibition, and sleep. *Electroencephalography & Clinical Neurophysiology, 23,* 509–520.

Shagass, C. (1972). Electrical activity of the brain. In N. S. Greenfield & R. A. Sternbach (Eds.), *Handbook of psychophysiology*. New York: Holt, Rinehart, & Winston.

Silver, B. V., Blanchard, E. B., Williamson, D. A., Theobald, D. E., & Brown, D. A. (1979). Temperature biofeedback and relaxation training in the treatment of migraine headaches. *Biofeedback & Self-Regulation, 4,* 359–366.

Slade, P. (1982). Towards a functional analysis of anorexia nervosa and bulimia nervosa. *British Journal of Clinical Psychology, 21,* 167–179.

Steptoe, A., Godaert, G., Ross, A., & Schreurs, P. (1983). The cardiac and vascular components of pulse transmission time: A computer analysis of systolic time intervals. *Psychophysiology, 20*(3), 251–259.

Steptoe, A., Smulyan, H., & Gribbin, B. (1976). Pulse wave velocity and blood pressure change: Calibration and applications. *Psychophysiology, 13,* 488–493.

Sterman, M. B., & Friar, L. (1972). Suppression of seizures in an epileptic following sensorimotor EEG feedback training. *Electroencephalography & Clinical Neurophysiology, 33,* 89–95.

Sterman, M. B., LoPresti, R. W., & Fairchild, M. D. (1969). *Electroencephalographic and behavioral studies of monomethylhydrazine toxicity in the cat.* Technical Report AMRL-TR-69-3, Wright-Patterson Air Force Base, Ohio.

Sterman, M. B., Macdonald, L. R., & Stone, R. K. (1974). Biofeedback training of the sensorimotor EEG rhythm in man: Effects on epilepsy. *Epilepsia, 15,* 395–416.

Sternbach, R. A. (1966). Individual response stereotypy. In R. A. Sternbach (Ed.), *Principles of psychophysiology*. New York: Academic.

Strupp, H. H., Levenson, R. W., Manuck, S. B., Snell, J. D., Hinrichsen, J. J., & Boyd, S. (1974). Effects of suggestion on total respiratory resistance in mild asthmatics. *Journal of Psychosomatic Research, 18,* 337–346.

Weinman, J. (1967). Photoplethysmography. In P. H. Venables & I. Martin (Eds.), *A manual of psychophysiological methods*. Amsterdam: North-Holland.

Williamson, D. A., & Blanchard, E. B. (1979a). Effect of feedback delay upon learned heart rate control. *Psychophysiology, 16,* 108–115.

Williamson, D. A., & Blanchard, E. B. (1979b). Heart rate and blood pressure biofeedback: I. A review of the recent experimental literature. *Biofeedback & Self-Regulation, 4,* 1–34.

Williamson, D. A., & Blanchard, E. B. (1979c). Heart rate and blood pressure biofeedback: II. Recent findings and theoretical considerations. *Biofeedback & Self-Regulation, 4,* 35–50.

Williamson, D. A., Epstein, L. H., & Lombardo, T. W. (1980). EMG measurement as a function of electrode placement and level of EMG. *Psychophysiology, 17,* 279–292.

Williamson, D. A., Kelley, M. L., Davis, C. J., Ruggiero, L., & Veitia, M. C. (1985). The psychophysiology of bulimia. *Advances in Behavior Research & Therapy, 7,* 116–172.

Williamson, D. A., McKenzie, S. J., & Goreczny, A. J. (in press). Biofeedback. In J. C. Witt, S. N. Elliott, & F. M. Gresham (Eds.), *Handbook of behavior therapy in education*. New York: Plenum.

Williamson, D. A., Waters, W. F., Bernard, B., Faulstich, M., & Blouin, D. (1985, March). *Test-retest reliability of psychophysiological assessment*. Paper presented at the sixth annual scientific session of the Society of Behavioral Medicine, New Orleans.

Williamson, D. A., Waters, W. F., & Hawkins, M. F. (in press). Physiological variables. In R. D. Nelson & S. C. Hayes (Eds.), *Conceptual foundations for behavioral assessment*. New York: Guilford.

Wyrwicka, W., & Sterman, M. B. (1968). Instrumental conditioning of sensorimotor cortex EEG spindles in the waking cat. *Physiology & Behavior, 3,* 703–707.

6

Neuropsychological Assessment of Children

THOMAS J. BOLL

The neuropsychological assessment of children differs, in a number of identifiable ways, from standard clinical child psychological assessment. None of these differences are absolute. Within the general approach to any patient population, there will always be substantial degrees of similarity. Such similarity involves the use of psychological tests themselves and many of the underlying theoretical notions that pertain to such procedures. Areas of similarity with regard to clinical style and method cannot be overlooked. It is also important to point out that, whether or not the child has a known neurological condition, a suspected neurological disorder, or a behavioral problem, the patient is still a child and the patient's world is still the world of children. That means that issues of family relationships, development of peer contacts, and competence in school and school-related environments must be dealt with. These are rather different issues than those typically raised for adult patients, and they require a different level of expertise that is specific to dealing with children. For that reason, no matter what the nature of the referral question, a clinical child neuropsychologist must be both a neuropsychologist and a clinical child psychologist. A whimsical way of stating this might be that a clinical child neuropsychologist is not just a small adult neuropsychologist. I will focus on some areas that distinguish clinical neuropsychological assessment of children from standard clinical psychological assessment without attempting to claim uniqueness or total nonoverlap for either procedure.

Neuropsychological assessment of children differs with regard to the patient population. Most patients referred for neuropsychological evaluation come from a medical–surgical referral network. Such patients most commonly have been identified as suffering from some form of brain disorder or impairment. Such children are those for whom questions have been raised with regard to the adequacy or integrity of brain functions; this may be reflected in some behavioral distress or disorganization, for which an etiology and explanation are sought.

Neuropsychological evaluation with known neurological conditions is influenced by a number of factors related to the kind of brain impairment that is most likely to be experienced during the developing years. Children's brain damage is, in the main, more likely to be diffuse and generalized rather than focal, chronic rather than acute, and static rather than progressive. It is caused by factors such as hypoxia, infection, and trauma more often than by stroke, tumor, or degenerative disease. Children can have cerebral vascular accidents, brain tumors, and even degenerative neurological disorders; but even here, the location and type of these conditions often differ from those of adults. Children are more likely to have strokes secondary to congenital abnormalities, often found below the cerebral hemispheres, and are more likely to have extracerebral than intracerebral neoplasms. Children may suffer from all (or almost all) afflictions known in adulthood, but the preponderance of disorders is somewhat different for children than for adults. This has an influence on the type of neuropsychological symptom and, therefore, the type of neuropsychological examination most commonly applied.

The types of disorders that are most frequently experienced by children are those more likely to impair higher cognitive functions to a greater degree, and lower, simpler psychological processes (such as motor and sensory functions) to a lesser degree. Brain disorders that produce a frank aphasia are less common than are brain disorders that result in a diminished capacity to learn and develop new language skills (Boll, 1984). On the other hand, during childhood, it is far more necessary that one be able to learn new information, and less possible to rely on utilization of previously learned data. Therefore, subtle deficits in knowledge acquisition capacity, as might be expressed through diminished attentional functions, reduced short-term and intermediate-term memory capacity, and impaired language manipulational skills, would be far more devastating to a child in the active learning years than to an adult with similar intellectual capacity. Adults are more in need of intact abilities to utilize previously learned skills than abilities to acquire an entirely new knowledge base.

The most common cause of death and disability in childhood is head injury. In fact, head injury is ahead of the next three leading causes of disability *combined* for children ages 1 to 14. It is common medical lore that children weather the effects of brain injury far better than adults. With regard to their actual medical survival, this is indeed the case. Children will often come through accidents producing unbelievable physical devastation, and appear, months later, in remarkably good physical condition. While children's bodies are definitely more resilient than those of adults, it is not entirely clear that this is always and necessarily the case with regard to brain functions. Both adults and children have been known to survive what would appear to be a devastating illness and regain a substantial amount of neurocognitive process and enjoy a continuing recovery period that lasts for many years. On the other hand, however, it is true that children who appear superficially normal and whose physical condition seems robust have been reported in great numbers to experience substantial decline in ability to perform mental processes. Even children with very minor head injuries (from a medical point of view) have been reported to experience years of neuropsychologically measurable recovery and a significantly elevated incidence of school failure and special education class placement (Klonoff, Low, & Clark, 1977). Particularly at the minor end of the severity spectrum, children are at considerable risk for being overlooked with regard to the sequelae of their injury. Thus they go not just untreated, but rather actively *mistreated* through the misunderstandings that develop when these apparently normal-looking individuals begin to function abnormally, both academically and behaviorally.

The need for increased neuropsychological diagnostic workup and the cost-effectiveness of intervention aimed at secondary prevention with this single group alone would very probably justify the entire neuropsychological enterprise within the health care system and, indeed, warrant a substantial expansion of these activities.

Children who have suffered serious and acute medical disorders such as cerebral vascular accidents or who have undergone treatment for intracranial neoplasms are a small but nevertheless important population of children for whom ongoing neuropsychological monitoring is essential. The ability of these children to take up their normal set of social and academic activities can only be adequately judged through careful neuropsychological evaluation. No amount of conversational contact can provide an adequate appreciation of the child's cognitive structure and the changes it may have undergone.

Children with serious but not *currently* life-threatening neurological disorders (such as epilepsy, spina bifida, hydrocephalus, and the sequelae from a variety of significant cerebral trauma, anoxia, and infectious conditions) comprise yet another population (Sabatino & Cramblatt, 1969; Stevenson, Stone, Dillard, & Morgan, 1974). Competent neuropsychological evaluation provides the best means for assessing adequacy of outcome and quality of survival, specifically as these relate to the variety of requirements that children face in their day-to-day life. Changes in neurocognitive structure here, as elsewhere, are unlikely to be fully appreciated during standard medical interactions with the patients, or even in more careful but nevertheless incomplete evaluations performed by non–neuropsychologically trained child clinicians. There is a substantial difference between simply appreciating a pattern of strengths and weaknesses that characterizes a child's ability structure and appreciating the relationship of that pattern to the specific brain disorder in question. It is through that latter step that specific and useful evaluation of outcome, assessment of prognosis, and development of intervention strategies are most likely to emerge.

Children whose behavior suggests the possibility of decline in mental process are often referred for neuropsychological evaluation. It is not uncommon that such children have medical conditions that are not traditionally associated with neurology but that have, nevertheless, known neurological consequences. This represents a wide spectrum of medical disorders, including diabetes, a variety of childhood cancers, some forms of cardiac disease, muscular dystrophy, and burns (Ack, Miller, & Weil, 1961; Drash, 1971; Knights, Hinton, & Drader, 1973; Mohnot, Snead,

& Benton, 1982; Mulhern, Crisco, & Kun, 1983). This also includes a population of children who may not initially be recognized as having suffered central nervous system consequences from such causes as exposure to toxic substances and near drowning (Needleman et al., 1979; Saigal, Lunyk, Larke, & Shernesky, 1982).

Questions are often raised about such children when they are perceived as performing less well academically and developmentally than they did prior to their illness. These questions may also be formulated on the basis of performance of other family members, superficial facade of the child's intellectual competence, and inconsistent evidence of better ability. That this population may well be a subset of those individuals identified as having a learning disability is simply another way of saying that many factors contribute to inconsistent and less than genetically planned cognitive development in intellectual performance. It is not possible in every instance to demonstrate that the kinds of cognitive deficits present are specifically related to the etiologic agent under suspicion. It has been possible to demonstrate the presence of negative effects. It may be sufficient to gain a more complete appreciation of a child's overall cognitive strengths and weaknesses, and to monitor these during development. In other conditions, such as tumor and head injury, the knowledge of the natural history and of typical interventions allows for assessment of changes in mental status specifically tied to the patient's overall medical situation (Boll & Barth, 1981).

Children with or without questions of neurological or medical disorder who are doing less well in school than their apparent ability often benefit from neuropsychological evaluation as well. It is not uncommonly found that children whose basic IQ structure is relatively unremarkable will, in the course of a more comprehensive and demanding neurocognitive examination, reveal areas of cognitive irregularity that go specifically to the nature of the child's expressed academic problems. In fact, it has been through a series of systematic neuropsychological investigations that such clinical scientists as Satz and Morris (1981) and Rourke (1981) have postulated subtypes of learning disabilities that are characterized by different neurocognitive profiles. These lead to an understanding of the differential performance of students in their several subjects. These in turn lead to a more individualized intervention approach than would a less specific delineation of the child's overall cognitive structure.

NEUROPSYCHOLOGICAL EVALUATION

Neuropsychological evaluation has underlying it a different basis upon which behavior is understood. The traditional clinical child psychological assessment approaches patients from one or a number of theoretical points of view, integrates them where necessary, and comes to an understanding of a child's mental functions that is dependent to a greater or lesser extent on these understandings alone. It would be foolhardy to attempt to take on a clinical neuropsychological practice without recognizing that the patient who has behavioral problems due to (or even in addition to) neurological problems comes to the consultation room with a multifaceted personality. This personality includes a learning history, a background of interpersonal interactions, and a set of predisposing mental attitudes that will affect substantially his or her reaction to neurological impairment. The ability to cope with any deficits that are attendant to that impairment and the ability to participate in a helpful way in any intervention program depend on this background. The clinical neuropsychologist, however, brings an additional perspective on human behavior to the clinical situation. Neuropsychology assumes that the brain is the organ of the mind and the organ of human behavior. This is not in any sense a reductionist point of view. It is one that recognizes that the behavior an individual emits and the responses that one is likely to be able to elicit from him or her are determined to a substantial degree by the biological limits of that individual's brain function. An individual cannot learn in school, no matter how nonanxious and conflict free, how devoid of fears, hostility, and aggression, if her brain cannot absorb, organize, retain, and produce language and language-based concepts. A child, no matter how reinforced for reading, cannot accomplish this task if his brain cannot process perceptual stimuli sufficiently well to allow him to recognize one letter from another. A child, no matter how healthy her motivation, cannot perform adequately in school if her brain does not provide a sufficiently mature level of neurological control and inhibition to permit her to remain in an attentive state for an appropriate period of time.

Many factors impinge upon a child's ability to do anything. Ignoring any one of them is a perilous business. It is unfortunately true, however, that, in the field of clinical psychology and clinical child psychology as well, the role of the brain in behavior has been the one factor more likely ignored than any other. This discussion is designed not to downplay the significance of multiple factors, but rather to enhance the significance of one factor that has substantial impact, requires particular and special training to understand, and has far broader relevance than has commonly been recognized. This applies to individuals in whom the brain has been compromised and to individuals with normal brain functions.

Rutter (1977) has postulated a series of factors that describe very well the effect of brain impairment and its attendant consequences upon human behavior, in general terms. Rutter rejects a vulnerability model as failing to fit the mass of data that has been accumulated regarding the increased incidence of psychological difficulty in children with brain injury. Instead, he postulates an additive model, which does not require premorbid susceptibility within either the patient or the patient's environment. Thus his theory is applicable to patients who not only come from situations of risk and disadvantage but appear to sustain psychological disruption after brain injury, even though their premorbid histories suggest entirely adequate adjustment and support systems. Rutter identifies five aspects of brain injury that can be predicted to have a negative influence on the patient and the patient's overall psychological adjustment: (1) abnormal brain activity, which, when present, can clearly disrupt all aspects of psychological functioning; (2) cognitive deficits that are produced by brain damage, reducing general coping and specific capabilities; (3) direct effects, such as irritability and lowered frustration tolerance, common to brain damage, which appear to produce a direct personality change; (4) effects of treatments, including but not limited to hospitalization, medication regimes, the reduction in and restriction of physical and social activities, and change in appearance; and (5) responses of the environment itself to the brain-injured individual. This last aspect involves particularly the family, but clearly goes beyond that to include a variety of significant others who may experience anxiety and uncertainty and demonstrate both oversolicitousness and rejection due to their fear of doing the wrong things. This also includes long-standing stereotypes about what brain injury means, and what an individual with brain injury may be like. All of these are likely to be more unhelpful than helpful to the patient and, in fact, to his or her entire environmental situation.

Denial of injury (be it in the extreme form of refusing to admit that a limb is paralyzed or in the much more common form of denying the need for restrictions) may well be conceptualized in psychodynamic terms. Nevertheless, it is also the case that certain specific kinds of brain injury produce a recognizable syndrome of failure to recognize a variety of aspects of one's external and internal environment (Berent, 1986). Failure to recognize even familiar individuals (prospagnosia) and failure to identify either the nature or the severity of one's illness (agnosagnosia) can be present and can produce substantial disruptions in coping with the patient, even though these symptoms may be present in relatively mild form. Continuing efforts to teach such patients that they are in fact unable to do something are as ineffective (and counterproductive) as would be continuing attempts to convince receptive aphasics that they can really understand. It is critical to the entire diagnostic and treatment enterprise to know what it is that is being treated and understand its external manifestations. Without that knowledge, treatment modalities are established that ignore a substantial portion of what may be wrong. They therefore not only deny the patient appropriate treatment but also provide inappropriate and very likely harmful efforts to induce changes in behavior. This may well result in failure, frustration, and discouragement on the part of the patient and his or her support system. Certain kinds of brain injury have a well-known recovery curve, during which interventions have a specific timeliness, and this kind of misunderstanding can result in not just treatment delayed, but treatment denied.

The most frequent cause of changes in children's brain function is head injury. This neurological disorder has come to receive substantial attention recently for several reasons. One of these reasons is that head injury, along with all other forms of accidental injury, is the most common cause of death and disability during the childhood and early adult years. The behavioral consequences of head injury result from actual changes in brain function (Generelli, Adams, & Graham, 1985). Work on this condition provides an elegant model from which understandings of other previously ignored conditions producing subtle changes in brain integrity can be approached. It is now well understood that patients who have even relatively minor brain injuries that produce brief loss of consciousness and no obvious physical disability or abnormality on traditional neurological examination sustain actual neurological damage to areas of the brain not identified by traditional techniques. Moreover, these areas of neurological damage produce significant, predictable, and identifiable behavioral changes. These changes have a known recovery pattern and provide considerable explanation for the types of difficulties experienced by these patients, which heretofore have gone without understanding or have been subject to misunderstanding (Boll, 1984; Rimel, Giordani, Barth, Boll, & Jane, 1981).

CLINICAL NEUROPSYCHOLOGICAL ASSESSMENT OF CHILDREN

Clinical neuropsychological assessment of children is accomplished for reasons that can be differentiated from those for which children are referred for standard clinical child evaluation. The most common of these referral questions requires that neuropsychology address the potential connection between a specific neurological disorder and either a specific or a general problem in behavior. It is therefore for the neuropsychologist to be able to make explicit reference to the type of neurological damage involved, its location, and other aspects of its nature, as this may or may not be relatable to a particular pattern of behavioral deficit (Hale & Saxe, 1983). It is not sufficient to say that a child has had brain injury and the child has cognitive or behavioral deficits and therefore they must be associated. It is, instead, entirely necessary to know whether or not the particular deficits are in fact associated with the neurological syndrome or disorder. It may be that they are associated with some other preexisting or independent source of difficulty.

Oftentimes, careful investigation demonstrates that difficulties that appear to have been initiated by neurological insult were present, at least in lesser degree, prior to the neurological event. Such alleged changes as those involving a decline in school performance, increase in irritability, or failure of adequate behavior control, while recognizable as consequences of neurological injury, also occur in patients with no known neurological injury. Therefore, neuropsychologists must be sufficiently trained in general clinical skills to allow for investigation and identification of preexisting difficulties. These may continue to coexist independently or may be acted upon or exacerbated by the current neurological state of the patient (Seidel, Chadwick, & Rutter, 1975).

A similar referral question involves the possibility of consequences from a neurological event that have not yet become manifest. Many patients following head injury, tumors, vascular accidents, infections, and so forth appear psychologically normal to bedside examination. This examination is notoriously undemanding, as is the general environment of the hospital itself. Therefore, questions about the patient's ability to perform successfully in the more demanding environments of school, work, and home would not receive adequate answers. Many times, subtle deficits in memory structure, attentional mechanisms, or problem-solving capacity, while not apparent in many aspects of a child's or adult's environment, can produce critical mischief in just those areas of functioning that are most central to adequate life progress. Knowledge of these deficits, understanding of their association to the condition involved, and appropriate intervention are critical for adequate overall care. There is nothing more disheartening to parents and patient alike than to find that a child is suddenly performing poorly and to have no known explanation. Such changes are often attributed to emotionally based causes. Recognition is increasing that a broad variety of neurological and general medical disorders represent such conditions of risk for a child's neurocognitive apparatus (Boll, 1983; Golden, Strider, Ariel, & Golden, 1986). Such recognition provides the impetus necessary to request neuropsychological evaluation, which is the only proper way fully to address this potential problem.

The experience of cognitive change, no matter how temporary, produces its own reactions in the patient (Boll, 1981). The loss of ability to perform usual and accustomed tasks is enormously disconcerting. This is true whether those tasks are simple ones of daily living or those that require the highest cognitive skills. Loss of capacity to perform simple tasks obviously suggests a greater degree of severity of the overall sequelae. Loss of more complex mental capacity often produces a decrease in performance capacity in just those areas the patient has self-identified as critical to his or her existence. Such tasks include the capacity to perform well in complex academic situations or in situations that demand a substantial degree of social acuity dependent upon reasonable cognitive processes (such as attention, memory, and rapid processing of subtle information). After all vestiges of such deficits have disappeared, it may nonetheless take a substantial period of time and not infrequently some degree of formal reassurance to gain a level of confidence that characterized the patient prior to the illness (Boll & Barth, 1983). In many settings, confidence can be as big a part of success as actual mental capacity. Therefore, disability can persist even in the face of apparent return to full cognitive capability. Furthermore, it must be pointed out that, even when cognitive capacity has apparently returned (even when this apparent return is based on judgments from careful neuropsychological examination), a patient may still be vulnerable, on a neurological basis, to a cognitive decline in some conditions not well measured by the usual neuropsychological examination procedures. Ewing, McCarthy, Gronwall, and Wrightson (1980) followed students who had sustained brain injury and clear-cut cognitive impairment but who then recovered well enough successfully to pursue their academic curricula. Placed in a hyperbaric chamber with simulated altitude of 3800 feet, this relatively intact group of students demonstrated significant decline in mental capabilities. These changes exceeded those noted in matched colleagues who were not previously brain injured. More common challenges to higher central nervous capacity, such as fatigue, marked emotional stress, and substances with a depressing effect on the central nervous system, often produce disproportional decline in patients who may otherwise appear clinically normal.

It is not uncommon to find that, following a relatively mild neurological event, patients experience consequences that appear at first glance to be out of proportion to the severity of the disorder. For such patients, one explanation may be the presence of a previous neurological insult from which recovery was so good that neither the patient nor the other attending doctors were predisposed to make the connection. It was pointed out two decades ago that central nervous damage is, in fact, cumulative (Symmonds, 1962). It is also necessary to note here that patients over the age of 50 have a substantially less positive prognosis than do younger patients with the same injury, producing yet another opportunity for the occurrence of apparently disproportionate age–sequelae relationships (Boll, 1981).

Patients currently undergoing treatment of a variety of medical conditions, particularly when the treatments are in the experimental phase, are often provided routine neuropsychological monitoring. Childhood brain cancer treatment protocols not uncommonly include neurological surgery, multiple types of chemotherapy, and substantial amounts of radiation therapy. Clinically, it is important to know the child's outcome at any point in the treatment course (Mulhern et al., 1983). It is important to know whether the quality of this outcome is improving or deteriorating. It is also important to know the relationship between the quality of outcome and the specific treatment protocol, including type, dosage, relationship to other treatments, and stage of the disease course at initiation of the treatment. In most instances related to childhood cancers, for example, this continues to represent an area under scientific investigation and, therefore, one that requires the most careful and sophisticated scientific scrutiny by neuropsychologists who are prepared to undertake this demanding longitudinal type of research.

Children now survive conditions that produce multiple congenital abnormalities and go on to apparent developmental normality (Hallert & Astrom, 1983; Stevenson et al., 1974; Taren, 1967; Willerman, 1970). Such advances in medical survival raise questions about the possibility of subtle impairments that may express themselves later in life as learning or other difficulties. For such conditions, the question arises as to the need for a research effort to produce more effective interventions that will not simply allow the child to survive without serious sequelae, but will prevent more subtle behavioral disturbances from being a necessary part of their long-term development. A case in point is the lingering suspicion regarding the consequences of birth with congenital virus, such as cytomegalovirus (Saigal et al., 1982). It is, of course, necessary to determine whether or not the suspicion of increased incidence of neurocognitive difficulties is, in fact, correct. In a careful longitudinal study, Conboy was able to document that such patients in the main are not at risk, despite the common perception to the contrary (Conboy et al., 1987). Such findings not only serve as scientifically validated sources of reassurance, but also serve to eliminate the need for additional treatment protocols. Investigation of subpopulations found to carry the burden of risk previously thought to apply to all is now in order. Such subgroupings as primary versus acquired infections and those with hearing impairments that appear to carry a burden of risk not shared with the majority of children with congenital asymptomatic cytomegalovirus can now receive the focus of attention. As mentioned previously, it is important, in order to do this sort of evaluation, to know what the associations are between neurological consequences and their behavioral expressions.

Myths abound in this area. One common misconception is that children who sustain brain injury are likely to become hyperactive (Boll, 1983). Barkley (1981) has provided an excellent discussion of what is and what is not hyperactivity. He indicates that even the fundamental manifestations of this condition are often incorrectly understood. When considering etiology, it is important to note that the most common consequence following neurological impairment is no change in motor activity. The next most common consequence is hypoactivity, or reduced motor competence. A number of studies with neurologically impaired patients, including a population study of the Isle of Wight, found that hyperactivity following neurological impairment occurs in no more than 2 percent of patients studied. This may suggest that, even in those patients, hyperactivity preexisted the neurological illness (Rutter, 1977).

Many individuals with some neuropsychological knowledge, including school personnel, continue their concern with the relationship between Verbal–Performance inconsistencies on the Wechsler Intelligence Scale and lateralized brain injury. It has been documented that neurologically impaired children are more prone to have a statistically significant Verbal–Performance discrepancy than are non–neurologically impaired children. The fact is, however, that no relationship between presence or absence of lateralized brain impairment and/or side of lateralization and direction of Verbal–Performance split has been consistently developed (Black, 1974; Boll, 1981; Boll & Berent, 1977; Kohn & Dennis, 1974). The most common pattern for children with any sort of neurological impairment who have a Verbal–Performance split is for the Verbal IQ to be higher than the Performance IQ. This has been reported to occur in up to 85 percent of all instances of Verbal–Performance splits in children with lateralized, as well as generalized, neurological impairment (Boll & Berent, 1977). It should also be pointed out that the magnitude of Verbal–Performance split has in no instance been associated with an increasing likelihood of neurological impairment.

On the other side of the coin, experiments have shown that sensory and motor functions are closely associated with neurological sequelae (Reed & Reitan, 1969). While this may seem obvious, it is important for two reasons. First, it presents information, through behavioral signs, of neurological sequelae. Second, it provides an area of surprising association between simple psychological functions, such as speed and strength, and a variety of higher cognitive performance areas (Boll, 1971). It has also been demonstrated that relatively subtle tactile perceptual impairments (also associated with the presence of neurological dysfunction) are highly correlated with adequacy of development of more sophisticated psychological processes (Boll, Berent, & Richards, 1977; Boll, Richards, & Berent, 1978).

Because of the degree of variability that is associated with the normal developmental process, changes in the relative strength or weakness within a child's behavioral repertoire are quite normal. An initially slow talker may emerge as a "chatty Cathy." These fluctuations are often seen in the most complex tasks requiring simultaneous mental operations. Sensory and motor tasks, on the other hand, are less subject to this degree of developmental uncertainty. The ability of even the youngest child to recognize, or at least discriminate among, nonverbal tactile cues is quite stable, at least from age 4 or 5. Therefore, a pattern of tactile deficits has a high level of association with central nervous system functions and general intellectual and academic development (Boll, 1974a; Reitan, 1974). This is true for brain-impaired and also for normally developing non–brain-impaired children (Boll et al., 1977; Boll et al., 1978).

That these tasks, which are less sensitive to developmental and environmental factors, have such a strong association with psychological functions underscores the value of a clinical neuropsychological examination. Examples of such motor tasks are those measuring speed (finger oscillation, Reitan, 1974), strength (Boll, 1981), motor persistence (Joynt, Benton, & Fogel, 1962), coordination (grooved pegboard, Boll, 1981), tactile and kinesthetic learning capacity (Reitan, 1974), and unimanual and bimanual upper extremity coordination (marching test, Reitan, 1974). Examples of sensory perceptual measures include the ability to recognize parts of the body when touched (finger agnosia), the ability to recognize numbers or shapes when drawn on a part of the body (fingertip number writing perception, fingertip symbol writing perception), and the ability to recognize and/or identify geometric shapes when presented through the tactile modalities (tactile form recognition). These procedures have been demonstrated to have neurological and behavioral validity (Boll, 1974a; Reitan, 1970). Such measures have been found useful in discrimination between primary emotional difficulties and cognitive dysfunction caused by neurological disorders (Boll, 1974b). They have also been found to be useful in identification of a neurocognitive versus environmental etiology of intellective dysfunctions (Reitan & Boll, 1973).

It is not sufficient, however, to consider these tests as aids in increasing the associational capacity between potentially lateralizable higher cognitive functions such as language or perceptual tasks on the one hand and actual states of brain integrity on the other. Rather, it is important in itself to know the motor, tactile, and kinesthetic capacity of a child. Frequently, in situations of identified disorders of learning and development, multimodal interventions, such as purely motor learning tasks, kinesthetic activities (such as acting out the shapes of letters), and tactile stimuli (such as the use of sandpaper, sand, and other shapes and tactile features) are employed. These are intended to aid the child in developing associations to the particular symbols involved. Such programs will thrive or fail, depending on the child's relative strength or weakness in these often unevaluated areas. Supplementing a learning program with a set of activities pitched to a child's *areas of deficit* can be seen as a substantially different situation than one in which the child's learning program is supplemented by activities pitched to his or her *areas of strength*. A teacher who performs such remedial activities without knowledge of whether or not they are designed to provide the child an increasingly more understandable or an increasingly less understandable set of stimuli is likely to be at a serious disadvantage with regard to predicting the child's reactions and progress.

THE NEUROPSYCHOLOGICAL EXAMINATION

The neuropsychological examination is likely to be somewhat more comprehensive than the standard clinical child psychological examination. This does not imply that the neuropsychological examination of a child is going to be unduly lengthy or unpleasant in any way. Rather, it is more often the case that a complete neuropsychological examination, involving a broad coverage of higher and lower psychological functions, can be completed in half a day. Such activities, because they are one to one, rapidly moving, widely varied in the kinds of tasks demanded, and with an adult providing individual attention, are perceived by the child in highly favorable manner. It is common for parents to report that their usually taciturn adolescent talked more about the neuropsychological evaluation than any other topic in the last 2 years.

It is quite possible to select a battery of tests to tap such standard as well as nontraditional functions as intelligence, attention and concentration, language skills, learning across several modalities (including verbal and nonverbal), memory, motor and sensory skills, auditory, visual, and tactile perceptual capacity, mental speed, abstraction and reasoning skill, and specific fund of general and academic knowledge. It is also standard procedure to include measures of emotional functioning, which, with children, typically involve a clinical interview and some form of direct testing. This may involve projective techniques, inventory data, or data obtained from family members and/or significant others in the child's environment.

One reason for the comprehensive nature of neuropsychological testing is an appreciation of the fact that neurological disorders express themselves in no single pattern or array. It is quite possible for a neurological condition to allow many cognitive functions to be performed quite normally, while producing mild, or even serious, disruption to other mental activities. While it is possible to develop hypotheses about the likelihood of greatest area of impact of any particular type of neurological function, it is, in fact, the task of neuropsychology to test those hypotheses by the broadest possible investigation, rather than taking the easy way out and simply assuming that one's hypotheses are correct. It is the case that some conditions have been investigated sufficiently well that knowledge adequate to direct a neuropsychological examination is available. An individual with a left cerebral hemisphere vascular accident is far more likely to have substantial attention paid to language repertoire and relatively less to perceptual–spatial capacities. Individuals with relatively mild and minor head injury are unlikely to have severe motor or sensory deficits and, therefore, less attention need be paid to those areas. Conversely, they are much more likely to have subtle cognitive difficulties in the areas of mental speed, resilience, short-term memory functions, and complex mental processing. Therefore, additional attention to those types of activities is appropriate. It is common practice, then, in neuropsychology to utilize somewhat different types of procedures when approaching patients with different types of problems. It is equally common practice, however, to attempt, as far as possible, to include some amount of standardization within the overall examination activity. It would be extremely difficult to develop any increase in clinical competence if one never did the same thing twice, thereby providing no background of learning against which to make better judgments in the future.

The primary reason for doing a more rather than less comprehensive examination relates to the clinical value to the patient. It is important to know not only what the patient cannot do but also areas of the patient's strengths. Selective search for neurological pathology may be appropriate in a medical context. But selective search for cognitive pathology is not appropriate because of the rather different aims and goals of neuropsychology. The purpose of a neuropsychological evaluation is not simply to guess the patient's lesion, nor is it simply to document areas of the patient's cognitive deficit that are related to the lesion. In addition to that task, it is important to understand the patient's overall psychological situation, so that adequate intervention can be developed. Furthermore, a more complete understanding of the patient allows for adequate education of the patient and significant others as to the actual consequences of the disorder. Most patients following neurological disorder can and do function well in one or many areas. Ignoring those would present an unduly bleak and, even more important, unduly unhelpful picture of the patient's overall symptom picture.

A term such as *clinical validity* perhaps should be coined to reflect the degree of congruence between the neuropsychologist's understanding of the patient and the patient's perception of his or her situation. Absence of face validity can make it difficult for nonpsychologists to accept the value of tests that possess other more important but more difficult types of validities. So, too, absence of clinical validity can make it less likely that a patient will benefit from what may be a validated description of his or her condition, simply because it does not "ring true." Obviously, some patients are influenced in their perception of their condition by psychologically and neurologically based denial. Nevertheless, many patients can and do appreciate the kinds of difficulties they are having. These patients respond, sometimes with substantial improvement in their overall condition, to an adequate explanation of the relationship between their subjective difficulties and their actual neurocognitive situation. In fact, in many instances this type of educational intervention is the first therapeutic activity the patient will experience. Upon such intervention rests the capacity of the patient and significant others to alter activities of an educational, social, and other nature to correspond to the patient's actual capacities and disabilities. Appropriate recommendations for all forms of intervention require appreciation of what the patient can do. Therapeutic interventions cannot be well established if they are based exclusively on an understanding of the patient's deficits, with no information about those areas the patient can effectively utilize for competent performances.

A third reason for more rather than less comprehensive examination is the often-asked question about the relationship between the emotional and cognitive impact on overall psychological functioning. While it is often asked in an "either–or" fashion, it is the case that neurological impairment can produce significant primary and secondary disruption of both cognitive and affective mechanisms. It is true, particularly in children, that little specificity has been developed between type or location of neurological disorder and emotional reactions. It is the case, nevertheless, that children with neurological impairment are more likely to experience emotional disorders than are non–neurologically impaired children. They are, in fact, more likely to experience emotional impairment than are non–neurologically impaired but physically handicapped peers (Shaffer, 1974; Shaffer, Chadwick, & Rutter, 1975). The incidence of emotional disruption in children with neurological impairment has been rated as high as six times more frequent than that seen in normal children (Rutter, 1977). The nature of this deficit is nonspecific. The emotional disturbances of children with neurological impairment closely resemble emotional disturbances of primarily emotionally disordered children, and do not appear to be specific to any neurological or emotional syndrome (Ernhart, Graham, Eichman, Marshall, & Thurston 1962). Nevertheless, the interaction between cognitive deficits and emotional pathology, both of primary and of secondary nature, is sufficiently important that no neuropsychological evaluation can afford to ignore this area.

Utilization of multiple tests also provides increased opportunity for employment of multiple inferential methods for their interpretation. Most psychologists employ a *level of performance model*, based on normative data and developmental understanding of children, to determine whether a child has done as well as might be expected. This information can be exceptionally helpful in placing the child in an appropriate context for academic competition, or for making assessments about the appropriateness of special placement in gifted or handicapped programs. It has the singular advantage of being able to provide evidence about relative degrees of excellence. It is not limited to identification of presence or absence of pathology, as are most other ways of looking at patients. It is also true, however, that this method of inference creates many questions. It is not possible, from a level of performance evaluation of data alone, to determine whether a patient has been substantially better in the past. Nor can one tell whether the patient is in the middle of a recovery process from a more disabled point. It may be possible, on the basis of analysis of past academic, occupational, and other historical records, to make that judgment, but the data do not reveal that information precisely. Therefore, it is not possible to tell whether a patient is stable enough to begin a remedial program, or is likely to be substantially changed in the near future. One cannot be sure whether patients will have to content themselves with functioning in a manner considerably different than that they were accustomed to at some previous time. Obviously, the presence of a requirement for that kind of adjustment could represent a major emotional challenge that would suggest the need for psychological intervention. In order to determine the presence of this kind of a circumstance, additional methods of inference are required. A common second method of inference is *pattern of performance*. It is often possible, on the basis of analysis of relative strengths and weaknesses, to determine whether an individual has sustained some change in cognitive structure. Certain types of inconsistencies are often incompatible with adequate functioning, which may have characterized the patient at some previous time. Furthermore, use of pattern analysis allows for additional data points, through comparison of one test with each additional test. If tests are administered in a relatively standard fashion, these multiple data points can allow for correlations between various patterns and identifiable neurological and behavioral conditions.

A third method of inference is a *specific pathognomonic sign* of deficit. Certain behaviors, such as sensory suppressions, aphasic errors, and motor impairments, among others, are essentially incompatible with normal development and normal functioning. Mere identification of these does not give a very rich understanding of the patient's overall neuropsychological profile. They do provide, however, quite helpful information in the context of other neurocognitive deficits. This information, when connected with information from other inferential methods in the context of a complete neuropsychological evaluation, can be exceptionally helpful in appreciating the significance of the data derived elsewhere.

A fourth method of inference involves the comparison of the *functional efficiency* of the two sides of the body. Children even as young as 4 years of age have a relatively stable preference for one side of the body. This preference is manifest not only in unimanual choice but also in unimanual increase in competence. Speed, strength, and certain coordination tasks are performed better with the preferred rather than the nonpreferred hand. There is no evidence that motivation or emotional pathology influences this relationship. Therefore, absence of expected performance can, like information from specific pathognomonic sign, provide substantial understanding about the presence and nature of the child's neurocognitive pathology, which greatly adds to the interpretability of other developmental data obtained through level and pattern analysis.

Assessment of *performance over time* represents yet another important inferential strategy. Seeing patients during their recovery phase, with the initial evaluation begun at the earliest possible moment to establish an appropriate baseline, can be crucial in appreciating the actual deficit the patient has sustained. Seeing a patient initially 3 or 4 months after a head injury allows one less opportunity to appreciate the kinds of difficulties with which he or she may have had to cope. The attendant stresses that may have been present to produce secondary cognitive and emotional pathology are often missed. Early evaluation not only provides an important baseline against which to judge future recovery, but also provides the earliest possible opportunity to begin intervention. An understanding on the part of the patient and family members of the areas of deficit and strength, the kinds of behaviors to be expected, and the steps to take that would be most helpful is far more likely to prevent secondary sequelae than any known intervention strategy is to treat it effectively.

Yet another factor in dealing with the technical aspects of neuropsychological examination, one that goes beyond the areas of psychological coverage, is the nature of the actual test instruments. Test instruments, both of a standard clinical and of a specific neuropsychological nature, vary widely across a number of dimensions, and there are many tests from which to choose. Some considerations that might aid in test selection would be as follows: (1) the test's availability in alternative forms; (2) its objective scorability; (3) its portability; (4) its cost; (5) its ability to evaluate simultaneously a variety of integrated human abilities; (6) its ability to tap a single human ability, uncontaminated by requirements for other skills; (7) its adequacy of standardization; (8) its adequacy of validation; (9) its ability to assess both multiple materials and multiple modalities of psychological function; (10) its appropriateness to a specific or a broad age range; (11) its demonstrated reliability; (12) its appropriateness to the physical and/or emotional limitations of a patient (blindness, depression, paralysis); (13) its recognized use and acceptance in the field for the purposes intended; and (14) its applicability for group or computer-assisted administration. Such a list, although lengthy, is obviously not comprehensive, but rather is representative of the multiple sorts of considerations that are part of the development of any neuropsychological examination procedure.

The validity of neuropsychological evaluation must be established in a context rather more challenging even than that required for the validity of tests designed for use in psychiatric populations (Heaton, 1976). In addition to the substantial primary mental disruption (often seen in psychiatric as well as neurological patients), other factors specific to neurological disorder are commonly encountered. Such factors include significant physical debility, pain, use of multiple medications, anxiety related to preparations for surgery, disruptions in physical and mental function due to having just undergone surgery, mild to significant physical handicaps, and the life-threatening nature of many progressive neurological disorders. It is necessary for neuropsychological procedures to be a type that can be administered to patients with any or all of these difficulties. The data obtained must reflect more than the undifferentiated distress or dysfunction that these patients demonstrate. The tests must cut through that type of noise in the system and pick up the "signal." The signals in this case are the specific behavioral consequences of the neurological event in question, rather than the diffuse behavioral consequences of the condition of generalized illness or disability. That is has been possible to establish this kind of validity in children is well documented in multiple reviews (Boll, 1974, 1978, 1981; Reed, Reitan, & Klove, 1965; Reitan, 1974; Satz, 1966; Smith, 1975; Teuber & Rudel, 1962; Tsushima & Towne, 1977; Willerman, 1970). The precise relationship between site, size, and type of neurological function and behavioral deficit has not been worked out as well as it has in adults. Such information continues to be the focus of many ongoing research investigations. It is, nevertheless, true to say that substantial validity has been established for the neuropsychological enterprise with children for both frank neurological conditions (Boll, 1981) and conditions of a more neurodevelopmental sort (Boll, 1986; Kinsbourne, 1981; Wilson, 1986).

SCIENTIFIC VALIDITY OF NEUROCOGNITIVE AND NEUROPSYCHOLOGICAL TREATMENT

The scientific validity of neurocognitive and neuropsychological treatment has been subject to several reviews in the last several years (Barth & Boll, 1980; Diller & Gordon, 1980; Grimm & Bleiberg, 1986). The unfortunate situation is one of essential lack of validation of any form of program to improve the *speed* with which brain recovers or to improve the *degree* to which brain recovers. There is no question but that recovery following brain injury occurs. It would also appear to be the case that, without appropriate treatment, recovery can be interfered with by a variety of physical, cognitive, and emotional factors, which makes intervention activity of a variety of sorts important in any overall treatment program. Furthermore, it has now been documented that intervention aimed at prevention of sequelae following neurological impairment is most likely to be of help to the largest percentage of neurologically impaired children and adults (Barth et al., 1983; Rimel et al., 1981).

It is very often the case immediately following neurological injury that the patient (and even the family) is unaware of the nature of the difficulties or their extent. While he or she is recuperating in a hospital or rehabilitation facility the structure is sufficiently clear and the demands sufficiently limited that no real opportunity is provided for the patient to test his or her full range of behavioral operations. Therefore, it is often only after discharge that patient and family alike come face to face with the actual nature of the consequences of the patient's brain injury. If this confrontation occurs without preparation, misunderstandings are more commonly than not the result. These difficulties set into motion an increasing spiral of difficulties that are not actually part of but are intimately related to the original neurocognitive problem. On the other hand, when patients and family are well prepared, difficulties encountered, while still providing a source for stress, are far more manageable. Furthermore, difficulties that arise within the context of a well-informed and prepared situation are much more likely to be brought to the attention of the treating professional (Conboy, Barth, & Boll, 1987).

Teachers are ill prepared by their formal training programs to deal with children who sustain neurological impairment. In fact, they are ill prepared to know that, in most instances, neurologically impaired children are far more like than unlike normal children. This leads to failure to provide the appropriate care that the neurological condition demands. It also leads to treatment that is different from that of other children in circumstances where no differences are required. This failure of adequate treatment can easily be seen to produce mischief, over and above whatever difficulties the child may already experience due to his or her actual neurological and neurobehavioral impairments. Therefore, simply treating the environment to manage the child in an appropriate fashion often has a substantially ameliorating effect on the overall situation. This is so even though the actual neurobehavioral syndrome and its underlying cause have not been altered at all. Education of patient, family, and other important environmental agents is quite likely the most important psychological intervention that can be provided for the treatment of brain-injured children. The patient's dysfunction may become as related to the way his or her condition is handled as it is to the condition itself. This is obviously far more true in situations of mild cerebral impairments than in situations of devastating neurological damage and profound neurocognitive loss. It is true, however, that patients with mild neurological syndromes outnumber patients with severe neurological damage by more than a thousand to one. It is such patients who are most likely encountered on a day-to-day basis. These patients are encountered not only in situations where they are identified as neurologically impaired, but often in situations where their deficits go unexplained and therefore are mistreated for that reason as well. This mistreatment is not willful, but rather, is due to the lack of preparation of individuals in a variety of environmental contexts for dealing with neurological or behavioral impairments (Conboy et al., 1987).

Intervention following neuropsychological evaluation is probably more directly tied to the data than any other form of clinical psychological endeavor. This is initially true because the cognitive structure being evaluated is dependent upon a biological entity. Patients who are doing poorly in language functions due to impairment in brain-related structures can be led to an understanding of the relationship between their behavioral difficulties and the condition of their brain. This potential understanding is well within the grasp of individuals who make up the general patient population. Second, the intervention activities themselves are more specifically relatable to the area of deficit than is typically the case for most types of psychological interventions. Sometimes, because of this direct relationship, failure to comply results in predictable and undeniable consequences. These have the effect of alerting the clinician to the patient's or family's lack of compliance. They alert the patient or family to this lack of compliance as well (Conboy et al., 1987).

The course of neurological disorders, be they ones with a progressively worsening prognosis or ones with a known course of neurological and cognitive improvement, also allows for accurate predictions about behavioral changes. Furthermore, through use of subsequent neuropsychological evaluations, increasing refinements in interactions, and continued accurate predictions of future behavioral developments, appropriate adjustments are indicated in the intervention program to fit the current status of the patient. Such a known course also allows for the kind of predictive descriptions to be provided to patient and family. This, in turn, allows them to understand and adjust to the altered requirements of a changing central nervous system. Such changes, even positive ones, may still represent a burden. Special education school facilities are aimed at a category of children who are not characterized by substantial change in their condition over the course of several months or even a year, in most instances. Children with rapidly resolving neurological dysfunctions, such as that often produced following anoxia, toxic exposure, infections, and head injury, may well require the services of a variety of special education experts. These experts, however, must be aided to realize that the child's learning capacities today may be dramatically different than those that will characterize him or her in 2 weeks or 2 months. Therefore, simply categorization as "learning disabled" or "mildly retarded" for placement in a class for such children may be appropriate for a very brief period of time, but may soon require adjustment and alteration. It is not uncommon to begin intervention with homebound instruction and, at a later date, combine this with a gradual return to school. These may go on simultaneously until an appropriate level of stability of in-class performance has been achieved. It is necessary to determine that the child will, in fact, be able to manage over a reasonable period of time in a single setting. Often, then, the neuropsychologist must have substantial understanding of and willingness to interact with school personnel, school policies, and educational issues. This is necessary to be perceived as helpful and to provide information that is likely to pertain to the child's academic situation. The specifics of the intervention program may be placed in the hands of the rehabilitation expert or the special educator. The structure of the patient's intellect, as this relates to his or her ability to learn, solve problems, attend, concentrate, organize material, process information, utilize knowledge already obtained, manage perceptual stimuli, and express and comprehend the cognitive as well as the emotional content of communication, is the province of the neuropsychologist. Continued consultation with the school, including periodic reexaminations of the child, represents a frequent and effective type of neuropsychological intervention for individuals with mild and moderate neurocognitive impairments.

The fact that neuropsychologists deal with medical populations, medical personnel, and medical conditions presents a specific challenge with regard to the nature of their training, which differs identifiably from the training of a non–medically oriented clinical psychologist (Costa, Matarazzo, & Bornstein, 1986). The validity demands and the issues of technical composition of the neuropsychological examination itself, while sufficiently well developed to allow for a recognizable "state of the art" in clinical child neuropsychology, nevertheless continue to be in a state of flux (Boll, 1978, 1981; Matthews, Shaw, & Klove, 1966; Reitan, 1974). Recognition of medical disorders with neurological correlates, the ability of medical science to allow children to survive with neurologically impairing conditions, and the increased interest in the rehabilitation of neurologically impaired patients and the prevention of neurological disorders or their sequelae all represent continuing frontier issues demanding increased research and clinical sophistication on the part of the field of neuropsychology (Boll, 1986). The impact that this clinical field has already had on quasi-neurological disorders of learning and development testifies to the high demand for immediate application of even the most current research in this field (Rourke, 1981; Wilson, 1986). The extremely high interest on the part of a multitude of employers in obtaining the services of a well-trained clinical neuropsychologist is in considerable contrast to the currently extremely limited availability of such individuals, further putting a premium of attractiveness on the field as a whole, both for those currently engaged and those considering career choices (Costa et al., 1986). New developments, such as positron emission tomography and magnetic resonance imaging, suggest at least one area in which future advances, with regard to criterion data for improved understanding of brain behavior relationships, are likely to emerge. The confluence of increased quality of criteria, lowered threshold for the recognition of neurological sequelae in neurological and nonneurological disorders, the increase in survivability of patients with "at-risk" conditions, and the great availability of research opportunities in this relatively new field mark neuropsychology as a growth area in both the science and the profession of psychology throughout the end of this century.

References

Ack, M., Miller, I., & Weil, W. B. (1961). Intelligence of children with diabetes melitus. *Pediatrics, 28*, 764–770.

Barkley, R. B. (1981). Hyperactive children. New York: Guilford.

Barth, J., & Boll, T. J. (1981). Rehabilitation and treatment of central nervous dysfunctions: A behavioral medicine perspective. In L. A. Bradley & C. Prokop (Eds.), *Medical psychology: A new perspective*. New York: Academic.

Barth, J. T., Macciocchi, S., Giordani, B., Rimel, R., Jane, J., & Boll, T. J. (1983). Neuropsychological sequelae of minor head injury. *Neurosurgery, 13*, 529–532.

Berent, S. (1986). Psychopathology and other behavioral considerations for the clinical neuropsychologist. In S. B. Filskov & T. J. Boll (Eds.), *Handbook of clinical neuropsychology* (Vol. 2). New York: Wiley.

Black, P., Shepard, R. H., & Walker, A. E. (1975). Outcome of head trauma: Age and post-traumatic seizures. In R. Porter & D. Fitzsimmons (Eds.), *Outcome of severe damage to the central nervous system* (CIBA Foundation Symposium). Amsterdam: Elsevier.

Black, F. W. (1974). Patterns of cognitive impairment in children with suspected and documented neurological dysfunction. *Perceptual & Motor Skills, 39*, 115–120.

Boll, T. J. (1971). Correlation of WISC with motor speed and strength for brain-damaged and normal children. *Journal of Psychology, 77*, 169–172.

Boll, T. J. (1974a). Behavioral correlates of cerebral damage in children aged nine–fourteen. In R. N. Reitan & L. A. Davison (Eds.), *Clinical neuropsychology: Current status and applications*. Washington, DC: V. H. Winston.

Boll, T. J. (1974b). Psychological differentiation of patients with schizophrenia versus lateralized cerebral vascular, neoplastic or traumatic brain damage. *Journal of Abnormal Psychology, 83*, 456–458.

Boll, T. J. (1978). Diagnosing brain impairment. In B. Wolman (Ed.), *Diagnosis of mental disorders: A handbook*. New York: Plenum.

Boll, T. J. (1981). The Halstead-Reitan neuropsychology battery. In S. B. Filskov & T. J. Boll (Eds.), *Handbook of clinical neuropsychology*. New York: Wiley.

Boll, T. J. (1983). Neuropsychological assessment of the child: Myths, current status and future prospects. In C. E. Walker & M. C. Roberts (Eds.), *Handbook of clinical child psychology*. New York: Wiley.

Boll, T. J. (1983). Minor head trauma in children: Out of sight but not of mind. *Journal of Clinical Child Psychology, 12*, 74–80.

Boll, T. J. (1984). Psychological consequences of head injury in children. In R. Glow (Ed.), *Advances in the behavioral measurement of children*. Greenwich, CT: JAI.

Boll, T. J. (1984). Pediatric neuropsychological assessment. In P. McGrab (Ed.), *Psychological and behavioral assessment: Impact on pediatric care*. New York: Plenum.

Boll, T. J. (1986). Nontraditional and threshold considerations in neuropsychological assessment. In S. B. Filskov & T. J. Boll (Eds.), *Handbook of clinical neuropsychology* (Vol. 2). New York: Wiley.

Boll, T. J., Berent, S., & Richards, H. (1977). Tactile–perceptual functioning as a factor in general psychological abilities. *Perceptual & Motor Skills, 44*, 535–539.

Boll, T. J., Richards, H., & Berent, S. (1978). Tactile–perceptual functioning in academic performance in brain-impaired and unimpaired children. *Perceptual & Motor Skills, 47*, 491–495.

Boll, T. J., & Barth, J. (1981). Neuropsychology of brain damage in children. In S. B. Filskov & T. J. Boll (Eds.), *Handbook of clinical neuropsychology*. New York: Wiley.

Boll, T. J., & Barth, J. (1983). Mild head injury. *Psychiatric Developments, 3*, 263–275.

Conboy, T. J., Barth, J. T., & Boll, T. J. (1987). Treatment and rehabilitation of mild and minor head injury. *Rehabilitation Psychology, 31*, 203–215.

Conboy, T. J., Pass, R. F., Stagno, S., Britt, W. J., Alford, C. A., McFarland, C. E., & Boll, T. J. (in press). Intellectual development in school-aged children with asymptomatic congenital cytomegalovirus infection. *Pediatrics*.

Costa, L. D., Matarazzo, J. D., & Bornstein, R. A. (1986). Issues in graduate and post-graduate training in clinical neuropsychology. In S. B. Filskov & T. J. Boll (Eds.), *Handbook of clinical neuropsychology* (Vol. 2). New York: Wiley.

Diller, L., & Gordon, W. A. (1981). Rehabilitation and clinical neuropsychology. In S. Filskov & T. J. Boll (Eds.), *Handbook of clinical neuropsychology*. New York: Wiley.

Drash, A. (1971). Diabetes melitus in childhood: A review. *Journal of Pediatrics, 78*, 919.

Ernhart, C. B., Graham, F. K., Eichman, P. L., Marshall, J. M., & Thurston, D. (1962). Brain injury in the pre-school child: Some developmental consideration: II. Comparison of brain-injured and normal children. *Psychological Monographs, 574*, 17–33.

Ewing, R., McCarthy, D., Gronwall, D., & Wrightson, P. (1980). Persisting effects of minor head injury observable during hypoxic stress. *Journal of Clinical Neuropsychology, 2*, 147–155.

Generelli, T. A., Adams, G. H., & Graham, D. I. (1985). Acceleration-induced head injury in the monkey: The model, its mechanical and physiological correlate. *Acta Neuropathologica* (Supplement).

Golden, C. J., Strider, N. A., Ariel, R., & Golden, E. E. (1986). Neuropsychology and medical disorders. In S. B. Filskov & T. J. Boll (Eds.), *Handbook of clinical neuropsychology* (Vol. 2). New York: Wiley.

Graham, F. K., Ernhart, C. B., Thurston, D., & Craft, M. (1962). Development three years after perinatal anoxia and other potentially damaging newborn experiences. *Psychological Monographs* (No. 76, p. 522).

Graham, P., Rutter, M. L., Yule, W., & Pless, I. B. (1967). Childhood asthma: A psychosomatic disorder question mark. Some epidemiological considerations. *British Journal of Preventive & Social Medicine, 21*, 78–85.

Grimm, B. H., & Bleiberg, J. (1986). Psychological rehabilitation in traumatic brain injury. In S. B. Filskov & T. J. Boll (Eds.), *Handbook of clinical neuropsychology* (Vol. 2). New York: Wiley.

Gronwall, D., & Wrightson, P. (1975). Cumulative effects of concussion. *Lancet, 2*, 995–997.

Hale, R. L., & Saxe, J. E. (1983). Profile analyses of the Wechsler Intelligence Scale for Children-Revised. *Journal of Psychoeducational Assessment, 1*, 155–162.

Hallert, C., & Astrom, J. (1983). Intellectual ability of adults after life-long intestinal malabsorption due to celiac disease. *Journal of Neurology, Neurosurgery & Psychiatry, 46,* 87–89.

Joynt, R. L., Benton, A. L., & Fogel, M. L. (1962). Behavioral and pathological correlates of motor impersistance. *Neurology, 12,* 876–881.

Kinsbourne, M. (1981). The development of cerebral dominance. In S. Filskov & T. J. Boll (Eds.), *Handbook of clinical neuropsychology* (Vol. 1). New York: Wiley.

Klonoff, H., Low, M. D., & Clark, C. (1977). Head injuries in children: A prospective five-year follow-up. *Journal of Neurology, Neurosurgery, & Psychiatry, 40,* 1211–1219.

Knights, R. M., Hinton, G. G., & Drader, D. (1973). Changes in intellectual ability with Duchene muscular dystrophy. *Research Bulletin No. 8.* Department of Psychology, Carleton University, Ottawa, Canada.

Kohn, B., & Dennis, M. (1974). Patterns of hemispheric specializations after hemidecortication for infantile hemiplegic. In M. Kinsbourne & W. L. Smith (Eds.), *Hemispheric disconnection in cerebral function.* Springfield, IL: Charles C. Thomas.

Matthews, C. G., Shaw, D. J., & Klove, H. (1966). Psychological test performances in "pseudoneurologic" subjects. *Cortex, 11,* 244–253.

Mohnot, D., Snead, O. C., & Benton, J. W. (1982). Burn encephalopathy in children. *Annals of Neurology, 12,* 42–47.

Mulhern, R. K., Crisco, J. J., & Kun, L. E. (1983). Neuropsychological sequelae of childhood brain tumors: A review. *Journal of Clinical Child Psychology, 12,* 66–73.

Needleman, H. L., Gunnoe, C., Leviton, A., Reed, R., Peresie, H., Maher, C., & Barrett, P. (1979). Deficits in psychologic and classroom performance of children with elevated dentine lead levels. *New England Journal of Medicine, 300,* 689–695.

O'Leary, D., & Boll, T. J. (1984). Neuropsychological correlates of early generalized brain dysfunction in children. In R. C. Almli & S. Finger (Eds.), *Early brain damage: Volume 1. Research orientations and clinical observations.* New York: Academic.

Reed, J. C., & Reitan, R. M. (1969). Verbal and Performance differences among brain-injured children with lateralized motor deficits. *Perceptual & Motor Skills, 29,* 747–752.

Reed, H. B. C., Reitan, R. M., & Klove, H. (1965). Influence of cerebral lesions and psychological test performance in older children. *Journal of Consulting Psychology, 29,* 247–251.

Reitan, R. M. (1974). Methodological problems in clinical neuropsychology. In R. M. Reitan & L. Davison (Eds.), *Clinical neuropsychology: Current status and application.* Washington, DC: V. H. Winston.

Reitan, R. M., & Boll, T. J. (1973). Neuropsychological correlates of minimal brain dysfunction. *Annals of the New York Academy of Science, 205,* 65–88.

Reitan, R. M. (1964). Psychological deficits resulting from cerebral lesions in man. In J. N. Warren & K. Akert (Eds.), *The frontal granular cortex in behavior.* New York: McGraw-Hill.

Reitan, R. M. (1970). Sensory motor functions, intelligence and cognition and emotional status in subjects with cerebral lesions. *Perceptual & Motor Skills, 31,* 275–284.

Reitan, R. M. (1974). Psychological effects of cerebral lesions in children in early school age. In R. M. Reitan & L. A. Davison (Eds.), *Clinical neuropsychology: Current status and applications.* Washington, DC: V. H. Winston.

Rimel, R. W., Giordani, B., Barth, J. T., Boll, T. J., & Jane, J. A. (1981). Disability caused by minor head injury. *Neurosurgery, 9,* 221–228.

Rourke, B. T. (1975). Brain–behavior relationships in children with learning disabilities. *American Psychologist, 30,* 911–920.

Rourke, B. T. (1976). Issues in the neuropsychological assessment of children with learning disabilities. *Canadian Psychological Review, 17,* 89–102.

Rourke, B. T. (1981). Neuropsychological assessment of children with learning disabilities. In S. Filskov & T. J. Boll (Eds.), *Handbook of clinical neuropsychology.* New York: Wiley.

Rourke, B. T., & Orr, R. R. (1977). Prediction of the reading and spelling performances of normal and retarded readers: A four-year follow-up. *Journal of Abnormal Child Psychology, 5,* 9–10.

Rutter, M. (1977). Brain damage syndromes in childhood: Concepts and findings. *Journal of Clinical*

Childhood Psychology & Psychiatry, 18, 1–21.

Rutter, M., Graham, P., & Yule, W. (1970). A neuropsychiatric study in childhood. *Clinics in Developmental Medicine* (Nos. 35 & 36). London: Simp/Seiman.

Sabatino, D. A., & Cramblatt, H. (1969). A longitudinal study of children with learning disabilities subsequent to hospitalization for viral encephalitis. II. *Journal of Learning Disabilities, 2,* 124–135.

Saigal, S., Lunyk, O., Larke, R. P. B., & Shernesky, N. A. (1982). The outcome of children with cytomegalovirus infection. *American Journal of Diseases of Childhood, 136,* 896–905.

Satz, P. (1966). Specific and non-specific effects of brain lesions in man. *Journal of Abnormal Psychology, 71,* 65–70.

Satz, P., & Morris, R. (1981). Learning disabilities subtypes: A review. In F. J. Pirozzolo & M. C. Wittrock (Eds.), *Neuropsychological and cognitive processes in reading.* New York: Academic.

Seidel, U. P., Chadwick, O. D., & Rutter, M. (1975). Psychological disorders in crippled children. A comparative study of children with and without brain damage. *Developmental Medicine & Child Neurology, 17,* 563–573.

Selz, M., & Reitan, R. M. (1979). Neuropsychological test performance of normal, learning-disabled and brain-damaged older children. *Journal of Nervous & Mental Disease, 167,* 298–302.

Shaffer, D., Chadwick, O., & Rutter, M. (1975). Psychiatric outcome of localized head injury in children. In R. Porter & D. Fitzsimmons (Eds.), *Outcome of severe damage to central nervous system* (CIBA Foundation Symposium 34). Amsterdam: Elsevier.

Shaffer, D. (1974). Psychiatric aspects of brain injury in childhood: A review. In S. Chess & A. Thomas (Eds.), *Annual progress in child psychiatry and child development.* New York: Brunner/Mazel.

Smith, A. (1975). Neuropsychological testing in neurological disorders. In W. J. Friedlander (Ed.), *Advances in neurology* (Vol. 7). New York: Raven.

Stevenson, J. G., Stone, E. F., Dillard, D. H., & Morgan, B. C. (1974). Intellectual development of children subjected to prolonged circulatory arrest during hypothermic open heart surgery in infancy. *Circulation, 50,* 54–59.

Swift, C. R., Seidman, F., & Stein, H. (1967). Adjustment problems in juvenile diabetes. *Psychosomatic Medicine, 20,* 555–571.

Symmonds, C. (1962). Concussion and its sequelae. *Lancet, 1,* 1–5.

Taren, L. M. (1967). Problems in management of rheumatic disease in children. In L. M. Taren (Ed.), *Collected works on rheumatic fever.* New York: International Professional Publications.

Teuber, H.-L., & Rudel, R. G. (1962). Behavior after cerebral lesions in children and adults. *Developmental Medicine & Child Neurology, 4,* 3–20.

Tsushima, W. T., & Towne, W. S. (1977). Neuropsychological abilities of young children with questionable brain disorders. *Journal of Consulting & Clinical Psychology, 45,* 757–762.

Tymchuck, A. J., Knights, R. M., & Hinton, G. C. (1970). Neuropsychological test results of children with brain lesions, abnormal EEGs and normal EEGs. *Canadian Journal of Behavioral Science, 2,* 322–329.

Willerman, L. (1970). Fetal head position during delivery and intelligence. In C. R. Angel & E. A. Bering (Eds.), *Physical trauma as an etiological agent in mental retardation.* Bethesda: National Institute of Neurological Diseases and Stroke.

Wilson, B. C. (1986). An approach to the neuropsychological assessment of the preschool child with developmental deficits. In S. B. Filskov & T. J. Boll (Eds.), *Handbook of clinical neuropsychology* (Vol. 2). New York: Wiley.

7

Assessment of Children's Temperament

RONALD SEIFER

The assessment of temperament in children has become increasingly popular in basic and applied research settings, and to a lesser extent in applied clinical settings. Early studies were explicitly designed to determine causal links between manifestations of individual differences in temperament and subsequent problems in adjustment. The material that follows will examine the utility of current constructs of temperament (and associated measurement instruments) in the context of a variety of applied settings. This will include discussion of various definitions of temperament, methods of measurement, adequacy of these measurement techniques, the costs and benefits of obtaining such information, and the place of temperament in a larger clinical picture. In addition, a theoretical perspective that defines temperament in the context of overall family systems will be presented.

HISTORY AND DEFINITIONS

Less than 30 years ago, Thomas and Chess (Thomas, Chess, Birch, Hertzig, & Korn, 1963) began their New York Longitudinal Study (NYLS) of temperament in infants who have subsequently been followed into young adulthood (see also Chess & Thomas, 1984; Thomas & Chess, 1977; Thomas, Chess, & Birch, 1968). This study has been most influential because it popularized the long dormant construct of *temperamental individuality* and extended the idea downward to apply to infants and children. Since that time, temperament has become a basic consideration of researchers and clinicians who work with varied childhood populations.

Thomas and Chess, from the start of their research program, have discussed temperament both as a specific content area and as an illustration of more general developmental processes. They defined the specific area as the *behavioral style* of an individual across the range of contexts he or she might encounter. They refer to temperament as the *how* of behavior, in contrast to ability and motivation constructs (the *what*, *why*, or *how well* of specific behaviors). In terms of developmental processes, Thomas and Chess emphasize that children make an active contribution to their own development as opposed to existing as passive receptors of their social context, that there is a dynamic interaction between individual child constitution and parent behaviors, and that the *goodness of fit* between parents and children is a major determinant of the child's developmental outcome.

This type of formulation of individual temperament has many clear implications. First, it is assumed that individuals exhibit substantial stability in how they behave across different settings. This is the fundamental assumption of temperament: that there is a behavioral style that describes each individual in all or most situations. A second implication from the Thomas and Chess approach is that this behavioral style has stability over time. The final implication of importance is that individual differences and contexts must be clearly and consistently specified.

It may already be apparent that Thomas and Chess have laid the groundwork for a theory of behavior that may be incorporated into a traditional behavior genetics perspective, as evidenced by constitutional individual differences that endure over place and time. Thomas and Chess, however, make no strong claims for intergenerational transmission of temperamental characteristics via genetic material, although others have strongly followed this path. For example, Buss and Plomin (1975, 1984) explicitly define temperament as the *inherited component of personality*, and have devoted most of their research efforts to demonstrating this single point.

A prominent theoretical perspective on temperament that does not incorporate the construct of behavioral style has been advanced by Rothbart (1981; Rothbart & Derryberry, 1981, 1982). She rejects the notion of style as being inherently vague, resulting in overgeneralization of temperament characteristics (see also Sroufe & Waters, 1977). Rothbart proposes that temperament be viewed as a *behavioral manifestation of more microscopic processes* such as arousal level or perceptual speed.

Despite differences in theoretical perspectives, questionnaire instruments designed to measure temperament in children exhibit remarkable similarity. All attempt to gather information from parents or other informants about the way that children usually behave in a variety of contexts. The specific classes of behavior include emotional expression, activity level, responses to people, intensity of responses, and reaction to novel events. Where the instruments differ is in their approach to obtaining this information, which may be more or less behaviorally specific (as opposed to asking informants to make broad generalizations), or in the degree of detail in which context and time frame are specified in individual items (Bates, Freeland, & Lounsbury, 1979; Carey & McDevitt, 1978; Fullard, McDevitt, & Carey, 1978; Goldsmith & Campos, 1982; Rothbart, 1981; Seifer & Sameroff, in press).

Characteristics of Specific Temperament Instruments

In this section I will describe features of specific instruments in order to provide a flavor of the options available for use in applied settings. However, this summary is designed not to be exhaustive, but merely to highlight some differences among the most popular sets of instruments. The emphasis is on the most prominent families of instruments that have relied on parent reports, because these are most likely to be employed in applied settings, and because they have had the most extensive use and psychometric scrutiny.

Carey Temperament Questionnaires. Perhaps the most widely used instruments are those developed by Carey and associates for use with infants (Carey & McDevitt, 1978), toddlers (Fullard et al., 1978), and children 3 to 7 (McDevitt & Carey, 1975). These instruments share in common the use of nine scales that were originally developed during the NYLS by Thomas and Chess: Activity, Rhythmicity, Approach Adaptability, Intensity of Behavior, Mood, Persistence, Distractibility (which changes from Soothability in infants to Level of Attention to Background Stimuli in older children), and Threshold to Stimulation. Indivudal items are scored by parents on 6-point scales that range from *almost never* to *almost always*. Each individual item describes a behavior (sometimes very specific, sometimes a more general class) and a style of response associated with that behavior, for example, "The infant accepts new foods right away, swallowing them promptly." The individual items do *not* specify specific time frames, specific contexts (the implicit context in most questions is the home), or detailed descriptions of behavior. The questionnaires contain between 95 and 100 items each.

Bates Characteristics Questionnaires. Bates and colleagues have developed a series of temperament instruments designed for use with children 6 months to 2 years of age Bates & Bayles, 1984; Bates et al., 1979; Lee & Bates, 1985). Unlike the Carey instruments and others based on the NYLS approach, the Bates instruments do not have the same set of scales at each assessment period. The main consistent scale at all three ages is Infant Difficulty. There is also some degree of overlap on scales for Unadaptable (to events and people) and Dull—Unexcitable. Other scales measure Regularity (6, 24 months), Persistence (13 months), and Non-Cuddly/Unstoppable (24 months). Most individual items require parents to make generalizations about specific classes of behavior, for example, "How well does your baby typically respond to being in a new place?" The response scale is different for each item but in all cases has 7 points that range from positive to negative types of response: for example, *very easy* to *difficult*; or *a great deal, really loves it* to *very little, doesn't like it much*. Some items on the scales specify detailed descriptions of behavior, response sets in counts of individual behavior, or detailed description of context, but most items are of a more general nature. The instruments contain between 24 and 32 items at the different ages.

Buss and Plomin's EAS. Buss and Plomin (1975, 1984) developed a set of instruments to be used as a self-report (adults), teacher-report, or parent-report measure from infancy to adulthood. The EAS acronym refers to the three scales on the instruments: Emotionality, Activity, and Sociability. The items are very general in nature, with little reference to specific of behavior, context, or time frame, for example, "Child is very sociable." All require broad generalizations to be made by the informant. The items for the parent- and teacher-report instruments are scored on a 5-point scale that ranges from *not characteristic or typical of your child* to *very characteristic or typical of your child*. For the adults, the scale is the same with the referent being *you*. Each instrument has 20 items, with a great deal of overlap in the two child instruments.

Rothbart Behavior Questionnaire. Rothbart (1981) developed a parent-report scale to assess temperament in children during the first year of life. Scales include Activity Level, Smiling and Laughter, Fear, Distress to Limitations, Soothability, and Duration of Orienting. Of all the parent-report measures, this is the most behaviorally specific, and the one that most clearly specifies context and time frame, for example, "During the last week, how often did the baby protest being put in a confining place (infant seat, play pen, car seat, etc.?" The items are scored by the parent on a 7-point scale of frequency ranging from *never* to *always*. The instrument contains 87 items.

Lerner's Dimensions of Temperament. Another set of instruments that are based on the NYLS are the Dimensions of Temperament Surveys (DOTS), which have both parent-report and self-report versions (Lerner, Palermo, Spiro, & Nesselroade, 1982). The instruments were developed to cover the age range from preschool through college. The five scales on the instruments are Activity Level, Attention Span/Distractibility, Adaptability/Approach, Rhythmicity, and Reactivity. The first four scales have labels (or combinations) that correspond with the NYLS; the fifth scale contains items related to NYLS dimensions of Activity, Intensity, and Threshold. The response scale on all instruments is *true* versus *false*. The three instruments (child [parent-report], child [self-report], adult [self-report]) all contain the same 34 items.

Similarities and Differences among Instruments. As noted earlier all of the instruments summarized here are parent-report measures (although some have self-report versions), so in that respect they have at least one common feature. A second common feature is that all require generalizations about children's behavior over a time period, although that time frame is almost always unspecified; terms such as "usually" or "during feeding" are characteristic of the instruments rather than an emphasis on "during the past 24 hours" or "in the previous month." A third similarity is that they share some core constructs across the different scales. For example, activity, adaptability to people and events, and quality of affect show up in one form or another on most of the instruments.

A property of the set of instruments and the field of inquiry that they represent is that they are focused more on the younger age range of children (infancy and early childhood). This probably stems from the fact that the first several reports of the NYLS were from these early age periods, and others attempting to replicate and follow up on their work chose the age range that was in existing studies.

Despite these similarities in their approach to the problem of measuring individual differences in temperament, there are definite differences in the instruments that would influence one's choice regarding their use in a specific setting. The most obvious differences are the size of the instruments and the age groups to which they apply. The shortest instrument is the Buss and Plomin EAS, which contains 20 multiple-choice items, compared with the Carey instruments, which contain up to 100 items. In general (although there is certainly not a one-to-one correspondence) the tradeoff in using shorter instruments is in decreased behavioral, contextual, and time-frame specificity. However, there is no clear evidence that the instruments with more specific items are necessarily better measures of temperament than others. With respect to age appropriateness, there is only one family of instruments that is designed to be used from infancy through adulthood—the Buss and Plomin EAS. The DOTS instruments of Lerner and colleagues also have a wide age range, but they cannot be used with infants. Note that these sets of instruments are both relatively small in terms of the item set size and the number of temperament dimensions measured.

A less obvious difference in the instruments involves whether they hypothesize a single set versus multiple sets of temperament dimensions over their specified time frame. For example, the Carey instruments were specifically developed to measure the nine temperament dimensions that were defined by the NYLS investigators, and as a result they have, by definition, the same set of scales in every form. The DOTS, which is also derived from the NYLS framework, determined at the outset that all forms of the instrument would have the same set of scales (although the scales do not exactly match the NYLS framework). In addition, both Buss and Plomin's EAS and Rothbart's IBQ have the same set of scales at each age. The exception to this pattern is the Bates ICQ instruments, which vary from form to form on the scales included. However, there is still a large conceptual overlap in the various versions.

A final difference that should be noted is that all of the instruments, with the exception of the Carey questionnaires, were developed primarily for research purposes. Even the Carey instruments, however, while originally used and standardized in a pediatric practice, have not undergone careful development within diverse clinical populations.

MEASUREMENT CHARACTERISTICS OF TEMPERAMENT INSTRUMENTS

An important consideration in deciding whether to use a specific instrument is the degree to which is has been demonstrated to measure what it claims to measure, as well as the consistency of those measurements across time and across individuals. In the case of all temperament instruments this is a nontrivial issue that is currently under much debate.

Utility of Parent Reports

The first major issue with temperament instruments is their primary reliance on parental report. Although there are some measures that employ direct observation of individuals (e.g., Rothbart & Goldsmith, 1985), these are more appropriate for basic research applications in the laboratory than for use in applied clinical settings. The most heated controversy is whether parent reports of their children's temperaments reflect more the concerns of the parents or the behavior of the children. Those questioning the validity of parent reports have noted that measures of parental anxiety, beliefs about children in general, prenatal conceptions of their own child, or social status explain more variance in temperament measures than do observations of actual child behavior (Bates et al., 1979; Daniels, Plomin, & Greenhalgh, 1984; deVries & Sameroff, 1984; Sameroff, Seifer, & Elias, 1982; Vaughn, Bradley, Joffe, Seifer, & Barglow, 1987; Vaughn, Deinard & Egeland, 1980; Zeanah, Keener, Stewart, & Anders, 1985). Bates and Bayles (1984) argued that parent-report instruments contain both *objective* child behavior and *subjective* parent cognition components that have the potential for being empirically distinguished. In contrast, Carey (1983, 1985) has emphatically argued that current temperament instruments do, in fact, accurately measure child behavior and that observation procedures used to validate the procedures are the main source of the problem (see Thomas, Chess, & Korn, 1982).

Relation to External Measures

Another important aspect of validation is the demonstration that parent-report instruments are, in fact, related to the specific child behavior in question. This has been an especially difficult issue in the field of temperament. Since temperament is defined as a set of dimensions that characterize behavior across time and setting, some have claimed that any validation study must include observations that are comprehensive in examining children in multiple settings over substantial time periods (Carey, 1983, 1985). In addition, Carey has argued that the observations should be specifically tailored to yield the same scales that appear on parent-report temperament instruments.

Most studies that have compared parent reports with observations of children have been restricted to either home or laboratory settings, and a time frame of a few days or a week. These studies have uniformly found small to moderate relationships between parent reports and observational measures (i.e., correlations in the range of .2 to .5). These observational measures have not generally been identical to those found on the parent-report instruments, but have been closely related (e.g., amount of crying and laughter rather than quality of mood). Those criticizing parent-report methods have emphasized that these observations should yield more substantial relationships with temperament instruments, while others have claimed that the observations are inadequate to test the validity hypotheses (Seifer & Sameroff, 1986).

However this dispute about validation is eventually resolved, there has, to date, been no definitive demonstration of substantial relationship between parent-report measures and observed child behavior. Whether a different type of observation will yield such relationships is still an open question. For those concerned with employing current temperament instruments, the possibility must be entertained (and all current evidence supports this possibility) that the *parental reports are strongly biased*, containing a large proportion of subjective factors.

Reliability of Instruments

The aspect of psychometric quality that is least disputed is in the area of reliability, where the temperament instruments appear strongest (Hubert, Wachs, Peters-

Martin, & Gandour, 1982; Seifer & Sameroff, 1986). Measures of test–retest reliability over short time frames (a few days or weeks) show high stability. That is, when asked to describe their child's behavior on two different occasions using the same instrument, a parent will give very similar reports.

Reliability of individual scales, that is, the degree to which each item on a scale is related to the whole scale, is also adequate or better for current instruments. The major issue here concerns whether temperament is best described by a smaller number of factors (Buss & Plomin, 1984; Seifer, 1983) or whether more detailed schemes like the nine-factor NYLS are most appropriate (Carey, 1985; Daniels et al., 1984). There is conflicting evidence on this issue, with only a small number of studies that may be compared. In general, there has been little careful factor-analytic work in the development stage of temperament instruments that would address this point, with most factor studies occurring post hoc. (The Lerner et al. [1982] DOTS development is a notable exception.)

A final issue that is often discussed in the context of reliability is the stability of temperament measures over longer time periods, that is, months or years. There has been a fair amount of research in this area, and the best summary is that the relationships have been small to moderate in size, and that some aspects of temperament (difficulty, activity, adaptability) have been more stable than others (Hubert et al., 1982; Seifer & Sameroff, 1986). The lack of large stability coefficients should not be interpreted as a necessary deficiency of the instruments. It may only mean that the children's temperaments are undergoing change over the longer time periods involved in these studies, in which case theories of temperament must include provision for development of temperament patterns over time, rather than reliance on simple notions of high stability, and even strong inheritance, in individuals.

COSTS AND BENEFITS ASSOCIATED WITH TEMPERAMENT ASSESSMENTS

For those working with children in clinical settings, the crucial question is: What are the benefits, and what are the costs, of obtaining temperament information? When considering this question, any answer must be evaluated in light of the measurement properties of current instruments just described. The present discussion, however, will assume for the moment that adequate measurement is possible.

The first, and most obvious, cost of obtaining temperament assessments is the time involved. The clinical settings where children most often participate are routine pediatric examinations, school evaluations, and referral to a medical or psychology–psychiatry setting for assessment or treatment. In all of these settings time devoted to assessment is limited, perhaps most so during routine pediatric exams. Also, temperament per se is rarely a reason for referral of a child (although behavioral problems like disruptive levels of activity clearly have a temperamental component). Thus one must determine that the utility of temperament information will justify the percentage of precious assessment time that it requires.

A second cost must be considered when temperament surveys are used as a screening tool, as recommended by Carey (1985). Since temperament instruments require some time to score, it is generally not possible to evaluate the parent report until after the initial clinical visit. If the temperament assessment should reveal some cause for concern, a follow-up visit is then required, with obvious associated costs to the clinical service.

The final cost to be considered is the degree to which completion of the temperament instrument might affect the parent. The 10 to 25 minutes required to complete a temperament instrument is probably not a burden to any reasonable adult; when a temperament instrument is combined with a battery of other questionnaires, which may occur in some settings, each assessment must be carefully considered so as not to overload the informant and create a situation where he or she is either hostile to the clinician or simply providing bad information because of the overload.

For the most part, the costs of administering temperament assessments in questionnaire format are minimal. The question in many cases will then be: What are the benefits in a clinical setting of having the obtained information? The first part of the answer lies in the clinical conditions that have been associated with temperament variations. The most striking characterization of this literature is that for any particular clinical condition there are a small number (usually one) of individual studies. In some instances one can document that patterns of temperament are substantially related to a specific clinical entity. More details are given in a later section.

Utility of Temperament Assessments in Clinical Practice

To summarize the previous sections on costs and benefits, most assessments of temperament are easy to administer, take up a small amount of time for the informants, and require some time for the clinician for scoring, interpretation, and, in some cases, follow-up visits. There are also many studies that indicate relationships between temperament profiles and various clinical conditions. Thus on the surface it appears that temperament assessments might be recommended as a general procedure in a variety of clinical settings. However, there is still a crucial question that remains unanswered: Do temperament assessments provide *unique* material that is unavailable from other widely used assessment instruments and that will provide additional screening or diagnostic information?

The answer to this question is complex, has been the subject of little discussion in clinical literature, and has been subject to even less empirical investigation. Thus the answer provided here will represent my own most informed judgments on the matter, with references to appropriate research and theory where appropriate.

Temperament as a Clinical Condition. The first part of this discussion will address the most fundamental part of the question of clinical utility: Is difficult temperament (or any other negative temperament description) itself to be considered a clinical condition? One simple way of answering this question is to refer to DSM-III (American Psychiatric Association, 1980) and note that no disorders defined there resemble behavior that is assessed by temperament instruments. The closest match would be between levels of activity or distractibility measured on temperament instruments and parts of the DSM-III diagnosis of attention deficit disorder. However, comparing temperament assessments with DSM-III classification is simply setting up a straw man to be knocked down. Many child clinicians agree that the classification scheme for diagnosis in DSM-III is, at best, a bare-bones approach to issues of mental health in children that does little to highlight the subtleties and unique aspects of assessing developing children. Further, where temperament assessment is most comprehensive, that is, during infancy and early childhood, DSM-III is probably weakest. As such, a more thorough discussion of defining variations in temperament as clinical conditions is warranted.

One way of rephrasing this question is to ask whether individual children are referred to clinical settings because of extreme variations in one or more temperament dimensions or because of unusual profiles. If one merely examines the titles of temperament scales, the answer would be, in some instances, yes. For example, extreme variations in such dimensions as Activity, Distractibility, Impulsivity, Sociability, Mood, and Rhythmicity certainly identify types of children who have clinically significant problems.

For example, as noted earlier, the DSM-III category of attention deficit disorder substantially overlaps with several NYLS temperament categories. Further, it is entirely conceivable that a child would be referred to a clinical setting for high activity level, low persistence, and high impulsivity. At the opposite end of the spectrum, children might be referred for a pattern of low activity, high withdrawal, and negative mood. This latter set of characteristics may correspond less closely with a DSM-III diagnosis in children, but certainly indicates a possible need for intervention.

However, this affirmative answer regarding the characterization of extreme temperament patterns as clinical conditions must be tempered by the fact that little is known about how sensitive the existing temperament instruments are for (1) detecting variability that is in the clinical range and (2) differentiating clinical conditions from normal variability. It must be remembered that temperament instruments were originally designed to measure variability in behavior within the normal range, and have been standardized exclusively on normal populations. Obviously, the intent of some major studies has been the examination of behavior problems (Thomas & Chess, 1977). However, even in studies of behavior disorders, the assessments of temperament were used not as an assessment of pathology, but as indicators of normative variance. Further, many of the major theorists regard difficult temperament as a problem only when there is a bad fit between parent and child. Thus to conclude that temperament itself is a clinical condition seems unwarranted at this time given current definition and assessment of temperament. In situations where a temperament dimension is of particular interest, for example, in assessing hyperactivity, there generally exist specific instruments that have been normed on clinical populations and have empirical evidence regarding their ability to distinguish clinical from nonclinical conditions (e.g., Conners, 1969, in the area of hyperactivity).

Temperament Associations with Clinical Conditions. If temperament variability itself (as measured by existing instruments) is not to be considered as having specific clinical implications, then the next issue is whether variations in temperament are often associated with other clinically significant conditions. Stated another way, is it useful to know, for diagnostic or treatment purposes, whether there are certain types of variance of behaviors in the normal range that may be associated with a particular clinical condition.

A review of studies that examine temperament as a consequence and a precursor of a variety of clinical conditions may be found in Carey (1985). As noted earlier, there are almost no instances where several well-executed studies examine a single temperament–clinical condition relationship.

There is some folklore that perinatal insult or other congenital conditions result in difficult temperament. There is, however, little evidence to support such a notion. In fact, most studies find no differences between children who have a variety of such characteristics (e.g., low birth weight, Down syndrome, small for gestational age) and normal children (Carey, 1985). More evidence exists that environmental insults such as poor nutrition or toxins may have consequences for child temperament (Carey, 1985; Rutter, 1980).

With respect to temperament as a predictor of clinical conditions, the best evidence is in the area of minor behavior disorders of childhood. The clearest evidence is from Thomas and colleagues (1968), with several other studies finding similar results (Carey, 1985; Graham, Rutter, & George, 1973). Such behavior disorders tend to be of an externalizing (Achenbach & Edelbrock, 1981) variety, including attention deficit disorder types of behavior. Carey (1985) also presents a set of intriguing findings, usually from single studies, that difficult temperament is related to more physician visits during early childhood, more accidents, abdominal pain, and more preschool absences.

A closely related issue is whether children who are at risk for clinical conditions have different patterns of temperament. To date, there is little evidence that children at risk because of perinatal status, maternal emotional disorder, or social–cultural factors have distinct temperament patterns (Carey, 1985; McNeil & Kaiji, 1987; Sameroff, Seifer, & Zax, 1982). However, in their longitudinal study Werner and Smith (1982) identify temperamental factors of activity, sociability, and low impulsivity (among many other contextual factors) as related to good developments in children identified initially as at substantial risk for poor outcomes.

To summarize the material just presented: (1) The costs of administering currently available temperament instruments are minimal, though not entirely trivial; (2) the benefits would *not* often be in detecting clinical conditions; (3) some clinical conditions are defined, at least in part, in terms of temperamentlike features, although current temperament instruments are not necessarily designed to detect such distinctions; and (4) there are some clinical conditions that appear to be consistently related to specific patterns of temperament. Thus the most prudent use of temperament instruments would be (1) to detect variation within normal ranges of functioning; (2) to screen large populations in a preventive manner, perhaps detecting early maladaptive patterns before they become clinically significant; and (3) to aid in assessment of the larger family system.

Perhaps the most striking characteristic of studies relating temperament to clinical conditions (as well as those examining normative aspects of temperament) is that they examine temperament solely as it relates to child behavior. The role of parents or other factors in the child's environment is not considered. This body of empirical work stands in contrast to the influential theoretical perspective of Thomas and Chess, which emphasizes the importance of *goodness of fit* between child behavior and environmental context. Recall that there were minimal differences in form and content among the many instruments used to measure temperament despite some strong theoretical differences among those who developed the questionnaires. In the sections to follow, the impact of the construct of goodness of fit on temperament definitions is more thoroughly explored, with implications for the assessment and interpretation of temperament in clinical practice.

THEORETICAL CONSIDERATIONS REGARDING GOODNESS OF FIT

The utility of the concept of temperament has been considered under three headings by Rutter (1982): demonstrations that (1) children exhibit individual differences, (2) these differences arise from constitutional factors, and (3) these differences can be used to predict developmental disorder or vulnerability to stressful situations. These issues have been considered in our discussions of various temperament theories. The first notion of individual differences is not controversial. The second issue of constitutional factors is not universally accepted (particularly by this writer), but this is probably of minimal interest in everyday clinical practice. The third topic, however, gets to the core of practical applications of the information gained from temperament research. The discussion in previous sections introduced a number of issues relevant to the ultimate clinical utility of the temperament concept. These themes will be integrated later to suggest an agenda that will lead to a more fruitful application of the temperament concept in the future.

At issue here is the basic way in which professionals have conceived of temperament. Implicit through previous sections of this chapter has been the notion that temperament is defined as a property of individual children, and that variations in temperament assessments reflect individual constitutional differences in specific classes of behavior across many settings. This is the essence of an explanation of human behavior in terms of *trait*. Such traits might then be predisposing factors to specific clinical conditions. However, such notions have not gone unchallenged (Seifer & Sameroff, 1986).

A brief digression to the area of adult personality is taken here to consider the ideas of theorists who have, over the years, most carefully considered issues of trait and contextual explanations of behavior. This will highlight how a theoretical controversy, analogous to the one described for temperament, is currently perceived. The issue is whether there are stable traits in personality or whether most of the variation in individual behavior can be explained by differences in the situations people encounter. Not surprisingly, the answer is that the results depend on the question asked.

> Why has there been such confusion in the person–situation debate? The answer is that situationists and trait theorists can both prove that they are right. The problem is that each group believes that because it is right, the other group must be wrong. The paradox lies in the fact that the following three statements are all true: (a) Behavior is situationally specific; (b) behavior is cross-situationally general; and (c) there are stable, broad response dispositions, or traits. (Epstein, 1983, p. 183)

> There seems to be general consensus both about the existence of behavioral stabilities and consistencies, on the one hand, and the occurrence of cross-situational discriminativeness in behavior, on the other. The significance, nature, and ways to conceptualize and pursue these coherences and the discriminative patterns—not the reality of either one—remain at issue and need to be our focus. It is encouraging that current work seems to be focusing more on the clarification of the psychological structure, organization, and construction of behavioral consistencies and of person–situation interactions, and less on debating their existence. (Mischel & Peake, 1983, p. 394)

> The controversy has served its purpose: Psychologists understand better than they did before how much consistency exists in human behavior, how to accentuate individual

> differences for study (aggregate across situations), and how to accentuate situational effects for study (aggregate across individuals). There seems to be little need to argue further whether personality "exists" or is "overwhelmed by situations," or about whether situations or persons are more deserving of being treated as "error"; such arguments are as between straw men, and more constructive issues remain to be explored. (Funder, 1983, p. 289)

The consensus just described indicates that notions of trait and context are both useful in understanding human personality. Difficulty arises when one approach is used to exclude the possibility of the other. The task of behavioral researchers is not to demonstrate that either trait or context is the only explanation of human behavior, but to formulate theories that successfully integrate the aspects of behavior that appear best explained by one or the other construct.

As was true for adults, when children are measured in a large number of situations, or when a large number of different children are measured in the same situation, consistencies in behavior are found to reflect either child or situational variables respectively. On the other hand, when we want to predict what a child will do in a given situation, or with a particular set of parents, we have to know something about the parents, as well as the way these parents interact with this particular child. The problem is even more complex because children naturally change in behavior as they grow, and these changes in behavior alter the ways that their parents interact with them (Chess & Thomas, 1984).

The major distinction between adult personality and child temperament is that adult personality is less obviously a developmental phenomenon. The more static notions commonly applied to adult personality lend themselves to interpretation in terms of stable within-the-individual traits, or constant interaction between specific individuals and specific settings. When personality characteristics are viewed in a more developmental perspective, however, the ongoing relationship between individuals and their contexts becomes the primary focus. We are thus left with four difficult issues to consider simultaneously: (1) the degreee of consistency in behavior patterns exhibited within individuals (trait); (2) the degree to which immediate contexts affect the expression of behavior (situationism); (3) the degree to which there are nonadditive interactions between individual and situational characteristics (interactionism); and (4) the degree to which the meanings of behaviors, settings, and their relationships change over time (development).

Organizational Construct of Temperament

Attempts to integrate these apparently conflicting interpretations of behavior have employed approaches best described as theories of hierarchically ordered systems (Bronfenbrenner, 1977; Sameroff, 1982, 1983). To digress briefly once again, Sroufe and Waters (1977), in the context of attachment theory, have developed such a systems theory to explain developmental phenomena that occur during infancy and early childhood. Describing the nature of the affective bond between parents and their young children poses many of the same problems of trait, situational, and developmental explanations found in temperament theory. Should attachment be considered a characteristic of the child, of the situation with the parents, or of the interaction between the two?

Sroufe and Waters addressed this problem by introducing an *organizational construct* to explain early parent–infant attachment relationships, and emphasized the goal-directed nature of the development and maintenance of strong attachment bonds (see also Ainsworth, 1972; Bowlby, 1969). Sroufe and Waters contend that specific behavior patterns such as maintaining proximity or interacting with other adults must be interpreted in the context in which the behavior occurs and the effect it has on the parent–child system, that is, the degree to which the observed action achieves the purpose of attachment relationships—to maintain security in a variety of settings. This theoretical approach, with its focus on the purpose of behavior in maintaining a relationship, permits the flexible interpretation of specific behaviors so that their meaning corresponds to specific settings and developmental periods.

Seifer and Sameroff (1986) have asserted that, in order fully to understand the concept of infant and child temperament, a similar organizational construct should be formulated. Although a full-scale organizational theory is not proposed (there is not enough basic information to do this at the present time), an outline for how such a formulation might proceed is given.

The aspect of this formulation most relevant to clinical concerns is the definition of the system. In existing temperament formulations, the system has been defined as the individual child. Temperament is conceived of as a property of the person, that is, as a constitutional trait. The concept of purpose is not considered in the temperament system. Rather, temperament is viewed more as an incidental stylistic aspect of other behavior systems.

To reconcile many of the conflicts that arise from current conceptions of temperament, it is proposed that the system of interest be redefined and the organizational properties of that system, most notably its goals or adaptations, be made explicit. From the perspective of a clinically useful construct, temperament must be viewed not just as a property of the child, but as a property of the child *in a specific context*. For young children the context is most importantly the family.* The family system thus becomes central to the definition and assessment of temperament. Furthermore, the goal of this system, that is, the regulated state to which behavior is directed, may be defined as the *well-adapted family*. Within the family, the best behavioral style for the child is one that most closely fits the needs, attitudes, beliefs, and values of the family, for example, the one that maximizes ease of caretaking, realization of parental aspirations for an individual child, and the ability to use one's preferred parenting style. On the other hand, children whose characteristics do not fit such familial expectations may be defined as *difficult children* independently of their scores from temperament questionnaires of the type currently used. For example, a child who requires extensive behavioral limits at home may be a bad fit for a parent who rigidly adheres to a laissez-faire philosophy of child rearing.

This general perspective on temperament is derived from the Thomas and Chess concept of goodness of fit. However, rather than as a derived description of families

* The family is identified here as the primary context so that presentation of basic ideas may be accomplished in the space available. This is not meant to imply that other contexts outside of the family are unimportant. To the contrary, it is assumed that nonfamily contexts such as schools and peer groups provide essential socializing experiences, where children's behavior often has unique characteristics. However, in most clinical settings the child and family are the people involved. Careful assessment of other contexts is important and should be considered in the overall clinical picture.

that are more likely to produce well-adjusted children, goodness of fit is employed here as a fundamental property of the temperament system under study. To elaborate, there are three basic components of the model: (1) child behavioral style; (2) parent qualities (behavior, cognition); and (3) goodness of fit between parent and child. Where Thomas and Chess equate temperament with behavioral style (thereby locating it in the child), the proposal here is to equate temperament with goodness of fit (locating it within the family system).

This approach to temperament is similar to that employed by Sroufe and Waters (1977) in the area of attachment. Where the question for attachment theory was originally posed as: How attached is child *A* to his or her parent? (child-centered definition), Sroufe and Waters modified the question to: What is the nature of the attachment relationship? (relationship-centered definition). With respect to temperament, the proposal is to modify the current question, How does child *A* behave most of the time? (child-centered definition), to How does child *A*'s behavior style affect relationships within the family? (relationship-centered definition). The implications of this shift in basic definition for integrating trait, situational, interactional, and developmental explanations are discussed through several examples.

Interpretation of Behavior in Organizational Theory

One feature of all current temperament theories is that they attempt to define a single set of temperament categories that will be applicable from early infancy through childhood and even into adulthood. The results of studies that might support such a theory have been mixed. Attempts to demonstrate substantial short- or long-term stability of individual temperaments, or to demonstrate factorial invariance across time, have been equivocal (Hubert et al., 1982; Seifer & Sameroff, 1986). The one construct that has shown resiliency across time and setting is the difficult (or easy) child (Bates, 1980). However, the problem with current measurement tools is that they attempt to measure difficulty in the same manner in all settings and ages.

When the definition of temperament is formulated from the perspective of an organizational construct of the *well-adapted family caregiving system*, individual behavior categories that show little stability across time, or little intercorrelation, may be reinterpreted to support a more general temperament construct at each specific developmental period. To exemplify how current and proposed formulations differ, I present a series of behavior examples in terms of how they may or may not be salient at different developmental stages. For ease of presentation, this discussion is restricted to the well-known categories of the NYLS (Thomas et al., 1963) and to family adaptation in terms of ease of caretaking.

Temperament and Development. During the newborn period (one rarely considered in temperament studies) the most salient features for ease of caretaking would be rhythmicity, particularly of sleep patterns, less so of eating patterns (especially if demand feeding is the style employed by parents), and least so for toileting. The other major temperament feature would be distractibility, usually defined by soothability items during infancy. New parents will be more comfortable with infants who will quiet quickly when distressed than with infants who maintain crying and fussiness over sustained periods. Other temperament categories, like activity, approach, and adaptabality, are less important in newborns who do not locomote and who make only rudimentary discriminations among caregivers and settings.

When these infants are about 6 months of age, other temperament categories become more relevant. Rhythmicity may still be an important issue, but feeding may be the dominant aspect, since this is a time when solid foods are often introduced and more attempts are made to have families eat together. Also, as infants begin to crawl and are awake for much longer periods, activity level becomes a central issue. An infant's strong attention to exploring the object world during this period would be emphasized in categories like approach, persistence, and intensity.

Still later in development, at about 2½ years, very different behaviors and categories will be salient. Rhythmicity may still be a major concern, but the focus might well be on elimination, as parents begin to institute toilet-training procedures. Toddlers who walk and run will vary in their activity level, but the larger gross motor behaviors may now be the most relevant. Object play is still important, but older children not only manipulate and explore but also engage in complex problem solving when playing with challenging toys. The parameters of persistence, approach, and intensity will be much different than at 6 months. Further, a child's exploration of the world will involve many more complex social situations at this age than at 6 months. Where infants have a small repertoire of behaviors with which to engage others, toddlers have sophisticated social skills and interact with a wider variety of adults and peers. Issues of approach and adaptability may be much more important in the domain of social interaction during this period.

Finally, during the school years still other behavior domains will become most salient for evaluating difficult temperament. For example, rhythmicity may again be most important in the areas of eating and sleeping as the coordination of school schedules with other family schedules takes on increasing importance. Also, sociability issues are much more focused on peers, and upon establishing an *enduring* relationship with a single nonfamily adult (teacher). Finally, issues of self-control that include the maintenance of quiet behavior, sustained attention, and low activity in classroom settings will affect how temperament dimensions such as activity, persistence, and distractibility are measured and interpreted.

As is evident in the examples just given, children change with development in the aspects of their personality that are most relevant to ease of caretaking. One should also expect some degree of individual variation in the manner in which such developmental patterns are manifest. Also, these examples can be extended to other aspects of the family system, such as conformity to parental expectations, that influence the way that child behavioral style affects family adaptation.

Temperament and Context. As just described, normal child developmental processes affect both the expression of temperament behavior and the interpretation of these behaviors. Another important factor is the immediate context in which behavior is expressed. One clear example can be seen by contrasting familial behavior in the home when the family is relaxed with behavior when the family is eating at a quiet but crowded restaurant. A child's expressions of two temperaments, for example, poor mood and low distractibility (soothability), have very different implications for ease of caretaking in these two settings. If a 1-year-old child, or for that matter a 10-year-old child, has an extended bout of crying in the home, parents might react in several ways. One widely used and effective strategy is to let the child cry for an extended period without receiving any attention from the parents, who then respond positively when the child achieves a better mood. Even if this occurs with some frequency, the parents may still feel that this particular child is easy to care for. While the behavior is not in itself pleasant, the course is predictable and the ultimate outcome acceptable.

In contrast, should the same behavior occur in a restaurant, the same parenting strategy is unacceptable to most parents due to the demands of the social context. The same parents who are effective in caring for the crying child's needs at home may be totally ineffective in soothing the child in the restaurant. They may not possess an effective alternative strategy to accomplish a prompt quieting on the part of the child. In this case, the interpretation by the parent, and by an observer, would be that this child is difficult to care for. Thus the goodness of fit with respect to temperament depends not only on the behavior of the child and parents, but also on the context in which the behavior is expressed. The extent to which families effectively manage this interaction between the child's needs and behavior, the parents' needs and behavior, and overall context will determine their success at establishing goodness of fit.

Subjective Parental Considerations. In addition to the more objective aspects of developmental chance and context of behavior, the more subjective aspects of parent interpretation must be considered. Bates (1980) clearly articulated the differences between subjective and objective factors that influence temperament reports made by parents. Bates's position, however, was that the subjective aspect of parents' reports should be treated as a factor that experimental methods should seek to eliminate, that is, as error variance. In contrast, the concept of temperament proposed here treats this subjective aspect as an integral component of measurement and interpretation. The reason for this is that the central issue of concern is goodness of fit among the components of the temperament system. While objectivity in measuring behavior is, of course, considered essential, the subjective experience of that behavior by the parent is no less important in interpreting the status of an individual family system.

An anecdote from one of our studies is very illustrative. Sameroff, Seifer, and Elias (1982) found that social status was substantially related to temperament ratings as measured by the Carey (1972) Infant Temperament Questionnaire. Specifically, low-SES Blacks more often rated their children as having what is traditionally interpreted as a difficult temperament than did high-SES Whites. However, when discussing their children, the low-SES Black mothers interpreted the high activity level, robust crying, and so forth as indications of healthy, feisty, and competitive children. Thus a behavior pattern often interpreted out of context as having a negative impact on goodness of fit was considered by a subsample of parents to be positive, apparently because of subcultural differences in the perception of positive development.

Carey (1983) has noted, in fact, that many mothers whose questionnaire ratings of temperament indicate that they have difficult children do not themselves classify their children as difficult when asked directly about ease versus difficulty of caretaking on a single question. Also, Carey (1982) has stated that a difficult temperament profile does not necessarily indicate a stressful parent–child interaction.

> Diverse parental expectations and coping capacities strongly affect the environment with which the child interacts. Therefore, intervention programs, intended to prevent emotional problems by early screening for difficult temperament alone, are destined to failure. (p. 195).

Despite such occasional acknowledgments in the temperament literature that the questionnaires do not measure goodness of fit, there is in fact almost no work that directly examines these issues.

In a contrasting stance, Chess (1982) qualifies Carey's point by noting that, as discussed by Carey, some infants and toddlers who were rated as being difficult according to the temperament categories were rated positively by their mothers when queried directly. However, as the children reached 3 or 4 years of age, the mothers became less positive in their overall ratings of the child. The problem with Chess's example is that she discussed only those children who were ultimately defined as difficult based on their scores during the first 5 years of life. It did not apply to those children who may have been rated as difficult during the first year or so, but who later received different temperament ratings.

Implications of the New Definition for Clinical Practice

The direct result of defining temperament as proposed here (in the context of an organizational construct that emphasizes the goal of achieving a well-adapted family system) is to force investigators and clinicians simultaneously to consider all objective, subjective, individual, and contextual sources of information. Despite the changing functions of specific behaviors and the salience of different aspects of temperament during the course of development, as observed in different environmental contexts and as interpreted by different parents, these factors may all be interpreted within the unifying organizational construct. If the goal of the behavioral system is a well-adapted, caregiving family, then the focus of assessment should be less on the frequency or duration of specific behaviors, and more on the implications of these behaviors within the caretaking pattern of the individual family.

One obvious change is that the use of 15-minute questionnaires that tap only individual behavioral qualities will no longer be applicable. Various methods that might be applied (e.g., questionnaires, observations, diaries, or Q-sorts) would no longer simply compare children on how often and how long they behaved in a particular way. Rather, the specific behaviors would be interpreted (by parents or observers) in the context in which they were observed, and for the implications they had for the caretaking system. Thus a much more comprehensive view of the family system would be involved in a temperament assessment.

Where does all of this ultimately lead? First, such assessments would probably be too extensive and costly for routine screening in normal populations (e.g., in a well child pediatric setting). In contrast, such a battery, because of its comprehensive systematic nature, might be an appropriate basis for examining high-risk populations, or some identified families, by providing information about normative functioning and information that is perhaps related to clinical conditions.

Measurement Issues. The previous discussion focused on resolving some basic theoretical problems existing in current conceptions of temperament. There are also difficult technical problems associated with confirming the validity of current measures, problems that were discussed in detail in previous sections and fully elaborated elsewhere (Hubert et al., 1982; Seifer & Sameroff, 1986). One important question is whether the proposed reformulation of the concept of temperament would seriously affect the psychometric properties of measurement tools. There is reason to believe that validity problems would be less complicated with the proposed approach. With current instruments, the major validity issue centers around determining, by objective means, whether the reports made by parents about long-term behavior patterns are accurate by normative standards. Given definitions of temperament that focus on individual behavioral stability over time and setting, there is great importance attached to whether parent reports do, in fact, accurately describe how a child behaves in most settings over extended time frames compared to normative standards. Subjective aspects of the reports are considered errors that must be weeded out by investigators, a task that has not yet been accomplished.

In the proposed reformulation, subjective aspects of the parental report would be an integral part of measuring the adaptive state of the temperament system. The focus would be on long-term interpretations made by the parents of the specific child behaviors in specific contexts. The strategy of measurements would focus not necessarily on obtaining accurate summaries of frequency and duration of child behavior, but on reports of how such behavior affects the parent–child caregiving system. Specific measures could involve more short-term, easily validated reports of child behavior. The long-term interpretations of child behavior made by the parents should also be more valid since the parents are being asked to make a generalization about *themselves* rather that about their child.

The emphasis on the impact of temperament behaviors on the family system is not meant to imply that careful documentation of infant or child behavior is unimportant. To the contrary, it is the child's behavior in context that is the immediate stimulus to which parents respond, and that is an important component of the behavioral substrate that develops within the family environment. What is proposed is that the question asked by researchers change from "*On the average*, does the child express *more or less* of a particular behavior?" to "When a particular behavior occurs, *what is its effect on the family system*?" The reformulated question is obviously more complex, but it generates information that directly addresses the fundamental issues inherent in child personality research. Further, each bit of information should be easiesr to validate since it is much more situationally specific. Thus the behavior is easier for clinicians and researchers to observe directly, and it requires fewer comparative assessments be made by parent informants.

The proposed concept of temperament addresses both theoretical and practical concerns in research methods, but the fundamental issue is whether this new proposal will more effectively answer the key questions that initially motivated temperament researchers. One of the goals of the proposed formulation is to provide a temperament concept that is consistent with current thinking on the issues of trait, context, and interaction as conceived by other personality researchers. The notion of relatively static traits, a main characteristic of existing temperament theories, is not sufficient to explain adult personality, and by implication will not be sufficient to explain the even more complex phenomena associated with development of personality in children. With respect to childhood behavior disorders, the most influential theory is Thomas and Chess's approach of goodness of fit. By incorporating this approach into the fundamental concept of temperament, researchers may more directly address the issues at the level of measurement and data reduction.

CLINICAL CONSIDERATIONS REGARDING GOODNESS OF FIT

In the review of theories at the beginning of this chapter, several areas of inquiry are identified. Chief among them are: (1) determining the roots of adult personality; (2) determining the roots of childhood behavior disorders; (3) identifying biobehavioral determinants of temperament; and (4) describing factors that modulate social contexts. Discussion of these issues was related to analogous theoretical issues pertaining to defining adult personality structure. For the clinician, however, the most important issue is the assessment and treatment of childhood behavior disorders. The implications of an organizational temperament construct based on gooodness of fit may best be seen in its application to assessment and treatment.

Assessment

With respect to assessment, there are three important domains to consider, which correspond to essential components of the organizational construct described earlier: (1) goodness of fit between (2) child behavior style and (3) parents' cognitive and behavioral qualities.

The first domain concerns how the child's behavior is related to the parents within the family system, an area almost totally ignored in past clinical applications. The direct interaction of specific child behavior with particular parents must be assessed and interpreted. Also, careful consideration of the variety of caretaking contexts that naturally occur (e.g., alone at home, with friends, in public places) must be integrated into the assessment and interpretation. Skilled clinicians routinely interpret child behavior in its appropriate context. The proposal regarding temperament given earlier would simply extend this type of contextual interpretation of child behavior to an area that had previously been thought of as a constitutional trait.

Second, we must directly assess the child's behavior. Reliance on parental reports as a primary source of data for the objective behavior will most likely lead to substantial psychometric measurement problems. Further, the specific child behaviors to measure are still in question (e.g., whether one should be brief and simple or attempt to measure the widest possible range of behavior). Regardless of the strategy, the important consideration here is to develop sound, objective measures of children's behavioral styles to be interpreted within the context of goodness of fit. The emphasis here will not be on stability of individual behaviors across time and setting. Instead, it will be on obtaining valid measure of child behavior that form the basis for parental evaluations, and thus goodness of fit. Such behaviors may be more situationally and temporally specific, perhaps even single instances of behavior. The important issue will be not the child's behavioral style in all situations, but the impact of specific child behaviors on family systems. It may be low-frequency behaviors, or behaviors in very specific settings, that prove to be the most relevant for establishing temperamental goodness of fit.

The third of these domains concerns parental cognitive perspectives, that is, how parents perceive and interpret a specific child behavior in a specific context. These perspectives include attitudes, values, beliefs, and agendas that parents hold for each of their children. Some of these perspectives are related to cultural and socioeconomic factors (Sameroff & Feil, 1985), while others are more personal in origin. Assessments are needed that more squarely focus on the parents' subjective experience of their children's behavioral style. This is the area that is currently least considered in child clinical settings, partially due to the lack of well-validated assessment instruments specifically designed for such settings.

For the clinician currently in practice, these perspectives on temperament may provide little immediate assistance (although it is hoped that they provide some guidance in interpreting information). An ambitious strategy for defining, assessing, and interpreting children's temperament is proposed, with little in the way of concrete assessment tools to use. However, in using parent report instruments that are currently available for the measurement of child traits, many cautions regarding interpretation are provided. For example, scores indicating difficult temperament may be unduly colored by subjective parental factors, or they may represent no significant concern if the parent has successfully adapted to the child's behavior. Current instruments should, at best, be used *to begin* an assessment of issues related to goodness of fit.

Treatment

Assuming that these complex assessment issues will be solved, attention must then focus on the prevention, intervention, or treatment of serious disturbances related to temperament. First, one must keep in mind that temperament is probably best considered outside the realm of clinical disturbance. However, poorly adapted temperament systems are candidates for treatment because they may be precursors to more serious disturbances (prevention); because they may be unwanted byproducts of other existing clinical conditions; or because families may wish to achieve better states of adaptation to improve quality of life, independent of any severe clinical concerns. There are two basic approaches to such intervention, about which clinicians will probably always disagree: attempting to change specific child behavior, or focusing on modifying characteristics of the family system.

Most temperament theorists assume that there are sets of child behaviors that are more or less desirable in the daily interaction between parents and children. To the extent these behaviors are inherited and under biological control, they may be less susceptible to change; the degree to which they are socialized may influence how much they may be modified by environmental intervention. Within such a trait perspective, any behavioral intervention will be directed at specific child behaviors.

As discussed earlier, the same child behavior styles may be interpreted in vastly different ways by parents holding differing perspectives on development. Thus to promote a well-adapted family system, a potentially successful approach may be to increase the flexibility of parents' attitudes, beliefs, values, and agendas regarding their own child's behavior. Parents' ability to adapt flexibly to a variety of child behaviors increases the likelihood that an acceptable family system will be attained. Such flexibility may include (among many other examples) simply observing child behavior more accurately, understanding that negative behavior is not necessarily personally targeted or malicious, especially in younger children, adjusting one's beliefs about the role of a parent, reevaluating expectations for a particular child in light of what an individual presents, and developing effective strategies for coping with, and decreasing the frequency of, negative behavior.

One intriguing research finding illuminates this point of parental context and goodness of fit. An aspect of the context of parents that has received theoretical examination is the degree to which their social supports enhance their ability to be effective parents (Crnic, Greenberg, & Slough, 1986). Along these lines, Crockenberg (1981) found that among mother–infant dyads where the infant was described as irritable, the amount of social support available to parents determined the success that the dyads had at achieving a secure attachment relationship. This effect was not found within a group of nonirritable infants. This study highlights the interaction among infant temperamental qualities and variation in parental context in determining the adaptive status of the family system.

Whichever of the parent-centered or child-centered approaches proves to be successful is in the long run not particularly important so long as effective treatments are established. (The most prudent prediction would be that a combination of child-centered and parent-centered treatment will prove most effective.) What is essential is that theorists and clinicians work jointly to develop the strategies that will serve to improve the functioning of poorly adapted family systems, that is, to improve the temperament relationship. The systems-oriented temperament formulation proposed here is a step in that direction.

References

Achenbach, T. M., & Edelbrock, C. S. (1981). Behavioral problems and competencies reported by parents of normal and disturbed children aged four through sixteen. *Monographs of the Society for Research in Child Development*, *46* (Serial # 188).

Ainsworth, M. D. S. (1972). Attachment and dependency: A comparison. In J. Gewertz (Ed.), *Attachment and dependency*. Washington, DC: Winston.

American Psychiatric Association (1980). *Diagnostic and statistical manual of mental disorders* (3rd ed.). Washington, DC: Author.

Bates, J. E. (1980). The concept of difficult temperament. *Merrill-Palmer Quarterly*, *26*, 299–319.

Bates, J. E., & Bayles, K. (1984). Objective and subjective components in mothers' perceptions of their children from age 6 months to 3 years. *Merrill-Palmer Quarterly*, *30*, 111–132.

Bates, J. E., Freeland, C. A., & Lounsbury, M. L. (1979). Measure of infant difficultness. *Child Development*, *50*, 794–803.

Bowlby, J. (1969). *Attachment*. New York: Basic.

Bronfenbrenner, U. (1977). Toward an experimental ecology of human development. *American Psychologist*, *32*, 513–531.

Buss, A. H., & Plomin, R. (1975). *A temperament theory of personality*. New York: Wiley.

Buss, A. H., & Plomin, R. (1984). *Temperament: Early developing personality traits*. Hillsdale, NJ: Erlbaum.

Carey, W. B. (1972). Measuring infant temperament. *Journal of Pediatrics*, *81*, 414–418.

Carey, W. B. (1982). Clinical use of temperament data in pediatrics. In R. Porter & G. M. Collins (Eds.), *Temperamental differences in infants and young children* (Ciba Foundation Symposium 89). London: Pitman.

Carey, W. B. (1983). Some pitfalls in temperament research. *Infant Behavior & Development*, *6*, 247–254.

Carey, W. B. (1985). Interactions of temperament and clinical conditions. *Advances in Developmental & Behavioral Pediatrics*, *6*, 83–115.

Carey, W. B., & McDevitt, S. C. (1978). Revision of the Infant Temperament Questionnaire. *Pediatrics, 61*, 735–739.

Chess, S. (1982). Discussion. In R. Porter & G. M. Collins, (Eds.), *Temperamental differences in infants and young children* (Ciba Foundation Symposium 89). London: Pitman.

Chess, S., & Thomas, A. (1984). *The origins and evolution of temperament*. New York: Brunner/Mazel.

Conners, C. K. (1969). A teacher rating scale for use in drug studies with children. *American Journal of Psychiatry, 126*, 152–156.

Crnic, K. A., Greenberg, M. T., & Slough, N. M. (1986). Early stress and social support influences on mothers' and high-risk infants' functioning in late infancy. *Infant Mental Health Journal, 7*, 19–33.

Crockenberg, S. B. (1981). Infant irritability, mother responsiveness, and social influences on the security of infant–mother attachment. *Child Development, 52*, 857–865.

Daniels, D., Plomin, R., & Greenhalgh, J. (1984). Correlates of difficult temperament in infancy. *Child Development, 55*, 1184–1194.

deVries, M. W., & Sameroff, A. J. (1984). Culture and temperament: Influences on infant temperament in three East African societies. *American Journal of Orthopsychiatry, 54*, 83–96.

Epstein, S. (1983). The stability of confusion: A reply to Mischel and Peake. *Psychological Review, 90*, 179–184.

Fullard, W., McDevitt, S. C., & Carey, W. B. (1978). *Toddler Temperament Scale*. Department of Educational Psychology, Temple University, Philadelphia.

Funder, D. C. (1983). Three issues in predicting more of the people: A reply to Mischel and Peake. *Psychological Review, 90*, 283–289.

Goldsmith, H. H., & Campos, J. (1982). Toward a theory of infant temperament. In R. N. Emde & R. J. Harmon (Eds.), *The development of attachment and affiliative systems*. New York: Plenum.

Graham, P., Rutter, M., & George, S. (1973). Temperamental characteristics as predictors of behavior disorders in children. *American Journal of Orthopsychiatry, 43*, 328–339.

Hubert, N. C., Wachs, T. D., Peters-Martin, P., & Gandour, M. J. (1982). The study of early temperament: Measurement and conceptual issues. *Child Development, 53*, 571–600.

Lee, C. L., & Bates, J. E. (1985). Mother–child interaction at age two years and perceived difficult temperament. *Child Development, 56*, 1314–1325.

Lerner, R. M., Palermo, M., Spiro, A., & Nesselroade, J. R. (1982). Assessing the dimensions of temperamental individuality across the life span: the Dimensions of Temperament Survey (DOTS). *Child Development, 53*, 149–159.

McDevitt, S. C., & Carey, W. B. (1975). The measurement of temperament in 3–7-year-old children. *Journal of Child Psychology & Psychiatry, 19*, 245–253.

McNeil, T. F., & Kaiji, L. (1987). Swedish high-risk study: Sample characteristics at age 6. *Schizophrenia Bulletin, 13*, 373–381.

Mischel, W., & Peake, P. K. (1983). Some facets of consistency: Replies to Epstein, Funder, and Bem. *Psychological Review, 90*, 394–402.

Rothbart, M. K. (1981). Measurement of temperament in infancy. *Child Development, 52*, 569–587.

Rothbart, M. K., & Derryberry, D. (1981). Development of individual differences in temperament. In M. E. Lamb & A. L. Brown (Eds.), *Advances in developmental psychology* (Vol. 1). Hillsdale, NJ: Erlbaum.

Rothbart, M. K., & Derryberry, D. (1982). Theoretical issues in temperament. In M. Lewis & L. T. Taft (Eds.), *Developmental disabilities: Theory, assessment, and intervention*. New York: Spectrum.

Rothbart, M. K., & Goldsmith, H. H. (1985). Three approaches to the study of infant temperament. *Developmental Review, 5*, 237–260.

Rutter, M. (1980). Raised lead levels and impaired cognitive/behavioral functioning: A review of the evidence. *Developmental Medicine & Child Neurology, 22* (Supplement), 1–26.

Rutter, M. (1982). Temperament: Concepts, issues, and problems. In R. Porter & G. M. Collins (Eds.), *Temperamental differences in infants and young children* (Ciba Foundation Symposium 89). London: Pitman.

Sameroff, A. J. (1982). Development and the dialectic: The need for a systems approach. In W. A. Collins (Ed.), *Minnesota symposium on child psychology* (Vol. 15). Hillsdale, NJ: Erlbaum.

Sameroff, A. J. (1983). Developmental systems: Contexts and evolution. In W. Kessen (Ed.), History, theory, and methods, Vol. 1 of P. H. Mussen (Ed.), *Handbook of child psychology*. New York: Wiley.

Sameroff, A. J., & Feil, L. A. (1985). Parental concepts of development. In I. Sigel (Ed.), *Parental belief systems: The psychological consequences for children*. Hillsdale, NJ: Erlbaum.

Sameroff, A. J., Seifer, R., & Elias, P. K. (1982). Sociocultural variability in infant temperament ratings. *Child Development, 53*, 164–171.

Sameroff, A. J., Seifer, R., & Zax, M. (1982). Early development of children at risk for emotional disorder. *Monographs of the Society for Research in Child Development, 47* (Serial Number 199).

Seifer, R. (1983). The structure of infant temperament: An examination of the Infant Temperament Questionnaire. In A. J. Sameroff (Chair), *Parent report instruments of infant temperament: What is being measured?* Symposium presented at the Society for Research in Child Development meeting, Detroit.

Seifer, R., & Sameroff, A. J. (1986). The concept, measurement, and interpretation of temperament in young children: A survey of research issues. In M. L. Wolraich & D. Routh (Eds.), *Advances in developmental and behavioral pediatrics* (Vol. 7). Greenwich, CT: JAI.

Sroufe, L. A., & Waters, E. (1977). Attachment as an organizational construct. *Child Development, 48*, 1184–1199.

Thomas, A. (1983). First discussant's comments. In A. J. Sameroff (Chair), *Parent report instruments for the assessment of infant temperament: What is being measured?* Symposium presented at the Society for Research in Child Development meeting, Detroit.

Thomas, A., & Chess, S. (1977). *Temperament and development*. New York: Brunner/Mazel.

Thomas, A., Chess, S., & Birch, H. G. (1968). *Temperament and behavior disorders in children*. New York: New York University Press.

Thomas, A., Chess, S., Birch, H. G., Hertzig, M. E., & Korn, S. (1963). *Behavioral individuality in early childhood*. New York: New York University Press.

Thomas, A., Chess, S., & Korn, S. (1982). The reality of difficult temperament. *Merrill-Palmer Quarterly, 28*, 1–20.

Vaughn, B. E., Bradley, C. F., Joffe, L. S., Seifer, R., & Barglow, P. (1987). Maternal characteristics measured prenatally predict ratings of temperamental "difficulty" on the Carey Infant Temperament Questionnaire. *Developmental Psychology, 23*, 152–161.

Vaughn, B. E., Deinard, A., & Egeland, B. (1980). Measuring temperament in pediatric practice. *Journal of Pediatrics, 96*, 510–514.

Werner, E. E., & Smith, R. S. (1982). *Vulnerable but invincible: A longitudinal study of resilient children and youth*. New York: McGraw-Hill.

Zeanah, C. H., Keener, M. A., Stewart, L., & Anders, T. F. (1985). Prenatal perception of infant personality: A preliminary investigation. *Journal of the American Academy of Child Psychiatry, 24*, 204–210.

8

Cognitive–Behavioral Assessment of Children in Health Settings

JULIA L. EISENSTEIN
ANNE P. COPELAND

INTRODUCTION

In recent years, increasing recognition has been paid to the cognitive aspects of problems that had previously been considered purely behavioral, medical, or emotional. In this chapter, we discuss several of these cognitive factors as they relate to children's medical disorders. Though the disorder may remain primarily medical (as in insulin level maintenance or tumor remission) or behavioral (as in dietary compliance), cognitive processes function to affect children's cooperation, recovery time, adjustment, emotionality, and a host of other outcome concerns. In some cases, children's cognitions are assessed and modified directly. In other cases, the focus in treatment is on behavioral rather than cognitive change, but cognitive changes may accompany these behavioral changes in an indirect and important manner. We will first briefly review the theoretical foundations of this literature, then focus on those cognitive factors that have been found to be particularly relevant to pediatric problems.

Theoretical Background

Bandura (1977) has posed a model to unify various explanations of psychological changes that result from treatment interventions. In this model he emphasizes person variables, that is, outcome expectations, self-efficacy, and cognitions, in the understanding of behavior. The term *outcome expectation* refers to how a person anticipates the results of intervention. Here the focus is on the contingencies of the situation itself rather than on the person's perceived own ability to act. Outcome expectations will affect the activities in which one decides to participate. For example, those situations in which an individual believes the outcome will be negative will be avoided. This avoidance may be physical, or when physical exit is impossible, may be psychological (Carver & Scheier, 1982). Individuals are more likely to enter into those situations that are expected to have positive outcomes. In addition, attempts at coping are likely to be repeated in the face of adversity when expectations are for favorable results. Outcome expectations will also affect emotional response. Expectations for an unfavorable outcome produce negative affect, while expectations for a favorable outcome produce positive affect (Carver & Scheier, 1982).

Outcome expectations are affected by several factors. If others have negative expectations of outcome, the individual is likely also to hold negative expectations of outcome, and the same is likely to be true for positive outcomes. This is particularly the case when there are expert opinions involved. Outcome expectations are also influenced by the kind of opportunities the environment poses for outcome. An environment that is restrictive will partially determine the kind of outcome that can be expected just by limiting the possible range of outcomes. In the same way, an environment that provides a wealth of opportunities for positive outcomes will raise outcome expectations. Finally, outcome expectations are influenced by the goal that is involved (Carver & Scheier, 1982). Expectations of positive outcome are associated with goals that are readily attainable, while expectations of negative outcome are associated with goals that are unrealistic. Further, negative outcome expectations may change when goals that seem unattainable are broken down to component goals that are easier to read (Carver & Scheier, 1982).

The second person variable posed in this model is *self-efficacy*, "the conviction that one can successfully execute behavior required to produce outcomes" (Bandura, 1977, p. 193). Here, the person's belief about his or her own ability is the focus. The strength of these convictions will affect coping behaviors. For example, people will avoid situations they believe will exceed their coping skills and engage in those activities they feel capable of handling. The amount of effort expended and how long efforts will be sustained under adverse circumstances are also affected by efficacy expectations. According to Bandura (1977), one source of efficacy information is past performance accomplishments. Past successes tend to raise efficacy expectations while past failures tend to lower them. A second source of efficacy information is vicarious experience. Seeing others perform activities that result in positive outcomes is likely to generate feelings of self-efficacy, an "I can do it" attitude. A third source is verbal persuasion. People are led to believe, through suggestion, that they can cope effectively, thus raising efficacy expectations. A fourth source is emotional arousal. People's perceptions of their ability to cope are partially determined by their state of physiological arousal. Expectations of success may be higher when individuals are not in situations that cause physiological manifestations of tension or anxiety.

The third person variable to which Bandura refers is the *cognitive appraisal* made by the person about a situation. The specific role of cognitive appraisal in the processing of self-efficacy information is the focus here. The social, situational, and temporal circumstances under which efficacy information is received will enter into an individual's processing of such information. Because of this, information regarding performance may or may not influence already held efficacy beliefs. In addition, the cognitive appraisal of the causes of performance outcome, that is, what an individual attributes performance outcome to, is also a factor in affecting efficacy beliefs.

Other aspects of cognition that are especially relevant are cognitive competencies, those abilities, capacities, talents, or strengths the child has to draw upon to cope with stressful events. The kind of cognitive strategies the child employs in the organization of information may play a role in his or her behavior. These strategies may be long-standing modes of processing and/or may be influenced by a child's developmental level (Wassserman, 1983). A final aspect of cognition as a person variable to be considered is the self-imposed set of standards the child has. These may be quite maladaptive and thus may provide obstacles to intervention that are difficult to overcome.

Consistent with this social learning viewpoint, and extending it into the intervention realm, is a cognitive–behavioral perspective. Here the emphasis is on the direct assessment and modification of a person's cognitions. Meichenbaum (1976), for example, suggested that individuals' cognitions, what they say or don't say to themselves as well as the images they create, play a crucial role in their presenting complaint. Thus the individual's appraisals, attributions, expectations, and self-evaluations are the focal point, not only for describing behavior, as Bandura (1977) emphasized, but for helping people as well. Coping abilities can be increased by altering what people say to themselves in difficult situations (Meichenbaum, 1977). For example, cognitive self-instruction is one approach to altering maladaptive cognitions. This procedure involves one person modeling overt verbalizations, then having the subject copy these verbalizations overtly and then covertly. Cognitive self-instruction emphasizes the importance of cognitive processes on overt action and the voluntary control of behavior. It involves the modification of overt behavior by modifying accompanying cognitions. It also helps to shape specific expectations and aspects of self-efficacy. Many other cognitive–behavioral interventions have been described (see following sections for examples of those used with pediatric patients); what they share is a focus on cognitive change as a method of bringing about behavioral change.

Cognitive Assessment

As these notions about the importance of cognitive process have become more incorporated into views of behavior and intervention, cognitive assessment has become an integral part of planning and treatment evaluation. Before treatment, the role of cognitive assessment is to determine the degree to which cognitions are influencing the problem. Cognitive assessment is necessary "to study relationships among covert phenomena and their relationship to patterns of behavior and expressions of emotion" and "to study the role of covert processes in the development of distinct psychopathologies and to examine their role in the behavioral patterns associated with coping" (Kendall, 1982, p. 56). Thus cognitive assessment is used to determine those variables that are likely to impinge on the child's ability to cope with medical interventions and comply with medical instructions. These variables include outcome expectations, self-efficacy, and cognitions, as previously outlined.

Following treatment, the role of cognitive assessment is to evaluate the effects of treatment procedures (Kendall & Korgeski, 1979). It may also be concerned with evaluating the generalization of treatment effects on cognitions across varying situations and on the long-term effects of treatment on cognitions.

In summary, the range of cognitive–behavioral approaches to the treatment of medical disorders is quite broad. Some programs focus on increasing children's compliance with treatment regimes, some on eliminating the disorder altogether, some on diminishing children's anxiety and/or pain. Across the specific goals, however, cognitive changes either are manipulated directly or can be assumed to take place as a result of treatment. We have found it useful to organize our discussion around these cognitive changes rather than around treatment technique or medical disorder. In some cases, the placement within the discussion is somewhat arbitrary inasmuch as several cognitive processes are occurring in each treatment program or study. In other cases, it could be argued from a less cognitive theoretical position that treatment effectiveness is due only secondarily to cognitive change. With these caveats, however, treatment programs are presented in terms of cognitive processes assumed to accompany them. No attempt has been made to include every relevant study; rather, examples of treatment approaches are used to illustrate processes of change. Assessment approaches have been described in the literature for many of the cognitive factors, and these are presented in each section; suggestions for the development of assessment tools where they do not exist are made as well.

OUTCOME EXPECTATIONS

One important focus of cognitive assessment with children with medical problems is how they understand the contingencies of what is happening to them, or the "rules of the game." This is different from how they understand their own power or role in altering the course of the medical problem, or their feelings of self-efficacy (see next section). Here the emphasis in assessment is on understanding what the child sees as the given facts of the case. Included are topics like children's understanding of the prognosis of their disease or their views of the likelihood of success of a treatment. By understanding what the child sees as true, we can be focused in our attempts to modify misunderstandings and tailor treatments to individual differences.

Expectations About Medical Disorder

If children have misconceptions about the cause and expected course of the illnesses that confront them, we can expect that their response to prevention and treatment interventions may be hampered. A child's not understanding the role of diet in the control of diabetes, for example, forces compliance with dietary restriction to be in the hands of an overseeing, policing adult, whereas having a way of understanding why it is so important to regulate eating refocuses the problem on the diet, not the adult.

As background to understanding the impact of sick children's knowledge about their diseases, some investigators (e.g., Bibace & Walsh, 1980; Perrin & Gerrity, 1981; Redpath & Rogers, 1984; Simeonsson, Buckley, & Monson, 1979) have studied the ways in which healthy children of different developmental levels understand illness. Young children (i.e., 4 to 6 years old) are generally found to have an immature understanding of what different illnesses mean, how people get sick, how medicine works; their level of understanding is typically found to be consistent with their overall level of cognitive functioning, so this is not surprising. As children get older and develop more sophisticated levels of reasoning in general, their understanding of illness and health improves as well. Bibace and Walsh (1980) make important suggestions about how to describe illness to sick children while being sensitive to their developmental level of understanding. For example, illnesses can be described at the child's level (e.g., using terms like *bug*) while being reframed in a nonnegative and reassuring manner ("I know about this kind of bug, and it can only bite once") or described at one (but only one) level above the child's current level of functioning, in order to promote growth.

The *effects* of understanding or misunderstanding illness were not specifically tested in these studies. Less attention has been paid to this issue to date, though it is clearly important. Related studies are enlightening, nevertheless, and suggest that the approach of providing accurate information about disease should be continued. For example, Slavin, O'Malley, Koocher, and Foster (1982) report that children who received early notification and information about their own cancer diagnosis had better long-term adjustment than those who were told of their diagnosis after a delay, or learned of it on their own. Potter and Roberts (1984) approached the problem somewhat differently by assessing the attitudes and knowledge of children about chronic illness that might afflict a friend. Outcome measures focused on children's acceptance, comprehension, and ratings of attractiveness of an imaginary friend with a disease. Children who received explanatory rather than descriptive information about a disease showed increased comprehension of the disorder, though they did not necessarily rate the imaginary friend as more attractive. (Rated attractiveness was more a function of the observability of the disorder.) Thus the demonstration that young, healthy children do have illness misconceptions and that their understanding follows a predictable developmental course provides an important lesson to professionals concerned with providing health care to this population. Assessment of a child's understanding of the nature and causes of an illness should help the professional choose a level of discussion and prescription that can be understood by the child.

Expectations About Treatment

If children misunderstand illness, do they also misunderstand treatment? If children are utterly confused, and therefore frightened, by the equipment and procedures that are part of a treatment, we can expect them to be at least less cooperative and potentially less responsive to the effects of the treatment as well.

The less surprising and overwhelming the treatment can be made, presumably, the less the children will be distracted and frightened by it.

The nature of children's understanding of treatment has not been extensively assessed, although one exception is a study by Redpath and Rogers (1984), who found healthy children's understanding of hospitals, medical personnel, and operations to be developmentally related, according to the Piagetian interview approach described earlier. Several other investigators have simply assumed (probably correctly) that misunderstanding occurs and have taken the approach of specifically teaching children what to expect during the course of treatment. An example of this approach is the study and follow-up reported by Siegel and Peterson (1980, 1981). These investigators worked with three groups of child dental patients. One group received no special pretreatment except contact with an experimenter. A second received training in self-control coping skills like relaxation, breathing, imagery, and calming self-directed speech. The third (and most relevant here) was given sensory information about what would be happening to them. Typical physical sensations were described, as well as the sights and sounds that the child would encounter during the course of dental treatment. Both the self-control and the sensory information training resulted in less anxiety on the part of the children, as measured by behavioral ratings of cooperation and anxiety and pulse rate (Siegel & Peterson, 1980), and these effects were maintained at a second, follow-up visit to the dentist (Siegel & Peterson, 1981).

Similarly, Wolfer and Visintainer (1975) worked with children 3 to 14 years old who were facing minor surgery. The experimental group was given accurate information about the sequences of events and sensory experiences they would encounter, expectations about their and others' roles, and what appropriate responses would be. Several coping strategies were also taught (e.g., counting, relaxation, crying) and the children were given a choice about which to use. The experimental group was rated as more cooperative and less upset than the no-treatment control. Similar findings were reported by Melamed and her colleagues (Melamed, Meyer, Gee, & Soule, 1976; Melamed & Siegel, 1975; Melamed, Weinstein, Hawes, & Katin-Borland, 1975; Melamed, Yurcheson, Fleece, Hutcherson, & Hawes, 1978), who prepared children for hospitalization and surgery by describing or demonstrating some of the experiences that the children would encounter, and by Johnson, Kirchoff, and Endress (1975), who prepared children for orthopedic cast removal by providing information about sensory experiences to be encountered, about the procedure itself, or no information at all. Johnson and colleagues posited that these three conditions represented to the child decreasing levels of discrepancy between expected and experienced physical sensations, and hypothesized that the group with the least discrepancy (i.e., the sensory information group) would show the least distress during cast removal. The hypothesis was supported.

On the flip side, outcome expectations have been successfully manipulated to produce improvement even using placebo treatments. Alford, Zegiob, and Briston (1982) used a "placebo machine" to treat a 10-year-old girl referred for headaches, nightmares, and enuresis. This patient was told the machine would "draw out and remove" her symptoms. None of the target behaviors were exhibited after the fourth treatment session or at the 24-month follow-up. The effects can reasonably be attributed to the girl's expectations that the machine would be effective in her treatment.

Assessment of Knowledge About Medical Disorders and Treatment

These demonstrations of the effectiveness of providing accurate information about illness and treatment experiences are compelling evidence that children are indeed apprehensive due to ignorance; if it were not so, the interventions would not result in such differences in outcome. Still, little attention has been paid in the literature to accurately assessing children's expectations and/or knowledge. How do children understand their medical problems? How misunderstood are the treatments? What are children's baselines of knowledge? More precise information about an individual child's level of understanding would help us provide tailored and efficient interventions.

Expectations About the Effect One's Behavior Would Have on Health

Besides having knowledge about the nature and causes of disease and the nature and progression of treatment, it is important to understand children's beliefs about how their own behavior might influence health outcomes. This issue is distinct from that of self-efficacy, discussed in the following section. *Self-efficacy* refers to an individual's belief that he or she can do what needs to be done to effect an outcome. Here, we discuss an individual's belief that outcome can be influenced by behavior. For example, a group of adults 20 to 39 years old were more likely to view exercise as disease preventative, while a group of adults over 60 tended to see avoiding physical exertion as more effective in preventing heart attack and lung cancer (Prohaska, Leventhal, Leventhal, & Keller, 1985). Assessment of the nature of a child's behavior–outcome beliefs logically precedes attempts to modify such beliefs.

One area of investigation that has included both assessment of and treatments designed to change children's beliefs about the impact of behavior on outcome, and can be used as a model to illustrate this issue, is that of cigarette smoking prevention. Children's (i.e., 4-, 7-, and 11-year-olds) understanding of the consequences of smoking has been shown to be related to their cognitive developmental level, with older children showing more formal logical and younger children more prelogical reasoning (Meltzer, Bibace, & Walsh, 1984). In reviewing different components of smoking prevention treatment programs for adolescents, McCaul and Glasgow (1985) conclude that smoking prevention programs have generally been most successful in increasing the amount of knowledge that adolescents have about short- and long-term effects of smoking, that is, their understanding of how their smoking behavior would influence their health. Twelve of 13 studies reviewed reported an increase in knowledge about the effects of smoking. Unfortunately, the relationship between knowledge and actual smoking was unclear and/or not very strong in these studies. The studies reviewed were less effective in altering adolescents' attitudes about smoking, although the authors suggest that reported attitudes may have been at a very negative level at the beginning, allowing little room for change. In general, however, the correlations between attitudes toward smoking and actual smoking were distressingly low. Thus while knowledge and attitudes about the consequences of smoking may be fundamentally important, perhaps even necessary (though not sufficient) for behavior change, other factors such as adolescents' perceptions about peer reactions, social competence to refuse, and the factors that influence intention to smoke must also be considered.

SELF-EFFICACY

A second important area of cognitive assessment is the degree to which treatments, whatever their nature, make lasting changes in children's attributions about their ability to have an impact on a desired outcome, or their self-efficacy (Bandura, 1977). Distinct from *outcome efficacy*, in which we are interested in children's understanding (accurate or not) of what is alterable or modifiable, *self-efficacy* refers to children's beliefs about their own abilities. Cognitive–behavioral treatment programs that address this issue, it could be argued, are designed around the assumption that children have inadequate levels of self-efficacy, or at least could benefit from increases in self-efficacy; thus the programs are focused on bolstering these levels. Little attention is paid in these studies to the assessment of actual self-efficacy levels; the outcome variable in these programs is usually on some measure of degree of adjustment. For example, children with disorder *X* needing treatment *Y* are assumed to have skill deficiencies and, perhaps, lower than optimal levels of self-efficacy. Coping skills, which probably yield improvements in self-efficacy along with other more direct skill levels, are taught, and improvement in disorder *X* or an increase in cooperation with treatment *Y* is assessed. Self-efficacy usually remains an invisible and unassessed moderator of effects. In the following sections, we first describe several methods that have been used to assess self-efficacy, and then, as we describe some of the approaches that have been used with children with medical disorders, we focus on how self-efficacy may be being altered through the treatment.

ASSESSMENT OF SELF-EFFICACY

For the most part, assessment of this construct has been done on an individual basis, using a questionnaire, rating scale, or other method that is tailor-made to the case or type of disorder under study. An exception, in which some more general notion is tapped, is the Generalized Self-Efficacy (GSE) Scale, designed for use with college students (Tipton & Worthington, 1984). Students with higher GSE scores were found to achieve at a physical task and to strive toward higher goal attainment than students with lower GSE scores.

A more common approach with children is to ask them to report their expectations for their own success. This can be done simply by asking them to rate on a scale how likely they think they are to succeed at coping with some medical treatment or at showing medical improvement. Sometimes a less direct approach is taken in order to understand more about the content of the self-efficacy belief. Nelson (1981), for example, felt that an 11-year-old girl's dental phobia was due to her expectations about her ability to cope (as well as her expectations about treatment); so she asked the patient to close her eyes and image and describe in detail a recent visit to the dentist. Nelson used the specific content of the images and negative self-statements produced by the girl to plan the treatment. Similarly, Weinstein (1976) taught a 10-

year-old burn victim to relax, then visualize and describe positive, calming experiences, ones in which he presumably was efficacious. Again, the child's individually designed images about self-efficacy were used in treatment.

Increases in Self-Efficacy Through Performance Accomplishments

If children can be helped to have some success experience, they are more likely to believe that they can succeed again. Conversely, failure experiences may teach a child that success is beyond reach. Thus some treatment approaches are designed to help children succeed where they have not succeeded before. For example, in the case study of an 11-year-old girl with dental anxiety just described, Nelson (1981) assumed that cognitions and images from a prior traumatic dental visit played a determining role in her present problem. Nelson used an imagery assessment technique to focus on the girl's internal dialogue. From the images and negative self-statements produced, she was taught to emit more adaptive self-statements, thus enhancing cooperation in the current dental situation. The negative earlier experience, then, was assumed to have produced in the girl the subsequent aversion and the assumption that she would "fail" (i.e., not be able to cope with the dental visit). Treatment focused on successfully changing this negative lesson by teaching positive coping statements.

Treatment approaches involving in vivo desensitization may also be contributing to a child's self-efficacy by providing positive performance histories. Weinstein (1976) worked with a 10-year-old burn victim who had developed a phobia to bathing, a critical component of the treatment to remove accumulation of scar tissue. The child's self-reported positive images were used during actual bathing episodes, accompanied by trained relaxation, to help the child cope with the bath. Incidents of screaming, hitting, and other phobic responses all diminished. While some combination of components may be functioning (including the effects of the child's medication and the physical effects of relaxation), it is reasonable to assume that, having once had a less traumatic bath, the child would incorporate more positive beliefs about his own ability and that this would contribute to future success and treatment maintenance.

Simple attribution about performance accomplishments may also be influential is affecting outcome. Chambliss and Murray (1979a, 1979b) gave placebo pills to adolescents trying to stop smoking and to women trying to lose weight, respectively. Half the subjects were later told that the pill had been a placebo, and that any change that had occurred had been due to their own efforts (the self-efficacy condition); the other half was allowed to continue attributing success to the pill. The self-efficacy group showed greater improvement than the drug attribution group, suggesting that feeling a sense of accomplishment about one's performance was indeed helpful.

Performance accomplishments can also be provided to children prior to, and thus preventing, the development of adjustment problems. Cassell (1965) exposed 20 children 3 to 11 years old to puppet therapy prior to cardiac catheterization procedures, and compared their response to 20 same-aged children in a control group. Puppets were provided to children in the treatment group for the roles of doctor, nurse, boy, girl, mother, and father, as was miniature equipment that resembled real medical equipment, for example, table, red lights, surgical masks, hospital gowns. The child and therapist acted out the entire catheterization procedure from both the child's and doctor's roles, including giving a shot, putting on a hospital gown, listening to the heart, having arms and legs restrained, applying antispetic, giving stitches, taking blood pressure, and so on. Children in the therapy group showed significantly less distress during the actual catheterization procedure and were significantly more willing to return to the hospital for follow-up treatment than were the children in the control group. While real performance was not included and while knowledge about treatment was probably also increased in the puppet therapy group, the author argued that children in the therapy group had been given a mastery experience through the puppet play, and that that was in turn related to better adjustment during the procedure.

Increases in Self-Efficacy Through Vicarious Experience

Related approaches to helping children are those that expose children to models who successfully cope with medical treatment. Here, the assumption is that, even if children do not experience success themselves, they learn that they could be successful by watching others succeed. A series of studies that illustrate this approach has been reported on the preparation of children for dental work or surgery (e.g., Ferguson, 1979; Melamed et al., 1976; Melamed et al., 1975; Melamed et al., 1978; Melamed & Siegel, 1975; Peterson & Shigetomi, 1981; Roberts, Wurtele, Boone, Ginther, & Elkins, 1986). The basic paradigm is that one group of children who are actually facing surgery or dental appointments are shown a peer modeling film prior to the medical care. The child in the film is shown to be facing the same medical setting and/or equipment that the subjects will be facing. He demonstrates coping strategies and successfully deals with the medical intervention. A second group of children is given some comparison treatment (e.g., a control film, or the same film at a different time) and the adjustment to treatment is measured, usually rated fear and anxiety, maladaptive behavior, pulse, and/or temperature. Peer modeling treatments have generally been quite successful in positively affecting treatment adjustment. The details of one such study will be given as an example of this approach.

Melamed and Siegel (1975) worked with 60 children 4 to 12 years old who were facing elective surgery that would involve a hospital stay of 2 to 3 days. On the day of admission, one group of children saw a 16-minute peer modeling film about a child being hospitalized and going through surgery; a second group saw a 12-minute unrelated control film about a nature trip. The peer modeling film, *Ethan Has an Operation*, showed a 7-year-old boy in various scenes encountered during admission for a hernia operation (e.g., having a blood test, or being separated from his mother), and various scenes in which the child described his fears and successful coping strategies. Adjustment to the hospitalization was found to be better for children in the film group, as assessed in a number of ways: children's self-report of anxiety, observers' ratings of the children's anxiety and adjustment, the Palmar Sweat Index, and mothers' reports of behavior problems following discharge.

Thus while self-efficacy was not specifically addressed in this study, one can argue that the children who saw a filmed peer successfully cope "learned" that they, too, would be likely to cope with hospitalization. It would be theoretically important to confirm that self-efficacy is indeed the moderator of this type of treatment, if this argument is to continue being made. For that, attributions of self-efficacy would have to be *assessed prior to and following* the peer modeling film, and shown to be related to amount of adjustment during and following hospitalization.

Increases in Self-Efficacy Through Verbal Persuasion

In a sense, most treatment procedures probably include some component of verbal persuasion, a "come on, I know you can do it" or "this treatment is really going to work now" message, even though this is seldom the focus of the treatment or its report in the literature. Verbal persuasion itself was emphasized in a study by Weinberg, Hughes, Critelli, England, and Jackson (1984), however, in their work with children, adolescents, and adults trying to lose weight. Self-efficacy manipulations were carried out by the therapist's periodic assertions during each treatment session of the subject's specially selected capabilities for success. The therapist would label task completion as exceptional and attribute those behaviors to the client's previously unrecognized capacity for self-control. Indeed, those subjects high in manipulated self-efficacy lost more weight over time than did those in the nonmanipulated self-efficacy group.

Increases in Self-Efficacy Through Reduction in Emotional Arousal

Problems in response or adjustment to medical intervention with children are often assumed to be rooted in fear or anxiety. Some treatment approaches are based on the assumption that reducing emotional arousal will facilitate better response or adjustment. For example, Russell and Carter (1978) trained a group of children to decrease their levels of EMG activity. Ten standard measures of classroom achievement showed significant improvement, in comparison with a group of untrained control group children. The authors concluded that, as the children became more relaxed, they learned more effectively. In the same way, heightened levels of arousal are also likely to interfere with treatment in the hospital. Thus a number of approaches have successfully demonstrated that training children to relax, whether by biofeedback, imagery, symbolic desensitization, or other approaches, helps them cope with stressful medical interventions.

Induction of self-efficacy need not be posed as the sole mechanism by which these treatments work, as it is seldom clear exactly how relaxation-based techniques function, that is, whether they have a physical effect on bodily functioning and/or whether there is a cognitive component wherein patients conclude from successfully calm episodes that they are effective copers. Even if multiply determined, however, the effectiveness of these approaches has been clearly demonstrated. Several examples can illustrate this point.

First, a different aspect of one study already described (Siegel & Peterson, 1980) can be highlighted. Forty-two young dental patients were assigned to one of three groups: an adult-contact-only control, a sensory information group, and a self-control coping skills training group. This last group is the relevant one here: The training consisted of teaching children relaxation skills, breathing, using relaxing cue words like *calm* or *nice*, pleasant imagery, and calming self-talk. The two treatments were more effective in reducing stress in the children than the control condition, as measured by dentist and observer ratings of cooperation and anxiety and, for the coping skills group, children's pulse rates. Thus training relaxation was effective in reducing stress. Whether children conclude, consciously or not, that they are more self-efficacious remains to be tested.

In a review of studies of relaxation therapy for the treatment of asthma, Erskine-Millis and Schonell (1981) suggest that relaxation therapy is based on the notion that emotional arousal can act as either a precipitator or an exacerbator of asthma. Relaxation is seen as the opposite of arousal and may interrupt the cycle between emotional and physical symptoms. The authors conclude that muscular relaxation alone appears to be ineffective in the treatment of asthma, but that *mental relaxation* techniques such as meditation, autosuggestion, and autogenic training seem to produce clinically and statistically significant improvements in pulmonary function.

Roberts and Gordon (1979) used systematic desensitization to help eliminate a fire-related phobia in a 5-year-old girl who had been burned in an accident. Exposure to magazine pictures of fires was paired with playing with a favorite toy; exposure could gradually be increased from 15 seconds to a minute. The phobia diminished and was still absent at a 6-month follow-up. Thus through symbolic, not in vivo, desensitization, the girl's emotional arousal was lowered, with beneficial effects.

As a final example, Zeltzer, Dash, and Holland (1979) hypnotized two adolescents with sickle cell disease, instructing them to imagine increasing bodily warmth and comfort, their blood vessels dilating and allowing the sickled cells to pass along with the "good, rich, healthy red cells." The authors reported a decrease in the frequency and intensity of pain crises, need for heavy analgesia, number of emergency room visits, and frequency and length of hospitalization for pain. Importantly, both adolescents also reported feeling more "in control" of their bodies and less reliant on external agents for help.

Thus it can be argued that children who are relaxed are learning the message, by observing themselves in a calm mode, that they can handle the situation facing them. To the extent that this is true, these approaches function by increasing feelings of self-efficacy.

Assessment of Emotional Arousal. The level of emotional arousal is often assumed to be a mediator of treatment outcome, and thus is important to assess carefully. Generally, measures are taken both before and after medical treatment, with the expectation that children who received help of one sort or another will show less arousal than those in comparison groups. Several different approaches have been taken to the measurement of arousal and can be broadly fit into one of three categories: physiological, self-report, and observational measures.

Children's arousal during medical procedures has been operationalized by measuring a number of physical changes: muscle tension (Ferguson, 1979), pulse rate (Johnson et al., 1975; Peterson & Shigetomi, 1981; Venham, Bengston, & Cipes, 1977), body temperature (Peterson & Shigetomi, 1981), fluid and food consumption following surgery (Peterson & Shigetomi, 1981), latency to void following surgery (Peterson & Shigetomi, 1981), and the Palmar Sweat Index (Melamed et al., 1976; Melamed & Siegel, 1975). While these are not measures of emotional arousal per se, and while the agreement among various physiological measures is often poor (Glennon & Weisz, 1978), these particular variables have been found to be related to experimental treatments and in the expected direction.

The accuracy of self-reports of psychological state may be problematic for any group of people, and this is particularly true for children. Several innovative techniques have been described, however, that appear to tap children's feelings of anxiety about specific medical issues. A general Fear Survey Schedule for Children (Scherer & Nakamura, 1968) was modified by Melamed and Siegel (1975) by taking the eight items from its Medical Fears subscale and adding eight other items with face validity and several filler items, to form what the authors called the Hospital Fears Rating Scale. Children rate their fear for each item on a "thermometer" from 1 (none) to 5 (high). Venham and colleagues (1977) developed a Picture Test to assess anxiety in children at dental visits. The test consists of eight drawings of pairs of boys, each depicting a different emotion (e.g., one smiling, one crying) or reaction (e.g., one sitting in a chair, one running away from a chair). Children are to choose the boy in each pair who feels most the way they feel. Finally, the specific content of children's anxiety has been assessed by asking them to imagine and describe past scenes that have been evocative for them. In one case study (Smith & Sharpe, 1970), a child was not able to say exactly what was anxiety producing about a phobic situation, so he was asked to describe in minute detail a typical scene while the therapist watched for flushing of the skin, an increase in bodily movements, muscular tension, vocal tension, and tears. The parts of the imagined scene that were accompanied by these signs of tension became the focus of successful intervention.

A final approach has been to ask others—parents, technicians, doctors, researchers—to observe a child for signs of arousal. In some cases, medical personnel are asked merely to rate on a 5- or 7-point scale the child's anxiety or cooperation during a medical procedure (Peterson & Shigetomi, 1981; Siegel & Peterson, 1981; Venham et al., 1977). In other cases, more detailed and specific coding has been done, often by researchers or trained observers. In general, these coding systems have provided reliable, valid, and practical information, but they are very time-consuming. For example, Melamed and colleagues (1975) developed a Behavior Profile Rating Scale for use in a dental office, consisting of 4 items concerning the child's separation from mother (e.g., "refuses to leave mother," "bodily carried in") and 23 items concerning the office behavior (e.g., "refuses to open mouth," "attempts to dislodge instruments"). Each item was weighted according to how disruptive dentists found it; a child's score consisted of the frequency of each behavior multiplied by the weighting factor per 3-minute interval. Children in this study were 5 to 9 years old; an observation system for preschoolers has also been described that appears to have adequate reliability and validity (Glennon & Weisz, 1978). Behavioral signs of distress relevant to particular medical procedures have also been reported. Katz, Kellerman, and Siegel (1980) observed children undergoing bone marrow aspirations and rated behavioral items such as verbal expressions of pain, crying, muscular rigidity, screaming, needing to be carried, requesting termination, and refusing to stay in the required position. Johnson and colleagues (1975) observed children during orthopedic cast removal and rated behavior such as saying "stop," holding the doctor's hand, and kicking.

COGNITIVE APPRAISAL

Finally, it is important to remember that information about both outcome expectations and self-efficacy may be moderated by a child's cognitive appraisals (Bandura, 1977). For example, older children may incorporate information differently than do younger children. Information that contradicts long-standing beliefs or styles may be incorporated more slowly than noncontradictory information. Children's beliefs about why they behave as they do may affect the power of treatments designed to alter efficacy. Or distorted beliefs may be intransigent obstacles to efforts at change. Several studies have noted the importance of assessing these cognitive variables.

Developmental Level

Wasserman (1983) presents a convincing argument, in his review of cognitive-behavioral interventions, for the necessity of assessing a child's cognitive developmental level before trying to apply these techniques. He suggests that many cognitive–behavioral treatments require skills that would not be expected to be present in younger children in the normal course of development. Therefore, the use of these techniques may be ineffective. For example, Wasserman notes that self-instructional techniques may be useful for younger children only on highly specific tasks, because the ability to generalize from this training may not occur developmentally until much later. Modeling may be quite useful for younger children, on the other hand, since it requires not language skills, but just the ability to represent experience through images and to reproduce these images in their original form. Imagery as a therapeutic device may not be beneficial for younger children until they can process and relate imagery to overt behavior, such as occurs in the development of formal operational thought. Finally, techniques that require linguistic processing skills as the basis for change may only be useful for those children who are cognitively advanced.

A number of studies, mentioned in the earlier section on outcome expectations, have addressed the question of how different-aged children understand illness (Bibace & Walsh, 1980; Perrin & Gerrity, 1981; Redpath & Rogers, 1984; Simeonsson et al., 1979). These studies often use a Piagetian (1929, 1930) model to organize their findings from interviews with children. Both models describe children as using cognitive, logical reasoning that is fundamentally and qualitatively different from that of adults. As children develop, their approach to reasoning changes, reflecting increasing levels of differentiation; that is, their understanding of concepts becomes more refined, and their understanding of self versus other becomes clarified.

For example, Bibace and Walsh (1980) interviewed 72 normal, well children who were 4, 7, or 11 years old. Children were asked a series of questions about the definitions (e.g., "What is a . . . ?") and causes (e.g., "How do people get . . . ?") of different common illnesses like colds, headaches, and measles. Children's responses were placed into one of six categories, which in turn fell into one of three levels: prelogical, concrete logical, and formal logical explanations. Older children were more likely to use the higher levels of reasoning. Prelogical explanations (phenomenism and contagion) are characterized by children's descriptions of immediately contiguous, concrete events that accompany illness and that are linked inexplicably, or by magic, to outcome ("people get colds by being outside—they just do, that's all"). In concrete logical explanations (contamination and internalization), the child can distinguish between what is internal and what is external to the self. Causes of illness are described as external and the effects as internal, though both are still nonspecific ("people get colds by breathing in too much cold air and the bacteria get in and make the lungs soft and it goes to the nose"). In formal logical explanations (physiological and psychophysiological) children have a more sophisticated understanding of the differentiation between the internal and external world, and understand that the source of illness may be a combination of external agents and internal states ("people get colds when there are more germs than platelets" or "people have heart attacks when they are all wracked up and worried too much").

Assessment of Developmental Level of Understanding. For the most part in clinical practice, developmental level is inferred from a child's chronological age: children 4 to 6 years old function at a prelogical level of reasoning, children 7 to 10 at a level of concrete logical reasoning, and adolescents at a more abstract level of reasoning. Studies that have confirmed that medical understanding conforms to these guidelines have often done so by comparing children's level of understanding of illness with their understanding of more general phenomena (Perrin & Gerrity, 1981; Redpath & Rogers, 1984; Simeonsson et al., 1979). It is from a fuller understanding of a child's general cognitive level that we can predict—and address—children's misinformation about illness and treatment.

Piagetian tasks (1929, 1930) have been useful in revealing important aspects of cognitive level. A Concept Assessment Kit exists for the assessment of conservation. (See Simeonsson et al., 1979, for an example of using it to assess both conservation and children's understanding of illness.) Understanding of the causes of illness has been compared with children's notions about physical causality in general by interviewing children about the origin of night and the mobility of clouds (Perrin & Gerrity, 1981; Redpath & Rogers, 1984; Simeonsson et al., 1979). Understanding of various aspects of illness has similarly been compared to understanding of egocentrism (Simeonsson et al., 1979), transformation (Perrin & Gerrity, 1981), and abstract thinking (Perrin & Gerrity, 1981). If a child is suspected of functioning at a cognitive level lower than that predicted by his or her chronological age, some of these items could be administered in conjunction with direct questions about the child's understanding of illness, with less time and effort and probably with more useful results than administering an IQ test. Results could be used to guide the level of interview with the child about his or her understanding of the illness.

Cognitive Styles and Long-Standing Beliefs

Long-standing modes or styles of thinking also provide a backdrop for children's response to our interventions. Understanding how these may influence or interact with treatment will improve the efficiency of our attempts. For example, Hart (1984) studied adolescent and adult patients who suffered from headaches. The subjects were placed in either a biofeedback group or a relaxation training group. Hart found that those patients with high scores on a cognitive measure of preference for structure (e.g., clear goals, guidelines, and procedures) were more likely to benefit from a structured relaxation training approach than from a relatively unstructured biofeedback task, thus demonstrating the importance of understanding a person's cognitive style.

In addition, the degree to which a child attributes outcomes to luck, fate, chance, or other external sources versus personal or internal sources is also a relevant dimension of cognitive style. The issue of the relationship of control and adjustment with illness among adults has been addressed more frequently than it has with children. Taylor (1982) discusses hospital patient behavior as a function of reaction, helplessness, and control. Specifically, the depersonalization and bureaucracy inherent in hospitals are posed as being conducive to feelings of loss of control, as are the fact of being sick in the first place and the frequent differing opinions of medical staff. Pennebaker (1982) has reported that adults who have no control over aversive stimuli report more symptoms than adults who do have control. This issue of control over the illness was also addressed by Felton and Revenson (1984). Adults with types of illnesses that either provided few opportunities for control (e.g., arthritis, cancer) or were responsive to individual or medical control (e.g., hypertension, diabetes) were compared for levels of adjustment. In addition, the adults were classified as using either an information-seeking or a wish-fulfilling fantasy approach to coping. The information-seeking strategy was found to be related to better adjustment than the wish-fulfillment approach, but no effects were found for controllability. On the other hand, Auerbach, Kendall, Cuttler, and Levitt (1976) manipulated the use of specific versus general information about treatment for dental patients and found that adults with internal loci of control responded better to specific information, while those with external loci responded better to general information. Thus with adults at least, control over illness and/or treatment has been found to be a salient feature of adjustment and recovery.

Kellerman, Zeltzer, Ellenberg, Dash, and Rigler (1980) compared healthy adolescents with those with serious or chronic diseases (from oncology, cardiology, diabetes, cystic fibrosis, nephrology, and rheumatology clinics) on measures of anxiety, self-esteem, and locus of control. The major finding of the study was that the ill groups, especially those with rheumatism, were generally more external in their perceptions of control than the healthy groups, although this was not true for the ill children with diabetes or cystic fibrosis. The authors suggested that children seemed to be more external when this was in fact more realistic, and more internal when, as with diabetes or cystic fibrosis, the course was somewhat under their own control, through diet or self-administered medication.

That control may be important in children's adjustment to surgery was also suggested by Wolfer and Visintainer (1975), who included as part of their preparation-for-surgery treatment a component in which the child was given the choice about which coping strategy (e.g. to count, to cry, to use muscle relaxation) to use. The treatment group showed better adjustment than the comparison group, although the control component was not tested separately from the rest of the preparation.

Assessment of Perceived Control. Several standardized measures of children's perceived control over their environment exist in the literature. They differ in the age of child for which they are appropriate (e.g., the Stanford Preschool Internal-External Scale [Mischel, Zeiss, & Zeiss, 1974], the Nowicki-Strickland Internal-External Scale [1973] for school-age children) and in whether they have a specific focus (e.g., Intellectual Achievement Responsibility [Crandall, Katkovsky, & Crandall, 1965], the Health and Locus of Control Scale [Wallston, Wallston, Kaplan, & Mardes, 1976]) or a general one (Nowicki & Strickland, 1973). All these measures involve close-ended questions (either yes–no or forced-choice items) and may be subject to distortion by social desirability (Weisz & Stipek, 1982), response set (Stephens & Delys, 1973; Weisz & Stipek, 1982), or the child's verbal and memory ability

(Gorsuch, Henighan, & Barnard, 1972; Weisz & Stipek, 1982). Nevertheless, they have been useful in helping to understand children's perceptions of control.

Distorted or Maladaptive Cognitions

Distorted and maladaptive beliefs about the self or the world have been posed as the basis for many disorders (Beck, 1976), and, even if they are not considered fundamental, they certainly can be expected to affect the outcome of treatment. Garner and Bemis (1982) have discussed the role of cognitive factors in the development and maintenance of anorexia nervosa, for example. Distorted thoughts and beliefs are often verbalized by patients even after weight gain. Among these beliefs is the idea on the part of the anorexic that she (or he) must be thin. The assessment of anorexic cognitions reveals a variety of other distortions in the processing and interpretation of events. These distortions may take several forms: selective abstraction (or basing conclusions on isolated details while ignoring contradictory and more salient evidence), overgeneralization (or extracting a rule on the basis of one event and applying it to other dissimilar situations), magnification (or the overestimation of the significance of undesirable events), dichotomous reasoning (or thinking in extreme or absolute terms), personalization (or the egocentric interpretation of impersonal events), and superstitious thinking (or believing in cause–effect relationships among noncontingent events). Fairburn (1981) suggests that the same kinds of misconceptions are involved in the development and maintenance of bulimia. Ollendick (1979) treated a 16-year-old male for anorexia nervosa. Prior to treatment, a 3-day observation period revealed that anxiety associated with weight gain and negative peer criticism maintained the boy's anorectic behavior. Treatment consisted of six phases. In the first phase, the boy was weighed and given feedback regarding his weight. Deep muscle relaxation training and systematic desensitization were also employed. The second phase was a feedback-only phase. The third and fourth phases were the same as the first and second, feedback and desensitization, followed by feedback only. The fifth phase introduced cognitive restructuring along with the feedback. The subject monitored his thoughts about weight gained, capabilities, excuses, and peer perceptions between therapy sessions. During sessions, maladaptive thoughts were analyzed and restructured. The sixth phase again consisted of feedback only. Results showed that weight gain was not maintained except after the introduction of cognitive restructuring. Eighteen months later, weight gain had remained stable. At 24 months, weight loss was evident and maintenance sessions resulted in rapid weight recovery. Thus the alteration of maladaptive cognitions was, in this case, the critical factor in improvement.

Bruenlin (1980), in treating a 46-month-old boy for eliminative disturbance, emphasized the importance of a multimodal approach to assessment and treatment. He assessed seven interdependent and interactive modalities of functioning: behavior, affect, sensation, imagery, cognition, interpersonal relationships, and drugs. Affect, imagery, and cognition are the modalities that are specifically cognitive in nature. Affects assessed included fears and anger regarding elimination. Imagery and cognition included misconceptions and irrational beliefs regarding the toilet and the eliminative disturbance. Breunlin's interventions were successfully applied specifically to each of the seven areas assessed. Cognitively based interventions consisted of the recognition and validation of expressed affect, direct cognitive appeal aimed at dispelling irrational beliefs, and mutual story telling for targeting images.

In a study of gastric output in males 16 to 28 years old, Sigman and Amit (1982) noted that increases in acid secretion may be more closely related to cognitive rather than somatic activity. Eleven of their 14 subjects reported feeling physically relaxed, yet 7 of them had increased levels of acid, possibly due to spontaneous anxious thoughts. Maladaptive cognitions, then, clearly can interfere with treatment effectiveness.

Assessment of Dysfunctional Cognitions. Kendall and Korgeski (1979) emphasize the importance of assessing both functional and dysfunctional cognitions in order to understand their role in the development of disorders and the process of coping, as well as to confirm the effects of treatment on cognitions. While many of the assessment techniques they describe have been used primarily with adults, the approaches could be modified and applied to assessment in children as well. For example, in vivo thought sampling involves asking the subject to record thoughts and feelings whenever a beeper sounds. This technique is particularly useful in understanding the frequency and content of pervasive or non–situation-specific cognitions, as might be the case with distorted or maladaptive thoughts. In guided imagery, subjects are asked to think about some assigned topic of relevance to the treatment, and to report cognitions that occur to them; the Nelson (1981) and Weinstein (1976) case studies described earlier are good examples of this approach with pediatric patients. Finally, some attempts have been made to assess standard lists of self-statements thought to be common in people with similar problems. With children, however, more individually designed approaches are more common.

SUMMARY

A variety of psychological approaches to the treatment of pediatric problems have been described within a structure that emphasizes cognitive changes that occur in children as a result of intervention. Any single treatment program probably functions in a number of ways, including the alteration of a number of cognitive characteristics in the children. Treatments may be effective in their manipulation of children's outcome expectancies; that is, they may focus on expectations about the medical disorder itself, about how or whether a treatment will work, or about the effect one's behavior would have on health. Some treatment programs also probably affect children's sense of self-efficacy by providing them with performance accomplishments, vicarious experience, attempts at verbal persuasion, or reductions in emotional arousal. Others attempt to alter, or at least be sensitive to, children's cognitive appraisal characteristics, including their developmental level, their long-standing beliefs and styles, and any maladaptive cognitions that may exist. All of these cognitive changes are important to assess if we are to evaluate the basis of improvement accurately and plan future interventions efficiently. Assessment tools that have been used in prior studies have been described, as have the many needs for new tools that exist in this field.

References

Alford, G. S., Zegiob, L., & Briston, A. K. (1982). Use of instructions and apparatus-enhanced suggestion in treating a case of headaches, nightmares, and nocturnal enuresis. *Psychotherapy: Theory, Research & Practice, 19,* 110–115.

Auerbach, S. M., Kendall, P. C., Cuttler, H. F., & Levitt, N. R. (1976). Anxiety, locus of control, type of prepatory information, and adjustment to dental surgery. *Journal of Consulting & Clinical Psychology, 44*, 809–818.

Bandura, A. (1977). Self-efficacy: Toward a unifying theory of behavioral change. *Psychological Review, 84*, 191–215.

Beck, A. T. (1976). *Cognitive theory and the emotional disorders*. New York: International Universities Press.

Bibace, R., & Walsh, M. E. (1980). Children's conceptions of illness. *Pediatrics, 66*, 912–917.

Breunlin, D. C. (1980). Multimodal behavioral treatment of a child's eliminative disturbance. *Psychotherapy: Theory, Research & Practice, 17*, 17–23.

Carver, C. S., & Scheier, M. F. (1982). An information processing perspective on self-management. In P. Karoly & F. H. Kanfer (Eds.), *Self management and behavior change: From theory to practice*. New York: Pergamon.

Cassell, D. (1965). Effect of brief puppet therapy upon the emotional responses of children undergoing cardiac catheterization. *Journal of Consulting Psychology, 29*, 1–8.

Chambliss, C. A., & Murray, E. J. (1979a). Cognitive procedures for smoking reduction: Symptom attribution versus efficacy attribution. *Cognitive Therapy & Research, 3*, 91–96.

Chambliss, C. A., & Murray, E. J. (1979b). Efficacy attribution, locus of control and weight loss. *Cognitive Therapy & Research, 3*, 349–354.

Crandall, V. C., Katkovsky, W., & Crandall, V. J. (1965). Children's beliefs in their own control of reinforcements in intellectual-academic achievement situation. *Child Development, 36*, 91–109.

Erskine-Millis, J., & Schonell, M. (1981). Relaxation therapy in asthma: A critical review. *Psychosomatic Medicine, 43*, 365–372.

Fairburn, C. (1981). A cognitive–behavioral approach to the treatment of bulimia nervosa. *Psychosomatic Medicine, 11*, 707–711.

Felton, B. J., & Revenson, T. A. (1984). Coping with chronic illness: A study of illness controllability and the usefulness of coping strategies on psychological adjustment. *Journal of Consulting & Clinical Psychology, 52*(3), 343–353.

Ferguson, B. F. (1979). Preparing young children for hospitalization: A comparison of two methods. *Pediatrics, 64*, 656–664.

Garner, D. M., & Bemis, K. M. (1982). A cognitive–behavioral approach to anorexia nervosa. *Cognitive Therapy & Research, 6*, 123–150.

Glennon, B., & Weisz, J. R. (1978). An observational approach to the assessment of anxiety in young children. *Journal of Consulting & Clinical Psychology, 46*, 1246–1257.

Gorsuch, R. L., Henighan, R. P., & Barnard, C. (1972). Locus of control—An example of dangers in using children's scales with children. *Child Development, 43*, 579–590.

Hart, J. D. (1984). Predicting differential response to EMG biofeedback and relaxation training: The role of cognitive structure. *Journal of Clinical Psychology, 40*, 453–457.

Johnson, J. E., Kirchoff, K. T., & Endress, M. P. (1975). Altering children's distress behavior during orthopedic cast removal. *Nursing Research, 24*, 404–410.

Katz, E. R., Kellerman, J., & Siegel, S. E. (1980). Behavioral distress in children with cancer undergoing medical procedures: Developmental considerations. *Journal of Consulting & Clinical Psychology, 48*, 356–365.

Kellerman, J., Zeltzer, L., Ellenberg, L., Dash, J., & Rigler, D. (1980). Psychological effects of illness in adolescence: I. Anxiety, self-esteem, and perception of control. *Journal of Pediatrics, 97*, 126–131.

Kendall, P. C. (1982). Behavioral assessment and methodology. *Annual Review of Behavior Therapy: Theory & Practice, 8*, 39–81.

Kendall, P. C., & Korgeski, G. P. (1979). Assessment and cognitive–behavioral intervention. *Cognitive Therapy & Research, 3*, 1–21.

McCaul, K. D., & Glasgow, R. E. (1985). Preventing adolescent smoking: What have we learned about treatment construct validity? *Health Psychology, 4*(4), 361–388.

Meichenbaum, D. (1976). A cognitive–behavior modification approach to assessment. In M. Hersen & A. S. Bellack (Eds.), *Behavioral assessment: A practical handbook*. New York: Pergamon.

Meichenbaum, D. (1977). *Cognitive–behavior modification: An integrative approach.* New York: Plenum.

Melamed, B. G., Meyer, R., Gee, C., & Soule, L. (1976). The influence of time and type of preparations on children's adjustment to hospitalization. *Journal of Pediatric Psychology, 1*(4), 31–37.

Melamed, B. G., & Siegel, L. J. (1975). Reduction of anxiety in children facing hospitalization and surgery by use of filmed modeling. *Journal of Consulting & Clinical Psychology, 43*, 511–521.

Melamed, B. G., Weinstein, D., Hawes, R., & Katin-Borland, M. (1975). Reduction of fear-related dental management problems with use of filmed modeling. *Journal of American Dental Association, 90*, 822–826.

Melamed, B. G., Yurcheson, R., Fleece, E. L., Hutcherson, S., & Hawes, R. (1978). Effects of film modeling on the reduction of anxiety-related behaviors in individuals varying in level of previous experience in the stress situation. *Journal of Consulting & Clinical Psychology, 46*, 1357–1367.

Meltzer, J., Bibace, R., & Walsh, M. E. (1984). Children's conception of smoking. *Journal of Pediatric Psychology, 9*(1), 41–56.

Mischel, W., Zeiss, R., & Zeiss, A. (1974). Internal–external control and persistence: Validation and implications of the Stanford Preschool Internal-External Scale. *Journal of Personality & Social Psychology, 29*, 265–278.

Nelson, W. M. (1981). A cognitive–behavioral treatment for disproportionate dental anxiety and pain: A case study. *Journal of Clinical Child Psychiatry, 10*, 79–82.

Nowicki, S., & Strickland, B. (1973). A locus of control scale for children. *Journal of Consulting & Clinical Psychology, 40*, 148–154.

Ollendick, T. H. (1979). Behavioral treatment of anorexia nervosa: A five year study. *Behavior Modification, 3*, 124–135.

Pennebaker, J. W. (1982). *The psychology of physical symptoms.* New York: Springer-Verlag.

Perrin, E. C., & Gerrity, P. S. (1981). There's a demon in your belly: Children's understanding of illness. *Pediatrics, 67*, 841–849.

Peterson, L., & Shigetomi, C. (1981). The use of coping techniques to minimize anxiety in hospitalized children. *Behavior Therapy, 12*, 1–14.

Piaget, J. (1929). *The child's conception of the world.* New York: Harcourt Brace.

Piaget, J. (1930). *The child's conception of physical causality.* London: Kegan Paul.

Potter, P. C., & Roberts, M. C. (1984). Children's perceptions of chronic illness: The roles of disease symptoms, cognitive development, and information. *Journal of Pediatric Psychology, 9*, 13–28.

Prohaska, T. R., Leventhal, E. A., Leventhal, H., & Keller, M. L. (1985). Health practices and illness cognition in young, middle aged and elderly adults. *Journal of Gerontology, 40*, 569–578.

Redpath, C. C., & Rogers, C. S. (1984). Healthy young children's concepts of hospitals, medical personnel, operations, and illness. *Journal of Pediatric Psychology, 9*(1), 29–40.

Roberts, M. D., Wurtele, S. K., Boone, R. R., Ginther, L. J., & Elkins, P. E. (1986). Reduction of medical fears by use of modeling: A preventative application in a general population of children. *Journal of Pediatric Psychology, 6*, 293–300.

Roberts, R. N., & Gordon, S. B. (1979). Reducing childhood nightmares subsequent to a burn treatment. *Child Behavior Therapy, 1*, 373–381.

Russell, H. L., & Carter, J. L. (1978). Biofeedback training with children: Consultation, questions, applications, and alternatives. *Journal of Clinical Child Psychology, 7*, 23–25.

Scherer, M. W., & Nakamura, C. Y. (1968). A fear survey schedule for children (FSS–FC): A factor analytic comparison with manifest anxiety (CMAS). *Behaviour Research & Therapy*, pp. 173–182.

Siegel, L. J., & Peterson, L. (1980). Stress reduction in young dental patients through coping skills and sensory information. *Journal of Consulting & Clinical Psychology, 48*, 785–787.

Siegel, L. J., & Peterson, L. (1981). Maintenance effects of coping skills and sensory information on young children's response to repeated dental procedures. *Behavior Therapy, 12*, 530–535.

Sigman, M., & Amit, Z. (1982). Progressive relaxation exercises and human gastric acid output: A study using telematic instruments. *Behaviour Research & Therapy, 20*, 605–612.

Simeonsson, R., Buckley, L., & Monson, L. (1979). Conceptions of illness causality in hospitalized children. *Journal of Pediatric Psychology, 4*, 77–84.

Slavin, L. A., O'Malley, J. E., Koocher, G. P., & Foster, D. J. (1982). Communication of the cancer diagnosis to pediatric patients: Impact on long-term adjustment. *American Journal of Psychiatry, 139,* 179–183.

Smith, R. E., & Sharpe, T. M. (1970). Treatment of a school phobia with implosive therapy. *Journal of Consulting & Clinical Psychology, 35,* 239–243.

Stephens, M., & Delys, P. A. (1973). A locus of control measure for preschool children. *Developmental Psychology, 8,* 55–65.

Taylor, S. E. (1982). Hospital patient behavior: Reactance, helplessness, or control? In H. S. Friedman & M. R. DiMatteo (Eds.), *Interpersonal issues in health care.* New York: Academic.

Tipton, R. M., & Worthington, E. L., Jr. (1984). The measurement of generalized self-efficacy: A study of construct validity. *Journal of Personality Assessment, 48,* 545–548.

Venham, L., Bengston, D., & Cipes, M. (1977). Children's response to sequential dental visits. *Journal of Dental Research, 56,* 454–459.

Wallston, B. S., Wallston, K. A., Kaplan, G. D., & Mardes, S. A. (1976). Development and validation of the Health and Locus of Control scale. *Journal of Consulting & Clinical Psychology, 44,* 580.

Wasserman, T. H. (1983). The effects of cognitive development on the use of cognitive behavioral techniques with children. *Child & Family Behavior Therapy, 5,* 37–50.

Weinberg, R. S., Hughes, H. H., Critelli, J. W., England, R., & Jackson, A. (1984). Effects of pre-existing and manipulated self-efficacy on weight loss in a self-control program. *Journal of Research in Personality, 18,* 352–358.

Weinstein, D. (1976). Imagery and relaxation with a burn patient. *Behaviour Research & Therapy, 14,* 481.

Weisz, J. R., & Stipek, D. J. (1982). Competence, contingency and the development of perceived control. *Human Development, 25,* 250–281.

Wolfer, J. A., & Visintainer, M. A. (1975). Pediatric surgical patients' and parents' stress responses and adjustment. *Nursing Research, 24,* 244–255.

Zeltzer, L. K., Dash, J., & Holland, J. P. (1979). Hypnotically induced pain control in sickle cell anemia. *Pediatrics, 64,* 533–536.

9

Personality and Social Skills Assessment of Children, with Special Reference to Somatic Disorders

STEVEN BECK
LAURA K. SMITH

Melissa is a 7-year-old, newly diagnosed insulin-dependent diabetic. Since her discharge from the hospital, her mother reports that Melissa appears less interested in peers. Melissa's mother is concerned about the deleterious effects the illness may have upon Melissa's interest toward her playmates.

Jacob is a 9-year-old child who has polyarticular-onset arthritis. His mother indicates that Jacob has had previous difficulty with peer relationships. His teacher reports he has problems maintaining friends because of his aggressiveness and bossiness with children. However, prior to Jacob's illness, his mother believed he was beginning to play better with neighborhood children. Jacob's mother worries that his medical condition is going to cause him to react in a more aggressive manner toward peers.

Mary is an 8-year-old severely asthmatic child. Her parents have recently heard children making fun of her wheezing and intermittent coughing. Although these taunts do not appear to upset Mary, her parents are concerned that her illness and its side effects are affecting her self-esteem.

These brief vignettes and parental issues are not unfamiliar to mental heatlh practitioners in health settings. The parental concerns require some form of systematic assessment of the child's current peer relationships as well as the child's relationships prior to his or her medical condition. The purpose of this chapter is to discuss various methods and strategies available for assessing the effects of chronic disorders, particularly somatic disorders, upon children's peer relationships and personality.

THE IMPORTANCE OF PEERS

Considerable attention has been directed toward the examination of children's peer relationships. Traditional theories of social development were usually predicated on the assumption that early experiences with parents laid the foundation for later friendships, and that the mother–child relationship was the prototype of all later meaningful relationships (Bowlby, 1969; Freud, 1965; Kagan, 1958). More recent theoretical speculation has it that, while a secure and effective parent–child relationship may be a critical condition for a child's acquisition of a positive orientation to the social world, it is the actual opportunity of relating with age-mates that allows skillful and satisfactory peer relationships to develop (Hartup, 1976, 1979). Hartup has argued for the importance of peers in their own right, and has noted that they serve as significant agents of socialization. For example, school-age children strongly identify with and are influenced by same-sex peers, develop more verbal as opposed to physical strategies in peer interpersonal exchanges, and learn mutual, reciprocal relationships that are more egalitarian than adult–child relationships. Peer relationships play a major role in sex-role learning, moral development, and the expression and control of aggression (Hartup, 1979).

DEVELOPMENTAL CONSIDERATIONS

Besides recognition that peers are important socializing agents, appreciation and knowledge of developmental factors are important in understanding children's relationships and the effects a chronic illness may have on children's social development. Erikson's (1963) psychosocial stages serve as a heuristic model for understanding the relationship between themes that occur during developmental stages and the effects a chronic disorder may have upon developing social behavior. For example, during the *autonomy stage* (1½ to 3 years) physical illness may result in restricted physical activity and environmental exploration that can be disruptive to the child's developing sense of confidence, mastery, and independence. During this stage, children will begin to open doors, drawers, and cabinets, turn on the television set, and feed and dress themselves. In short, they learn to do things on their own. Major social themes may not be developed during this stage for a chronically ill child who is frequently at home sick, or is too weak, or is isolated (physically and psychologically) from peers. For example, delays may occur in the ability to learn the reciprocity or sequence of social exchanges that occurs between rapidly maturing children. Also, the gradual shift toward relating predominantly with peers, and the lessening of an exclusive maternal attachment, may be delayed in children who have fewer opportunities to play with other children.

During the *initiative stage* (from 3 years to about 6 years of age) children begin assuming responsibility for their care and hygiene, their toys and pets, and perform certain duties such as keeping their rooms clean. Parents facilitate children's sense of initiation by stimulating their curiosity and applauding their efforts. According to Erikson's model, the overprotective and restrictive parent of a chronically ill child is likely to produce a sense of guilt in the child for attempting to initiate activities with peers.

During the *industry stage* (6 years of age to the beginning of puberty) children start to turn away from the family setting to seek an identity among their school-age peers. According to Erikson, the cornerstone of this developmental stage is the child's cognitive and social endeavors with school and peers. This is an era of intense social comparison; members of the peer group begin to "measure" themselves against one another to determine who they are and of what they are capable. There are a myriad of interrelated social skills that may be hampered for chronically ill children who are either absent from school or kept from interacting with peers on a consistent basis. During this developmental stage children begin learning to rely almost exclusively on verbal as opposed to physical strategies for controlling the ongoing social exchange. Children learn to respond effectively to more than one peer during this stage, and begin responding less to adult structure and more to peer direction.

The next developmental stage is adolescence, called the *identity stage* in Erikson's psychosocial theory of development. Erikson suggests that puberty is a remarkable and somewhat disturbing event for the developing child, given the physical, hormonal, and societal changes that accompany adolescence. During this stage an adolescent's identity begins to take shape by the trying on of values, ideologies, and interests. Many of these issues are dealt with through intense peer relationships. Daily friendship interactions take up a substantial portion of the adolescent's free time (Crockett, Losoff, & Peterson, 1984; Montemayer, 1982), and adolescents report spending more time talking to peers than in any other activity (Csikszentmihalyi, Larson, & Prescott, 1971). The chronically ill child may not have the opportunity to establish enduring peer relationships due to the restrictions inherent in his or her illness or its treatment. Furthermore, according to Erikson's model, the chronically ill adolescent is likely to rebel against the expectations of parent and health practitioners by failing to adhere closely to necessary medical regimens in hopes that such a rebellion may help to crystallize an emergent identity.

CHILDREN DEFICIENT IN PEER RELATIONSHIPS

A critical factor influencing the quality of children's relationships is the actual social skill repertoire that permits children to relate to each other in a personally and mutually beneficial manner (Combs & Slaby, 1977). Research comparing children who are viewed as well liked by peers to children who are neglected or disliked by peers can provide valuable insights for clinicians working with chronically ill children. Although chronically ill children may not fit neatly into social status groups of popular, rejected, or neglected children, the following studies allow for a conceptual framework from which to view chronically physically disordered children and their social behaviors.

For example, Gottman, Gonso, and Schuler (1976) found that elementary-age children with few friends, compared to children who had many friends, were deficient concerning knowledge of how to make friends and performed more poorly on a task that involved the ability to take the perspective of another person.

Dodge, Coie, and Brakke (1983) found that third and fifth grade children who were disliked by their peers displayed more aggressive behaviors and less classroom on-task behaviors compared to popular children. Similarly, children who had minimal positive or negative contact with peers and were generally ignored by peers displayed relatively good-on-task classroom behaviors, but initiated interactions with peers infrequently. Asarnow and Callan (1985) reported that problem solving of fourth- and sixth-grade boys with peer problems tends to be ineffective, unique, unsophisticated, and predominantly impulsive and aggressive. Children rejected by peers generated fewer alternative solutions, proposed fewer assertive and mature solutions, generated more intense aggressive solutions, showed less adaptive planning, and evaluated physically aggressive solutions more positively and positive prosocial responses more negatively than popular children. Similarly, Richard and Dodge (1982) found that neglected and aggressive boys were able to generate only one effective solution to hypothetical problem situations, while popular children generated several prosocial solutions to each situation. In summary, children with problematic peer relationships appear to be deficient in the cognitive problem-solving skills of generating prosocial solutions to ambiguous or conflictual peer encounters.

While there is an emerging picture of children who have problematic peer relationships in the school setting, there are virtually no empirical studies about the effects of children's chronic illness upon their peer relationships. In addition, premorbid personality and temperamental traits would almost certainly be important child characteristics related to adjustment or maladjustment to a chronic illness, yet there has been a scarcity of direct empirical evidence to support such a relationship (Pless, 1983). There are, however, a number of studies that suggest that children with chronic physical disorders are at some increased risk for psychological maladjustment (Pless, 1983). Simply put, there is a greater association between childhood adjustment problems and chronic illness than one would expect in a healthy population. However, these studies generally display an overreliance on subjective assessment measures and lack suitable control groups. For obvious reasons, experimental manipulations are not feasible when studying chronically ill children, and problems of measurement are exaggerated by the absence of any reasonable standards for comparison. For example, is it or is it not appropriate to use standardized, objective measures derived from a sample of nondisabled children as normative guidelines when evaluating chronically ill children?

With these limitations in mind, this chapter discusses available assessment strategies for evaluating children's personality and socialization. The chapter gives emphasis to the characteristics of physically ill children with the chronic somatic disorders of asthma, arthritis, and juvenile diabetes. Children with mild chronic conditions do not experience severe physical symptoms, nor do they usually need to cope with demanding treatments on a daily basis. Consequently, they may have life-styles very similar to those of physically healthy children, except for their need to cope with activities such as visits to physicians and periodic medical regimens.

In fact, Parmelee (1986) suggests that minor common childhood illnesses can have a beneficial effect upon a child's development. He argues that children with minor illnesses can develop a greater sense of competency by developing autonomy and differentiation from others. Children with minor illness have the opportunity to gain knowledge about their bodies as well as to develop coping strategies (e.g., maintaining social relationships) in order to reduce their temporary feelings of distress. On the other hand, children with chronic and protracted illnesses face daily reminders of their disease and require additional resources to adapt to their condition.

ISSUES SPECIFIC TO SOMATIC ILLNESSES

Much of the writing on children's disorders focuses upon specific illnesses rather than chronic illness in general. These studies have been helpful in isolating some of the problems and stressors inherent in these illnesses. This section will briefly describe three common somatic childhood chronic disorders and the special problems associated with each illness.

Asthma

Asthma is characterized by hyperresponsiveness of the bronchi and bronchioles of the lungs to various stimuli, such as allergens, exercise, respiratory infections, and other airway irritants such as cold air and dust. When the asthmatic's respiratory system becomes overly stimulated, changes in the bronchi and bronchioles (including the secretion of thick mucus, mucosal edema, and contraction of bronchial smooth muscles) lead to a reduction in airway passages. Overt symptoms of an asthmatic episode will include wheezing, shortness of breath (dyspnea), coughing, and excessive mucus production. In status asthmaticus, the dyspnea becomes so severe and constant that it is potentially life threatening. Nevertheless, the airway obstruction experienced during attacks of asthma is completely reversible, and the asthmatic experiences normal pulmonary functioning between attacks. Asthmatics vary widely in terms of the stimuli that provoke attacks and the severity of attacks.

Asthma is the most common pediatric chronic disorder. This disease is the most frequent cause of limitation of activity in children under the age of 17, and accounts for almost one-quarter of school days missed due to chronic illness (National Center for Health Statistics, 1971). Approximately 5 to 7 percent of the U.S. population either have suffered from asthma in the past or currently suffer with this disorder. Two to 4 percent of the U.S. population currently suffer from asthma (Purcell & Weiss, 1970). Prevalence rates vary from study to study, with approximately 5 to 10 percent of children below the age of 15 having the disorder (Fritz, 1983). Boys are three times more likely to have asthma as children, but sex ratios start to even out around adolescence (Fritz, 1983). Up to 75 percent of asthma sufferers will experience complete or partial remission of symptoms within 5 years after diagnosis (Smith, 1971), while 40 percent of childhood asthmatics will experience a spontaneous and complete remission of their asthma by adulthood (Alexander, 1983).

A great deal of psychological literature has been devoted to asthma, and much of it has centered on the controversy over whether asthma is *caused* by physiological or psychological factors. One of the most influential papers on this topic was written by French and Alexander in 1941. They suggested that asthma represents the suppression of an intense emotion—a suppressed cry for the mother. Following the publication of their paper, a number of theories were put forward in which the child's asthma was attributed to a pathological child-rearing style on the part of the mother (Wright, Schaefer, & Solomons, 1979). Research is also currently being conducted on the emotional expressiveness of asthmatics. Such studies often find that asthmatic children show less emotional reactivity and suggest a causal link between emotional suppression and asthma. Currently, the dominant view among many psychologists is that there is no evidence of abnormality in the parent–child relationships of asthmatics and no personality style that predisposes an individual to develop the disease (Alexander, 1980; Creer, 1982; King, 1980). The decreased emotional expressivity of asthmatics has been attributed to the child's need to suppress emotions for fear of bringing on an attack (Creer, 1982). In this view, emotional expression—not its suppression—leads to attacks. The debate over the etiologic role of emotional suppression is not over, as evidenced by a recent study in which a negative correlation was found between duration of emotional expression and difficulty in breathing (Hollaender & Florin, 1983).

Another important issue involves defining subclasses of asthma: The population of asthmatics is very heterogeneous. A number of methods for classifying asthmatics have been described. Many writers describe differences between extrinsic (allergy induced) and intrinsic (non–allergy induced) asthma. Not all children can be classified using this simple distinction, however. Thus more elaborate systems have been devised (King, 1980). Wright and colleagues describe four classes of asthma: (1) a more or less purely allergic type; (2) a primarily allergic type; (3) a primarily emotional type; and (4) a purely emotional type. While a specific classification system for asthma has not been devised, it has become increasingly clear that a very individualized approach in assessment and treatment is especially important for these children.

Alexander (1980) has stated that many of the problems common among asthmatics can be seen in children with other chronic illnesses. These problems include a poor self-concept, impaired academic and social development, use of the illness to manipulate others, and ambiguity concerning the extent to which the child can safely engage in certain activities. Other problems more specific to asthma include panic responses to stimuli that are associated with asthma attacks, hyperventilation, and excessive ("psychogenic") cough. Some serious problems for asthmatic children can be attributed to absences from school. Twenty-five percent of all school days lost due to chronic illness can be attributed to asthma (Schiffer & Hunt, 1963). Children who have frequent absences may be at an increased risk for failing to form good friendship bonds with peers and may be especially prone to having social skill as well as academic deficits.

Arthritis

Arthritis is a term used to refer to the presence of joint inflammation with concomitant swelling, pain, and impaired functioning in one or more joints. In actuality, such symptoms can occur in conjunction with a large number of diseases. The most common arthritic disease is juvenile rheumatoid arthritis (JRA), which is characterized by continuous pain, swelling, warmth, and redness in one or more joints for more than 6 weeks (Williams, 1981). Within children suffering from JRA, there is much variation in terms of the severity of symptoms and the extent of disability experienced. Gregg (1971) distinguishes among three types of JRA according to mode of onset. Acute-onset JRA accounts for 5 to 25 percent of all JRA, and most frequently begins by the age of 3. This type of arthritis is often preceded by a fever and rash. Other symptoms (e.g., abdominal pain, pericarditis, and lymphadenopathy) may be present along with the joint inflammation. Polyarticular-onset arthritis involves painful swelling of at least four joints, usually in the upper or lower extremities, but occasionally in the spinal column as well. Fever, impaired appetite, and lethargy may also occur. This type of JRA accounts for approximately 50 percent of the cases, and its mean age of onset is 7 years. The monarticular type of JRA onset usually involves only one joint, most often the knee. The mean age of onset for this type of JRA is also 7, but it seems to have a bimodal distribution with peak incidences in the age range from 1 to 3 years and from 11 to 13 years.

It is difficult to make an estimate of the overall incidence of arthritis because it occurs in conjunction with so many different diseases, although it is estimated that from 175,000 to 250,000 cases per year are reported, with females being afflicted two to three times more often than males (Calabro, 1969).

Like many chronically ill children, arthritic children have been reported to suffer from their inability to conform with their peer group. For example, Kornreich, Kostes, and Hanson (1973) report that adolescents have an especially difficult time dealing with arthritis and may refuse certain aspects of treatment such as crutches and steroids (which can cause obesity). Growth retardation often accompanies arthritis (Wright et al., 1979). Short stature has been associated with emotional problems (e.g., poor self-concept) and can increase feelings of being different from peers.

A number of studies have attempted to document emotional problems in arthritic children (Cleveland, Reitman, & Brewer, 1976; Hooks, 1971). As with many other studies that assess emotional factors such as depression and self-esteem in chronically ill children, inconsistent findings have been obtained, with many studies finding few or no differences between arthritic children and healthy controls (Wright et al., 1979).

An interesting study by McAnarney, Pless, Satterwhite, and Friedman (1974) found that mildly affected arthritics had more serious disturbances on a number of measures (including self-esteem and school achievement) than severely affected children. The authors observed that parents of the least severely affected arthritics often denied that the arthritis had any impact on their children's current behavior, but at the same time were less likely to expect that their arthritic children would attend college (compared to their other children). The arthritic child thus received mixed messages from his or her parents about what he or she could accomplish. McAnarney and his colleagues also discuss the concept of marginality, which involves children who are only mildly affected by a disease or disability and who consequently face ambiguity and uncertainty concerning the behavior expected of them. These children often have difficulty accepting the reality of their disability.

Juvenile Diabetes

One of the distressing problems for the diabetic child is having to cope with the most complex and demanding treatment regimen of any common disease. Diabetic children are likely to experience problems in their peer relationships due to the many treatment-related activities that set them apart from their friends (Johnson, 1980). They may experience the fear of social embarrassment due to mood swings and the ever-present possibility of an insulin reaction (Hamberg, 1983). Gross and Johnson (1981) have suggested that many of the interpersonal problems experienced by juvenile diabetics may stem from the fact that they rarely have observable models from which to learn effective ways of dealing with their disease-related social stresses. Consequently, Gross and Johnson posit that many diabetic children suffer from deficits in social skills. These investigators suggest that the social skill deficit and the stress diabetics suffer as a consequence play a large role in the onset of adjustment problems frequently reported in diabetics. Gross, Heimann, Shapiro, and Schulty (1983) also suggest that diabetics who are deficient in social skills may be in poorer metabolic control. They cite research that indicates a link between stress and elevated blood glucose levels, and posit that metabolic control may be improved through social skills training because such training improves one's ability to deal with stress.

Diabetes usually appears as Type I, or insulin-dependent diabetes mellitus (IDDM), or Type 2, or non–insulin-dependent diabetes mellitus (NIDDM). Non–insulin-dependent diabetes is the less severe form of the disorder and can be controlled through weight reduction and diet, since the pancreas continues to produce some insulin (Wing, Epstein, Nowalk, Koeske, & Hagg, 1985). In contrast, IDDM is characterized by an eventual complete pancreatic failure; daily insulin replacement by injection is necessary for survival.

Type I IDDM diabetes usually manifests between infancy and 35 years of age. In children, two peaks of incidence have been noted, around 5 to 6 years of age and also in the age group of 11 to 13 years old (Drash, 1979). The prevalence of Type I IDDM in children is about one child per thousand (Dahlquist et al., 1982), although in recent years the incidence has been increasing (Fishbein, Faich, & Ellis, 1982).

ASSESSMENT STRATEGIES

This section describes three general assessment methods useful for gathering information about a chronically ill child's personality and social skills. The strategies described in this section are not exhaustive, but are considered the best assessment armamentarium for clinicians examining children's personality and peer relationships. The flowchart in Figure 9.1 provides the reader a schematic view of the major assessment questions addressed by the strategies described in this section.

THE INTERVIEW

Interviewing the Referring Adult. Clinical interviews typically serve as the major source of information about a client's problem. The clinical interview is usually the starting point from which the clinician begins to collect information about the presenting problem(s). Since a child with a chronic illness being seen in a health care setting rarely refers himself or herself to a clinician for assessment and treatment, adults serve as the primary source of information about a child's social interactions. Due to the fact that the identified child is not referring himself or herself, is it not

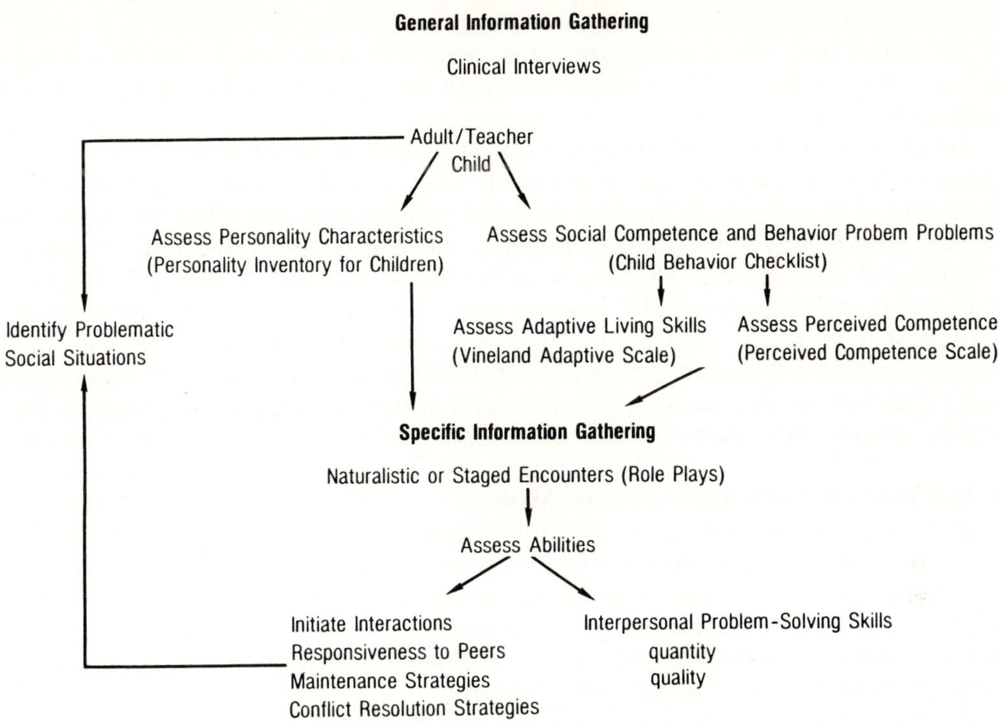

FIGURE 9.1. Process of assessment for the chronically ill child with potential peer relationship problems.

uncommon for the child and the referring adult (usually the parent or medical personnel) to disagree over the existence of the presenting problem. When these differences in opinion exist, the clinician must exhibit sensitivity in collecting information from both the child and the referring adults and rely on developmental and normative information to make judgments regarding the quality of the child's personality and peer relationships.

When collecting information from adults about a child's potential relationship problems, the following questions need to be asked. (When important, expectations for children's developmental age will be delineated.) First of all, the therapist should determine how the child may have changed since the illness began, in terms of his or her temperament and relations with friends. The therapist needs to be cognizant of the fact that the child's typical response to the initial onset of a chronic disease, such as insulin-dependent diabetes, is characterized by mild sadness, feelings of friendlessness, occasional apprehension or fear, crankiness, and somewhat decreased socialization with family and friends (Kovacs et al., 1985). However, studies suggest that the majority of these mild adjustment problems dissipate 3 months after an initial diagnosis of a chronic illness is made (Kovacs et al., 1985; Pless & Perrin, 1985).

Determining the onset of a chronically ill child's peer relationship problems in relation to the onset of the child's illness is critical. Children who do not adjust to their chronic illness after a short period of time are likely to exhibit withdrawal or increased argumentativeness with peers, teachers, and family members. The severity of the child's peer relationship difficulties cannot be appreciated until the clinician has a notion of the child's relationship with others prior to his or her medical diagnosis.

Adults should be asked how many close friends the child has, realizing that for children under the age of 7 the number of "close friends" is heavily influenced by proximity of similar-age children in their neighborhood or extended family. By the second grade, however, children begin to develop friendships based more on dispositional characteristics and less on such contextual factors as proximity (Furman & Bierman, 1984). For a child 7 years of age or older, a problem in peer relations may exist if an adult surmises that the child has no close friends or only one. Similarly, children 8 years of age or older typically belong to at least one organization (e.g., Cub Scouts) or team (e.g., soccer), and appear to enjoy participating in this activity. For the chronically ill child, sports participation may obviously be restricted; however, these children can still be expected to be involved in social organizations if their medical condition is not debilitating.

If the interviewed adult has the opportunity to observe the identified child interacting with other children, questions can be asked regarding the frequency and quality of the identified child's initiations and responsiveness toward peers, as well as the child's ability to maintain interactions with other children and to avoid or minimize conflicts with peers. Further information about these specific social skills is presented in the next section.

For preadolescent or older children the quality of their relationships with peers can be indirectly assessed by asking how often the preadolescent or adolescent visits or is visited by friends, or how often he or she phones or is called by friends. Adults can also be asked how often the chronically ill child complains of being lonely or bored. Elementary-age children who are either neglected or rejected by peers will occasionally complain of loneliness. Children often complain of being bored at home or on weekends with nothing to do, when in fact the primary problem is their lack of friends.

Interviewing the Teacher. While parents' perceptions of their children are obviously important, teachers provide several unique perspectives of children's social functioning. Teachers are in an excellent position to observe children's social skills and peer relationships. Teachers observe and interact with children in a somewhat standardized social environment that allows direct comparisons among children of similar developmental levels.

A child's social skills can be assessed by inquiring about his or her social interactions with peers (e.g., "Does she have many friends?" "Does he initiate activities with other children?", "How does she respond to peers' initiations toward her?"). Teachers can be very astute at identifying children who are rejected, neglected, or popular with their peers (Green, Vosk, Forehand, & Beck, 1981).

Teachers can also be asked to what degree they believe that children's illness interferes with their social functioning and academic work. Given that 25 percent of all school days lost to chronic illness can be attributed to asthma Schiffer & Hunt, 1963), questions to a teacher about a severely asthmatic child's academic and social functioning would be critical. Pless (1975) reviewed a number of studies that report lower academic achievement in chronically ill children. An obvious set of questions to ask in this area include: "Does the child's illness interfere with his ability to do the work?" "Are assignments completed on time?" "Relative to classmates, how would you evaluate her performance in math, language, arts, and so on?" "Does he require more time to complete assignments than the other children?" "Does she have difficulty staying on a task?"

Finally, the interview with the teacher should result in an assessment of the willingness of the teacher to assist in an intervention program. As noted by Gross (1984), teachers are generally very interested in the performance of their students. A clinician who consults with a child's teacher and exhibits a sincere appreciation for his or her observations is likely to elicit a cooperative teacher response.

Interviewing the Child. While adult informants and behavioral observations can generally provide very complete and accurate information about a child's behavior, clinical interviews with children regarding their peer relations should be considered integral parts of the overall assessment (Bierman, 1983). The manner in which the chronically ill child conceptualizes and perceives peer relations and responds to the therapist in terms of motivational and affective states can provide potential hypotheses about the quality of the child's peer relationships. The manner in which a child maintains eye contact with the clinician, offers spontaneous speech, and responds to the therapist's questioning can provide clues regarding how the child may similarly respond to new peers.

Due to the lack of normative data for chronically ill children (particularly regarding the quantitative and qualitative aspects of a chronically ill child's peer relationships), the clinician needs to be cognizant of global clinical and developmental guidelines when interviewing a child about his or her peer relationships. Emotionally disturbed children often show less differentiation and less integration in explaining their interpersonal relations than do nondisturbed children. Research by Selman and his colleagues (Selman, 1980; Selman & Jacquette, 1977) has shown that institutionalized boys with emotional and behavioral disorders are likely to show less mature and more variable reasoning in areas such as conceptions of friendships and interpersonal relationships. Elementary-age chronically ill children with poor peer relationships may use logic more characteristic of a younger child. They may view peers in either–or extreme terms (e.g., a 7-year-old with insulin-dependent diabetes reporting that all of his classmates are "very mean"). Such children may conceptualize emotions in global, exaggerated ways (e.g., a 9-year-old child with arthritis reporting that she has "the best friend in the whole world").

As mentioned earlier, by the early grade school years, children begin to identify prosocial actions, such as liking, helping, and sharing, as the prominent characteristics of friendships (Furman & Bierman, 1984). Preadolescents identify friends as those persons with whom they have established a relationship based upon such ideals as loyalty and trustworthiness. Adolescents can construct complex social worlds in which multiple and mixed motivations are recognized and understood. For example, a 14-year-old adolescent can recognize and tolerate the fact that his best friend often "talks behind his back" about the genuineness of his chronic illness.

When interviewing children, the clinician must adapt to the developmental level of the particular child, and this may require substantial modification in the clinician's usual interview and questioning behavior. For young children (under the age of 6) an introductory play period is often necessary to ease the child into a fact-finding situation and to allow the child to become more comfortable with the clinician. Since preschool children conceive of others in simple evaluative and concrete terms, carve the world into rigid "good" and "bad" categories, and usually lack the words or organizational skills to describe their thoughts or feelings, a therapist may have to employ such concrete stimuli as dolls, puppets, or pictures of familiar situations to obtain information about their peer relationships. Once the child has become more relaxed in the situation, the interviewer can set up with dolls, puppets, or drawings of various situations involving typical peer interactions (e.g., playing in a sandbox, swinging on a swing set) and can simplify the interview by modifying questions to make them less threatening and more understandable. L. J. Yarrow (1980) describes several ways to modify questions addressed to young children. The clinician can suggest that other children feel a certain way (e.g., "One kid I know told me he wished more kids liked him. Do you ever feel that way?"). The clinician can give two alternatives (e.g., "Do you ever wish you had more friends or do you think you have enough friends?"). The clinician can soften negative choices or phrase questions to imply negatives (e.g., "What kinds of things do you and your brother fight about?" rather than "Do you ever fight with your brother?").

Grade school children may not require an introductory play period, but may feel more comfortable if some task orientation is provided in the interview (Bierman, 1983). The clinician might suggest that they begin working on a paper or construction task, such as Lego or dominoes, and then gradually begin to ease into questions concerning friends. For example, initially asking questions like "What grade are you in?" or "Who are some of the kids you like the most in your class?" and then gradually asking the child to elaborate on his or her thoughts or feelings expressed in the initial answers will allow the clinician to explore more complex and difficult areas.

If performed with sensitivity and an understanding of developmental considerations, interviewing chronically ill children about their thoughts and feelings concerning their peer relationships can be a valid and reliable means of assessment.

PAPER-AND-PENCIL MEASURES

The following list of paper-and-pencil measures is certainly not exhaustive of the available checklists or self-report measures for evaluating children's personality and socialization. However, the four measures to be discussed are recommended because of their comprehensiveness, clinical utility, and acceptable psychometric properties. The Personality Inventory for Children and the Child Behavior Checklist are considered the two best empirically developed scales for assessing dimensions of children's personality and for globally differentiating behaviorally and emotionally disturbed children (Beck, 1987). The Vineland Social Maturity Scale, while most commonly associated with assessing developmentally handicapped children and adults, can be a useful instrument for evaluating a chronically ill child's day-to-day functioning. Since there are reasons for assuming that a child with a chronic disorder is likely to experience changes in his or her self-concept, a self-report measure of self-concept may be desired by the clinician. The only self-report measure described in this chapter is the Perceived Competence Scale, which assesses a child's perceived competence in four clinically relevant domains.

The Personality Inventory for Children

The Personality Inventory for Children (PIC) is a 600-item true–false instrument designed to assess childhood psychopathology (Wirt, Lachar, Klinedinst, & Seat, 1977). The PIC is completed by an adult informant, usually the child's mother. The PIC yields multidimensional data for children and adolescents, with separate norms and profiles for males and females, ages 3 to 5 and 6 to 16. A manual providing T-score conversions similar to the MMPI and interpretations of the profiles is published by Western Psychological Association (Wirt et al., 1977). The original creators of this instrument, Wirt and Broen (1958), used a methodological approach similar to that employed by Hathaway and McKinley (1951) in developing the MMPI. The PIC yields 3 validity scales that detect response tendencies toward exaggerating or minimizing symptoms, 1 screening scale for assessing general adjustment, 12 clinical scales to evaluate the presence of pathology in the child, and 17 supplemental scales created to convey information about specific areas of parental concern (see Table 9.1).

The PIC scales were developed using either an empirical or a rational–content strategy. The empirical approach tested PIC items utilizing criterion groups, and has been proven of value in the identification of children classified as psychotic, hyperactive, delinquent, developmentally delayed, and learning disabled (Lachar & Wirt, 1981). The remaining scales were constructed using clinicians' judgments of what content items are clinically relevant. Two scales, the Withdrawal and Social Skills scales, important for the specific identification of peer relationship problems, have been derived using the rational–content strategy. The Withdrawal scale identifies children who avoid social contact, desire to remain isolated, have few friends, and

TABLE 9.1. SCALES IDENTIFIED ON THE PERSONALITY INVENTORY FOR CHILDREN (PIC)

Validity Scales	Clinical Scales	Supplemental Scales
Lie	Adjustment	Adolescent Maladjustment
F	Achievement	Aggression
Defensiveness	Intellectual Screening	Asocial Behavior
	Development	Cerebral Dysfunction
	Somatic Concerns	Delinquency Prediction
	Depression	Ego Strength
	Family Relations	Excitement
	Delinquency	Externalization
	Withdrawal	Infrequency
	Anxiety	Internalization
	Psychosis	Intraversion–Extraversion
	Hyperactivity	K
	Social Skills	Learning Disability Prediction
		Reality Distortion
		Sex Role
		Social Desirability
		Somatization

distrust others, while the Social Skills scale assesses children's effective social relations, active participation in socialized activities, and skills and poise in social situations.

The original norms for the PIC were not systematically selected so as to be nationally representative, and little information is available about the norm groups in either the 1977 or the newer 1982 PIC manual (Naglieri & Genshaft, 1985). The PIC was normed on a sample of 2390 equally divided males and females at each age level between the ages of 6 and 16 and on a sample of several hundred children between the ages 3 and 5, mostly Minneapolis public school children. A number of reliability and validity studies have been conducted by Wirt and his colleagues. Test–retest reliability in a clinical sample has been shown to be very stable, achieving a mean correlation of .89, with only the scale for Somatic Concerns obtaining a test–retest correlation below .80 over a 2-week period (Wirt & Lachar, 1981). In terms of validity, Gdowski (1977) reported that the 12 clinical scales, with the exception of Somatic Concerns, were able to differentiate groups of emotionally and behaviorally disturbed children and adolescents.

The *Revised Format Administration Booklet* of the Personality Inventory for Children presents the original 600 inventory items in a rearranged order to permit the clinician to administer fewer than the 600 original items while still allowing valid interpretation of the results. The Revised PIC items are placed in one of four sections or parts of the administration booklet (Lachar, 1982). In part one, scores from the four broad-based factor-derived scales (Undisciplined [poor self-control], Social Incompetence, Internalization/Somatic System, and Cognitive Development) can be derived from the first 131 inventory items. Lachar, Gdowski, and Snyder (1984) have indicated that health providers interested in giving the PIC as a screening measure should administer the first 131 items, which assess broad dimensions of psychological adjustment. If any factor scale is significantly elevated, the respondents may then complete the second, third, or fourth part, which would bring the total to 280, 420, or 600 items, respectively. Each additional part provides further information about the supplemental scales.

Assessment of Adaptive Behaviors

Adaptive behavior scales are a systematic method of obtaining objective information about a child's adaptive behavior, social maturity, and social development. Although adaptive behavior scales are most often associated with the assessment of developmentally disabled individuals, mental health practitioners working in a health setting may occasionally desire information about the developmental level at which a child was functioning prior to or after being diagnosed with a chronic illness. The best current measure of adaptive behavior appears to be the revision of the Vineland Social Maturity Scale called the Vineland Adaptive Behavior Scale (VABS; Sparrow, Balla, & Cicchetti, 1984). This new measure of adaptive functioning is a major revision of the 1953 Vineland with an excellent standardization sample and promising psychometric qualities (Naglieri & Genshaft, 1985).

Information about a child's level of functioning on the VABS is obtained through an interview administered to the child's primary caregiver. The Vineland interview is an organized series of questions designed to elicit information from an informant regarding the child's daily functioning. According to Sparrow and colleagues (1984), adaptive functioning is defined as the ability of individuals to exercise personal independence and social responsibility.

The VABS contains three forms: a survey form, an expanded form, and a classroom edition. Both the survey and expanded forms are norm referenced according to the child's chronological age, and provide standard scores and individual profiles of adaptive behavior strengths and weaknesses. The classroom edition is a criterion-referenced measure designed to provide material for educational planning (see Kratochwill & Roseby, Chapter 10, this volume). Within these forms, adaptive functioning is organized into several areas, called domains and subdomains. These domains are measured at every age level and scores are combined to yield a separate as well as an overall standard score of adaptive behavior comparable to well-known tests of intelligence, with a mean of 100 and a standard deviation of 15.

There are five domains assessed in the VABS. The Communication domain involves questions about how the individual uses verbal, nonverbal, symbolic, and written means of communicating with others. The second domain, Daily Living Skills, examines children's behavior in a number of areas vital to performance of everyday activities, such as eating, toileting, and dressing. The Socialization domain assesses children's interactions with peers and adults, willingness to follow rules in games, participation in social events, control of anger, and so forth. The fourth domain, Motor Skills, is administered only to children 8 years old and younger and aims to determine how they manipulate objects, walk, write, run, and so forth. The final area of assessment is the Maladaptive Behavior domain, which is intended to measure the kinds of behaviors commonly viewed as inappropriate for children above 4 years of age. Included are such behaviors as bed-wetting, level of activity, and aggressiveness.

For clinicians, the survey form of the VABS will be used most frequently since it comprises 140 items and is organized into the five adaptive behavior domains. The expanded form contains more than 500 items (in the five domains) and is primarily intended to gather a maximum amount of information about handicapped children and adults.

The Child Behavior Checklist (CBCL)

The CBCL (Achenbach, 1966; Achenbach & Edelbrock, 1978, 1983) is a standardized checklist containing 20 social competence items and 118 behavior problem items as reported by a child's parent(s). The CBCL is unique because it assesses adaptive competencies as well as behavior problems and has separate norms for boys and girls at ages 4 to 5, 6 to 11, and 12 to 16. These age ranges were chosen because Achenbach and Edelbrock believe that children make important transitions in cognitive, physical, educational, and social–emotional development during these age periods (Achenbach & Edelbrock, 1983).

The CBCL contains three social competence scales. The Activity scale taps the extent and quality of children's participation in sports, nonsports hobbies, activities, games, and jobs and chores. The Social scale assesses children's membership and participation in organizations, the number of friends and contacts with them, and behaviors with others and alone. The School scale assesses the amount and quality of the children's school experiences, placement in a regular or special class, and whether they have repeated grades or displayed school problems. The Behavior Problem scale dimensions are divided into two empirically derived broad-band groups, labeled externalizing and internalizing factors. Several narrow-band syndromes of behaviors are also empirically derived for each sex and age grouping.

Although the narrow-band syndromes are analogous to syndromes found in the DSM-III-R (American Psychiatric Association, 1987), such as attention deficit disorder, conduct disorders, and anxiety disorders, no scale is meant to be directly equivalent to a clinical diagnosis, nor is it intended to be used for conferring a diagnostic label (see Table 9.2).

To facilitate a comparison of how a child's problems and competence compare with those of children of similar age and sex, raw scores are converted to T-scores and are placed on the Child Behavior Profile. T-scores have a mean of 50 and a standard deviation of 10, and normalized scores are provided on the Child Behavior Profile for statistical and research purposes.

The norms for the CBCL appear to be fairly good. The scales were constructed from analyses of parent ratings of 2300 clinic-referred children from various public and private mental health centers and 1300 nonreferred children from randomly selected homes in the Washington, D.C. area. This sample appears fairly representative in terms of race and socioeconomic status.

Comparisons of clinical and nonclinical samples generally show significant differences on the competence and behavior problem scores for each sex and age

TABLE 9.2. BEHAVIOR PROBLEM SCALES IDENTIFIED ON THE CHILD BEHAVIOR CHECKLIST

Group	Internalizing Syndromes	Mixed Syndromes	Externalizing Syndromes
Boys 4 to 5	Depressed Immature Social withdrawal Somatic complaints	Sex problems	Aggressive Delinquent Schizoid
Girls 4 to 5	Depressed Schizoid or anxious Social withdrawal	Obese	Aggressive Hyperactive Sex problems
Boys 6 to 11	Depressed Obsessive–compulsive Schizoid or anxious Somatic complaints Uncommunicative	Social withdrawal	Aggressive Hyperactive Delinquent
Girls 6 to 11	Depressed Schizoid–obsessive Social withdrawal Somatic complaints		Aggressive Cruel Delinquent Hyperactive Sex problems
Boys 12 to 16	Immature Obsessive–compulsive Schizoid Somatic complaints Uncommunicative	Hostile withdrawal	Aggressive Delinquent Hyperactive
Girls 12 to 16	Anxious–obsessive Depressed withdrawal Schizoid Somatic complaints	Hyperactive Immature	Aggressive Cruel Delinquent

grouping (Achenbach, 1978). Test–retest reliabilities of scale scores for competence and behavior problems for each sex and age grouping at 1-week, 3-month, and 6-month intervals are on the average .89, .70, and approximately .60, respectively. The profile appears to be sensitive to stabilities as well as to changes in children's behaviors. The CBCL is already widely respected and is likely to become the checklist from which similar instruments are compared, given its emphasis on empirical classification of behavior problems, attention to children's social competence, and its use of large clinical and nonclinical norms broken down by sex and at least three different age groups (Beck, 1987).

The Perceived Competence Scale

The three paper and pencil measures described so far are completed by informants knowledgeable about the chronically ill child's behavior and temperament. Yet the most popular assessment method in clinical psychology is the self-report measure (Kazdin, 1981). However, children's self-report measures have not been given much emphasis in the assessment literature for the same reason that children's interviews have been minimized: Children are not viewed as capable of accurately reporting their psychological states. However, it is now recognized that a child's perception of his or her problems is critical for a more complete understanding of the child's current adjustment.

Given the concern about chronically ill children's self-esteem, one self-report measure that has the potential to be widely used by clinicians in health settings is the Perceived Competence Scale (PCS) (Harter, 1982). The PCS is a self-report measure that differs from other self-esteem measures (most notably the Piers-Harris Children's Self-Concept Scale [Piers & Harris, 1969]) in that the PCS assesses a child's perceived competence across Cognitive, Social, and Physical domains. A fourth subscale, General Self-Worth, is also assessed, which is independent from the other three skill domains and not merely the cumulative total of all scores on the PCS.

The PCS can be used for children in third through ninth grade, although the measure will probably have to be read to children 8 to 10 years old who are poor readers. Means and standard deviations of PCS scores broken down by grade for more than 2000 children are presented by Harter (1982). However, these samples appear to have been assessed more by convenience than by a stratified sampling procedure. Three-month test–retest reliabilities of the PCS were .78, .80, 87, and .70 for the four subscales, and .78, .75, .80, and .69 after 9 months.

Harter and Pike (1984) also developed a Pictorial Scale of Perceived Competence and Social Acceptance for Young Children. There are two versions of this instrument, one for preschoolers and kindergartners and a second for first and second graders, each tapping the four domains assessed in the PCS. The psychometric properties of these two scales were found to be acceptable, although weak correlations were found between children's and teachers' judgment of perceived competence and social acceptance. Harter and Pike caution that these two measures appear to assess separate constructs in young children, namely, perceived competence and social acceptance.

Children with arthritis, juvenile diabetes, or asthma represent a unique subgroup of children that would appear to be particularly vulnerable to decrements in perceived competence in the four domains assessed by the PCS. Unfortunately, the lack of normative data and validity studies of the PCS for chronically ill children makes clinical judgments regarding high or low self-ratings of competence difficult to make. For example, without the availability of norms for similar asthmatic children, how does one determine whether high Physical domain scores (indicating that the child perceives himself or herself as capable in the realm of athletics) represent a child who is denying the reality of his or her disability or displaying resiliencies? Nonetheless, even without norms for chronically ill children, the PCS and its downward extension for young children appear to be potentially useful instruments for assessing a child's self-concept from a multifaceted perspective.

ANALOGUE ASSESSMENTS

Ideally, a child's social behavior should be observed in his or her natural setting, such as the classroom, school play ground, neighborhood, or back yard. The importance of such assessment is highlighted by the fact that the identification of particular social contexts, tasks, or situations in which the "incompetent" child displays his or her problematic behavior is necessary before remediation of deficits can begin (Dodge & Murphy, 1984).

Given the obvious difficulties for clinicians trying to conduct observations of children in naturalistic settings, analogue strategies can be employed and appear to be valuable for assessing children's social skills (Kendall & Braswell, 1985). Analogue strategies are a variety of simulated or staged encounters that are designed as close parallels to situations commonly encountered in "real life" (Bellack, 1979). For example, Gross and Johnson (1981) developed an eight-item role-play test that attempts to replicate "real-life" problems for preadolescents that were reported by college-age diabetics as having been stressful when they were younger. Role-play scenes involved such issues as having to explain their illness to peers or teachers, pressures to conform to peers by breaking adherence to their medical regimen, and responding to parental demands. Gross, Johnson, Wildman, and Mullett (1981) have completed preliminary research identifying socially unskilled diabetic preadolescents and providing social skills training centered on the problematic situations described above. Staged role-play scenes particularly relevant to asthmatic or arthritic children have yet to be developed. Nevertheless, this method of assessment appears to be a potentially useful strategy given the relative ease that children's role-play situations can be set up with a similar-age child or adult acting in a prescribed manner toward the target child.

While relevant problematic social situations have not been identified for chronically ill children, Dodge, McClaskey, and Feldman (1985) have developed an empirically based taxonomy of social situations that has successfully differentiated children identified by teachers as rejected from children rated as popular with peers. The 44-item Taxonomy of Problem Situations (TOPS) assesses a child's performance in five general social situations: entering a peer group, responding to a peer provocation, responding to a school failure or school success, conforming to social expectations, and finally, responding to teacher expectations. Results were similar to the findings reported by Asarnow and Callan (1985) that children with peer problems exhibit deficient problem-solving skills in problematic social situations; Dodge and his colleagues found that boys with poor peer relationships were less adaptive and displayed more aggressive behaviors in the five social situations identified in the TOPS.

In addition to inquiring about situations that would appear unique to chronically ill children (e.g., explaining their illness to uninformed peers, what to say to peers after a prolonged school absence), it would appear of value for clinicians to ask parents of chronically ill children how their child would respond to the situations identified in the TOPS. If serious concerns were raised by questioning the parents, or if the clinician suspected that a child might have difficulty relating to peers in an adequate fashion in specific situations, staged role-play scenes could be conducted. Keep in mind, however, that research by Beck, Forehand, Neeper, and Baskin (1982) suggests that role-play situations may elicit more social behaviors in children than are observed in similar but more naturalistic interactions (e.g., playing or watching a board game with other peers). These researchers hypothesize that interacting with an adult who provides social prompts in a staged role-play scene may be easier for some children than interacting with similar-age peers. While role-play scenes may present a more positive view of the targeted child's social abilities, they can still provide valuable information if one is concerned about how the child would behave under optimal conditions. For example, if an asthmatic child cannot adequately explain why he or she must occasionally use an inhaler to an adult in a staged scene, this may be a good indication that the child would have similar difficulty explaining this device to peers.

In addition to identifying specific social situations or tasks that elicit either prosocial or ineffective responses from children, a step in planning social skill intervention is assessing the critical skills in each of the problematic social situations (Dodge & Murphy, 1984). Some of the most critical behaviors are initiation skills, responsiveness to peers, the ability to maintain peer interactions, conflict resolution strategies, and, finally, peer social perceptions of the target child (Guralnick, Beck, Sanders, & McBride, 1985). Initiation skills are those critical behaviors that allow a child successfully to enter a group or an interaction with a peer. Putallaz and Gottman (1981) found that disliked elementary-age children use unsuccessful entry behaviors such as calling attention to themselves and not accurately assessing the tempo or content of an ongoing activity. Responsiveness to peers is how well a child responds to the social interactions of others. Socially skilled children are generally more receptive to peer initiations. Responsiveness to peers could be an important skill for chronically ill children who are frequently absent from school and need to integrate themselves back into their peer group.

Maintenance skills are how well the child is able to maintain an interaction with peers. Children who are on medication or who fatigue easily need to learn how to pace their playtime with peers, and also need to have the prerequisite skills for following the flow of an ongoing conversation or play theme. Conflict resolution is how the child resolves inevitable disagreements with other children. Skilled children tend to minimize potential conflicts by employing good problem-solving strategies (Asarnow & Callan, 1985; Dodge, Coie, & Brakke, 1983). Finally, social perceptions are personal characteristics or the prior history of a target child that affects peer peceptions and corresponding peer interactions with the child. A chronically ill child who is frequently absent from school or who is lethargic due to medication may be viewed by peers as fragile and sickly. Peers may also resent a chronically ill child because of his or her "vacations" from school. These perceptions can influence the manner in which peers relate to the child.

CONCLUDING REMARKS

Figure 9.1 shows a flowchart of assessment methods for evaluating chronically disordered children's potential personality and socialization difficulties. The figure depicts assessment as a multilevel phenomenon requiring use of different types of methods to produce different types of information. At the outset, the clinician will use a rather broad-band, low-fidelity approach, such as interviews, adult checklists, and child self-report measures. Specific behaviors to be modified in specific social situations will be isolated using more narrow-band, high-fidelity methods such as direct observations.

As any experienced clinician knows, assessing chronically ill children and using the assessment methods described in this chapter are fraught with potential problems. First of all, while the clinician is sensitized to the fact that chronically disordered children are considered high risk for adjustment problems, there is a dearth of objective, normative data for these groups of children. Furthermore, each assessment method described in this chapter has potential limitations. For example, checklists such as the Personality Inventory for Children and the Child Behavior Checklist completed by the child's parent(s) inherently assess adults' sensitivity and threshold for child behaviors. Some parents may be very sensitive or have a low threshold for children's behaviors, while other parents may underreport deviant or troublesome behaviors (Beck, 1987). A common remark by parents of chronically ill children is that deviant behavior is often the "result of the child's illness," and as such is not the child's "actual personality"; therefore the adult will minimize or underreport current problematic behaviors.

There are clear limitations for child self-report measures. These measures, by their very nature of asking children their subjective opinions, are vulnerable to distortions and socially desirable responses. Self-report measures, except perhaps the Pictorial Scale of Perceived Competence and Social Acceptance for Young Children (Harter & Pike, 1984), depend heavily upon reading and verbal skills. Finally, while direct observations of social behavior are vaunted as a narrow-band, high-fidelity assessment method (Cone, 1987), in reality the clinician must exercise extreme caution and sensitivity when inferring social competence based on naturalistic observation or structured role-plays. Direct observations of role-play tests are subject to potential artificiality, reactivity, and, at times, questionable validity (Van Hasselt, Hersen, & Bellack, 1981). The clincian must carefully select social situations relevant to the target child (e.g., Dodge et al., 1985) and use appropriate props and instructions in an effort to elicit realistic responses from the target child (Bellack, 1979).

The clinician working with chronically ill children must possess knowledge and sensitivity on a wide range of topics. The clinician needs to be well versed in the medical treatment and course of chronic disorders, be knowledgeable about the cognitive and social development of children from the age of 2 through adolescence, and possess an internal barometer to gauge when a child may be "adjusting" or "not adjusting" to a chronic illness. Globally determining a child's adjustment to a chronic disorder also must take into account the child's age at initial diagnosis and length of time the child has been diagnosed. Finally, the clinician must pick and choose assessment methods and make decisions gleaned from such strategies about the need for further assessment.

References

Achenbach, T. M. (1966). The classification of children's psychiatric symptoms: A factor analytic study. *Psychological Monographs, 80*(7, Whole No. 615).

Achenbach, T. M. (1978). The child behavior profile: I. Boys aged 6–11. *Journal of Consulting & Clinical Psychology, 46*, 478–488.

Achenbach, T. M., & Edelbrock, C. S. (1978). The classification of child psychopathology: A review and analysis of empirical efforts. *Psychological Bulletin, 85*, 1275–1301.

Achenbach, T. M., & Edelbrock, C. S. (1983). *Manual for the Child Behavior Checklist and Revised Child Behavior Profile*. Burlington, Vermont: Queen City Printers.

Alexander, A. B. (1980). The treatment of psychosomatic disorders: Bronchial asthma in children. In B. B. Lahey & A. E. Kazdin (Eds.), *Advances in child clinical psychology* (Vol. 3). New York: Plenum.

Alexander, A. B. (1983). The nature of asthma. In P. J. McGrath & P. Firestone (Eds.), *Pediatric and adolescent behavioral medicine* (Vol. 10). New York: Springer.

American Psychiatric Association (1987). *Diagnostic and statistical manual of mental disorders* (3rd ed., Revised). DSM-III-R Washington, DC: Author.

Beck, S. (1987). Methods of assessment II: Questionnaires and checklists. In C. L. Frame & J. L. Matson (Eds.), *Handbook of assessment in childhood psychopathology: Applied issues in differential diagnosis and treatment evaluation*. New York: Plenum.

Beck, S., Forehand, R., Neeper, R., & Baskin, C. H. (1983). A comparison of two analogue strategies for assessing children's social skills. *Journal of Consulting & Clinical Psychology, 50*, 596–597.

Bellack, A. S. (1979). A critical appraisal of strategies for assessing social skills. *Behavioral Assessment, 1*, 157–176.

Bierman, K. L. (1983). Cognitive development and clinical interviews with children. In B. B. Lahey & A. E. Kazdin (Eds.), *Advances in clinical child psychology* (Vol. 6). New York: Plenum.

Bowlby, J. (1969). *Attachment and loss: Vol. I. Attachment*. New York: Basic.

Calabro, J. J. (1969). Juvenile rheumatoid arthritis. *General Practice, 60*, 78–88.

Cleveland, S. E., Reitman, E. E., & Brewer, E. J. (1965). Psychological factors in juvenile rheumatoid arthritis. *Arthritis & Rheumatism, 8*, 1152–1158.

Combs, M., & Slaby, D. (1977). Social skills training in children. In B. B. Lahey & A. E. Kazdin (Eds.), *Advances in clinical child psychology* (Vol. 1). New York: Plenum.

Cone, J. D. (1987). Behavioral assessment with children and adolescents. In M. Hersen & V. B. Van Hasselt (Eds.), *Behavior therapy with children and adolescents: A clinical approach*. New York: Wiley.

Creer, T. L. (1982). Asthma. *Journal of Consulting & Clinical Psychology, 50*, 912–921.

Crockett, L., Losoff, M., & Peterson, A. C. (1984). Perceptions of the peer group and friendship in early adolescence. *Journal of Early Adolescence, 4*, 155–181.

Csikszentmihalyi, M., Larson, R., & Prescott, S. (1977). The ecology of adolescent activity and experience. *Journal of Youth & Adolescence, 6*, 281–294.

Dahlquist, G., Gustavson, H. K., Holmgren, G., Haglof, B., Larsson, Y., Nilsson, K. O., Samuelson, G., Sterky, G., Thalme, B., & Walls, S. (1982). The incidence of diabetes mellitus in Swedish children 0–14 years of age: A prospective study 1977–1980. *Acta Paediatrica Scandinavica, 71*, 7.

Dodge, K. A., Coie, J. D., & Brakke, N. P. (1983). Behavior patterns of social rejected and neglected preadoleslcents: The role of social approach and aggression. *Journal of Abnormal Child Psychology, 10*, 389–409.

Dodge, K. A., McClaskey, C. L., & Feldman, E. (1985). Situational approach to the assessment of social competence in children. *Journal of Consulting & Clinical Psychology, 53*, 344–353.

Dodge, K. A., & Murphy, R. R. (1984). The assessment of social competence in adolescents. In P. Karoly

& J. J. Steffen (Eds.), *Adolescent behavior disorders: Current perspectives*. Lexington, MA: D. C. Heath.

Drash, A. L. (1979). The child with diabetes. In B. Hamburg, L. F. Lipsett, G. E. Inoff, & A. L. Drash (Eds.), *Behavioral and psychosocial issues in diabetes* (NIN Publication No. 80, pp. 33–42). Washington, DC: U.S. Department of Health and Human Services.

Erikson, E. H. (1963). *Childhood and society*. New York: Norton.

Fishbein, H. A., Faich, G. A., & Ellis, S. E. (1982). Incidence and hospitalization patterns of insulin-dependent diabetes mellitus. *Diabetes Care, 5*, 63.

French, T. N., & Alexander, F. (1941). Psychogenic factors in bronchial asthma. *Psychosomatic Medicine Monograph, 4*, 2–94.

Freud, A. (1965). *Normality and pathology in childhood: Assessments of development*. New York: International Universities Press.

Fritz, G. K. (1983). Childhood asthma: Psychosomatic illness review: No. 13. *Pediatrics, 24*, 959–967.

Furman, W., & Bierman, K. L. (1984). Children's conceptions of friendships: A multimethod study of developmental changes. *Developmental Psychology, 20*, 925–931.

Gdowski, C. L. (1977). Typologies of childhood psychopathology and their relationship with the personality inventory for children. Unpublished doctoral dissertation, Wayne State University, 1978. *Dissertation Abstracts International, 38*, 5566–B.

Gottman, J. M., Gonso, J., & Schuler, P. (1976). Teaching social skills to isolated children. *Journal of Abnormal Child Psychology, 4*, 179–197.

Green, K. D., Vosk, B., Forehand, R., & Beck, S. (1981). An examination of differences among sociometrically identified accepted, rejected, and neglected children. *Child Study Journal, 4*, 117–124.

Gregg, S. (1971). Rheumatoid arthritis in childhood. *Arizona Medicine, 28*, 577–585.

Gross, A. M. (1984). Behavioral interviewing. In T. H. Ollendick & M. Hersen (Eds.), *Child behavioral assessment: Principles and procedures*. New York: Pergamon.

Gross, A. M., Heimann, L., Shapiro, R., & Schulty, R. M. (1983). Children with diabetes, social skills training and hemoglobin Alc levels. *Behavior Modification, 7*, 151–164.

Gross, A. M., & Johnson, W. G. (1981). The diabetes assertiveness test: A measure of social coping skills in preadolescent diabetics. *The Diabetes Educator, 7*, 26–27.

Gross, A. M., Johnson, W. G., Wildman, H., & Mullett, N. (1981). Coping skills training with insulin-dependent preadolescent diabetes. *Child Behavior Therapy, 3*, 141–153.

Guralnick, M., Beck, S., Sanders, T., & McBride, S. (1985). *The peer interaction assessment (PIA)*. Unpublished manuscript, the Ohio State University, Columbus.

Hamberg, B. A. (1983). Chronic illness. In M. B. Levine, A. C. Crocker, W. B. Carey, & R. T. Gross (Eds.), *Developmental-behavior pediatrics*. Philadelphia: Saunders.

Harter, S. (1982). The Perceived Competence Scale for Children. *Child Development, 53*, 87–97.

Harter, S., & Pike, R. (1984). The Pictorial Scale of Perceived Competence and Social Acceptance for Young Children. *Child Development, 55*, 1969–1982.

Hartup, W. W. (1976). Peer interaction and the behavioral development of the individual child. In E. Schopler & R. J. Peichler (Eds.), *Psychopathology and child development: Research and treatment*. New York: Plenum.

Hartup, W. W. (1979). The social worlds of childhood. *American Psychologist, 34*, 944–950.

Hathaway, S. R., & McKinley, J. C. (1951). *The Minnesota multiphasic personality inventory manual* (rev. ed.). New York: Psychological Corporation.

Hollaender, J., & Florin, I. (1983). Expressed emotion and airway conductance in children with bronchial asthma. *Journal of Psychosomatic Research, 27*, 307–311.

Hooks, W. C. (1971). Personality factors associated with juvenile rheumatoid arthritis. *Dissertation Abstracts International, 32B*, 3637–3638.

Johnson, S. B. (1980). Psychosocial factors in juvenile diabetes: A review. *Journal of Behavioral Medicine, 3*, 95–116.

Kagan, J. (1958). The concept of identification. *Psychological Review, 65*, 296–305.

Kazdin, A. E. (1980). *Research design in clinical psychology*. New York: Harper & Row.

Kendall, P. C., & Braswell, L. (1985). *Cognitive–behavioral therapy for impulsive children*. New York: Guilford.

King, N. J. (1980). The behavioral management of asthma and asthma-related problems in children: A critical review of the literature. *Journal of Behavioral Medicine, 3,* 169–189.

Kornreich, H., Kostes, K., & Hanson, V. (1973). The rheumatic diseases in adolescence. *Pediatric Clinics of North America, 20,* 911–931.

Kovacs, M., Feinberg, F., Paulauskas, S., Finklestein, R., Pollock, M., & Crouse-Novak, M. (1985). Initial coping responses and psychosocial characteristics of children with insulin-dependent diabetes mellitus. *Journal of Pediatrics, 106,* 827–834.

Lachar, D. (1982). *Personality Inventory for Children: Revised format manual supplement.* Los Angeles: Western Psychological Services.

Lachar, D., Gdowski, C. L., & Snyder, D. K. (1984). External validation of the Personality Inventory for Children (PIC) profile and factor scales: Parent, teacher, and clinician ratings. *Journal of Consulting & Clinical Psychology, 52,* 155–164.

Lachar, D., & Wirt, R. (1981). A data-based analysis of the psychometric performance of the Personality Inventory for Children (PIC): An alternative to the Achenbach review. *Journal of Personality Assessment, 45,* 614–616.

McAnarney, E. R., Pless, B., Satterwhite, B., & Friedman, S. B. (1974). Psychological problems of children with chronic juvenile arthritis. *Pediatrics, 53,* 523–527.

Montemayer, R. (1982). The relationship between parent–adolescent conflict and the amount of time adolescents spend alone and with parents and peers. *Child Development, 53,* 1512–1519.

Naglieri, J. A., & Genshaft, J. L. (1985). Recent advances in the psychological assessment of children. In S. I. Pfeiffer (Ed.), *Clinical child psychology: An introduction to theory, research and practice.* New York: Grune & Stratton.

National Center for Health Statistics. (1971). Chronic conditions and limitations of activity and mobility in the United States, July 1965–July 1967. *Vital & Health Statistics, 10* (61).

Parmalee, A. H. (1986). Children's illnesses: Their beneficial effects on behavioral development. *Child Development, 57,* 1–10.

Piers, E., & Harris, D. (1969). *The Piers-Harris Children Self-Concept Scale.* Nashville, Tenn.: Counselor.

Pless, I. B. (1983). Effects of chronic illness on adjustment: Clinical implications. In P. Firestone, P. J. McGrath, & W. Feldman (Eds.), *Advances in behavioral medicine for children and adolescents.* Hillsdale, NJ: Erlbaum.

Pless, I. B., & Perrin, J. M. (1985). Issues common to a variety of illnesses. In N. Hobbs & J. M. Perrin (Eds.), *Issues in the care of children with chronic illness.* San Francisco: Jossey-Bass.

Pless, I. B., & Pinkerton, P. (1975). *Chronic childhood disorder: Promoting patterns of adjustment.* Chicago: Yearbook Medical Publishers.

Purcell, K., & Weiss, J. H. (1970). Asthma. In C. G. Costello (Ed.), *Symptoms of psychopathology: A handbook.* New York: Wiley.

Putallaz, M., & Gottman, J. M. (1981). An interactional model of children's entry into peer groups. *Child Development, 52,* 986–994.

Richard, B. A., & Dodge, K. A. (1982). Social maladjustment and problem solving in school-aged children. *Journal of Consulting & Clinical Psychology, 50,* 226–233.

Schiffer, C. G., & Hunt, E. P. (1963). Illness among children: Data from United States national health survey (Children's Bureau Publication No. 405). Washington, DC: U.S. Government Printing Office.

Selman, R. L. (1980). *The growth of interpersonal understanding: Developmental and clinical analyses.* New York: Academic.

Selman, R. L., & Jacquette, D. (1977). Stability and oscillation in interpersonal awareness: A clinical-developmental analysis. In C. B. Keary (Ed.), *The Nebraska Symposium on Motivation* (Vol. 25). Lincoln: University of Nebraska Press.

Smith, J. M. (1971). A five-year prospective survey of rural children with asthma and hay fever. *Journal of Allergy, 47,* 23–30.

Sparrow, S. S., Balla, D. A., & Cicchetti, D. V. (1984). *Vineland Adaptive Behavior Scales.* Circle Pines, MN: American Guidance Service.

Williams, G. (1981). *Children with chronic arthritis.* Littleton, MA: PSG.

Wing, R. R., Epstein, L. H., Nowalk, M. P., Koeske, R., & Hagg, S. (1985). Behavior change, weight loss, and physiological improvements in Type II diabetic patients. *Journal of Consulting & Clinical Psychology, 53*, 111–122.

Wirt, R., & Broen, W. (1958). *Booklet for the Personality Inventory for Children*. Minneapolis: Authors.

Wirt, R. D., Lachar, D., Klinedinst, J. K., & Seat, P. D. (1977). *Multidimensional description of child personality: A manual for the Personality Inventory for Children*. Los Angeles: Western Psychological Services.

Wirt, R. D., & Lachar, D. (1981). The Personality Inventory for Children: Development and clinical applications. In P. McReynolds (Ed.), *Advances in psychological assessment* (Vol. 5). San Francisco: Jossey-Bass.

Wright, L., Schaefer, A. B., & Solomons, G. (1974). *Encyclopedia of pediatric psychology*. Baltimore: University Park Press.

Van Hasselt, V. B., Hersen, M., & Bellack, A. S. (1981). The validity of role play tests for assessing social skills in children. *Behavior Therapy, 12*, 202–216.

Yarrow, L. J. (1960). Interviewing children. In P. H. Mussen (Ed.), *Handbook of research methods in child development*. New York: Wiley.

10

Psychoeducational Assessment

THOMAS R. KRATOCHWILL
VIVIENNE ROSEBY

INTRODUCTION

Scope of Psychoeducational Assessment Activities

We view psychoeducational assessment in health care settings as a broad-based activity involving the collection of information for the purpose of decision making (Ysseldyke, 1979). Decision making involves several interrelated activities consisting of screening or identification, classification or placement, instructional planning, client evaluation, and program evaluation (Salvia & Ysseldyke, 1978, 1985). It is important to distinguish among these different categories of assessment activities since different assessment devices, procedures, and techniques will likely be involved in each.

Screening or identification as an assessment process typically involves collecting data that allow the psychologist or other mental health professional to determine

The authors express appreciation to Drs. Paul Karoly, Edward S. Shapiro, and James E. Ysseldyke for their comments on an earlier draft of this chapter. The authors also thank Ms. Karen Kraemer for word-processing the manuscript.

whether further and more comprehensive assessment is necessary. Typically, in the screening or identification process broad-band norm-referenced screening devices are administered to determine whether or not the health-impaired child is significantly different from a norm group on various academic or personality measures.

When classification or placement of the child is a primary concern, individuals involved in psychoeducational assessment must typically adhere to existing diagnostic or classification guidelines that are used to qualify children for special services. Two systems that are commonly used to make a diagnosis include the *Diagnostic and Statistical Manual of Mental Disorders* (DSM-III-R) (American Psychiatric Association, 1987) and Public Law 94-142. These two diagnostic systems differ on a number of important dimensions that often influence the nature of the assessment process when classification or placement in a special program is necessary. Neither system is as useful in instructional planning.

Assessment data are also gathered to develop or implement a special intervention program, although this has not been typical in more traditional assessment. In this assessment mode the health care psychologist typically will focus on assessment devices and procedures that allow a careful analysis of the specific deficits or of the skills that patients need to have in order to perform academic or social behaviors. In such cases it is often necessary to use assessment techniques and procedures that identify treatments, so that others can actually work with a child within an intervention context.

Individual pupil evaluation will also be an important focus of the assessment efforts so that individuals involved in implementing the intervention program can determine whether or not progress is actually being made (Kratochwill, 1980). A number of specific assessment procedures have been designed to monitor students and their progress in academic areas.

Finally, assessment data may also be gathered for the purpose of evaluating programs that have been implemented in applied health care settings (Maher & Bennett, 1984). Often the unit of analysis is a total or comprehensive program that has been implemented for purposes of facilitating academic or social skills in children and adolescents. For example, a special tutorial program established for children in a hospital might be evaluated in terms of its specific goals and objectives of helping children make a successful transition to public school. Obviously, psychoeducational assessment focused on this activity is quite different than that focused on screening or identification and classification and placement.

In the conduct of psychoeducational assessment in health care settings it is important to emphasize that different assessment strategies will be used at different phases of the child's assessment process. Typically, depending on the nature of the handicapping condition, assessment will begin with more global or broad-based strategies and move to more specific and narrower strategies (Elliott & Piersel, 1982; Hawkins, 1979). Figure 10.1 depicts an "assessment funnel" in which assessment techniques are arranged in a conceptual order based on the degree of relevance to diagnosis and educational programming. The psychoeducational assessment techniques described in the chapter should be considered within this context.

In this chapter we provide an overview of some of the major domains of psychoeducational assessment that can be used for decision making in medical settings. Our chapter provides readers with an overview of procedures and techniques that can be used during the first four phases of assessment. The reader interested in program evaluation should review Maher and Bennett (1984).

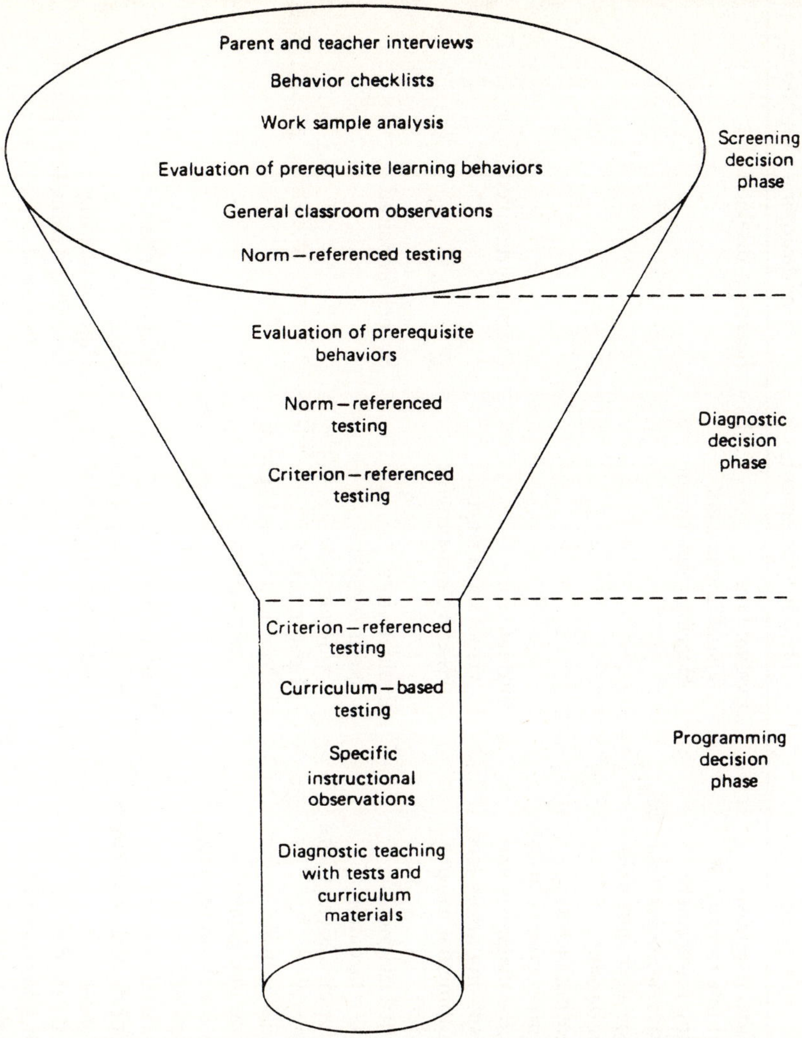

FIGURE 10.1. The assessment funnel. From "Direct Assessment of Reading Skills: An Approach Which Links Assessment to Intervention" by S. N. Elliott and W. C. Piersel, 1982, *School Psychology Review, 11*, pp. 267–280. Reprinted by permission.

Categories of Psychoeducational Assessment in Medical Settings

When psychoeducational assessment is called for in the medical setting the presenting problems are likely to fall into one of two broad categories:

1. Problems with primarily psychoeducational presentation and somatic features (see Table 10.1)
2. Problems with primarily somatic presentation and psychoeducational features (see Table 10.2)

TABLE 10.1. DISORDERS WITH PSYCHOEDUCATIONAL PRESENTATION—SOMATIC FEATURES

Primary Disorder	Predisposing Factors/Differential Diagnosis	Health Assessment	Possible PL 94–142 Educationally Handicapping Conditions
Developmental reading disorder	Differential diagnosis Visual impairment Hearing impairment Mental retardation (may be associated with mild retardation) Predisposing factors Poor instructional history	Evaluate for: Visual impairment Hearing impairment	Learning disabled
Developmental arithmetic disorder	Differential diagnosis and predisposing actors (see Developmental reading disorder)	Evaluate for: Visual impairment Hearing impairment	Learning disabled
Developmental articulation disorder	Differential diagnosis Mental retardation Developmental language disorder Infantile autism Hearing impairment Pervasive developmental disorder	Evaluate for: Neurological impairment Head trauma Disorders in oral speech mechanism	Speech impaired
Developmental language disorder Receptive and expressive types	Differential diagnosis Developmental articulation disorder Mental retardation Hearing impairment Infantile autism Pervasive developmental disorder Acquired aphasia	Evaluate for: Neurologic impairment Hearing impairment	Mentally retarded Deaf Hard of hearing Learning disabled or speech impaired

Attention deficit disorders With or without hyperactivity	Predisposing factors Mental retardation Neurologic impairment Chaotic environment Conduct disorder Schizophrenia Affective disorders	Evaluate for: Neurologic impairment	Learning disabled Mentally retarded or seriously emotionally disturbed
[a] Atypical stereotyped movement disorders	Prevalent in mentally retarded Developmental disorderd children Inadequate social stimulation	Evaluate for: Neurologic involvement	Mentally retarded Seriously emotionally disturbed
[a] Stuttering	Psychosocial stress may be predisposing factor	Evaluate for: Spastic dysphonia	Speech impaired
[a] Functional enuresis and encopresis	Psychosocial stress may be predisposing behavior	Evaluate for: Functional and/or structural urologic abnormalities	
[a] Asthma	Emotional tension may precede attack Conflict prevalent in families of asthmatics	Evaluate for: Cardiac and lung function [c] Pharmacological interventions	Other health impaired
Transient and chronic motor tic disorders	Psychosocial stress may be predisposing factor [b]	Evaluate for: Neurologic involvement	

[a] DSM-III-R.
[b] Schumer, 1983; Weiner, 1977.
[c] UW medical faculty.

TABLE 10.2. DISORDERS WITH SOMATIC PRESENTATION AND PSYCHOEDUCATIONAL FEATURES

Primary Disorder	Predisposing Factors/Differential Diagnosis	Health Assessment	Possible PL 94-142 Educationally Handicapping Conditions
Tourette's disorder	Differential diagnoses Schizophrenia Amphetamine intoxication Organic mental disorders Paresis Multiple sclerosis Cardiovascular accident	Evaluate for: Neurologic involvement or impairment Amphetamine intoxication Cerebrovascular accidents Multiple sclerosis	
Pica	Predisposing factors Mental retardation Mineral deficiency Poor supervision Differential diagnoses Infantile autism Schizophrenia	Evaluate for: Neurologic impairment (Klein-Levin syndrome) Systemic medical problem	Mentally retarded Seriously emotionally disturbed

Elective mutism	Differential diagnoses Mental retardation Pervasive developmental disorder Major depression Avoidant disorder Overanxious disorder Oppositional disorder Social phobia Inability to speak language		Mentally retarded Seriously emotionally distrubed
Infantile autism	Differential diagnosis Developmental language disorder Mental retardation Schizophrenia	Evaluate for: Hearing impairment Neurologic impairment	Other health impaired
Childhood-onset pervasive developmental disorder	Differential diagnosis Mentally retarded Schizotypal personality disorder Hearing impairment Developmental language disorder	Evaluate for: Hearing impairment Neurologic impairment	Mentally retarded

The psychoeducational assessment should encompass intellectual, achievement, adaptive behavior, and social or personality factors within the child's learning and living environments. The following framework may be applied to the child, taking into account the decision-making process noted in the previous section:

1. A working hypothesis regarding the way in which medical and psychoeducational variables interact with each other and with the presenting problem, to ensure that the total "gestalt" of the child is addressed, and to clarify, when possible, the most parsimonious point of intervention
2. Primary and differential diagnosis
3. Educational classification and placement decisions
4. Intervention planning
5. Evaluation of the intervention

Assessment of Psychoeducational Problems with Somatic Features. In some cases, referral data may identify the presenting problem as primarily psychoeducational. In such cases, diagnostic labels that might be considered include developmental reading, math, or language disorders, which are potentially classifiable as specific learning disabilities according to PL 94-142, or developmental articulation disorder, which may be classified as speech impaired according to PL 94-142 criteria. Attention deficit disorders with and without hyperactivity also occur in psychoeducational assessment domains and may be classified as handicapping conditions according to PL 94-142 as learning disabilities and/or serious emotional disturbance. Infantile autism and pervasive developmental disabilities may indicate more global impairment with significant deficits in all psychoeducational domains. Autism is classified according to PL 94-142 as "other health impaired" whereas pervasive developmental disability may be classified as mental retardation or "multihandicapped." Similarly, elective mutism and pica may be associated with significant psychoeducational deficits, and may suggest educational classification as seriously emotionally disturbed, mentally retarded, or learning disabled depending on the particular features of the individual diagnostic picture. In such instances, the psychoeducational clinician's tasks include the need to:

1. Validate diagnosis and check for differential diagnostic indices
2. Assess the extent, severity, and situational specificity of the disorder
3. Assess for stress factors within child's life that contribute to the cause and/or maintenance of the disorder
4. Assess for functional deficits in other domains that are suspected associated features of the primary disorder
5. Develop psychoeducational remedial approaches and objectives when appropriate

Sometimes referral data will identify or suggest specific psychoeducational deficits that have been noted but not assessed meaningfully in terms of the total diagnostic picture and remedial plan. In such cases the psychoeducational clinician's tasks extend to developing a primary diagnosis in medical and/or psychoeducational terms if appropriate and useful, and assessing the extent, severity, and situational specificity of the problem and its contribution to the primary problem. In such a case tasks 3, 4, and 5 remain the same.

Assessment of Somatic Problems with Psychoeducational Features. Primary disorders with somatic presentation and possible psychoeducational complications include: atypical stereotyped movement disorder; stuttering; functional enuresis and encopresis; transient and chronic motor tic disorders; Tourette's disorder, and asthma. In these cases the psychoeducational clinician may need to:

1. Assess for functional deficits in psychoeducational domains that may be associated features of the primary disorder
2. Assess (to the extent possible) the degree to which psychoeducational deficits are contributing to the cause and/or maintenance of the somatic symptoms
3. Assess for the existence of an educationally handicapping condition

Developmental Considerations

While it is impossible to provide an in-depth overview of the myriad issues surrounding diagnosis and classification of specific medically related disorders (see topical chapters in this volume for more coverage), developmental factors are especially noteworthy. Depending on the nature and type of health problem, the normal development process may be compromised (Magrab, 1984). This is especially the case of long-term hospitalization that may be needed for chronic illness. Magrab (1984) notes:

> In planning an assessment of a chronically ill child, one must understand not only the implicit developmental stages but also the developmental aspects of chronic illness. At different ages children have varying concepts of illness and death and different perceptions of and reactions to treatments and hospitalization, and these interact with age-appropriate psychological issues. The patient's understanding of the disease's etiology and the treatment processes may differ significantly depending on his or her level of development. For example, one 6-year-old hemodialysis patient believed there were bees causing the buzzing in her fistula (a surgically joined artery and vein for dialysis access); a very bright 7-year-old hypothesized that he had congenital kidney problems because his mom ate too many peaches when she was pregnant (he had overheard his father teasing her about this); and, a third child, a very religious, mildly retarded 15-year-old, became terrified that if she received a cadaver transplant its owner or the devil might come to haunt her. (p. 12)

In planning psychoeducational assessment, Magrab (1984) has provided a useful range of factors to consider for the developmental aspects of chronic illness. Table 10.3 provides a brief overview of the psychological issue, concept of illness, reaction to hospitalization, and perception of death at various developmental stages. While the information presented in the table is not all empirically based, it does convey issues to which the psychologist must be sensitive in planning the assessment and treatment process.

TABLE 10.3. DEVELOPMENTAL ASPECTS OF CHRONIC ILLNESS

Age	Psychological Issues	Concepts of Illness	Reaction to Hospitalization	Perception of Death
Infancy	Importance of parent–child bonding Need to be as close physically as feasible	Generalized perception of discomfort and pain Perceptions modulated by response of the environment	Need to have parents close by Parents' presence and reactions provide best support in handling fear, pain, and separation	Fear of separation
Preschool	Need to bolster sense of mastery Need to prepare for medical procedures, separation, etc. Possibility of regressions, fears	Illness seen as punishment for bad behavior Magical view, fullness Adults seen as omnipotent with power to cure the illness magically if they wish to Conceptualization characterized by incomprehension, phenomenalism, and contagion Simple explanations useful for maintaining trust	Presence of parents continues to be of primary importance Hospitalization perceived as rejection or punishment Fears of mutilation arise Treatment may be seen as hostile or punitive Concerns about bodily penetration aroused by surgery or injections	Death may be personified Death often seen as violent Death comes as retaliation for being bad Death may not be permanent Dead people continue to live Death may be confused with separation and sleep
School age	Need to continue to produce and learn Begins to utilize	Notions of self-causation of illness from disobedient or	Primary concern is lack of body control and mastery	Begins to understand irreversibility of death Death becomes more real,

	knowledge and understanding of the body, causation of illness, and the process of treatment Need for honest explanations Fear of loss of control and sense of body integrity	imprudent behavior still occur but may take longer to express Can begin to understand body processes and functions Conceptualization characterized by internalization and contamination	Feelings of inadequacy arise May become demanding or rebellious to maintain semblance of control Knowledge about illness effective in handling anxiety Separation from family and peers may interfere with developmental task mastery	final, universal, and inevitable Differentiation of living and nonliving
Adolescence	Begins to deal with problems of illness as an individual Relies less on family support Difficulty with compliance of medical regimes proposed by adults (rebellion that may jeopardize health) Intense preoccupation with body changes and sexuality exacerbated Concerns about being "different" heightened Illness may impair ability to plan for the future	Focus on discrete symptoms rather than overall impact of illness Ability to deal intellectually with information about illness May use denial of illness or overcompensation in areas not affected Conceptualization characterized by physiological and psychophysiological causes of illness	Seen as threat to independence Conflicts over control may become acute Concern about status in peer group after hospitalization	Able to acknowledge the fragility of life Death may be viewed as philosophical problem in life or challenged and denied by risk taking Idea that death is not permanent may recur (suicide seen as retaliatory but reversible)

Source: From "A Developmental Framework for Psychological Assessment of Pediatric Conditions" by P. R. Magrab, in *Psychological and Behavioral Assessment: Impact on Pediatric Care* (pp. 3–21) by P. R. Magrab (Ed.), 1984, New York: Plenum. Reprinted by permission.

Conceptual Framework for Assessment

The clinician involved in psychoeducational assessment typically operates within some type of conceptual framework when conducting the specific assessment task. Although there is a great deal of overlap between traditional and behavioral assessment methods, each holds some different perspectives on the nature of the assessment activity and what might ultimately be the focus of intervention efforts. This issue is discussed, since the way that the specific assessment methods are used will vary depending on the particular orientation or philosophy of the psychologist.

While both behavioral and traditional assessment are focused on hypothesis testing, traditional psychologists have tended to focus on underlying structures or causes of the problem within the organism. In contrast, behavioral assessors have typically focused on environmental or person–environment interaction constructs during assessment efforts (Hartmann, Roper, & Bradford, 1979). Generally, behavioral assessment is characterized by fewer inferential assumptions about the nature of the academic or psychological difficulty experienced by the child client. Most nonbehavioral approaches to assessment conceptualize the academic problem as relatively stable and enduring, and further relate learning and behavior disorders to internal processes or characteristics of the child. Within traditional models, assessment of only the overt behaviors or performance of the client is considered inadequate or insufficient to gain a full understanding of the problem. Rather, the assessor often relates internal components to the external manifestations of the difficulty. As a typical example, traditional assessors might use a variety of psychoeducational or psycholinguistic devices (e.g., Illinois Test of Psycholinguistic Abilities) or tests of perceptual motor functioning (Developmental Test of Visual Perception) to gain an understanding of the client's educational problems. Although there are many different options for conceptualizing learning problems within the traditional framework, the hypothesis-testing model of Kirk and Kirk (1971) provides an illustration of the traditional approach to psychoeducational assessment (pp. 54–55):

1. Determining whether a learning problem exists
2. Determining the behavior manifestations and the specific problems encountered by the child
3. Discovering the physical, environmental, and psychological correlates of the disability
4. Evolving a diagnostic hypothesis on the basis of behavioral analysis and the correlates
5. Organizing a systematic remedial program based on the symptoms and deficits and diagnostic hypotheses determined during the previous stages

The key difference between more conventional behavioral (i.e., applied behavior analysis) and traditional approaches lies in points 3 and 4 (Kratochwill, 1982). The term *correlates of the disability* refers to various physical processes (e.g., visual defects, an environmental traumatic experience, sensory deprivation) or some psychological process (difficulties with auditory discrimination or short-term memory) that may be hypothesized as responsible for the disorder.

Growing evidence exists that traditional models have spawned a variety of technically inadequate procedures that do not have major implications for the design and monitoring of intervention programs (see Ysseldyke et al., 1983). A major limitation of many traditional assessment strategies is that they often involve removing the child from the natural setting (i.e., classroom) where the problem may be occurring.

In contrast to traditional approaches, the conventional behavioral assessment format moves from steps 1 and 2 to the development of an intervention program. Typically, inferred causes of the disorder might be deemphasized; an analysis of the environment and the client's skills in interaction with environmental demands would be the primary focus.

While behavioral psychoeducational assessment has increased in sophistication and actual use in practice, many unresolved issues remain within this model of assessment. Among the more salient concerns are the manner in which target measures are chosen (Kratochwill, 1984), the lack of standardized and psychometrically sound devices in assessment, and the extensive cost and time needed to conduct comprehensive behavioral assessments.

Although it is beyond the scope of the present chapter to discuss the specific differences between behavioral and traditional assessment in great detail, it is important again to emphasize that the same assessment *methods* associated with the two different models might be employed. What is at issue is what model of understanding human behavior is actually being used to guide assessment efforts, interpret the data, and link them to an intervention program.

Assessment Standards

Psychoeducational assessment, especially the tests used in this process, is governed by the *Standards for Educational and Psychological Testing* (American Psychological Association, 1985). The recent volume includes technical standards for test construction and evaluation, professional standards for test use, standards for particular applications, and standards for administrative procedures. We present only a brief review of the technical standards; readers are advised to review them all.

Validity. Validity of a test "refers to the appropriateness, meaningfulness, and usefulness of the specific inferences made from test scores" (p. 9). Three types are considered important in establishing validity evidence. *Construct-related* validity focuses on the test score as representative of the construct of interest. *Content-related validity* refers to the degree to which the sample of the test (i.e., items, tasks, or questions) is representative of a domain of content. *Criterion-related validity* involves establishing evidence that various test scores are related systematically to one or more outcome criteria.

Reliability. In the most general sense reliability "refers to the degree to which test scores are free from errors of measurement" (p. 19). So-called errors of measurement are differences between scores from one form to another, or from one time to another, but not due to such factors as maturation, interventions, or other factors that might actually cause scores to change.

Test Development and Revision. *Standards for Educational and Psychological Testing* was developed to encourage the proper development, use, and revisions of tests. Clinicians are encouraged to read test manuals for evidence of reliability, validity, norming, and conditions of testing that facilitate proper test use.

Scaling, Norming, Score Comparability, and Equating. The primary means of test interpretation relates to available scoring scales and norms that assist the clinician in relating raw scores to well-defined distributions. Each test must be examined to determine the type of derived scales and norms (e.g., national, local) that are offered by the test publisher. Moreover, if multiple forms of a test are available, assessors should determine how comparable alternate forms are, or if methods have been used to equate alternate test form scores.

Technical Manuals and Users' Guides. Test publishers should make available a *technical manual* that will assist the assessor in appropriate use of the test. *Standards for Educational and Psychological Testing* includes 11 major recommendations for technical manuals and users' guides.

Educational and Psychological Testing in the Schools. The standards referring to educational and psychological testing in the schools are especially relevant to psychoeducational assessment by individuals working in medical settings. Table 10.4 includes the 12 standards that guide psychoeducational assessment in the schools. It is important that psychologists working in medical settings adhere as closely as possible to the standards, especially in use of norm-referenced tests that are used for diagnosis and classification. It is in this domain of use that major problems have been identified in their application.

METHODS OF PSYCHOEDUCATIONAL ASSESSMENT

A number of different conceptual frameworks have been employed in the literature for organizing psychoeducational assessment methods including tests, work samples, and a variety of other devices and procedures (see e.g., Stetson, 1985). Our conceptual framework in this chapter provides a general way of organizing the diverse strategies that might be used in psychoeducational assessment. However, compelling arguments could obviously be developed for using other organizational schemes. Generally, the methods of psychoeducational assessment that can be used in medical settings consist of *interviews, self-report, checklists and rating scales, direct observation* procedures, and a wide range of *analogue measures* including formal standardized and informal nonstandardized measures. Each of these is reviewed briefly, and examples are presented of typical psychoeducational assessments that might be employed in health care settings.

Interview Assessment

The interview is used routinely in psychoeducational assessment activities. The interview can be adapted to virtually any form of psychoeducational assessment and used during the various phases of assessment just outlined. The interview

TABLE 10.4. STANDARDS FOR EDUCATIONAL TESTING AND PSYCHOLOGICAL TESTING IN THE SCHOOLS

Standard	Description
Standard 8.1	Those responsible for school testing programs should ensure that the individuals who administer the tests are properly instructed in the appropriate test administration procedures and that they understand the importance of adhering to the directions for administration that are provided by the test developer. (primary)
Standard 8.2	Those responsible for school testing programs should ensure that the individuals who use the test scores within the school context are properly instructed in the appropriate methods for interpreting test scores. (primary)
Standard 8.3	If test results are used in making statements about the differences between aptitude for an individual student, any educational decision based on these differences should take into account the overlap between the constructs and the reliability or standard error of the difference score. (primary)
Standard 8.4	When a test is to be used to certify the successful completion of a given level of education, either grade-to-grade promotion or high school graduation, both the test domain and the instructional domain at the given level of education should be described in sufficient detail, without compromising test security, so that the agreement between the test domain and the content domain can be evaluated. (primary)
Standard 8.5	When a test is developed by a state or local district to be used for student promotion, graduation, or classification decisions, users' guides or technical reports should be developed and disseminated. (conditional)
Standard 8.6	Results from certification tests should be reported promptly to all appropriate parties, including students, parents, and teachers. The report should contain a description of the test, what is measured, the conclusions and decisions that are based on the test results, the obtained score, information on how to interpret the reported score, and any cut score used for classification. (primary)
Standard 8.7	When a test is used to make decisions about student promotion or graduation, there should be evidence that the test covers only the specific or generalized knowledge, skills, and abilities that students have had the opportunity to learn. (primary)
Standard 8.8	Students who must demonstrate mastery of certain skills or knowledge before being promoted or granted a diploma should have multiple opportunities to demonstrate the skills. (primary)
Standard 8.9	Relationships between predictors and criterion measures that are used in educational admissions should be described by regression equations and associated standard errors of estimate or by expectancy tables in addition to correlation coefficients. (primary)
Standard 8.10	The possibility that differential prediction exists in educational selection for selected groups should be investigated where there is prior evidence to suggest that positive results may be found and where sample sizes are adequate. (conditional)
Standard 8.11	Test users should not imply that empirical evidence exists for a relationship among particular test results, prescribed educational plans, and desired student outcomes unless such evidence is available. (primary)
Standard 8.12	In elementary or secondary education, a decision or characterization that will have a major impact on a test taker should not automatically be made on the basis of a single test score. Other relevant information for the decision should also be taken into account by the professionals making the decision. (primary)

Source: Adapted from *Standards for Educational and Psychological Testing,* Washington, D.C.: American Psychological Association, 1985 (pp. 52–54).

allows the clinician to gather a great deal of diverse data from the client with flexibility in types of questions asked, the format used for coding data, and the specific link to other assessment methods (Gross, 1985).

The interview should occur very early in the psychoeducational assessment process. In this regard, it has often been used as the method of promoting a personal relationship between the assessor and the client. To some extent the interview actually overlaps with other assessment methods, since a variety of stimuli and materials associated with a wide range of tests could be used as a basis for conducting an interview. For example, background history questionnaires commonly used as a self-report method of obtaining data could be used within an interview context to refine the assessment process further. Moreover, one could use responses to a standardized test as a basis for asking various questions during the interview process.

Generally, in assessment of psychoeducational problems, the clinician has the option of assessing parents or care providers, teachers, and the child himself or herself. Typically in the parental interview the clinician obtains demographic data and information related to the broad concerns the family may have with the child. Although not providing a specific standardized format for the interview, Barkley (1981) suggested that several specific areas need to be addressed during the clinical interview with parents of learning disabled children. These include:

1. Questions related to the parents involving the child on homework or in the general areas where the child is displaying a deficiency
2. Information on background features of the child such as pregnancy, delivery, developmental and medical histories, as well as seizure patterns
3. Comprehensive academic history of the child including such things as when school first began, the child's general progress in school, evaluations from school, as well as programming the child may have received from the school situation
4. An evaluation of parent and family variables, including such things as educational level, existence of learning problems in the family, and related difficulties (e.g., psychiatric, marital, financial, emotional problems)
5. The parents' perceptions of what caused the child's difficulty, and the expectations the family has in terms of the outcome of any evaluation and/or any intervention program
6. An assessment of reinforcers of the child that might be used during the intervention program

Other formats exist as well, such as the one outlined by Thompson and O'Quinn (1979), who provided an interdisciplinary case history outline that can help guide the interview efforts (see Table 10.5). As can be observed in the table, the interview includes a wide range of assessment content including birth history, physical and developmental data, speech and language, motor skills, nutrition, social and personal factors, educational factors, as well as a probe into various personality characteristics that could be related to the psychoeducational or developmental problems of the child (see also Beck & Smith, Chapter 9, this volume).

TABLE 10.5. INTERDISCIPLINARY CASE HISTORY INTERVIEW OUTLINE

I. Birth History
   A. *Pregnancy:* length, condition of mother, unusual factors
   B. *Birth conditions:* mature or premature, duration of labor, weight, unusual circumstances
   C. *Conditions following birth*

II. Physical and Developmental Data
   A. *Health history:* accidents, high fevers, other illnesses
   B. *Present health:* habits of eating and sleeping, energy and activity level, medications
   C. *Developmental history:* held head up, crawled, sat alone, walked, babbled, first words, (2-word) sentences, language difficulties

III. Speech and Language
   Parents' description of child's speech and language skills at the present time with regard to:
   A. *Sound production:* How easy is it to understand the child?
   B. *Sentence construction:*
      1. Sentence length
      2. Words in proper order
   C. *Grammar:*
      1. Usage of pronouns
      2. Usage of plurals
      3. Usage of verb tenses
   D. *Voice quality:*
      1. Nasality
      2. Hoarseness
      3. Breathiness
   E. *Rate and rhythm*
      1. Speaks too fast
      2. Speaks too slow
      3. "Stuttering" behavior
   F. *Language comprehension:* Does the child understand what is said to him or her?
      1. Does he or she follow instructions, with or without gestures?
      2. Can he or she answer questions appropriately?
      3. Does he or she relate verbally what has happened?
   G. Are the parents concerned about the child's speech and language skills?
   H. Are the child's speech and language skills as good as those of other children the same age?
   I. What languages are spoken at home?

IV. Motor Skills
   A. Clumsiness, awkwardness, lack of coordination and balance
   B. Ability to plan and execute skilled gross motor acts (ride a tricycle, put on clothing, etc.)
   C. Abnormal types of movements, abnormal muscle tone, or orthopedic problems
   D. Eye–hand coordination for fine motor tasks (using a pencil, cutting with scissors, putting toys together, etc.)

V. Nutrition
   A. Does the child have any unusual food habits? (e.g., pica, eating snacks only, eating no vegetables, etc.)

(*Table continues on p. 190.*)

TABLE 10.5. (*Continued*)

- B. Does the child have any difficulty in sucking, swallowing, chewing, or frequent drooling?
- C. Does the child frequently suffer from any of the following conditions: diarrhea, vomiting, constipation, colds, or fevers?
- D. Is the child excessively over- or underweight, or very pale?
- E. Does the child have rough, dry, or puffy skin?

VI. Social and Personal Factors
- A. Friends
- B. Sibling relationships
- C. Hobbies, interests, recreational activities (toy and play activities)
- D. Home and parent attitudes
- E. Acceptance of responsibilities
- F. Attitude toward learning problems
- G. Self-care activities (degree of independence in dressing, feeding, toileting, etc.)

VII. Educational Factors
- A. *Preschool education:* nursery school, kindergarten
- B. *School experience:* skipped or repeated grades, moving, change of teachers
  1. Teacher's report
  2. Child's attitude toward school
- C. Special help, if any, previously received

VIII. Personality Characteristics, especially regarding:
- A. Anxieties
- B. Fears
- C. Dependence
- D. Mood swings
- E. Aggression tantrums
- F. Reliability
- G. Enuresis

IX. Impressions

X. Recommendations

Source: From *Developmental Disabilities: Etiologies, Manifestations, Diagnoses and Treatment* (pp. 270–271) by J. R. Thompson, Jr., and A. N. O'Quinn, 1979, New York: Oxford University Press. Reprinted by permission.

Teacher Interview. It is essential for the clinician to conduct a teacher interview for a child experiencing any learning difficulties. Teachers have intense involvement with children and their academic performance. Also, if the child is hospitalized for an extended period, it will be necessary to help the child maintain academic assignments in the hospital and eventually make the transition to the school. Therefore, the clinician should conduct an interview with the teacher in the natural environment, if the child is to be understood within the context of usual academic expectations.

Again, there are relatively few standardized formats that have been developed for interview assessment of teachers. One semistandardized method of interviewing teachers has been developed in the consultation model presented by Bergan and Kratochwill (in press). The model provides the clinician with a systematic format for conducting the interview and consists of four stages, including problem identification, problem analysis, plan implementation, and problem evaluation. The interview format has been described elsewhere and will not be presented here (see Bergan & Kratochwill, in press, for examples).

Child Interview. Children are sometimes a neglected focus of interview assessment activities because it is sometimes assumed that they may not have insight into their own academic problems. However, an interview (both structured and unstructured) can be very useful in obtaining information surrounding the child's academic difficulties (Barkley, 1981).

Especially important in interviewing are a wide range of developmental factors that interact with the type and quality of information obtained from the child client. The reader is referred to Witt, Cavell, Heffer, Carey, and Martens (in press) for an overview of these issues. Some of the general areas that can be addressed in a child interview include the following domains: demographic information (e.g., age, address); academic performance (e.g., study habits, grades); classroom behavior (e.g., classroom rules, rewards); peer relations (e.g., number of friends, play activities); interests (e.g., free-time activities, sports); relations with parents (e.g., parental expectations); treatment preferences (e.g., reinforcer preferences, goals of treatment); and various other referral concerns. This broad-focus interview format also provides the clinician with an excellent opportunity to obtain information on whether there are any emotional factors that might be related to the child's difficulties. Emotional factors that relate to the child's learning difficulties outside the assessment situation should be differentiated from the effects of anxiety, misunderstanding, response sets, and demand characteristics within the interview. These distinctions are best made when the interviewer obtains and attends to a "child's eye view" of the situation before arriving at any diagnostic conclusions (Achenbach, 1978).

Self-Report

Self-report methods of assessment represent an indirect method of obtaining data on a client or others involved in the academic difficulties. While self-report has sometimes been regarded as unreliable due to the unstructured and open-ended nature of questions, a variety of self-report inventories might be used further to structure the situation. Self-report is particularly important in assessing cognitive processes and in obtaining the client's own perception regarding the nature of the problem. Self-report measures provide a relatively colorful picture of the client's objective and subjective experiences related to the problem he or she may be having.

It is important to distinguish between objective and subjective data obtained through self-report measures (Bellack & Hersen, 1977). With self-report methods that require an objective and publicly observable response, verification is possible (e.g., "How many pages of your reading text did you complete?"). On the other hand, more subjective questions (e.g., "Do you like school?") are not possible to verify via direct observation. These differences in the ways that scales are constructed have important implications for establishing validity.

A number of variables have been identified that influence the validity of self-report data, including whether the report is written or verbal, the form of the questions asked, the actual content of the questions, situational factors, operational specification of the terms among other factors (i.e., Haynes, 1978; Tasto, 1977).

A rather large number of self-report scales covering a wide range of childhood and adolescent disorders could be used in psychoeducational assessment. The reader is again referred to Witt and colleagues (in press) for a brief overview of some self-report scales that could be used in assessment of children and adolescents. Only some representative examples are presented here.

One measure that is often used in psychoeducational assessment is the child form of the Behavior Rating Profile (BRP; Brown & Hammill, 1978). The child form has 20 items in a true–false format and is standardized on children 6 to 13 years old. Since the complete scale is designed to be used by teachers, parents, and the child, a more comprehensive assessment is possible than if only one informant were used. The scale is also useful due to the focus on the situational specificity of the child's behavior.

Self-report forms that can be used for conducting a psychoeducational evaluation of children have also been presented by Cautela, Cautela, and Esonis (1983). A number of specific forms are included that can be used with children including those assessing assertive behavior, body tension, fear inventories, self-evaluation scales, and a variety of other forms that can be used over various phases of an intervention program. Among the more common examples of self-report forms are those used to sample various reinforcers that a child might like and that could possibly be used during an intervention program. Some common items used in a reinforcement survey schedule for children include the following:

Having a story told or read to me by

a. my mother
 not at all ________
 a little ________
 very much ________
 not done with my mother ________

b. my father
 not at all ________
 a little ________
 very much ________
 not done with my father ________

Getting help with my homework with

a. my mother
 not at all ________
 a little ________
 very much ________
 not done with my mother ________

b. my father
 not at all ________
 a little ________
 very much ________
 not done with my father ________ (Cautela et al., 1983, pp. 125–126)

Individuals employing self-report scales should always consider the psychometric data available on a particular scale when psychoeducational decision making is involved. Self-report scales should seldom be the primary assessment focus; nevertheless the scales can be useful when they are supplemented with other data.

Checklists and Rating Scales

A large number of checklists and rating scales are used in psychoeducational assessment of children. Select reviews of various aspects of this literature have been presented and the reader is referred to some of these original sources for a more detailed presentation (Edelbrock, in press; Hoge, 1983; Quay, 1979). The primary characteristic of rating scales and checklists is that they require adult informants to rate children's functioning on several different dimensions of behavior. In Hoge's (1983) review of teacher judgment measures, rating scales were categorized as (1) behavior measures; (2) aptitude measures; and (3) achievement measures. In behavior measures teachers and other care providers are asked to make judgments of some aspect of the child's behavior in the classroom setting (e.g., easily distracted). In contrast, aptitude assessment tends to focus on more general characteristics, or traits of the client (e.g., intellectual potential; arithmetic aptitude). Achievement measures include a rating of some aspect of the child's performance (e.g., reading or math achievement).

Several specific advantages of checklists and rating scales or informant reports can be identified (Edelbrock, in press). To begin with, these measures provide a list of the descriptors that form a common language for communication about a given client. This is an advantage since some type of standardized response format is introduced into the assessment process. Second, checklists and rating scales typically provide some type of format for the individual to rate the presence, frequency, or severity of the response mentioned (e.g., behavior, aptitude, or achievement). Such a rating format may reduce the subjectivity surrounding these judgments and increase reliability. Third, the standardized format used in rating scales allows the assessor to compare data across children. That is, similar target behaviors can be assessed using standard sets of items in rating formats. Fourth, standardized checklists and rating scales are relatively cost- and time-efficient relative to many other psychological or psychoeducational assessment measures. Fifth, these measures, largely because of their efficiency, have been applied to a wide range of clinical disorders. Especially beneficial in this context are the reliability, validity, and normative data that rating scales have provided for psychoeducational assessment.

A variety of checklists and rating scales have been developed, and it is impossible to provide a comprehensive review here. The interested reader is referred to some primary sources where this literature is reviewed in great detail (Achenbach & Edelbrock, 1978; Edelbrock, in press; Hoge, 1973; Quay, 1979). Tables 10.6 and 10.7 from Hoge (1983) provide a listing of the various checklists and rating scales that can be used in psychoeducational assessment across behavior and aptitude levels.

Based on a review of teacher-completed scales, Hoge (1983) concluded that results of an analysis of the behavioral measures supported a three-factor model consisting of personality adjustment, social adjustment, and academic competence. On the other hand, there was less support for a three-factor model in the case of aptitude measures.

There were some data also on discriminant validity for two of the aptitude measures and eight of the behavioral measures. With one exception, all indicated statistically significant levels of discriminant validity, therefore supporting reliance on the teacher as a source of information during assessment. With regard to criterion-

TABLE 10.6. DESCRIPTION OF BEHAVIORAL MEASURES

Measure	Reference	Focus[a]		Reliability[b]		Validity[c]		
		A-C	S-P	T-R	I-R	Con.	Disc.	C-R
1. Behavior Problem Checklist	Quay & Peterson	√	√	√	√	√	√	√
2. Behavioral adjustment ratings	Bolstad & Johnson (1977)		√					√
3. Child Activity Rating Scale	Lorion et al. (1975)	√	√			√	√	
4. Child Behavior Rating Scale	Kim et al. (1968)	√	√			√		√
5. Children's Behavior Questionnaire	Rutter (1967)		√	√			√	
6. Classroom Behavior Inventory	Blunden et al. (1974)	√	√		√	√		√
7. Conduct rating	Green et al. (1980)		√					√
8. Conners Teacher Rating Scale	Conners (1969)	√	√	√		√		√
9. Devereux Elementary School Behavior Rating Scale	Spivack & Swift	√	√	√		√	√	√
10. Health Resources Inventory	Gesten (1976)	√	√	√			√	√
11. Level of interaction ranking	Greenwood et al.		√	√				√

Measure	Source							
12. Pittsburgh Adjustment Survey Scales	Ross et al. (1965)	√	√			√		√
13. Assertion skills ratings	Reardon et al. (1979)		√					√
14. Preschool Behavior Questionnaire	Behar & Stringfield (1974)	√	√	√	√	√		√
15. Pupil Behavior Rating Scale	Lambert & Nicoll (1977)	√	√			√		√
16. Pupil Evaluation Inventory	Pekarik et al. (1976)	√				√		√
17. Rhode Island Pupil Identification Scale	Novack et al. (1973)							√
18. Problem Checklist & Social Competence Scale[d]	Kohn & Rosman (1972a)		√		√	√	√	√
19. Teacher Behavior Description Form	Seidman et al. (1979)	√	√			√		√
20. Teachers Social Behavior Rating Scale	Greenberg et al.		√	√		√		√
21. Teachers Observation of Classroom Adaptation	Kellam et al. (1975)	√	√	√			√	√
22. Walker Problem Behavior Checklist	Walker (1970)		√				√	

[a] A-C = academic cognitive focus and S-P = social-personality focus.
[b] T-R = test–retest reliability and I-R = interrater-agreement reliability.
[c] Con. = construct validity, Disc. = discriminant validity, and C-R = criterion-related validity.
[d] Scores from these two measures are generally combined.

Source: From "Psychometric Properties of Teacher Judgment Measures of Pupil Aptitudes, Classroom Behaviors, and Achievement Levels" by R. D. Hoge, 1983, *Journal of Special Education, 17*, pp. 401–429. Copyright by Pro-Ed, Inc. Reprinted by permission.

TABLE 10.7. DESCRIPTION OF APTITUDE MEASURES

Measure	Reference	Reliability[a]		Validity[b]		
		T-R	I-R	Con.	Disc.	C-R
	1. Multifacet Measures					
1.1 Academic and social aptitude ratings	Pedulla et al. (1980)					√
1.2 Academic and social aptitude ratings	Solomon & Kendall (1977)			√		√
1.3 Academic and social aptitude ratings	Stevenson et al. (1976a, 1976b)	√		√		√
1.4 Behavior-trait ratings	Schwartz et al. (1974)		√			√
1.5 Pupil Behavior Rating Scale	Myklebust (1971)				√	√
1.6 Schenectady Kindergarten Rating Scale	Conrad & Tobiessen (1967)				√	
	2. Measures of Specific Academic and Cognitive Aptitudes					
2.1 Academic skills rating	Dusek & O'Connell (1973)					√
2.2 Academic skills rating	Glazzard (1977)					√
2.3 Academic skills rating	Luce & Hoge (1978)					√
2.4 Academic skills rating	Mellon & Crano (1977)					√
2.5 Academic skills rating	Tokar & Holthouse (1977)					√
2.6 Academic skills rating	Farr & Roelke (1971)	√				√
2.7 Student Rating Scale	Feshbach et al. (1977)		√	√		√
2.8 Reading readiness rating	Keogh & Smith (1970)					√
2.9 Teacher Rating Scale	Reschley & Reschley (1979)					√
	3. Global Ratings of Academic Competence					
3.1 Academic competence rating	Evertson et al.					√
3.2 Academic competence rating	Perry et al. (1979)					√
3.3 Academic readiness rating	Brown (1976)					√
3.4 Expected achievement rating	Kapelis (1975)					√
3.5 Expected achievement rating	Morine-Derschimer (1978–1979)					√
3.6 Expected achievement rating	Willis (1972)					√

[a] T-R = test–retest reliability and I-R = interrater-agreement reliability.
[b] Con. = construct validity, Disc. = discriminant validity, and C-R = criterion-related validity.
Source: From "Psychometric Properties of Teacher Judgment Measures of Pupil Aptitudes, Classroom Behaviors, and Achievement Levels" by R. D. Hoge, 1983, *Journal of Special Education, 17,* pp. 401–429.

related validity, the majority of studies employed indices of academic achievement as a criterion. With both concurrent and predictive validity analyses there is a great deal of consistency in studies showing significant relations between rating measures and achievement indices. The majority of measures reviewed by Hoge display adequate levels of reliability, although some coefficients were below acceptable levels.

Although it is beyond the scope of the present chapter to review the many different parent ratings that have been used, a more comprehensive review of these rating scales can be found in Edelbrock (in press). One of the more common parent-completed rating scales is the Child Behavior Checklist (CBCL), a measure designed to tap a broad range of children's behavior problems and adaptive competencies (Achenbach, 1978; Achenbach & Edelbrock, 1979; Edelbrock & Achenbach, 1984). The CBCL is completed by parents and includes 20 social competence items including school performance, social relations, and amount and quality of participation in hobbies, activities, and sports. In addition, 118 items covering specific behavior problems are included. The parent rates items on a 0-1-2 scale corresponding to *not true, somewhat or sometimes true,* and *very or often true,* respectively. Parents also are requested to have a 6-month baseline for reporting children's behavior.

An important feature of the CBCL is that it is scored on a Child Behavior Profile. Profiles are developed and standardized separately for boys and girls ages 3 to 5, 6 to 11, and 12 to 16. Norms are available from 1300 randomly selected nonreferred children between the ages of 4 and 16 years (Achenbach & Edelbrock, 1981, 1983).

A teacher version of the CBCL has also been developed recently (Achenbach & Edelbrock, 1986; Edelbrock & Achenbach, 1984). The Teacher Checklist is similar in content and format to the CBCL, but contains items that are more relevant to the school setting.

When checklists and rating scales are employed it is important to take into consideration the various conceptual and methodological concerns that have been raised over their use in both research and practice (Anastasi, 1976; Ciminero & Drabman, 1977; Evans & Nelson, 1977; Walls, Werner, Bacon, & Zane, 1977). To begin with, checklists and rating scales are an indirect sample of performance. Data are typically gathered retrospectively; and the relation of these measures to actual occurrences of the problem behavior in natural settings may not be high. The ratings from these scales may even reflect "perceptions" that do not relate to actual occurrence of behavior. Second, the item content of the scale may provide a comprehensive overview of concerns in the psychoeducational realm, but seldom provides specific information for instructional planning. Instructions in administration of the scales sometimes differ across items and it is not always clear whether the person is rating frequency, intensity, or duration in the rating format. Despite these concerns, checklists and rating scales are very useful in overall psychoeducational assessment efforts of children and are to be recommended during early phases of the assessment process.

Self-Monitoring and Self-Assessment

Self-monitoring is a multistage assessment process. First, the child client must be aware of or discriminate the presence or absence of some response that is the focus of assessment. Second, the occurrence of the response must be recorded systematically. In contrast to discriminating, self-recording requires overt action on the part of the child to make a permanent record of the event. Both of these stages are considered essential to self-monitoring and, by some writers, are considered sufficient to describe the process (Nelson, 1977a; Nelson & Hayes, 1981). Other authors, however, believe that a third stage or self-evaluation is necessary in which the individual evaluates his or her own behavior against some standard (Kanfer, 1977; Mahoney & Arnkoff, 1978; Thoresen & Mahoney, 1974). Rather extensive applications of self-monitoring have occurred in the psychological and psychoeducational assessment of children. The reader is referred to Mace and Kratochwill (in press) for an overview of self-monitoring applications and issues in applied settings.

Self-monitoring is used for both assessment and treatment of various psychoeducational problems. Our focus will be on its applications in assessment. The reader interested in self-monitoring as a psychoeducational treatment should consult Hallahan, Lloyd, Kauffman, and Loper (1983) for a comprehensive review of its application to academic problems. Reviews of the applications of self-monitoring in other areas of clinical and applied psychology can also be found (e.g., Haynes, 1978; Mahoney, 1977; Nelson, 1977a,1977b).

When self-monitoring is used in psychoeducational assessment the client is requested to present data on his or her own performance either during the initial stage of assessment when trying to identify specific areas of problems or over the course of an intervention program where treatment progress is monitored. A teacher might also become involved in the self-monitoring process when there is a concern with analyzing his or her role in contributing to the academic environment.

Many different assessment devices and techniques have been developed for self-monitoring assessment, including record booklets, checklist forms, counters, timers, and meters, among others.

When self-monitoring is used in psychoeducational assessment a wide range of variables have been identified that could influence the data, in terms of both accuracy and reactivity. Table 10.8 provides an overview of the factors that could influence the accuracy and the reactivity of self-monitoring when it is employed in applied settings. The interested reader should consult McFall (1977, pages 200–204) as well as Mace and Kratochwill (in press) and Gardner and Cole (in press) for an overview of these and related factors that influence the self-monitoring process.

Self-monitoring is a useful strategy in psychoeducational assessment in applied settings for several reasons. First, it is a cost-efficient means of assessment, since it involves a client directly in a self-observational process. Self-monitoring may also be the only method of assessment available when the clinician is trying to obtain information on private activities or activities of rather low frequency. Self-monitoring can also help minimize sometimes obtrusive and subsequently reactive effects of assessment that could occur through other more direct strategies. Finally, self-monitoring can be especially useful in monitoring intervention programs. Despite the positive features of self-monitoring, the clinician must attend to the rather large range of variables in Table 10.8 that are known to influence the process of assessment. It is especially difficult to predict which factors will influence the assessment process.

Direct Observational Assessment

Direct observation of children and their performance in a natural environment is a very effective way to obtain information from which to design an intervention

TABLE 10.8. FACTORS INFLUENCING SELF-MONITORING ASSESSMENTS

Accuracy Factors	Reactivity Factors
1. *Training:* Clients should be trained in the use of SM. Training in SM will result in better accuracy (see Mahoney, 1977, for an example of training).	1. *Motivation:* Clients who are motivated to change their behavior prior to engaging in SM are more likely to demonstrate reactive effects.
2. *Systematic methods:* Systematic SM methods will typically result in more reliable and accurate outcomes than those methods that are more informal and nonsystematic.	2. *Valence:* Depending on how clients value a particular SM behavior, it may or may not change. Generally, positively valued behaviors are likely to increase, negatively valued behaviors are likely to decrease, and neutral behaviors may not change.
3. *Characteristics of the SM device:* A SM device such as a wrist counter, which is easy to use and does not depend on the client's memory, will usually provide more accurate data than when such a tool is not employed.	3. *Target behaviors:* The nature of the target behavior chosen for SM may influence reactivity.
4. *Timing:* Generally, the closer in time the actual SM act is to the occurrence of the target behavior, the more likely the data will be accurate.	4. *Goals, reinforcement, and feedback:* Specific performance goals, feedback, and reinforcement scheduled as part of SM could increase reactivity.
5. *Response competition:* When a client is required to monitor concurrent responses, his or her attention is divided. This may cause interference and thereby reduce the accuracy of the SM data.	5. *Timing:* Reactivity may vary as a function of the timing of SM. For example, recording prior to behavior act may be more reactive than recording subsequent to its occurrence.
6. *Response effort:* The more time and energy the client must spend on the SM activity, the less accurate the data may be. Thus aspects of "time" and "energy" may prove to be aversive.	6. *Self-monitoring devices:* Generally, the more obtrusive the recording device, the more reactive it tends to be (e.g., hand-held timer may be more reactive than one that is out of sight and "awareness").
7. *Reinforcement:* Contingent positive reinforcement for accurate recording tends to increase accuracy. Some external criterion is usually established for accuracy.	7. *Number of target behaviors:* As the number of target behaviors being monitored increases, reactivity may decrease.
8. *Awareness of accuracy assessment:* The clinician should monitor the client's data and make him or her aware that accuracy is being monitored. Such client awareness will typically increase accuracy.	8. *Schedule of self-monitoring:* Continuous SM may be more reactive than intermittent SM.
9. *Selection of target behaviors:* Since some behaviors are more salient, more easily discriminated, or more memorable, variations in accuracy will occur from differences in these dimensions. Generally, higher levels of accuracy have been established on motor behaviors (e.g., nail biting) than verbal behaviors (e.g., number of times the person says "ah"), and positively valued behaviors are more accurately recorded than those that are negatively valued.	

(*Table continues on p. 200.*)

TABLE 10.8. *(Continued)*

Accuracy Factors	Reactivity Factors
10. *Characteristics of clients:* Some clients are more accurate recorders than others. One would generally expect young children to be less accurate than older children, adolescents, and adults. However, individual variations will occur within ages.	

Source: Adapted from "Analogue Methods in Behavioral Assessment: Issues and Prospects" by R. M. McFall, in *Behavioral Assessment: New Directions in Clinical Psychology* (pp. 202–204) by J. D. Cone and R. P. Hawkins (Eds.), 1977, New York: Brunner/Mazel.

program. Direct observation consists of recording behavioral events in a natural setting when they occur, and not retrospectively. Typically, trained observers use codes that require minimal inference to record the actual events occurring (Jones, Reid, & Patterson, 1974).

In the initial stages of observation it is important to learn as much as possible about the structural components and interpersonal behaviors of others in the setting to which the child is expected to adapt. Sensitive assessment of the setting, as well as of the child, may yield new and/or unexpected information that will require flexibility and a willingness to reformulate the problem and/or its treatment. In addition, assessment of subjective, private events such as thoughts, feelings, and impressions is an important adjunct to behavioral observation. These covert factors may contribute significantly to the cause and maintenance of a disorder, and, if not addressed, may render interventions that focus exclusively on overt behavior ineffective.

In psychoeducational assessment it is useful to distinguish between direct observation of a rather informal nature and observation using some type of systematic code. Typically, in direct observational assessment, the clinician must first choose a specific target response or measure. This topic is a rather complex one and subject to a number of methodological and conceptual considerations (see Kratochwill, 1984, for an overview). Usually, direct observation is conducted as an ongoing assessment process where a target response is defined in some natural setting. When choosing a direct observational assessment, the clinician must decide on the response dimension to monitor. Several options are available, including frequency, duration, and response quality. Response frequency is an important dimension when the target measures are relatively discrete units. Response duration, on the other hand, is typically used when a temporal characteristic of a response is of primary interest. Duration measures will usually require some type of timing device to be used during the assessment. Finally, response quality is assessed when the target measures vary in intensity, accuracy, or acceptability (Cone & Foster, 1982).

Once dimensions of response measures have been identified for psychoeducational assessment, the clinician must select some type of observational procedure (Hartmann, 1984). Four different methods of observational recording techniques can be employed, each with its own advantages and limitations (see Table 10.9). Real-time observations involve recording event, frequency, and duration on the basis of actual occurrence in a noninterrupted or natural time flow. Event recording (also called frequency

TABLE 10.9. FACTORS TO CONSIDER IN SELECTING AN APPROPRIATE RECORDING TECHNIQUE

Method	Advantages and Disadvantages
Real-time recording	*Advantages:* Provides unbiased estimates of frequency and duration Data capable of complex analyses such as conditional probability analysis Data susceptible to sophisticated reliability analysis *Disadvantages:* Demanding task for observers May require costly equipment Requires responses to have clearly distinguishable beginnings and ends
Event or duration recording	*Advantages:* Measures are of a fundamental response characteristic (i.e., frequency or duration) Can be used by participant–observers (e.g., parents or teachers) with low rate responses *Disadvantages:* Requires responses to have clearly distinguishable beginnings and ends Unless responses are located in real time (e.g., by dividing a session into brief recording intervals), some forms of reliability assessment may be impossible. May be difficult with multiple behaviors unless mechanical aids are available
Momentary time samples	*Advantages:* Response duration of primary interest Time saving and convenient Useful with multiple behaviors and/or children Applicable to responses without clear beginnings or ends *Disadvantages:* Unless samples are taken frequently, continuity of behavior may be lost May miss most occurrences of brief, rare responses
Interval recording	*Advantages:* Sensitive to both response frequency and duration Applicable to wide range of responses Facilitates observer training and reliability assessments Applicable to responses without clearly distinguishable beginnings and ends *Disadvantages:* Confounds frequency and duration May under- or overestimate response frequency and duration

Source: From *Child Behavior: Analysis and Therapy* (2nd ed.) by D. M. Gelfand and D. P. Hartmann, 1984, Elmsford, NY: Pergamon Press. Copyright 1984. Adapted by permission.

or tally or trial observational assessment) is used to record discrete trial behavior when frequency is the response dimension of primary interest. Duration recording is used when the clinician is primarily interested in the actual length of a particular response. However, duration recording is not used as often as the frequency, which is regarded as the more basic response characteristic in recording.

Scan sampling (also called instantaneous time sampling, momentary time sampling, and discontinuous probe time sampling) is used when the clinician is interested in duration as a more meaningful response dimension than frequency. The procedure consists of scanning the client and then noting whether or not the behavior occurs at the instant of observation. Interval recording (or time sampling) is a commonly used procedure in which an observational session is divided into brief intervals. The clinician observes, records, and scores an interval if the target response of interest occurs throughout the interval or during any part of the interval.

When conducting observational assessments, a number of recommendations can be advanced to improve the measurement process. To begin with, individuals functioning as observers should be trained in the recording procedures and techniques that are to be employed. This is sometimes overlooked, because observation is often regarded as an informal assessment technique. However, the credibility of the procedure can be enhanced greatly by offering specific training to observers. Second, when possible, it is useful to establish the accuracy of the assessment process by having two or more individuals observe the criterion response simultaneously. Third, conditions for assessing the child should be maintained to establish consistent levels of agreement. Fourth, a number of potential observer effects must be eliminated or reduced (with the most common ones being reactivity, bias, drift, and cheating). Reactivity occurs when the client or individual being observed changes as a function of the recording process. Generally, observation should be conducted in an unobtrusive fashion to reduce the influence of an observer entering a classroom. Data must be monitored to note any changes that occur from the actual recording (see Hartmann, 1984, for specific examples of methods to eliminate the effects of, or to reduce reactivity in observational assessment). Observer bias is any systematic error associated with observer expectancies during the assessment process. Observer bias can be reduced by not communicating specific treatment plans or the focus of assessment to observers, including well-defined observational definitions of behavior, and ensuring that observers are well trained to conduct the assessments. Observer drift can also occur when an observer's accuracy of recording changes over time. That is, observers may drift from the original definition of the behavior that is being recorded.

Direct observational assessment is a very effective means of establishing natural occurrences of various behaviors. One of the most significant benefits of naturalistic observation is that the clinician can identify factors in the child's environment that may interfere with adaptation to the instructional setting. Within the context of observational assessment, a structured approach to assessing setting factors is to observe and record in sequence events most proximal to the onset and ending of the target behaviors of interest. This analytic system, deriving from early experimental psychology, is primarily associated with behavior analysis, and is called the functional analysis of behavior. In this paradigm, antecedent events (preceding the behavior) and consequent events (following the behavior) are interpreted within a behavioral framework (see Bijou, 1976).

The various facets of each ecological characteristic in interpersonal or academic behavior that could be observed in one setting at any one time are infinite. Clearly, if functional analysis is to be useful, it is crucial that the clinician establish a discrete set of events that are to be recorded before the observation takes place. One way to establish the priorities of evaluation is to specify a categorical system according to which events are observed or classified in the recording period.

A variety of other observational codes have been developed that can be used in psychoeducational assessment activities. These include codes appropriate for home settings (Patterson, Ray, Shaw, & Cobb, 1969); school settings (O'Leary, Romanczyk, Kass, Dietz, & Santogrossi, 1979; Saudargas, 1983); and home and school (Wahler, House, & Stambaugh, 1976). The code developed by Wahler and his associates (1976) provides for 24 possible categories of behavioral observation. The observer marks one of 6 types of events preceding some behavior, followed by an appropriate response category that corresponds to the behavior; thus scoring in multiple categories of behavior is possible. Wahler and associates' code has been used in several applied settings (Wahler, 1980; Wahler & Fox, 1980).

Another code by Saudargas (1983) was developed for use by school psychologists and enables the observer to record 15 different student and 6 teacher behaviors. The code is considered very useful in overall psychoeducational assessment efforts (Shapiro, in press; Shapiro & Lentz, 1986), and allows recording of a wide range of teacher and child behaviors. The recording sheet used in the Saudargas observational assessment is reproduced in Figure 10.2. As can be observed in the figure, relevant information regarding conditions occurring at the time of observation are recorded by the observer. The various behavior categories are abbreviated in the left-hand column with various states followed by events. Although the Saudargas code has been the subject of rather limited research, it is particularly useful for observing teacher and child behavior. Nevertheless, the code is designed primarily to be used in classroom settings where some type of academic instruction occurs. Thus it might be limited in terms of assessing a broader sample of childhood behavior in nonclassroom settings (Shapiro, in press).

In most cases it will be up to the clinician to determine the structure and content of an observational code. This decision (one that is vulnerable to the clinician's subjectivity, theoretical, or treatment biases) largely determines the clinical value of a careful functional analysis. Use of narrative records from pilot observations as well as consultation with the child and other care providers, as well as professionals in the child's setting, can help to preserve the objectivity of the observational psychoeducational assessment.

Functional analysis can provide invaluable information regarding which antecedents and/or consequences should be examined as potentially important in the treatment program carried out with the child. This type of assessment is essential to the design and monitoring of an intervention program across phases. Nevertheless, it must be regarded as one of a variety of dimensions of dysfunction that must be evaluated before the target of intervention is identified. Diagnosis and responsiveness to treatment may vary greatly as a function of variables not currently observed in a functional analysis of immediate behavior. Such variables may include severity, chronicity, and onset of target behavior, affect or cognitions, and contextual events such as family variables and other situationally or temporally remote stressors (Kazdin, 1983).

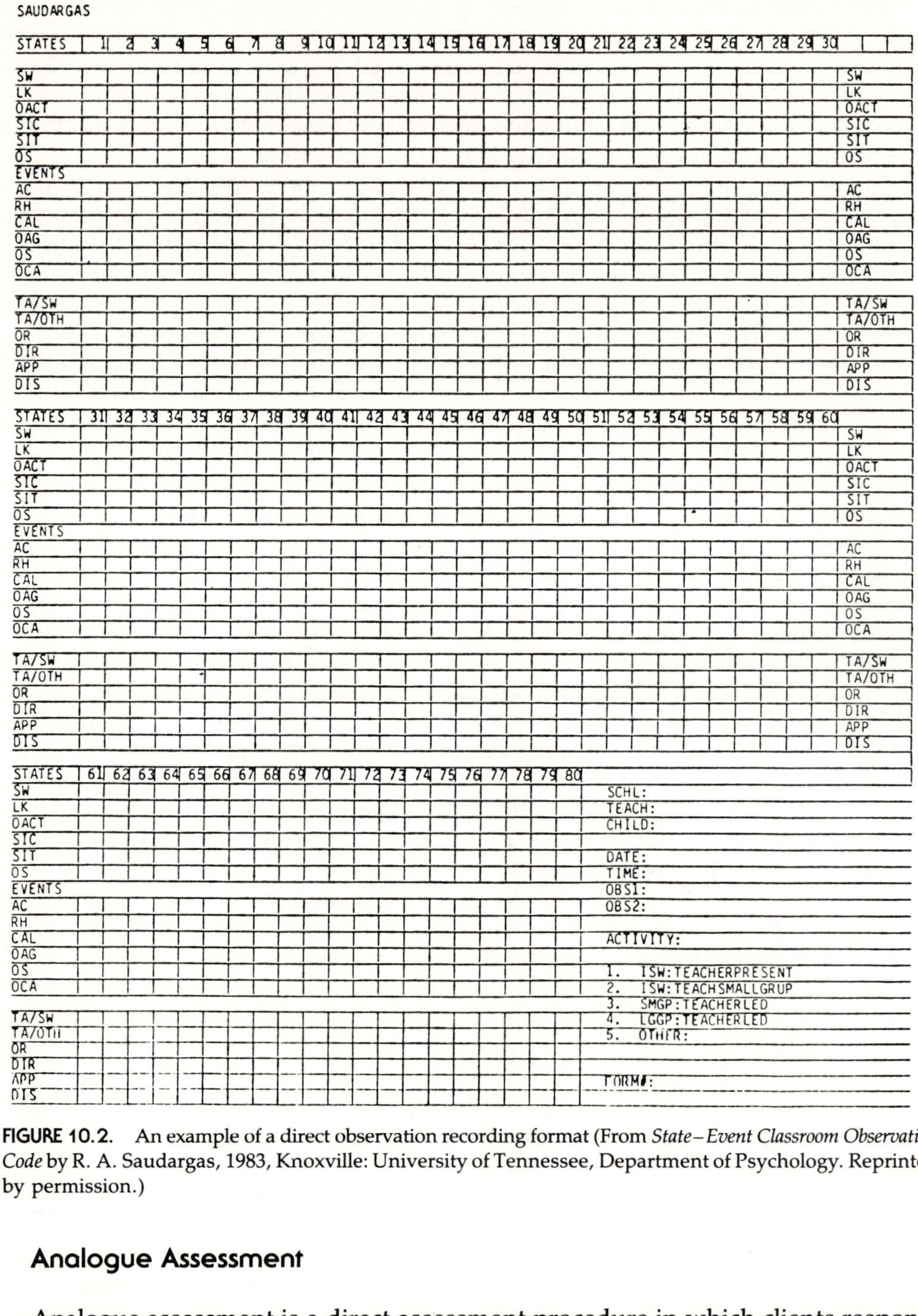

SAUDARGAS

STATES	1	2	3	4	5	6	7	8	9	10	11	12	13	14	15	16	17	18	19	20	21	22	23	24	25	26	27	28	29	30	
SW																															SW
LK																															LK
OACT																															OACT
SIC																															SIC
SIT																															SIT
OS																															OS
EVENTS																															
AC																															AC
RH																															RH
CAL																															CAL
OAG																															OAG
OS																															OS
OCA																															OCA
TA/SW																															TA/SW
TA/OTH																															TA/OTH
OR																															OR
DIR																															DIR
APP																															APP
DIS																															DIS

STATES	31	32	33	34	35	36	37	38	39	40	41	42	43	44	45	46	47	48	49	50	51	52	53	54	55	56	57	58	59	60	
SW																															SW
LK																															LK
OACT																															OACT
SIC																															SIC
SIT																															SIT
OS																															OS
EVENTS																															
AC																															AC
RH																															RH
CAL																															CAL
OAG																															OAG
OS																															OS
OCA																															OCA
TA/SW																															TA/SW
TA/OTH																															TA/OTH
OR																															OR
DIR																															DIR
APP																															APP
DIS																															DIS

STATES	61	62	63	64	65	66	67	68	69	70	71	72	73	74	75	76	77	78	79	80	
SW																					SCHL:
LK																					TEACH:
OACT																					CHILD:
SIC																					
SIT																					DATE:
OS																					TIME:
EVENTS																					OBS1:
AC																					OBS2:
RH																					
CAL																					ACTIVITY:
OAG																					
OS																					1. ISW:TEACHERPRESENT
OCA																					2. ISW:TEACHSMALLGRUP
																					3. SMGP:TEACHERLED
TA/SW																					4. LGGP:TEACHERLED
TA/OTH																					5. OTHER:
OR																					
DIR																					
APP																					FORM#:
DIS																					

FIGURE 10.2. An example of a direct observation recording format (From *State–Event Classroom Observation Code* by R. A. Saudargas, 1983, Knoxville: University of Tennessee, Department of Psychology. Reprinted by permission.)

Analogue Assessment

Analogue assessment is a direct assessment procedure in which clients respond to stimuli that simulate those found in the natural environment. Included within analogue assessment are a rather large number of psychoeducational tests, both norm-referenced and criterion-referenced, as well as a variety of curriculum-related assessment tasks that are developed to assess the child's specific problems in content areas. Analogue assessment procedures obviously vary a great deal in terms of the degree to which they match the actual natural setting in which the client functions. For example, some analogue assessment procedures, such as traditional IQ tests, may only indirectly sample the child's performance in the natural setting, since the task requirements do not necessarily match those found in the school curriculum, and the demand chracteristics of the testing situation (i.e., one-on-one testing) vary from what might be required in a normal classroom. On the other hand, analogue assessment measures, such as achievement tests or curriculum-based assessment, may more closely match the task requirements the child experiences in a normal classroom.

Relative to direct and naturalistic assessment in applied settings, analogue measures share several positive features. To begin with, analogue measures typically allow the clinician to structure the assessment situation to obtain more control of variables that might contaminate the assessment process. Many extraneous variables that operate in the natural environment (e.g., noise, interruptions from peers) can often be controlled in analogue assessment. Second, analogue assessment may allow the clinician to assess behaviors that are impossible to monitor in natural settings. Third, analogue assessment strategies may be less costly in terms of time and resources relative to direct observational measurement of behaviors in a classroom situation. Fourth, analogue assessment may help the clinician to simplify or reduce complex assessment concerns. Finally, analogue assessment allow the clinician a wide range of psychometrically validated strategies.

In analogue assessment, it is important to distinguish between norm-referenced and criterion-referenced tests. Norm-referenced tests, when used in psychoeducational assessment, allow the clinician to compare the individual's performance to that of a normative group. Consequently, norm-referenced tests typically yield grade equivalent percentile ranking and standard scores. These scores are often used to make decisions on whether or not the child deviates from the norm group used in the construction of the test. Norm-referenced test data, for example, are often used to determine grade placement and grade level, when used for grading instructional material, or in any situation in which the individual standing in relation to the *average performance* of a comparable sample of peers is relevant to the purposes of assessment. Across all norm-referenced tests, consideration of the appropriateness of the comparison of the assessed child with the normed group is essential. A rather large range of norm-referenced tests have been used in psychoeducational assessment (see Salvia & Ysseldyke, 1985, for a review).

In contrast to norm-referenced tests, criterion-referenced assessment has often been used in routine psychoeducational evaluations (Cancelli & Kratochwill, 1982; Hambleton, 1982). Glaser (1971) advanced the following definition of a criterion-referenced test:

> A criterion-referenced test is one that is deliberately constructed to yield measurements that are directly interpretable in terms of specified performance standards. Performance standards are generally specified by defining a class or domain of tasks that should be performed by the individual. Measurements taken are representative samples of tasks drawn from the domain, and such measurements are referenced directly to this domain for each individual. (p. 41)

Table 10.10 provides a comparison of norm-referenced and criterion-referenced achievement tests along several different areas of test construction and use.

TABLE 10.10. COMPARISON OF NORM-REFERENCED AND CRITERION-REFERENCED ACHIEVEMENT TESTS

Area	Norm-Referenced Tests	Criterion-Referenced Tests
Purpose	A norm-referenced test is constructed specifically to facilitate comparisons among examinees on the content area measured by the test. Age-, grade-, percentile-, and standard-score norms are available to assist in the accomplishment of the purpose. In addition, since test items can be referenced to particular objectives, objective-referenced score interpretations are possible.	A criterion-referenced test is constructed to assess an examinee's level of performance in relation to each of a set of objectives or competencies measured by the test. Scores may be used (1) for descriptive purposes, (2) to make decisions, and (3) to evaluate program effectiveness. Examinees (or groups) can be compared with one another but this is not a primary use of the scores.
Test development	A test blueprint is prepared and items are written to fit the blueprint. An important factor in item selection is the statistical properties of the test items (item difficulty and discrimination). In general, items of moderate difficulty (*p* values in the range .30 to .70) and high discriminating power (point biserial correlations over .30) are the most likely to be selected for inclusion in a test because they contribute substantially to test score variance. Test reliability and validity will, generally, be higher when test score variance is high.	In addition to a test blueprint, very clear objective statements (sometimes called "domain specifications" or "expanded objectives") are prepared along with test items that are valid indicators of the objectives. Items are only deleted from the available item pool if they are not judged to measure the objective they were written to measure. "Representative" samples of test items are usually selected for inclusion in the test. Item statistics may be used to construct parallel tests or to design a test to optimally discriminate in the region of a standard of performance on the test score scale.
Measurement scales	The norm-referenced test score scale is anchored in the middle (the average level of group performance).	For criterion-referenced test score scales, the anchor points are two in number and located at the ends of the scale (0% and 100%).
Test score generalizability	There is seldom interest in making generalizations from norm-referenced achievement test scores. Usually, the job is completed when test scores are compared to appropriate norms tables. Generalizations from examinee performance on aptitude and personality measures are, however, of considerably more interest than those from	With criterion-referenced test scores, the matter of generalizability is important. Seldom would anyone be content to interpret an examinee's score in terms of the specific items on a test. (Incidentally, this is all that can be appropriately done with scores obtained from objectives-referenced tests.). If the objective measured by a test is clear, and

TABLE 10.10. *(Continued)*

Area	Norm-Referenced Tests	Criterion-Referenced Tests
	achievement tests (e.g., it is common to generalize from a WISC-R score to "intelligence"). Still, while generalizations from nonachievement test scores are of considerable interest and import, the primary basis for test score interpretations is normative.	if items are selected to be representative of the content domain measuring the objective, examinee test performance on a set of items included in the test can be generalized to test performance in the larger domain of behaviors. Strong criterion-referenced test score interpretations of the kind just described are usually of interest to criterion-referenced test users.
Specificity of test score information	A norm-referenced test score provides a summary of a broadly defined area of achievement.	Users of criterion-referenced tests are endorsing the notion that important outcomes can be separated into discrete categories (referred to as objectives, skills, or competencies).
Reliability and validity	Test-retest, parallel-form, and internal consistency measures are useful ways for assessing score reliability. Approaches to validity depend on the intended uses of the scores.	Measures such as standard error of measurement and decision consistency are useful ways for assessing score reliability. Best methods for validity assessment depend on the intended uses of the scores. Since criterion-referenced test scores are used differently from norm-referenced scores, the kinds of validity investigations will differ also.
Norms	Essential for norm-referenced tests.	Norms can be of value when interpreting individual and group scores. For example, norms can be useful in setting realistic standards for examinee performance.

Note: While all criterion-referenced tests are achievement tests, some norm-referenced tests are not (e.g., intelligence tests). The comparisons in this table are between norm-referenced and criterion-referenced *achievement* tests.

Source: From "Advances in Criterion-Referenced Testing Technology" by R. K. Hambleton, in *Handbook of School Psychology* by C. R. Reynolds and T. B. Guthin (Eds.), 1982, New York: John Wiley & Sons. Reprinted with permission.

Criterion-referenced tests have been used for a wide variety of purposes within clinical settings, including diagnosing problem behavior, monitoring learning, and assessing readiness for a placement in prescribed educational programs (Bijou, 1976). We shall now provide a brief overview of some common assessment procedures that are used in psychoeducational evaluation of children. It should be emphasized that these are among some of the more common assessment instruments that have been employed in applied settings. No attempt is made to provide a comprehensive overview of the variety of tests that can be used, since there are literally thousands that might be employed in specific circumstances. Moreover, it is impossible to provide an adequate review of the psychometric creditability of all instruments that have been employed. Readers are referred to some basic sources on psychoeducational evaluation such as Salvia and Ysseldyke's (1985) text and *The Ninth Mental Measurements Yearbook* (Vols. 1 and 2) (Mitchell, 1985a, 1985b), which includes a comprehensive overview of the psychometric characteristics of various norm-referenced and criterion-referenced tests.

Analogue Assessment

Individually Administered Tests of Intelligence. An individually administered test of intelligence is typically used when a primary diagnosis of mental retardation is being considered. PL-94-142 specifies, however, that the measure of intelligence must be considered in conjunction with a measure of adaptive behavior before the child may be classified and placed in a special education program for the mentally retarded (see Shapiro, in press, for an overview of adaptive behavior measures).

When the presenting problem is a failure to achieve in one or more academic areas, a primary diagnosis of mental retardation or developmental reading, math articulation, or language disorder is often considered.

In the case of developmental learning disorders, PL 94-142 calls for a major discrepancy between expected achievement and ability before the child may be classified and placed in a special education program for the learning disabled. Ability is typically assessed by means of an individually administered test of intelligence. A test of intelligence is frequently administered when aspects of the presenting problem suggest the possibility of mental retardation, but careful differential diagnosis is required, as in Tourette's disorder, elective mutism, and attention deficit disorders with and without hyperactivity.

Finally, a test of intelligence is sometimes used to identify or rule out subaverage cognitive factors that may be an associated feature in primary disorders such as infantile autism, childhood-onset, pervasive developmental disorder, and pica.

Bias in IQ Tests. IQ tests are standardized, norm-referenced assessment instruments. The IQ score indicates the examinee's performance relative to a select representative sample of the population who, during the course of its development, completed the test under the standardized test administration conditions specified in the manual. Appropriate training in administration of the selected test is a prerequisite for obtaining valid information on all standardized tests of intelligence. In addition, it is important when selecting a test of intelligence to assess whether the characteristics of the individual examinee are similar enough to those of the norming sample to warrant the comparison that the IQ score suggests (described in the test manual). It has been argued, for example, that inappropriate comparisons with national norms and culturally biased test items have led to overrepresentation of ethnic minority children in programs for the mentally retarded. The reader interested in a more comprehensive discussion of bias in testing should read Reynolds and Brown (1984).

Test Modifications. A further consideration in the use of individually administered tests of intelligence is the effect of standardized administration conditions on the child's ability to produce maximal performance. Consideration of this question is not only basic to sensitive evaluation but specifically required by the PL 94-142 testing guidelines. In cases where vision, hearing, speech, language, motor, and/or attentional impairment is suspected, these functions should be evaluated before the IQ test is administered so that procedural modifications can be made or a more appropriate test selected. Examples of procedural modifications that do *not* break standardization might include testing in a distraction-free environment for short periods over several sessions for a child with attention deficits, or using extra lighting and enlarged test materials for a child with impaired visual acuity. Emotional factors such as anxiety or low motivation may also significantly impair test performance. Development of responsive and sensitive rapport is essential to protect the child from the encroachment of these factors on test performance. For a more complete discussion of modifications and alternative tests for specific handicapping conditions see Sattler (1981, pp. 68–95).

Finally, valuable information may be gained from readministration of a test of intelligence under nonstandardized conditions. For example, readministering a timed subtest without the usual time constraints for a separate evaluation of ability and speed may provide insights into how the child performs under these conditions.

Individually Administered Tests of Intelligence

Wechsler Intelligence Scale for Children—Revised. The Wechsler Intelligence Scale for Children—Revised (WISC-R) (Wechsler, 1974) is appropriate for testing children ages 6 to 16½ years. The test consists of 12 subscales, 6 of which comprise a Verbal scale and 6 a Performance (or Nonverbal) scale. Testing time may range from 1 to 2 hours, depending on the child's age, fluency, level of motivation, and other related factors. The WISC-R yields Verbal, Performance, and Full Scale IQ scores and has excellent psychometric properties.

The profile of a child's performance on the WISC-R allows for comparison of verbal and nonverbal scores and analysis of specific strengths and weaknesses indicated by clusters of performance variation among the 12 subtests. Kaufman's (1979) volume on WISC-R testing provides an in-depth discussion of the various approaches to interpreting performance on this intelligence test.

Stanford-Binet. The Stanford-Binet (S-B) (Fourth Edition) (Thorndike, Hagen, & Sattler, 1985) is appropriate for use with individuals from age 2 to adult. Testing time required for the S-B may range from ½ to 2 hours. Traditionally, the S-B was often preferred to the WISC-R when a diagnosis of mental retardation was being considered because the instrument was more sensitive to test performance in the lower scoring range. The current S-B samples a wide range of behaviors that can be used for clinical assessment of behavioral, emotional, physical, and motivational factors.

Wechsler Preschool and Primary Scale of Intelligence. The Wechsler Preschool and Primary Scale of Intelligence (WPPSI) (Wechsler, 1967) has a format similar to that of the WISC-R and was designed for use with children ages 4 to 6½ years. The WPPSI, like the WISC-R, yields a Verbal, Performance, and Full Scale IQ score. Careful attention should be paid to the test manual's discussion of floor and ceiling effects before the WPPSI is used for primary diagnosis of mental retardation (or giftedness) in this age range.

Tests of General Achievement

Wechsler Adult Intelligence Scale—Revised. The Wechsler Adult Intelligence Scale—Revised (WAIS-R) (Wechsler, 1981) also has a format similar to that of the WISC-R and yields Verbal, Performance, and Full Scale IQ scores. The test is appropriate for evaluating adolescents and adults ages 16 to 74. The WISC-R or the WAIS may be used with individuals 16 to 16½ years old. The WAIS-R is generally preferred, unless mental retardation is suspected, since the test items and presentation style may be more acceptable to an adolescent than those of the more child-oriented WISC-R.

Kaufman Assessment Battery for Children. The Kaufman Assessment Battery for Children (K-ABC) (Kaufman & Kaufman, 1983) is appropriate for testing children ages 2½ to 12½ years old. The test's authors define intelligence in terms of mental processing: The instrument yields scores of simultaneously sequential processing and achievement. The authors note that the K-ABC is "first and foremost a clinical instrument" that can be used to assess personality and learning style as well as intelligence of the examinee. The K-ABC has a version developed for Spanish-speaking children (not bilingual).

McCarthy Scales of Children's Abilities. The McCarthy Scales of Children's Abilities (MSCA) (McCarthy, 1972) is appropriate for assessing the cognitive abilities of children ages 2½ to 8½ years, and requires approximately 45 minutes to administer. The test yields a General Cognitive Index and a profile of abilities including verbal and nonverbal skills, short-term memory, and motor abilities. The test should not be used as a substitute for the psychometrically stronger Wechsler or Binet scales, particularly when classification and placement in special programs are being considered. A comprehensive review of the McCarthy scales can be found in Kaufman (1982).

System of Multicultural Pluralistic Assessment. The System of Multicultural Pluralistic Assessment (SOMPA) (Mercer & Lewis, 1978) is a test of children's cognition, perception, and motoric and adaptive behavior designed for White, Black, and Hispanic children ages 5 years, 0 months to 11 years, 11 months. The SOMPA attempts to eliminate "biased" testing in special education placements of minorities by limiting normative comparisons of children's performance to their own ethnic or racial group. The test requires 5 to 6 hours to administer and yields a "corrected" (for cultural and SES factors) WISC-R score labeled the child's Estimated Learning Potential. At this point it is unclear whether the SOMPA is a useful and unbiased measure of learning potential. The norming sample is restricted to California, so that application to children in other geographic regions is limited (Reschly, 1979). The correlation of SOMPA scores to school achievement has been found to be lower than the correlation of IQ scores to school achievement (Brown, 1979) and the test has been criticized for its lack of prescriptive information (Sattler, 1982).

Tests of General Achievement

Tests of general achievement are appropriate for screening purposes and may be used in the early stages of assessment when academic deficits are suggested but not specifically identified in the referral data. In particular, academic deficits may be associated with such primary disorders as elective mutism, transient or chronic motor tic disorders, asthma, stuttering, encopresis, or enuresis. Tests of general achievement are also appropriately used to screen achievement deficits that are typically associated features of primary disorders such as infantile autism, childhood-onset pervasive developmental disorder, attention deficit disorder with and without hyperactivity, and atypical stereotyped movement disorders.

When academic deficits and/or learning problems have been identified (in the referral data or during screening), domain-specific tests of achievement can provide a profile of skill strengths and weaknesses within the content area, and an opportunity to analyze individual learner characteristics as they are expressed in relation to the domain of interest.

Individual learner characteristics may include: a preference for auditory or visual learning, motor strengths and/or weaknesses, meaningful variations in levels of attention and/or motivation during different types of tasks, a tendency to respond reflectively or impulsively or to attend to the details more than the whole or vice versa. In some cases, retesting to assess these and related aspects of the learning processes may be useful. Careful analysis of the individual's skills and learning style is essential for sound instructional planning and represents the crux of meaningful assessment in any academic achievement domain.

Wide Range Achievement Test—Revised. The Wide Range Achievement Test—Revised (WRAT-R) (Jastak & Wilkinson, 1984) measures general achievement in reading, arithmetic, and spelling skills. Level I of the WRAT-R is appropriate for use with children 5 to 11 years, 11 months, and Level II is appropriate for adolescents and adults ages 12 to 75 years. The WRAT-R is a timed test requiring 15 to 30 minutes to administer. This revised version of the WRAT-R is based on a new national, stratified norming sample and is designed to yield an age-equivalent score. A large-print edition is available for examinees who require magnification of reading material.

Peabody Individual Achievement Test. The Peabody Individual Achievement Test (PIAT) (Dunn & Markwrandt, 1970) measures achievement in the areas of general information, reading comprehension, recognition, and mathematics. The PIAT is not timed, and takes approximately 30 to 40 minutes to administer under normal conditions. The test is appropriate for grades K through 12 and yields approximate grade equivalents, percentile ranking, and standard scores.

Woodcock Johnson Psychoeducational Battery. The Woodcock Johnson Psychoeducational Battery (WJPB) (Woodcock, 1977), measures Cognitive Ability (12 subtests such as memory and concept formation) Achievement (10 subtests including reading, spelling, capitalization, punctuation, and science) and Interest Level in reading, math, language, and physical and social activities. The battery is appropriate for children and adults beginning at age 3 years, and yields an Achievement Aptitude Profile that allows for comparison of Cognitive Ability and Achievement. It should be noted, however, that Cognitive Ability scores do not represent an acceptable substitute for WISC-R or Stanford-Binet scores.

Reading

Assessment in this domain may include evaluation of both oral and silent reading skills. Samples of oral reading allow the clinician to evaluate rate and accuracy, sight-word vocabulary, phonics skills (mastery of sound–symbol associations and blending), and characteristic error patterns that may form the focus of remediation. Oral reading is typically followed by questions to assess comprehension skills as well.

Silent reading tasks are used primarily to assess the student's level of reading comprehension, which may range from the most basic literal or factual understanding to deductive or interpretive, and finally, critical comprehension of the written material. Tests of general academic achievement such as the WRAT or the PIAT may be used to identify broad areas that require more fine-grained assessment of specific reading skills. Individual reading tests such as the Durrell Analysis of Reading Difficulty or the Gates-McKillop-Herowitz Reading Diagnostic Tests (or the Woodcock Reading Mastery Test) may be used to identify reading strengths and weaknesses more specifically.

When formal tests such as these are used to assess specific academic skills, it is important to note that the test title can only identify a general skill domain. It is the format of the test items that defines which subskills within that general domain are actually tapped by the test. For example, on a test of blending skills, the format may tap recognition (when the examiner says the blend and the examinee selects the blend from a number of visually similar choices), or production (in which the examinee sees and pronounces the blend). While both tests assess general phonics, each taps different and significant components of that skill. It is important, therefore, to select tests on the basis of item format as well as title.

An alternative approach to formal testing is the construction of an Informal Reading Inventory (IRI). In this assessment procedure, the clinician selects passages of approximately 100 words from a series of graded reading texts. The selected passages are read orally by the examinee and followed by comprehension questions. After noting the number of errors the clinician can estimate independent, instructional, and frustration reading levels according to the following criteria:

Independent reading level, at which the student can read without assistance, is defined by 99 percent word accuracy and 90 percent comprehension.

Instruction reading level, at which the student should receive reading instruction, is defined by 95 percent word accuracy and 70 percent comprehension.

Frustration reading level, that is, a level too difficult for the student to work from profitably, is defined by less than 90 percent word accuracy and less than 50 percent comprehension. As a general rule, the deficit is likely to be attentional, behavioral, or motivational when the examinee self-corrects more than 50 percent of his or her oral reading errors. When appropriate, the IRI may be read silently and followed by comprehension questions, in which case reading levels are determined on the basis of comprehension alone.

Arithmetic

Arithmetic is, in several ways, a hierarchical domain. Acquisition of arithmetic skills, for example, cannot occur without prerequisite cognitive–developmental achievements such as classification, one-to-one correspondence, ordering, flexible and reversible thinking, and conservation. Arithmetic skills that include computation (i.e., adding, dividing, etc.), concepts (i.e., time, measurement, etc.), and application (of computational skills and concepts to mathematical reasoning tasks) are also arranged hierarchically so that achievement depends on skills previously mastered in a logical, instructional sequence. Careful evaluation of the child's instructional history can, therefore, be useful in determining whether arithmetic skill deficits can be remediated through specific instruction in skill deficit areas.

Tests of general achievement may be used to determine the relative level of the child's arithmetic skills; however, diagnostic tests of arithmetic performance provide a more fine-grained analysis of specific deficits. Such tests include the Diagnostic Inventory of Basic Arithmetic Skills (Enright, 1983), which is appropriate for grades 1 through 9 and measures computation, fractions, and decimals; the Key Math Diagnostic Test (Connolly, Nachtman, & Pritchett, 1976), which is appropriate for grades K through 6 and measures content, computational operations, and applications; and the Stanford Diagnostic Mathematics Test (Beatty, Madden, Gardner, & Karlsen, 1976), which is appropriate for grades K through 12 and also measures numeration, computation, and application.

Information yielded by formal measures of arithmetic skills is, however, limited to the final work product, which is a composite of applied skills and problem-solving strategies. These components cannot be analyzed successfully without observing the problem-solving process and/or reviewing performance on a standardized test or classroom work product to determine exactly which skills and problem-solving strategies are deficient.

Writing

Assessment is this domain may focus on the mechanical or expressive qualities of writing. Spontaneous writing samples (in response to a concrete stimulus), dictated writing, and/or classroom work samples of content-specific writing may be used to evaluate mechanical skills such as handwriting, punctuation, and capitalization. Mechanics are critical determinants of the child's ability to use written language to communicate clearly and accurately. Failure to master these basics may indicate motoric and/or perceptual deficits. For these reasons, evaluation of the mechanical aspects of writing should not be overlooked. The potential therapeutic value of writing as a tool for children and adolescents who wish to clarify and express their thoughts and ideas in private records and/or communicate them to others should also be considered before writing mechanics are targeted for direct intervention.

The expressive quality of written content is determined by skills such as grammar, organization, word usage, and productivity, which may be evaluated according to relatively objective and measurable standards. On the other hand, qualities such as creativity, maturity and adequacy of theme, and degree of abstract versus concrete ideation lack objective standards. Therefore, evaluation of these skills may be influenced easily by prior knowledge of the child and must be conducted with care.

Formal approaches to evaluating writing skills include diagnostic tests such as the Picture Story Language Test (Mykelbust, 1965), which is appropriate for children and adolescents 7 to 17 years old. The test yields a spontaneous writing sample (produced in response to pictures) and measures productivity, syntax, and abstract–concrete meaning. The Test of Written Language (Hammill & Larsen, 1978) is appropriate for grades 2 through 12 and yields spontaneous and contrived writing samples. Handwriting, thought units, vocabulary, thematic maturity, word usage, grammar, punctuation, capitalization, and spelling are measured. The Test of Adolescent Language (Hammill, Brown, Larsen, & Widerholt, 1980) is appropriate for grades 6 through 12, yields both spontaneous and contrived writing samples, and measures vocabulary and grammar.

Informal spontaneous writing tasks, completed in the presence of the clinician, provide an opportunity to observe the writing process directly. In addition, the writing stimulus can be controlled and its effect on the child's writing (e.g., a high vs. low interest cue) can be evaluated. Similarly, even more contrived writing tasks can be developed to evaluate specific skills, such as use of a particular grammatic tense, or written expression of knowledge in a specific content area. Samples of writing produced in the classroom should be obtained routinely and compared to writing produced in other situations. Differences in the mechanical or expressive quality of the writing may be useful in identifying the source of the problem and/or defining appropriate instructional modifications.

Spelling

When assessing spelling skills it is especially important to evaluate the student's instructional and learning history. In many cases a failure to receive systematic spelling instruction will account for a deficit in this domain. Both formal and informal methods may be used to assess overall level of spelling skills. Formal measures include spelling subsections of general achievement tests, diagnostic instruments such as Diagnostic Spelling Potential Tests (Arena, 1982) and the Test of Written Spelling (Larsen & Hammill, 1986), and criterion-referenced measures such as the Diagnostic Screening Test: Spelling (Gnagey, 1979).

Formal tests of spelling skills typically use either a dictated word format (which relies more heavily on auditory skills) or a recognition format (which draws more on visual skills). In some cases both formats may be used to assess the child's processing strengths. In other cases, where one type of test has already been administered, the other may be administered to assess performance differences. The format that yields a significantly higher score may suggest an effective approach to spelling instruction.

An Informal Spelling Inventory (ISI) may be developed by selecting 15 to 20 words from each level of a basal spelling series. Words are dictated to the child until he or she reaches a ceiling of 7 errors. After noting the number of errors the clinician can estimate independent, instructional, and frustration levels, respectively defined as 0 to 2 errors, 3 to 6 errors, and 7+ errors on a 20-word list. Alternatively, the Mann-Suiter Developmental Spelling Inventory, which is commercially available, may be used.

Analysis of written work samples produced in a variety of learning situations can provide more direct assessment information regarding naturally occurring spelling skills. A *cloze procedure,* which involves filling in blanks in a paragraph, may also be used to assess spelling words used in context. The cloze procedure allows for analysis of specific types of errors since the spelling words called for in the blanks can be controlled.

Once a spelling sample is obtained, it is useful to differentiate the student's ability to spell phonetically regular and irregular words. Errors in phonetically regular words may suggest broader deficits in areas such as auditory discrimination, phonics, attention, or motivation.

Other Measures

A variety of other assessment strategies can be used to obtain information in a comprehensive psychoeducational evaluation of the child. These include test procedures such as diagnostic teaching, task analysis, error analysis, modified assessment, curriculum-based assessment, work sampling, and diagnostic instruction (Smith, 1983). Although it is impossible to cover each of these procedures in great detail, a more comprehensive discussion of the procedures can be found in Gettinger (in press).

Generally, *diagnostic or trial teaching* refers to an assessment strategy that involves viewing the child while he or she actually is taught some academic skills. The clinician focuses on an identification of effective instructional strategies while sampling material from the child's curriculum. This is followed by testing the student's level of mastery. If the instructional objective is not met, the instructional approach is modified or changed, and this process continues until the most effective approach to instruction has been identified. In this sense, trial or diagnostic teaching is designed to simulate classroom instruction, and focuses on a process analysis of what the child is actually doing. Trial teaching has been advocated by a number of individuals across a variety of curriculum areas (Bryant, 1966; Hunter, 1979; Hutson & Niles, 1974; Kratochwill, 1977; Kratochwill & Severson, 1977).

Task analysis is another approach to analogue assessment that involves conducting a careful analysis of the skills and subskills within a particular area of the child's academic curriculum (e.g., math or reading). Task analysis procedures allow the clinician to identify which subskills need to be taught before the overall tasks can be mastered. Task analysis generally focuses on breaking more complex instructional tasks into subskills or subtasks that then become the focus of instruction (Resnick, Wang, & Kaplan, 1973; Smith, 1980). Task analysis is designed to identify the skills the child may not possess in order to complete a task and develop a sequence of instructional objectives. Finally, task analysis is linked to an evaluation of the child's progress in the skill sequence.

Task analysis is sometimes done informally or through more formal procedures called *path-referenced assessment* (Bergan, 1981, 1986). Path-referenced assessment was developed by Bergan and his associates to examine progress along various academic paths of learning in particular content areas. Path-referenced assessment approaches assume that the child moves from more simple to more complex capabilities in a particular area of the academic curriculum. For example, a technology for path-referenced assessment evolved out of development of the Head Start Measures Battery (Bergan & Smith, 1984), in which a variety of path-referenced assessment instruments were developed for use in the Head Start program. In contrast to norm-referenced and criterion-referenced assessment, path-referenced assessment involves a description of student progress along empirically evaluated developmental tasks that reflect broader achievement of educational objectives. The path-referenced assessment tactic involves developing information about educational progress within a particular area of the curriculum. Through the method of path-referenced assessment the clinician is provided with quantitative scales for measuring educational progress, which is linked to an empirically validated developmental sequence. Thus path-referenced assessment combines information from criterion-referenced assessment and task analysis toward a description of path position and path progress in a curriculum. In addition, path-referenced assessment can be used with norm-referenced assessment data to make decisions about a child's position within a norm group. The interested reader is referred to Bergan (1981) for a more detailed description of path-referenced assessment.

Error analysis is another analogue method of assessment that allows the clinician to analyze a child's performance in a particular area of the curriculum. The clinician sets up an analogue task during which various areas of the curriculum are taken from the student's actual classroom curriculum. An error analysis is then conducted that involves an examination of the processes that a student employs to complete the task (Algozzine, Siders, & Beattie, 1982). The error analysis strategy is considered very useful for instructional planning since many standardized tests do not allow development of specific instructional objectives for the child. Based on an error analysis, the clinician is able to construct specific instructional objectives for the individual education plan for the child (Gettinger, in press).

Another major development in analogue assessment involves *direct and curriculum-based measurement*. Direct curriculum-based measurement is affiliated with a number of different approaches as represented in the work on the Resource/Consulting Teaching Model (Idol-Maestas, 1981, 1983a, 1983b), the Vermont Consulting Teaching Models (Christie, McKenzie, & Burdett, 1972), the directive teaching procedures affiliated with the work of Stephens (1977), exceptional teaching (White & Haring, 1980), and precision teaching (Lindsley, 1964) and data-based program modification (Deno, Marston, & Tindal, 1986; Deno & Mirkin, 1977). All of these models emphasize direct and frequent measurement of student performance in the curriculum, *and* typically employ a structured behaviorally oriented teaching system. It is not possible to review each of these particular models in great detail here, and the reader is referred to Deno and colleagues (1986) for an overview of curriculum-based assessment.

Personality: Affective Domain

In problems that have a primarily somatic or psychoeducational presentation, assessment of the child's personality and emotional well-being is often not considered essential to primary diagnosis and is omitted from the assessment battery. This is unfortunate, since affective variables clearly may contribute to, or result from, any of the disorders discussed (Magrab, 1984). In some cases, particularly those in which stress is a salient factor (such as enuresis, encopresis, stuttering, asthma, elective mutism, and attention deficit disorders), impaired emotional functioning may well be the most powerful cause or the most serious consequence of the problem.

In other cases, assessment for psychosis is essential to accurate differential diagnosis. This is particularly true in disorders such as pica, attention deficit disorders, Tourette's disorder, infantile autism, and pervasive developmental disorder. When considering elective mutism as a primary diagnosis, assessment for personality and affective disorders such as major depression, overanxious disorder, and social phobia is recommended.

When the relation of affective variables to the primary disorder cannot be specified precisely it will be clear to the clinician that once a problem has been identified, regardless of its label, emotional well-being is at risk and may already be significantly impaired. For these reasons, appropriate and relevant assessment of the affective or personality domain should be incorporated into psychoeducational assessment. Although extensive review of this important area is not within the purview of this chapter, a very brief list of assessment tools is presented for illustration and emphasis.

Personality Inventories for Broad Assessment of General Personality Attributes. The Personality Inventory for Children (PIC) by Lachar (1984) is a 600-item paper and pencil inventory for use with children ages 3 to 16 that evaluates personality "attributes" such as anxiety, social skills, somatic concerns, psychosis, depression, delinquency, and withdrawal. The California Psychological Inventory (CPI) by Gough (1975) is a 480-item paper and pencil measure of 18 socially desirable behavioral tendencies such as dominance, sense of well-being, communality, achievement via conformity, and achievement via independence. Such measures may provide a gross screening function and serve to alert the clinician to possible areas for further assessment.

Identification of Psychosis and Affective Disorders. The Schedule for Affective Disorders and Schizophrenia (SADS) by Endicott and Spitzer (1978) is a measure of recent psychopathology, consisting of over 200 scales. The examiner rates items according to data obtained from interviews with the subject, case record, and clinical evaluation. The SADS may be used with children older than 12 years of age and adults. SADS-C (by Endicott) includes 29 scales, measures symptom changes over the week preceding testing, and is appropriate for adolescents and adults. SADS-L (by Endicott) assesses clinical history of psychopathology and may be used with adolescents and adults. A children's version of the SADS was developed by Puig-Antich and Chambers (1978). It is appropriate for use with children ages 6 to 12. Use of all versions of the SADS requires extensive examiner training.

Projective Techniques. Koppitz (1982) notes that personality assessment of school children can serve at least four important functions: to determine the youngster's behavioral and learning styles; to discover his or her motives, attitudes, and modes of adjustment to school and school work; to explore the child's self-concept and ability to relate to others; and to find out whether the child shows evidence of undue anxiety, serious emotional disturbance, or thought disorders that require further evaluations and therapeutic intervention.

Projective techniques are often considered an important part of traditional personality assessment (Anastasi, 1982) and have been used in a number of assessment domains, such as in interviewing children (e.g., Bierman & Schwartz, 1986). It may be important to keep in mind Hertz's (1970) caveat that projectives cannot be employed to their fullest potentialities by those who lack broad scholarship, intensive training, and varied experience. Projectives may also elicit information that may be otherwise unobtainable from resistant, fearful, nonverbal, and/or hostile examinees (Prout & Farber, in press). In such cases, referral for assessment to appropriately trained clinicians may be warranted. However, projectives have not fared well when traditional psychometric criteria have been applied (Anastasi, 1982), and scholarly reviews of the literature on the use of projectives with children have been very pessimistic (Gittelman, 1978, 1980).

Measures of Specific Factors. A variety of specific scales have been developed to measure constructs that could be useful in treatment planning. The Piers-Harris Children's Self-Concept Scale (Piers, 1984) is an 80-item paper and pencil test that assesses aspects of a child's self-esteem including behavior, intellectual and school status, physical appearance and attributes, anxiety, popularity, happiness, and satisfaction. The scale is appropriate for use with children 9 through 18 years old. Children's Depression Inventory (CDI) was developed by Kovacs (1979) and consists of 27 items that measure "overt symptoms of childhood depression such as sadness, anhedonia, suicidal ideation, and sleep and appetite disturbance" (Kovacs, 1981, p. 309).

Children's Depression Rating Scale by Poznanski, Cook, and Carroll (1979) is designed for use with children 6 to 12 years old and consists of 15 items that are given a severity rating by the clinician during a clinical interview. The Revised-Children's Manifest Anxiety Scale by Reynolds and Richmond (1985) contains 28 items that measure physiological, worry and oversensitivity, and concentration types of anxiety in children from third through twelfth grade. The test is particularly useful in conjunction with a clinical interview. The assessment of a specific factor or construct should be guided by empirical support for the measure's psychometric properties as well as its contribution to treatment planning.

SUMMARY AND CONCLUSIONS

In this chapter we provided an overview of psychoeducational assessment that can be conducted by individuals working in medical settings. We noted that psychoeducational assessment should be aimed toward a broad-based decision-making process that takes into account screening and identification, classification and placement, instructional planning, client evaluation, and program evaluation. Assessment activities will usually begin at a general or broad-based level and proceed to a more specific or narrow strategy. Those who work in medical settings will likely encounter child clients with primarily psychoeducational problems and somatic features as well as children with primarily somatic problems with attendant psychoeducational difficulties. A conceptual framework for how these two somewhat different case presentations would be handled was presented.

Among the more common methods of psychoeducational assessment are interviews with care providers and the child, self-report methods, checklists and rating scales, self-monitoring, direct observational assessment, and a wide range of analogue measures. In the last category are traditional intellectual and achievement measures as well as more specific and curriculum-based assessment tactics.

In the overall decision-making process, the clinician working in medical settings should note at least two trends occurring within the mainstream of psychoeducational assessment (Reschly, 1986). First of all, there is greater emphasis on linking assessment with design and evaluation of interventions. While this was once true only for more behaviorally oriented assessors (Kratochwill, 1982), the trend appears to be emerging across many different orientations to psychoeducational assessment.

Second, there is a growing emphasis on assessment of the child in the natural environment, and by individuals who function in that environment, including teachers, parents, and the child. For the individual working in medical settings this means that assessment activities must occur outside the hospital or clinic, if a comprehensive picture of the child is to be obtained. Such assessment, when combined with methods that result in program planning and monitoring, will more likely be functional for the overall positive impact on the child and family.

References

Achenbach, T. M. (1978). The Child Behavior Profile: I. Boys aged 6–11. *Journal of Consulting & Clinical Psychology, 46,* 478–488.

Achenbach, T. M., & Edelbrock, C. S. (1978). The classification of child psychopathology: A review and analysis of empirical efforts. *Psychological Bulletin, 85,* 1275–1301.

Achenbach, T. M., & Edelbrock, C. S. (1979). The Child Behavior Profile: II. Boys aged 12–16 and girls aged 6–11 and 12–16. *Journal of Consulting & Clinical Psychology, 47,* 223–233.

Achenbach, T. M., & Edelbrock, C. S. (1983). *Manual for the Child Behavior Checklist and Revised Child Behavior Profile.* Burlington, VT: Author.

Achenbach, T. M., & Edelbrock, C. S. (1984). Psychopathology of childhood. *Annual Review of Psychology, 35,* 227–256.

Achenbach, T. M., & Edelbrock, C. S. (1986). *Manual for the teacher version of the Child Behavior Checklist and Profile.* Burlington, VT: Author.

Alessi, G. J., & Kaye, K. H. (1983). *Behavior assessment for school psychologists.* Kent, OH: National Association of School Psychologists.

Algozzine, B., Siders, J., & Beattie, J. (1982). Using assessment information to plan reading instructional programs: Error analysis and word-attack skills. *Reading Improvement, 19,* 156–163.

American Psychiatric Association (1987). *Diagnostic and statistical manual of mental disorders* (3rd ed., rev.). Washington, DC: Author.

American Psychological Association (1985). *Standards for educational and psychological testing.* Washington, DC: Author.

Anastasi, A. (1982). *Psychological testing* (5th ed.). New York: Macmillan.

Arena, J. (1982). *Diagnostic Spelling Potential Test.* Novato, CA: Academic Therapy Publications.

Barkley, R. A. (1981). Learning disabilities. In E. J. Mash & L. G. Terdal (Eds.), *Behavioral assessment of childhood disorders.* New York: Guilford.

Beatty, L. S., Madden, R., Gardner, E. F., & Karlsen, B. (1976). *Stanford Diagnostic Mathematics Test.* New York: Harcourt Brace Jovanovich.

Behar, L. B., & Stringfield, S. (1974). A behavior rating scale for the preschool child. *Developmental Psychology, 10,* 601–610.

Bellack, A. S., & Hersen, M. (1977). The use of self-report inventories in behavioral assessment. In J. D. Cone & R. P. Hawkins (Eds.), *Behavioral assessment: New directions in clinical psychology.* New York: Brunner/Mazel.

Bergan, J. R. (1977). *Behavioral consultation.* Columbus, OH: Charles E. Merrill.

Bergan, J. R. (1981). Path-referenced assessment in school psychology. In T. R. Kratochwill (Ed.), *Advances in school psychology* (Vol. 1). Hillsdale, NJ: Erlbaum.

Bergan, J. R. (1986). Path-referenced assessment: A guide for instructional management. *Special Services in the Schools, 2,* 29–41.

Bergan, J. R., & Kratochwill, T. R. (in press). *Behavioral consultation in applied settings.* New York: Plenum.

Bergan, J. R. (Ed.), & Smith, A. N. (1984). *Head Start Measures Battery.* Department of Health & Human Services, under contract No. HHS-105-81-C-008. Tucson, Arizona: University of Arizona.

Bierman, K. S., & Schwartz, L. A. (1986). Clinical child interviews: Approaches and developmental considerations. *Journal of Child & Adolescent Psychotherapy, 3,* 267–278.

Bijou, S. W. (1976). *Child development: The basic stage of early childhood.* Englewood Cliffs, NJ: Prentice-Hall.

Blunden, D., Spring, C., & Greenberg, L. M. (1974). Validation of the classroom behavior inventory. *Journal of Consulting & Clinical Psychology, 42,* 84–88.

Bolstad, O. D., & Johnson, S. M. (1977). The relationship between teachers' assessment of students and the students' actual behavior in the classroom. *Child Development, 48,* 570–578.

Brown, N. W. (1976). Non-cognitive characteristics in the prediction of reading readiness. *Educational & Psychological Measurement, 36,* 537–542.

Brown, L. L., & Hammill, D. D. (1978). *The Behavior Rating Profile: An ecological approach to behavioral assessments.* Austin, TX: Pro-Ed.

Bryant, N. D. (1966). Clinical inadequacies with learning disorders—The missing clinical educator. In J. Hellmuth (Ed.), *Learning disorders* (Vol. 2). Seattle: Special Child Publications.

Cancelli, A. A., & Kratochwill, T. R. (1981). Advances in criterion-referenced assessment. In T. R. Kratochwill (Ed.), *Advances in school psychology* (Vol. 1). Hillsdale, NJ: Erlbaum.

Cautela, J. R., Cautela, J., & Esonis, S. (1983). *Forms for behavior analysis with children.* Champaign, IL: Research Press.

Christie, L., McKenzie, H., & Burdett, C. (1972). The consulting teacher approach to special education: Inservice training for regular classroom teachers. *Focus on Exceptional Children, 5,* 1–10.

Ciminero, A. R., & Drabman, R. S. (1977). Current developments in the behavioral assessment of children. In B. B. Lahey & A. E. Kazdin (Eds.), *Advances in clinical child psychology* (Vol. 1). New York: Plenum.

Cone, J. D., & Foster, S. L. (1982). Direct observation in clinical psychology. In P. C. Kendall & J. N. Butcher (Eds.), *Handbook of research methods in clinical psychology.* New York: Wiley.

Conners, C. K. (1969). A teacher rating scale for use in drug studies with children. *American Journal of Psychiatry, 6,* 884–888.

Connolly, A. J., Nachtman, W., & Pritchett, E. M. (1976). *Key Math Diagnostic Arithmetic Test.* Circle Pines, MN: American Guidance Service.

Conrad, W. G., & Tobiessen, J. (1967). The development of kindergarten behavior rating scales for the prediction of learning and behavior disorders. *Psychology in the Schools, 4,* 359–363.

Darrell, D., & Catterson, J. (1980). *Durrell Analysis of Reading Difficulty* (3rd ed.). New York: Psychological Corporation.

Deno, S. L., Marston, D., & Tindal, G. (1986). Direct and frequent curriculum based measurement: An alternative for educational decision making. *Special Services in the Schools.*

Deno, S. L., & Mirkin, P. (1977). *Date-based program modification: A manual.* Minneapolis, MN: Leadership Training Institute/Special Education, University of Minnesota.

Dunn, L. M., & Markwardt, F. C., Jr. (1970). *Peabody Individual Achievement Test.* Circle Pines, MN: American Guidance Service.

Dusek, J. B., & O'Connell, E. J. (1973). Teacher expectancy effects on the achievement test performance of elementary school children. *Journal of Educational Psychology, 65*, 371–377.

Edelbrock, C. (in press). Informant reports. In E. S. Shapiro & T. R. Kratochwill (Eds.), *Behavioral assessment in the schools*. New York: Guilford.

Edelbrock, C., & Achenbach, T. M. (1984). The teacher version of the Child Behavior Profile: I. Boys aged 6–11. *Journal of Consulting & Clinical Psychology, 52*, 207–217.

Edelbrock, C., & Achenbach, T. M. (1985). *The teacher version of the Child Behavior Profile: II. Boys aged 12–16 and girls aged 6–11 and 12–16*. Manuscript submitted for publication.

Elliott, S. N., & Piersel, W. C. (1982). Direct assessment of reading skills: An approach which links assessment to intervention. *School Psychology Review, 11*, 267–280.

Endicott, J., & Spitzer, R. L. (1978). A diagnostic interview: The schedule for affective disorders and schizophrenia. *Archives of General Psychiatry, 35*, 837–844.

Enright, B. E. (1983). *Diagnostic Inventory of Basic Arithmetic Skills*. Woburn, MA: Curriculum Associates.

Evans, I. M., & Nelson, R. O. (1977). Assessment of child behavior problems. In A. R. Ciminero, K. S. Calhoun, & H. E. Adams (Eds.), *Handbook of behavioral assessment*. New York: Wiley.

Evertson, C., Brophy, J., & Good, T. (1972). *Communication of teacher expectations: First grade*. Austin: Report No. 91, Research and Development Center for Teacher Education, University of Texas at Austin.

Farr, R., & Roelke, P. (1971). Measuring subskills of reading: Intercorrelations between standardized reading tests, teachers' ratings, and reading specialists' ratings. *Journal of Educational Measurement, 8*, 27–32.

Feshbach, S., Adelman, H., & Fuller, W. (1977). Prediction of reading and related academic problems. *Journal of Educational Psychology, 69*, 299–308.

Gardner, W. I., & Cole, C. (in press). Self-monitoring. In E. S. Shapiro & T. R. Kratochwill (Eds.), *Behavioral assessment in the schools*. New York: Guilford.

Gesten, E. L. (1976). A health resources inventory: The development of a measure of the personal and social competence of primary-grade children. *Journal of Consulting & Clinical Psychology, 44*, 775–786.

Gettinger, M. (in press). Analogue measures. In E. S. Shapiro & T. R. Kratochwill (Eds.), *Behavioral assessment in the schools*. Hillsdale, NJ: Erlbaum.

Gittelman, R. (1980). The role of psychological tests for differential diagnosis in child psychiatry. *Journal of the American Academy of Child Psychiatry, 19*, 413–438.

Gittelman-Klein, R. (1978). Validity of projective tests for psychodiagnosis in children. In R. L. Spitzer & D. F. Klein (Eds.), *Critical issues in psychiatric diagnosis*. New York: Raven.

Glaser, R. A. (1971). A criterion-referenced test. In W. J. Popham (Ed.), *Criterion-referenced measurement: An introduction*. Englewood Cliffs, NJ: Educational Technology Publications.

Glazzard, M. (1977). The effectiveness of three kindergarten predictors for first-grade achievement. *Journal of Learning Disabilities, 10*, 95–99.

Gnagey, T. D. (1979). *Diagnostic Screening Test: Spelling* (3rd ed.). Ottowa, IL: Facilitation House.

Gough, D. (1985). *California Psychological Inventory*. Palo Alto, CA: Consulting Psychologists Press.

Green, K. D., Beck, S. J., Forehand, R., & Vosk, B. (1980). Validity of teacher nominations of child behavior problems. *Journal of Abnormal Child Psychology, 8*, 397–404.

Greenwood, C., Walker, H. M., Todd, N. M., & Hops, H. (1976). *Preschool teachers' assessments of social interaction: Predictive success and normative data*. Eugene, OR: Report No. 26, C.O.R.B.E.H.

Gross, A. M. (1985). Children. In M. Hersen & S. M. Turner (Eds.), *Diagnostic interviewing*. New York: Plenum.

Hallahan, D. P., Lloyd, J. W., Kauffman, J. M., & Loper, A. B. (1983). In R. J. Morris & T. R. Kratochwill (Eds.), *The practice of child therapy*. New York: Pergamon.

Hambleton, R. K. (1982). Advances in criterion-referenced testing technology. In C. R. Reynolds & T. B. Gutkin (Eds.), *Handbook of school psychology*. New York: Wiley.

Hammill, D., Brown, V., Larsen, S. C., & Widerholt, J. (1980). *Test of Adolescent Language*. Austin, TX: Pro-Ed.

Hammill, D., & Larsen, S. C. (1978). *Test of Written Language*. Austin, TX: Pro-Ed.

Hartmann, D. P. (1984). Assessment strategies. In D. H. Barlow & M. Hersen (Eds.), *Single case experimental designs: Strategies for studying behavior change* (2nd ed.). New York: Pergamon.

Hartmann, D. P., Roper, B. L., & Bradford, D. C. (1979). Some relationships between behavioral and traditional assessment. *Journal of Behavioral Assessment, 1*, 3–21.

Hawkins, R. P. (1979). The functions of assessment: Implications for selection and development of devices for assessing repertoires in clinical, educational, and other settings. *Journal of Applied Behavior Analysis, 12*, 501–516.

Haynes, S. N. (1978). *Principles of behavioral assessment*. New York: Gardner.

Hertz, M. (1970). Projective techniques in crisis. *Journal of Projective Techniques, 34*, 449–467.

Hoge, R. D. (1983). Psychometric properties of teacher-judgment measures of pupil aptitudes, classroom behaviors, and achievement levels. *The Journal of Special Education, 17*, 401–429.

Hunter, M. (1979). Diagnostic teaching. *Elementary School Journal, 80*, 41–46.

Hutson, B. A., & Niles, J. A. (1974). Trial teaching: The missing link. *Psychology in the Schools, 11*, 188–191.

Idol-Maestas, L. (1981). A teacher training model: The resource consulting teacher. *Behavioral Disorders, 6*, 108–121.

Idol-Maestas, L. (1983a). *A follow-up report on mildly handicapped students receiving direct reading instruction*. Unpublished manuscript.

Idol-Maestas, L. (1983b). *Special educator's consultation handbook*. Rockville, MD: Aspen.

Jastak, J. F., & Jastak, S. (1978). *The Wide Range Achievement Test* (rev. ed.). Wilmington, DE: Jastak.

Jones, R. R., Reid, J. B., & Patterson, G. B. (1974). Naturalistic observation in clinical assessment. In P. McReynolds (Ed.), *Advances in psychological assessment*. San Francisco: Jossey-Bass.

Kanfer, F. H. (1977). The many faces of self-control. In R. B. Stuart (Ed.), *Behavioral self-management strategies, techniques, and outcome*. New York: Brunner/Mazel.

Kapelis, L. (1975). Early identification of reading failure: A comparison of two screening tests and teacher forecasts. *Journal of Learning Disabilities, 8*, 638–641.

Kaufman, A. S. (1979). *Intelligent Testing with the WISC-R*. New York: Wiley-Interscience.

Kaufman, A. S. (1982). An integrated review of almost a decade of research on the McCarthy scales. In T. R. Kratochwill (Ed.), *Advances in school psychology* (Vol. II). Hillsdale, NJ: Erlbaum.

Kaufman, A. S., & Kaufman, N. L. (1983). *Kaufman Assessment Battery for Children*. Circle Pines, MN: American Guidance Service.

Kellam, S. G., Branch, J. D., Agrawal, K. C., & Ensminger, M. E. (1975). *Mental health and going to school*. Chicago: University of Chicago Press.

Keogh, B. K., & Smith, C. E. (1970). Early identification of educationally high potential and high risk children. *Journal of School Psychology, 8*, 285–290.

Kim, Y., Anderson, H. E., & Bashaw, W. C. (1968). Social maturity, achievement, and basic ability. *Educational & Psychological Measurement, 28*, 535–543.

Kirk, S. A., & Kirk, W. D. (1971). *Psycholinguistic learning disabilities: Diagnosis and remediation*. Urbana: University of Illinois Press.

Kohn, M., & Rosman, B. L. (1973a). Cognitive functioning in five-year-old boys as related to social-emotional and background-demographic variables. *Developmental Psychology, 8*, 227–294.

Koppitz, E. M. (1982). Personality assessment in the schools. In C. R. Reynolds & T. B. Gutkin (Eds.), *Handbook of school psychology*. New York: Wiley.

Kovacs, M. (1979). *Children's Depression Inventory*. University of Pittburgh School of Medicine, Department of Psychiatry.

Kovacs, M. (1981). Rating scales to assess depression in school-aged children. *Acta Paedopsychiatrica, 46*, 305–315.

Kratochwill, T. R. (1977). The movement of psychological extras into ability assessment. *Journal of Special Education, 11*, 299–311.

Kratochwill, T. R. (1980). Behavioral assessment of academic and social problems: Implications for the individual education program. *School Psychology Review, 9*, 199–206.

Kratochwill, T. R. (1982). Advances in behavioral assessment. In C. R. Reynolds & T. B. Gutkin (Eds.), *Handbook of school psychology*. New York: Wiley.

Kratochwill, T. R. (1985). Selection of target behaviors in behavioral consultation. *Behavioral Assessment, 7*, 49–61.

Kratochwill, T. R., & Severson, R. A. (1977). Process assessment: An examination of reinforcer effectiveness and predictive validity. *Journal of School Psychology, 15*, 293–300.

Lambert, N. M., & Nicoll, R. C. (1977). Conceptual model for nonintellectual behavior and its relationship to early reading achievement. *Journal of Educational Psychology, 69*, 481–490.

Larsen, S. C., & Hammill, D. D. (1986). *Test of Written Spelling*. Austin, TX: Pro-Ed.

Lindsley, O. R. (1964). Direct measurement and prothesis of retarded behavior. *Journal of Education, 147*, 62–81.

Lorion, R. P., Cowen, E. L., & Caldwell, R. A. (1975). Normative and parametric analyses of school maladjustment. *American Journal of Community Psychology, 3*, 291–301.

Luce, S. R., & Hoge, R. D. (1978). Relations among teacher rankings, pupil–teacher interactions, and academic achievement: A test of the teacher-expectancy hypothesis. *American Educational Research Journal, 15*, 489–500.

Mace, F. C., & Kratochwill, T. R. (in press). Self-monitoring: Applications and issues. In J. C. Witt, S. N. Elliott, & F. M. Gresham (Eds.), *Handbook of behavior therapy in education*. New York: Plenum.

Magrab, P. R. (1984). A developmental framework for psychological assessment of pediatric conditions. In P. R. Magrab (Ed.), *Psychological and behavioral assessment: Impact on pediatric care*. New York: Plenum.

Maher, C. A., & Bennett, R. E. (1984). *Planning and evaluating special education services*. Englewood Cliffs, NJ: Prentice-Hall.

Mahoney, M. J. (1977). Some applied issues in self-monitoring. In J. D. Cone & R. P. Hawkins (Eds.), *Behavioral assessment: New directions in clinical psychology*. New York: Brunner/Mazel.

Mahoney, M. J., & Arnkoff, D. (1978). Cognitive and self-control therapies. In S. L. Garfield & A. E. Bergin (Eds.), *Handbook of psychotherapy and behavior change: An empirical analysis* (2nd ed.). New York: Wiley.

McCarthy, D. A. (1972). *Manual for the McCarthy Scales of Children's Abilities*. New York: Psychological Corporation.

McFall, R. M. (1977). Analogue methods in behavioral assessment: Issues and prospects. In J. D. Cone & R. P. Hawkins (Eds.), *Behavioral assessment: New directions in clinical psychology*. New York: Brunner/Mazel.

Mellon, P. M., & Crano, W. D. (1977). An extension and application of multitrait-multimethod matrix technique. *Journal of Educational Psychology, 69*, 716–723.

Mercer, J. R., & Lewis, J. F. (1978). *System of multicultural pluralistic assessment*. New York: Psychological Corporation.

Mitchell, J. V., Jr. (1985a). *The ninth mental measurements yearbook* (Vol. I). Lincoln, NE: University of Nebraska Press.

Mitchell, J. V., Jr. (1985b). *The ninth mental measurements yearbook* (Vol. II). Lincoln, NE: University of Nebraska Press.

Morine-Dershimer, G. (1978–1979). The anatomy of teacher prediction. *Educational Research Quarterly, 3*, 59–65.

Mykelbust, H. R. (1965). *Development and disorders of written language: Vol. I.* Picture Story Language Test. New York: Grune & Stratton.

Mykelbust, H. R. (1971). *The Pupil Rating Scale: Screening for learning disabilities*. New York: Grune & Stratton.

Nelson, R. O. (1977a). Assessment and therapeutic functions of self-monitoring. In M. Hersen, R. M. Eisler, & P. M. Miller (Eds.), *Progress in behavior modification* (Vol. 5). New York: Academic.

Nelson, R. O. (1977b). Methodological issues in assessment via self-monitoring. In J. D. Cone & R. P. Hawkins (Eds.), *Behavioral assessment: New directions in clinical psychology*. New York: Brunner/Mazel.

Nelson, R. O., & Hayes, S. C. (1979). Some current dimensions of behavioral assessment. *Behavioral Assessment, 1*, 1–16.

Nelson, R. O., & Hayes, S. C. (1981). Theoretical explanations for reactivity in self-monitoring. *Behavior Modification, 5,* 3–14.

Novack, H. S., Bonaventura, E., & Merenda, P. F. (1973). A scale for the early detection of children with learning problems. *Exceptional Children, 40,* 98–105.

Nowick, S., & Strickland, B. (1973). A locus of control scale for children. *Journal of Consulting & Clinical Psychology, 40,* 148–154.

O'Leary, K. D., Romanczyk, R. G., Kass, R. E., Dietz, A., & Santogrossi. D. (1979). *Procedures for classroom observation of teachers and children.* Stony Brook, NY: Psychology Department, SUNY at Stony Brook.

Patterson, G. R., Ray, R. W., Shaw, D. A., & Cobb, J. A. (1969). *A manual for coding family interactions* (6th rev.). New York: ASIS National Auxiliary Publications Service, CCM Information Services, Document No. 01234.

Pedulla, J. J., Airasian, P. W., & Madaus, G. F. (1980). Do teacher ratings and standardized test results of students yield the same information? *American Educational Research Journal, 17,* 303–307.

Pekarik, E. G., Prinz, R. J., Liebert, D. E., Weintraub, S., & Neale, J. M. (1976). The pupil evaluation inventory: A sociometric technique for assessing children's social behavior. *Journal of Abnormal Child Psychology, 4,* 83–97.

Perry, J. D., Guidubaldi, J., & Kehle, T. (1979). Kindergarten competencies as predictors of third-grade classroom behavior and achievement. *Journal of Educational Psychology, 71,* 443–450.

Piers, E. (1984). *Piers-Harris Children's Self-Concept Scale.* Los Angeles, CA: Western Psychological Services.

Poznanski, E. O., Cook, S. C., & Carroll, B. J. (1979). A Depression Rating Scale for Children. *Pediatrics, 64,* 442–450.

Prout, H. T., & Ferber, S. M. (in press). Analogue assessment: Traditional personality assessment measures in behavioral assessment. In E. S. Shapiro & T. R. Kratochwill (Eds.), *Behavioral assessment in the schools.* New York: Guilford.

Puig-Antich, J., & Chambers, W. (1978). *The Schedule for Affective Disorders and Schizophrenia for School-Aged Children.* New York: New York State Psychiatric Institution.

Quay, H. C. (1979). Classification. In H. C. Quay & J. S. Werry (Eds.), *Psychopathological disorders of childhood* (2nd ed.). New York: Wiley.

Quay, H. C., & Peterson, D. R. (1975). *Manual for the Behavior Problem Checklist.* Unpublished manuscript.

Reardon, R. C., Hersen, M., Bellack, A. S., & Foley, J. M. (1979). Measuring skill in grade school boys. *Journal of Behavior Assessment, 1,* 87–105.

Reschly, D. J. (1986). Functional psychoeducational assessment: Trends and issues. *Special Services in the Schools, 2,* 57–69.

Reschly, D. J., & Reschly, J. E. (1979). Validty of WISC-R factor scores in predicting achievement and attention for four sociocultural groups. *Journal of School Psychology, 17,* 355–361.

Resnick, L. D., Wang, M. C., & Kaplan, J. (1973). Task analysis in curriculum. *Journal of Applied Behavior Analysis, 6,* 679–710.

Reynolds, C. R., & Brown, R. T. (Eds.). (1984). *Perspectives on bias in mental testing.* New York: Plenum.

Reynolds, C. R., & Richmond, B. O. (1978). What I Think and Feel: A revised measure of children's manifest anxiety. *Journal of Abnormal Child Psychology, 6,* 271–280.

Reynolds, C. R., & Richmond, B. O. (1985). *Revised Children's Manifest Anxiety Scale.* Los Angeles, CA: Western Psychological Services.

Ross, A. O., Lacey, H. M., & Parton, D. A. (1965). The development of a behavior checklist for boys. *Child Development, 36,* 1013–1027.

Rutter, M. (1967). A children's behavior questionnaire for completion by teachers: Preliminary findings. *Journal of Child Psychology & Psychiatry, 8,* 1–11.

Salvia, J., & Ysseldyke, J. E. (1978). *Assessment in special and remedial education.* Boston: Houghton-Mifflin.

Salvia, J., & Ysseldyke, J. E. (1985). *Assessment in special and remedial education* (2nd ed.). Boston: Houghton-Mifflin.

Sattler, J. M. (1981). *Assessment of children's intelligence and special abilities.* Boston, MA: Allyn & Bacon.

Saudargas, R. A. (1983). *State-event classroom observation code.* Knoxville, TN: University of Tennessee, Department of Psychology.

Schumer, F. (1983). *Abnormal psychology*. Lexington, MA: D.C. Heath.

Schwartz, J. C., Strickland, R. G., & Krolick, G. (1974). Infant day care: Behavioral effects at preschool age. *Developmental Psychology, 10*, 502–506.

Seidman, E., Rappaport, J., Kramer, J., Linney, J. A., Herzberger, S., & Alden, L. (1979). Assessment of classroom behavior: A multiattribute, multisource approach to instrument development and validation. *Journal of Educational Psychology, 71*, 451–464.

Shapiro, E. S. (in press). *Behavioral assessment in school psychology*. Hillsdale, NJ: Erlbaum.

Shapiro, E. S., & Lentz, F. (1986). Direct assessment of academic skills. In T. R. Kratochwill (Ed.), *Advances in school psychology* (Vol. 5). Hillsdale, NJ: Erlbaum.

Smith, C. R. (1980). Assessment alternatives: Non-standardized procedures. *School Psychology Review, 9*, 46–56.

Smith, C. R. (1983). *Learning disabilities: The interaction of learner, task, and setting*. Boston: Little, Brown.

Solomon, D., & Kendall, A. J. (1977). Dimensions of children's classroom behavior, as perceived by teachers. *American Educational Research Journal, 14*, 411–421.

Spivack, G., & Swift, W. (1967). *Devereux Elementary School Behavior Rating Scale Manual*. Devon, PA: Devereux Foundation.

Stanford-Binet (1985) (4th ed.). Chicago, IL: The Riverside Publishing Company.

Stephens, T. (1977). *Teaching skills to children with learning and behavior disorders*. Columbus, OH: Charles E. Merrill.

Stetson, E. (1985). Educational assessment of the child. In C. E. Walker & M. C. Roberts (Eds.), *Handbook of clinical child psychology*. New York: Wiley.

Stevenson, H. W., Parker, T., Wilkinson, A., Hegion, A., & Fish, E. (1976a). Longitudinal study of individual differences in cognitive development and scholastic achievement. *Journal of Educational Psychology, 68*, 377–400.

Stevenson, H. W., Parker, T., Wilkinson, A., Hegion, A., & Fish, E. (1976b). Predictive value of teachers' ratings of young children. *Journal of Educational Psychology, 68*, 507–517.

Tasto, D. L. (1977). Self-report schedules and inventories. In A. R. Ciminero, K. S. Calbourn, & H. E. Adams (Eds.), *Handbook of behavioral assessment*. New York: Wiley.

Terman, L. M., & Merrill, M. A. (1960). *Stanford-Binet Intelligence Scale*. Boston: Houghton Mifflin.

Thompson, J. R., Jr., & O'Quin, A. N. (1979). *Developmental disabilities: Etiologies, manifestations, diagnoses and treatment*. New York: Oxford University Press.

Thorndike, R. L., Hagen, E. P., & Sattler, J. M. (1985). *Stanford-Binet* (4th ed.). Chicago, IL: Riverside Publishing Company.

Thoresen, C. E., & Mahoney, M. J. (1974). *Behavioral self-control*. New York: Holt, Rinehart, & Winston.

Tokar, E. B., & Holthouse, N. D. (1977). The validity of the subtests of 1976 edition of the Metropolitan Readiness Tests. *Educational & Psychological Measurement, 37*, 1099–1101.

Wahler, R. G. (1980). The insular mother: Her problems in parent–child treatment. *Journal of Applied Behavior Analysis, 13*, 207–220.

Wahler, R. G., & Fox, J. J. III. (1980). Solitary toy play and time out: A family treatment package for children with aggressive and oppositional behavior. *Journal of Applied Behavior Analysis, 13*, 23–40.

Wahler, R. G., House, A. E., & Stambaugh, E. E. II. (1976). *Ecological assessment for child problem behavior: A clinical package for home, school, and institutional settings*. New York: Pergamon.

Walker, H. M. (1970). *Walker Problem Behavior/Identification Checklist*. Los Angeles: Western Psychological Services.

Walls, R. T., Werner, T. J., Bacon, A., & Zane, T. (1977). Behavior checklists. In J. D. Cone & R. P. Hawkins (Eds.), *Behavioral assessment: New directions in clinical psychology*. New York: Brunner/Mazel.

Wechsler, D. (1967). *Manual for the Wechsler Preschool and Primary Scale of Intelligence*. New York: Psychological Corporation.

Wechsler, D. (1974). *Manual for the Wechsler Intelligence Scale for Children-Revised*. New York: Psychological Corporation.

Wechsler, D. (1981). *Manual for the Wechsler Adult Intelligence Scale-Revised*. New York: Psychological Corporation.

Weiner, H. (1977). *Psychobiology and human disease*. New York: Elsevier.

White, O., & Haring, N. (1980). *Exceptional teaching*. Columbus, OH: Charles E. Merrill.

Willis, S. (1972). *The formation of teachers' expectation of students' academic performance*. Unpublished doctoral dissertation, University of Texas at Austin.

Witt, J. C., Cavell, T. A., Heffer, R. W., Carey, M. P., & Martens, B. K. (in press). Child self-report: Interviewing techniques and rating scales. In E. S. Shapiro & T. R. Kratochwill (Eds.), *Behavioral assessment in the schools*. New York: Guilford.

Woodcock, R. W. (1977). *Woodcock Johnson Psycho-Educational Battery: Technical Report*. Boston: Teaching Resources.

Ysseldyke, J. E. (1979). Issues in psychoeducational assessment. In G. Phye &. D. J. Reschly (Eds.), *School psychology: Perspectives and issues*. New York: Academic.

Ysseldyke, J. E., & Christenson, S. L. (1985). *TIES: The instructional environment scale*. Minneapolis, MN: University of Minnesota.

Ysseldyke, J. E., Thurlow, M. L., Graden, J. L., Wesson, C., Algozzine, B., & Deno, S. L. (1983). Generalizations from five years of research on assessment and decision-making: The University of Minnesota Institute. *Exceptional Education Quarterly*, 4, 75–95.

11

Family Systems Assessment

MARILYN A. McCUBBIN
HAMILTON I. McCUBBIN

The use of family assessment measures in child intervention is based on the premise that the family system interacts with its members, particularly children and adolescents, and consequently shapes them and is shaped by them in discernible and predictable ways. Additionally, while family social scientists, child developmentalists, adolescence scholars, epidemiologists, nurses, social workers, and physicians have pursued their research separately, we believe that the development of theories about and measures of family systems and their properties and function will enhance family practice across disciplines and ultimately advance our knowledge of the relationship between the family environment and child- and adolescent-related developmental, psychological, and physical health outcomes. This emerging interdisciplinary interest in family system influences child and adolescent health

This project was funded by Agriculture Experiment Station Project #3021, University of Wisconsin–Madison (H. McCubbin), and a grant from the Graduate School of the University of Wisconsin–Madison (M. McCubbin).

research: systems research on child and adolescent development; public health investigations; socioecological research; and psychosomatic research.

By focusing upon stress and child development, the outstanding anthology of Garmezy and Rutter (1983) brought to the forefront some of the most interesting and penetrating investigations on the linkage between the family and child development. In the traditional line of research and theory building, Michael Rutter, Norman Garmezy, Lewis Lipsitt, Jerome Kagan, and Eleanor Maccoby highlighted the importance of stressors, particularly loss and separation for children, the origins of coping, pointing to the defensive behaviors of infants as they seek to promote physiological integrity, the development of awareness and limitations through the experiencing of distress, and the linkage between transitional stressor events, vulnerability, and the emergence of coping from childhood to adolescence. Of greatest importance, the landmark publication included elements of family research. By focusing on children *at risk*, particularly children of divorce, Judith Wallerstein provided a process-oriented view of the impact of the family system upon children. In the final analysis, however, her exemplary work focused less upon the family system and more upon the developmental tasks of children of divorce. By focusing upon children with antisocial behavior, Gerald Patterson brought to center stage those interactional (dyadic) processes that appeared to be implicated in antisocial behavior in children. He emphasized the interaction pattern of escalating coercive regulatory interactions between aggressive child and mother, which seems amenable to behavior change in some families. This line of scientific inquiry, although limited in its emphasis upon the family system as a whole and its impact on child and adolescent development, was vitally important in facilitating family stress and coping research and the development of family system–oriented studies and measures.

Clearly, the *family system* is but one of a host of interrelated environmental influences that can and do have a profound impact upon the child and adolescent members and particularly their physical and psychological health status. But the research to substantiate these relationships is in an embryonic state of development. The jury remains in session deliberating the merits of current research in support of family research and the value of family interventions as a part of family-oriented health care. However, until such research has been accumulated to guide family in-the-clinic or in-home interventions, the training of family physicians, and family-based prevention-oriented interventions (i.e., changing family behaviors, family health-promoting practices, etc.), we will continue to operate on the basis of faith, experience, clinical insights, and unconfirmed hypotheses. By discussing the various self-report measures of family functioning for use in family systems and child-oriented research, we expect to reinforce extant investigations and encourage new and creative efforts in both instrument construction and hypothesis testing in this emerging arena of family systems, child and adolescent development, and health risk research.

CHALLENGES IN THE SELECTION OF MEASURES OF FAMILY SYSTEM FUNCTIONING FOR CHILD-ORIENTED ASSESSMENT

The selection of measures (and particularly self-report measures of family system functioning) linking the family system to child and adolescent outcomes is a major challenge for behavioral, social, and biosocial scientists and practitioners for several important reasons. First, there is the problem of conceptualization and definition. To the family scholar, child developmentalist, nurse scholar, practicing physician, and family therapist, the concept of family system functioning has heuristic value (and thus has meaning to everyone); after all, we all come from families and thus are family experts by experience. Yet as we observe family system functioning, this seemingly understandable phenomenon becomes increasingly slippery; we have many different definitions of family system functioning and each means different things to different professionals. Some would describe family functioning in terms of structure—single parents, two-parent, binuclear family, reconstituted family, gay family, lesbian family, and so on. Others would point to the interactional nature of families with an emphasis upon family communication, cohesion, adaptability, conflict, expressiveness, control, and affective involvement, to name a few. Others would describe family functioning in terms of its transactional processes, including coping, adaptation, social support, assimilation, and accommodation. Still other family specialists would emphasize the psychological characteristics of family members such as esteem, depression, and denial as indices of family functioning. Finally, others would focus on subsystems (mother–child, father–child, child–child, relatives–child, etc.) as important dimensions for study. The systematic assessment of family system functioning by self-report measures is limited by the lack of agreed-upon concepts and definitions. Consequently, we have narrowed our selection of family systems–oriented instruments to *those that have well-defined family systems–oriented constructs and appear to fit the broad range of concepts used to describe how families respond to change, stress, and their developmental tasks.*

Second, we are challenged by numerous family systems–oriented research propositions and hypotheses that have yet to be explored fully. Up to this point in the chapter we have referenced only one research question to be studied: the role of the family system in shaping the development of children and adolescents. There is reason to believe that family scholars, health professionals, and life span developmentalists might also be interested in the systematic assessment of: (1) family system functioning in response to children with acute illnesses; (2) family system functioning in shaping the adjustment of child or adolescent patients with specific medical conditions such as coronary bypass surgery and renal transplantation; (3) family system functioning in the long-term rehabilitation of child patients with chronic health conditions such as diabetes, cystic fibrosis, and cerebral palsy; (4) family system functioning in the care of terminally ill and handicapped children and adolescents; and (5) family system functioning in the child's or adolescent's adherence to the medical regimen in the home setting. These are but a very few of the more salient research issues relevant to the health care professional's research. It is important to determine what aspects of family system functioning are to be evaluated or assessed for the different research questions. Therefore we selected *self-report measures that encompass a range of dimensions associated with family functioning and that would be applicable to a wide range of relevant questions and hypotheses in child- and adolescent-oriented research and clinical assessment.*

Third, we are challenged by the methodological limitations and strengths of family systems measures and particularly self-report measures. Any review of the various methods of measuring families' systems would include the laundry list of difficulties associated with family systems–oriented self-report measures, which include: (1) distortion in the recall of family processes and interaction; (2) lack of objectivity in perceptions that guide the recording of family systems–oriented observations; and (3) the difficulty of deriving family level measures from individual assessments of family functioning. On the other hand, we are sensitive to the fact that self-report measures have unique and positive properties of interest to family- and child-oriented researchers. Specifically, self-report measures have the potential of capturing family dynamics across a period of time. Family members are called upon to sample their life experiences, across time and across events, and to use these recollections to describe, evaluate, and record their assessment of how the family typically behaves under a wide range of situations. Family processes, which may be viewed as an integral part of family functioning, can be described and documented, provided the responding family members consider how the family behaves across time and in response to a range of situations and circumstances. Therefore, in selecting self-report measures to be reviewed here, we focused on *those instruments that operationalized family dynamics, interpersonal properties, and processes that evolved over time, which we felt the self-report measures were best suited to capture.*

Fourth, if family scholars, developmentalists, and health care professionals are to build upon previous research and to maximize the accretion of research data and findings, it is vital that family systems–oriented theories be used to guide both the development of family systems measures and the design of child and adolescent research and practice. Idiosyncratic measures that are unique to a specific subsystem (marital dyad, parent–child, parent–adolescent) in the child or adolescent study will have immediate value to the family scholar or developmentalists, but may contribute but a little to a group of family professionals searching for common threads of evidence that point to the importance of the family system in child, adolescent, and health research. Instruments based on theories about family system functioning, particularly in relationship to child, adolescent, and health outcomes, have a greater potential of being refined and improved upon and still remain focused upon the family property or dimension being measured. This process of developing and refining family systems–oriented instruments is a vital and valued part of child and adolescent research and is enhanced by a strong linkage between the instrument and its theoretical underpinnings. Therefore, we limited our selection of family systems instruments to *those based upon a documented family systems–oriented theoretical framework.*

Fifth, we are challenged by the ever-present need to refine and confirm the strengths of family systems measures through standardized procedures establishing the instruments' reliability and validity. While this seems to be an obvious criterion in the selection of instruments, this matter takes on added complexity and importance in child-, adolescent-, and health-oriented research. Certainly, the standard psychometric procedures to confirm an instrument's reliability (i.e., test–retest, internal consistency, split-half, etc.) and validity (i.e., concurrent, discriminatory, construct, etc.) apply to family–child, family–adolescent, and family–health research. But we are also challenged by the need to validate these measures in relationship to specific health outcomes. We have need to accumulate evidence that confirms that measures of family functioning are sensitive to physiological changes, changes in health status, and medical conditions of family members. In this review we selected *those self-report measures that already have confirmatory statistics as to their link to child, adolescent, and health outcomes.* Additionally, recognizing that some of the strongest family systems self-report measures are now being used in child, adolescent, and health research, we selected *those we felt had the greatest potential of validation against criterion indices of child and adolescent psychological functioning, physiological changes, and health status.*

In the final analysis four comprehensive family systems instruments (multiple dimensions of the family system captured in a single tool) and two family systems typology instruments (i.e., groupings of instruments designed to create family types and to assess the same or different dimensions of family system functioning defined by the same theoretical framework or variations of the same instrument) were selected for this review. The comprehensive family systems instruments are: (1) Family APGAR (FAPGAR) (Smilkstein; 1978); (2) the Family Environment Scales (FES) (Moos, 1974); (3) the Family Assessment Device (FAD) (Epstein, Levin, & Bishop, 1976); and (4) the Family Assessment Measure (FAM I, II, III) (Steinhauer, Santa-Barbara, & Skinner, 1984). The family systems typology instruments are: (1) the Family Adaptability and Cohesion Evaluation Scales (FACES I, II, III) (Olson, Portner, & Bell, 1982; Olson, Portner, & Lavee, 1985); and (2) the Family Adjustment and Adaptation Measures (FILE, FIRM, FHI, FTRI, CHIP, and FCOPES) (H. McCubbin, A. Larson, & D. Olson, 1987; H. McCubbin & M. McCubbin, 1987; H. McCubbin, M. McCubbin, & Thompson, 1987; H. McCubbin & Patterson, 1981). Selection was guided by the five general criteria described earlier.

At the outset it is important to underscore the unique importance and value of each instrument or set of instruments in family systems– and child- and adolescent-oriented assessment. While this review may appear critical, and will reference apparent discrepancies between the ideal expectations and the limitations of each instrument, we also point to the embryonic nature of family system instrument development and testing. As already noted, the jury is still in session and is not likely to render any firm judgment until a sufficient body of empirical data is presented and reviewed. This chapter introduces six instruments or clusters of instruments with the intention of encouraging new and creative research with the ultimate goal of advancing our understanding of family relationships and its impact upon response to the health status of its members. In an effort to introduce the six self-report instruments (or sets of instruments) in a brief but meaningful manner we have introduced the appropriate conceptual frameworks, described the instruments and their major dimensions, and discussed their psychometric properties. Over time, we will accumulate the empirical verifications or refutations we seek about these self-report instruments. But until then we indicate our total support and appreciation of these six instruments, note their relative value to a wide range of research and practical questions, and acknowledge their contribution to this valuable line of inquiry.

THE FAMILY APGAR (FAPGAR)

Smilkstein (1978) of the University of Washington was challenged by the observation that, while a host of examinations and tests were available to the physician for evaluating a diseased organ's functional state, tools for evaluating the family unit of which the patient is a part were limited in number. Furthermore, while questionnaires and procedures existed to establish the state of functional integrity of the family, none had proven of practical value for daily use in the physician's office.

In response to this challenge, Smilkstein (1978, 1984) introduced a brief screening questionnaire called the Family APGAR or FAPGAR, which was designed to elicit a data base that would reflect a patient's view of the functional state of his or her family. The APGAR acronym was applied since the author felt that the name was already familiar to physicians involved in the evaluation of the newborn.

Since family structure and family function play a part in understanding and managing the complaint of the individual patient as well as of the family in trouble, Smilkstein (1978) focused upon the family unit as part of "medical" care and treatment. He defined the family as a psychosocial group consisting of the patient and one or more persons (children or adults) in which there is a commitment for members to nurture each other. This definition allows for a wide range of family life-styles, including the traditional nuclear family, communal groups, and nonmarried partners, whether heterosexual or homosexual. The process of nurturing included in the definition is equated with family function that promotes emotional and physical growth and maturation of its members.

Five basic components of family function were selected, defined, and operationalized in the development of the Family APGAR. These components and their definitions appeared to represent common themes in the social science literature that deals with families. These dimensions may also be likened to the body's organ system, in that each component has a unique function, yet each is interrelated to the whole. The family in health may be considered to be a nurturing unit that demonstrates integrity of the components of (1) *A*daptability, (2) *P*artnership, (3) *G*rowth, (4) *A*ffection, and (5) *R*esolve. The family systems model of the Family APGAR is outlined in Figure 11.1

The Family APGAR, a questionnaire that features five close-ended questions, is introduced by the author as a screening test to give a rapid overview of the components of family function. The questionnaire is designed so that it may be given to members

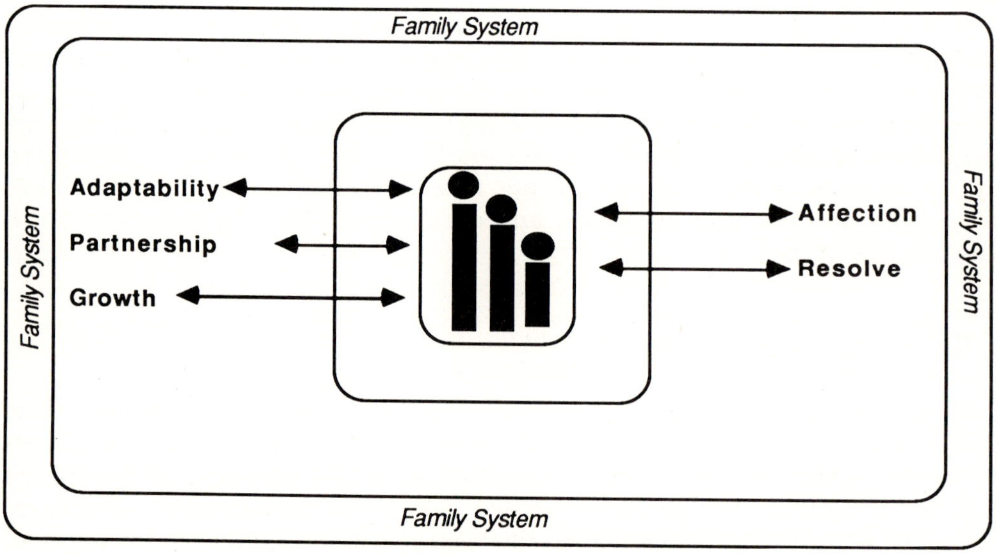

FIGURE 11.1. Family Systems Outline of the Family APGAR.

of either nuclear or alternative life-style families. The questions are designed to permit qualitative measurement of family members' satisfaction with each of the five basic components of family function. The functional components of the Family APGAR are: (1) adaptation—how resources are shared or the degree to which a member is satisfied with the assistance received when family resources are needed; (2) partnership—how decisions are shared, or the members' satisfaction with mutuality in family communication and problem solving; (3) growth—how nurturing is shared, or the members' satisfaction with the freedom available within the family to change roles and attain physical and emotional growth or maturation; (4) affection—how emotional experiences are shared, or the members' satisfaction with intimacy and emotional interaction that exists in a family; and (5) resolve—how time (and space and money) is shared, or the members' satisfaction with the time commitment that has been made to the family by its members.

Psychometric Properties

Statistical information regarding the reliability and validity of the Family APGAR was not available at the time of this writing. However, the author presents a strong and persuasive argument for the use of the Family APGAR in family practice. Through the use of medical case studies, Smilkstein (1978) points out the importance of family assessment in medical care and the viability of the Family APGAR in the conduct of these family-focused evaluations.

Smilkstein (1978) recommended that the Family APGAR be used as part of a broader data base to be collected regarding: (1) identifying and evaluating the family's crises, present and past; (2) the level of family function (through the use of Family APGAR); and (3) the family's resources. In support of this line of reasoning, the author proposes a modification in the problem-oriented record so that the format (data base, numbered problem list, titled plan, and follow-up) may be applied to the family.

THE FAMILY ENVIRONMENT SCALES (FES)

In elaborating upon environmental factors that impact on health, Moos (1979) introduced a comprehensive socioecological perspective designed to advance our understanding of and explain the complex but important linkage between the environment and health status. Specifically, Moos discussed the central importance of personal and environmental systems in determining the individual's health status. The personal system includes age, socioeconomic status, sex, intelligence, cognitive and emotional development, ego strength, self-esteem, attitudes, values, traits, and expectations. The environmental system includes the physical setting, organizational factors, the human aggregate, and the social climate. The family system, which is an integral part of the social climate, is characterized by the relationship dimension, the personal growth or goal orientation dimension, and the system maintenance and system change dimensions. The family systems model of the Family Environment Scales is presented in Figure 11.2.

The Family Environment Scale (FES) is a 90-item true–false questionnaire that focuses on the interpersonal relationships among family members, on the directions of personal growth emphasized in the family, and on the organizational structure of the family. It consists of 10 subscales that measure three domains of the family milieu: Relationship Dimensions (cohesion, expressiveness, conflict); Personal Growth or Goal Orientation dimensions (independence, achievement orientation, moral–religious emphasis, and intellectual–cultural and active recreational orientation); and Systems Maintenance and Change dimensions (organization, control). These three domains, which characterize a variety of settings, ranging from classrooms to work environments (Moos, 1974), provide the clinician with a conceptual framework to help organize many disparate observations about a family system (Eichel, 1978; Moos & Fuhr, 1982). The 10 FES subscales are shown in Table 11.1. A description of the logic underlying the FES, the steps involved in its construction, and its psychometric characteristics and a review of relevant research are provided elsewhere (Moos, 1974, 1979).

Psychometric Properties

In brief, an initial pool of 200 items was reduced to the final 90-item self-report questionnaire after analysis of the responses of a diverse sample of 285 families. The subscales have internal consistencies ranging from .64 to .79, 8-week test–retest reliabilities ranging from .68 to .86, and average intercorrelations of about .20. The scale has been used with more than 1600 families in more than 45 studies focused on its construct validity, its relationships to other dimensions of family functioning, and its implications for treatment outcome (Moos, Bromet, Tsu, & Moos, 1979; Moos & Moos, in press). Normative data are also available to the family physician to facilitate the identification of those at-risk families. There is a Real and an Ideal Form of the FES. Family members use the Real Form (Form R)

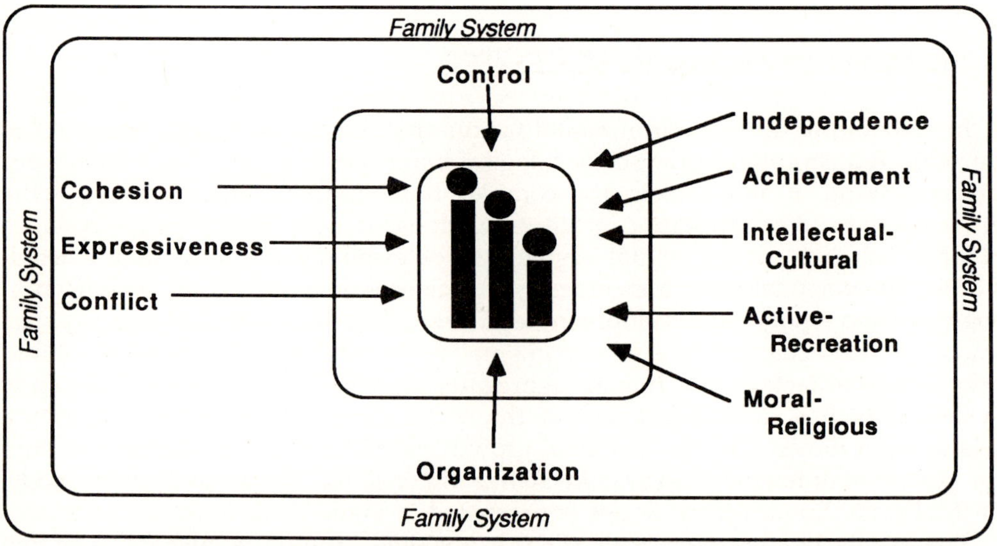

FIGURE 11.2. Family Systems Model of the Family Environment Scales.

TABLE 11.1. THE FAMILY ENVIRONMENT SCALE AND SUBSCALES

I. Relationship Dimensions	
1. Cohesion	Commitment, help, and support family members provide for one another
2. Expressiveness	How much family members are encouraged to act openly and to express their feelings directly
3. Conflict	The amount of openly expressed anger, aggression, and conflict among family members
II. Personal Growth Dimensions	
4. Independence	The extent to which family members are assertive, self-sufficient, and make their own decisions
5. Achievement	The extent to which activities (e.g., school and work) are cast into an achievement-oriented or competitive framework
6. Intellectual	The degree of interest in political, social, cultural, and intellectual activities
7. Active	The extent of participation in social and recreational activities
8. Moral	The emphasis on ethical and religious issues and religious values
III. System Maintenance Dimensions	
9. Organization	The importance of clear organization and structure in planning family activities and responsibilities
10. Control	The extent to which set rules and procedures are used to run family life

to describe the current family environment and the Ideal Form (Form I) to describe their preferred or ideal family.

In summarizing the clinical value of the FES, we can expand upon Fuhr, Moos, and Dishotsky's (1981) conclusions and argue that: (1) since the FES focuses on the present family situation, it can help shift attention from exclusive concern with medical problems of the "identified patient" to a consideration of family issues and concerns; (2) the FES can be used to organize and objectify the discussion of family issues in relationship to medical treatment; (3) through the use of the Ideal Form of the FES, family members can take an active part in shaping the nature of their goals, and it can be used to foster consensus on needed change, or, at minimum, clarify the nature and extent of discrepancies in family goals; and (4) the FES can be used to monitor the progress and outcome of family changes, particularly in relationship to improvements or deterioration in the patient's medical condition.

THE FAMILY ASSESSMENT DEVICE (FAD)

The McMaster Model of Family Functioning (MMFF) has evolved from studies of normal as well as clinical populations; it has developed over a period of 25 years. The initial research that contributed to the model's evolution was conducted in the late 1950s at McGill University. In the late 1960s and through the 1970s work on the model took place at McMaster University. Currently, research and theory-building activities are taking place at both McMaster and Brown universities.

The model is based on concepts from the family therapy literature, as well as from the authors' clinical, teaching, and research experience. Consequently, the model has been continually refined and reformulated. The concepts have been tested in clinical work, research, and teaching. Inconsistencies in observations and empirical invalidations became the basis for reformulations in the MMFF. The model has been used extensively in a variety of psychiatric and family practice clinics (Comley, 1973; Sigal, Rakoff, & Epstein, 1967; Westley & Epstein, 1960). The framework has also been used in a number of family therapy programs and found readily teachable (Bishop & Epstein, 1979).

As is true for all instruments discussed in this chapter, the MMFF is based on a systems perspective.

> The family is seen as an open system consisting of systems within systems (individual, marital dyad, etc.) and relating to other systems (extended family, school, industry, etc.). The unique aspect of the dynamic family group cannot be simply reduced to characteristics of the individual or interaction between pairs of members. Rather, there are explicit and implicit rules, plus action by members, which govern and monitor each other's behavior. (Epstein & Bishop, 1973, p. 176)

It follows that the basic assumptions of this systems model would emphasize that: (1) the parts of the family are interrelated; (2) one part of the family cannot be understood in isolation from the rest of the system; (3) family functioning cannot be fully understood by simply understanding each of the parts; (4) a family's structure and organization are important factors determining the behavior of family members; and (5) transactional patterns of the family system shape the behavior of family members (Epstein, Bishop, & Baldwin, 1982).

The McMaster model is based on the assumption that the primary function of today's family unit is to provide a setting for the development and maintenance of family members on the social, psychological, and biological levels (Epstein et al., 1976). In the course of fulfilling this function, families will have to deal with a variety of issues and problems, or tasks, which the authors group into three areas: basic tasks, developmental tasks, and hazardous tasks. The basic tasks are the most fundamental and involve the provision of food, money, transportation, and shelter. The developmental tasks encompass those family issues that arise as a result of development over time. These developments are associated with individual and family stages. The hazardous tasks involve the management of crises that arise as a result of illness, accident, loss of income, and other major and minor life events and changes. Families who are able to deal effectively with these three task areas are most likely to endure and thrive and less likely to develop clinically significant problems and/or chronic maladaptive problems. The family systems model of the Family Assessment Device is presented in Figure 11.3.

To advance the development of the MMFF around structure, organization, and transaction patterns of the family, the authors focused on six dimensions: Problem Solving, Communication, Roles, Affective Responsiveness, Affective Involvement, and Behavioral Control. The same MMFF dimensions served to guide the development of a self-report instrument called the Family Assessment Device.

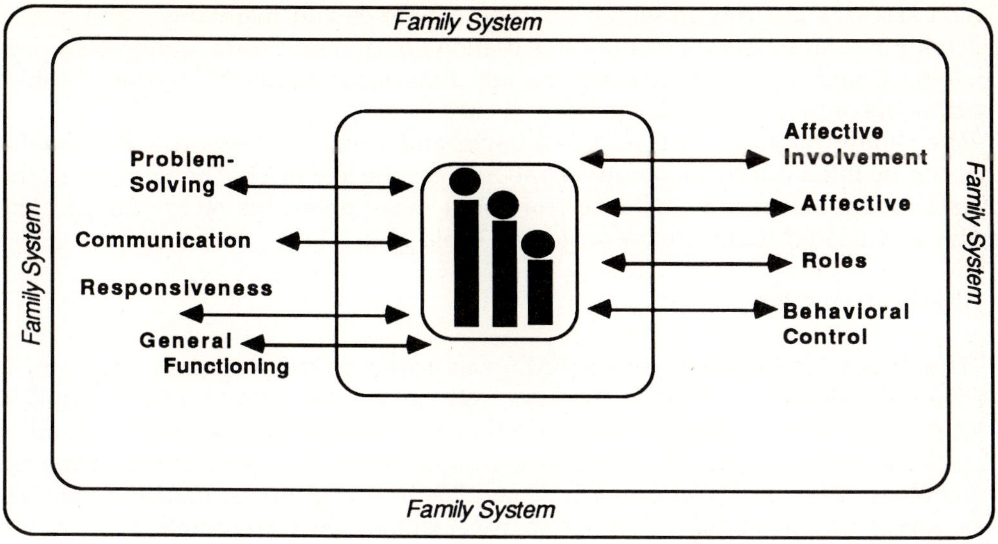

FIGURE 11.3. Family Systems Model of the Family Assessment Device.

The Family Assessment Device (FAD) was designed as a screening instrument to identify problem areas in the most simple and efficient fashion possible. The FAD measures structural and organizational properties of the family group and the patterns of transactions among family members that have been found to distinguish between healthy and unhealthy families. Specifically, in addition to a measure of General Functioning, FAD assesses six dimensions of family functioning. Problem Solving, the first dimension of the MMFF, refers to the family's ability to resolve problems (issues) to maintain effective family functioning. Seven steps of effective problem solving are identified. The second dimension of the MMFF is Communication, which is defined as the exchange of information among family members. The focus is on whether verbal messages are clear with respect to content and direct in the sense that the person spoken to is the person for whom the message is intended. The third dimension is Roles. Here the MMFF focuses on whether the family has established patterns of behavior for handling a set of family functions that include provision of resources, providing nurturance and support, supporting personal development, maintaining and managing the family system, and providing adult sexual gratification. In addition, assessment of the Roles dimension includes consideration of whether tasks are clearly and equitably assigned to family members and whether tasks are carried out responsibly by family members. The fourth dimension, Affective Responsiveness, assesses the extent to which individual family members are able to experience appropriate affect over a range of stimuli. Both welfare and emergency emotions (Rado, 1961) are considered. The fifth dimension, Affective Involvement, is concerned with the extent to which family members are interested in and place value on each other's activities and concerns. The healthiest families have intermediate levels of involvement, neither too little nor too much. The final dimension of the MMFF is Behavior Control, which assesses the way in which a family expresses and maintains standards of behavior of its members. Behavior in situations of different sorts (dangerous, psychological, and social) is assessed, as are different patterns of control (flexible, rigid, laissez-faire, and chaotic).

The Family Assessment Device is a paper and pencil, self-report questionnaire that can be filled out by all family members over the age of 12. The 53 items in the questionnaire are statements a person could make about his or her family. The scales and related items are presented in Table 11.2.

Psychometric Properties

The Family Assessment Device (FAD) was based on the responses of a sample of 503 individuals. Of these individuals, 294 came from a group of 112 families. This group includes 4 families of children in a psychiatric day hospital, 6 families of patients with a stroke rehabilitation unit, and 9 families of students in advanced psychology courses. The remaining 93 families in this group contained a member who was an inpatient in an adult psychiatric hospital. The total sample was selected

TABLE 11.2. FAMILY ASSESSMENT DEVICE MAJOR SUBSCALES AND SAMPLE ITEMS

Problem Solving
We usually act on our decision regarding problems.
After our family tries to solve a problem, we usually discuss whether it worked or not.

Communication
When someone is upset the others know why.
You can't tell how a person is feeling from what they are saying.
People come right out and say things instead of hinting at them.

Roles
When you ask someone to do something, you have to check that they did it.
We make sure members meet their family responsibilities.
Family tasks don't get spread around enough.

Affective Responsiveness
We are reluctant to show our affection for each other.
Some of us just don't respond emotionally.
We do not show our love for each other.

Affective Involvement
If someone is in trouble, the others become too involved.
You only get the interest of others when something is important to them.
We are too self-centered.

Behavioral Control
We don't know what to do when an emergency comes up.
You can easily get away with breaking the rules.
We know what to do in an emergency.

General Functioning
Planning family activities is difficult because we misunderstand each other.
In times of crisis we can turn to each other for support.
We cannot talk to each other about the sadness we feel.

so that it would contain individuals from families varying considerably at their level of functioning.

The reliability coefficients for the seven scales range from .72 to .92. The intercorrelations of the FAD subscales range from .4 to .6, indicating only a moderate degree of independence. However the authors reported that the partial correlations between the dimensions approach zero when General Functioning is held constant. The variance shared between the dimensions is for the most part accounted for by the variance that each shares with the General Functioning scale.

The authors report two general findings that suggest that the FAD has some limited validity. First, using data from a sample of 503 individuals, they compared the FADs for 218 nonclinic families and 98 clinical families in a discriminant analysis to determine whether family scores on FAD could predict whether the family came from the clinical or nonclinical group. Sixty-seven percent of the nonclinical group and 64 percent of the clinical group were correctly predicted. Second, they examined the retirement adjustment of 178 couples in their sixties. To assess concurrent validity they used regression analysis. The FAD explained 28 percent of the variance on couple marital satisfaction for both husbands and wives analyzed separately. The FAD also explained 22 percent of the variance in the morale scores for husbands and 17 percent of the variance for wives.

THE FAMILY ASSESSMENT MEASURE (FAM)

The Process Model of Family Functioning, upon which the Family Assessment Measure is based, differs from the McMaster Model of Family Functioning and their common source, the Family Categories Schema, by its increased emphasis on the dynamic interaction between the major dimensions of family functioning and by its emphasis on the interface between intrapsychic subsystems and the interpersonal dimension of the family system.

While recognizing that the McMaster Model of Family Functioning contributes to providing an organizing structure, Steinhauer and colleagues (1984) felt the need for a more process-oriented and dynamic model that satisfied four criteria: The model (1) would be capable of describing successful and unsuccessful patterns of family structure and functioning; (2) would allow a summary and integration of various clinical and research findings; (3) would provide a dynamic and process-oriented conceptual framework to guide clinical assessment and ongoing treatment; and (4) would encourage the generation of new and researchable hypotheses and insights into the structure and functioning of families.

The Process Model of Family Functioning (PMFF) is an attempt to meet these criteria. Consequently, the model emphasizes the dynamic interaction between the major dimensions of family functioning and the ongoing and interrelated development of individual and family. It goes beyond merely describing family structure to describing family process. Additionally, it systematically begins the task of integrating system theory with theories of individual psychopathology. It emphasizes the important linkage between the individual subsystems and the family system. Finally, the model emphasizes a systematic attempt to define the interface between the family and the greater social system of which it is but a part.

The Family Process Model of Family Functioning (FPMFF) underscores the basic assumption that the family and its members share common goals or objectives without which the family would not exist (Skynner, 1969; Tallman, 1970). The overriding goals of the family are to provide for the biological, psychological, and social development and maintenance of family members, thus ensuring the survival of both the family and the species (Ackerman, 1958; Murdock, 1960; Parsons & Bales, 1955). These overriding goals require the execution of certain tasks. The authors (Steinhauer et al., 1984) assume that these tasks may vary over the course of the family life cycle, but they involve the same basic skills and processes.

The central focus of the Process Model of Family Functioning is task accomplishment. Some of the family's tasks are culturally defined, while others are unique to an individual family and are determined by that family's norms and values. It is through successful task accomplishment that families achieve their biological, psychological, and social goals. Some of the basic goals include: ensuring the continuing development of all family members; providing reasonable security and autonomy for all; adapting usual patterns of functioning to meet environmental and developmental demands for change; and supplying the cohesion needed to hold the family together. The PMFF focuses upon three types of tasks to be accomplished. Basic tasks are those related to day-to-day survival (i.e., food, shelter, health care, etc.). Developmental tasks provide for the continuing development of all members evolving constantly over the course of the family's life cycle as members' developmental needs change. An index of the successful accomplishment of developmental tasks is a family's ability to perceive and adapt its responses to changing task requirements. Clearly, accomplishment of developmental tasks at one stage may facilitate but will not guarantee successful development at a later stage. Crisis tasks include the family's way of dealing with the periodic crises that result when the number and intensity of stressors confronting the family exceed the combined skills and resources (psychological, familial, and social) available to deal with them. In crisis situations, the family capacity for successful task accomplishment is undermined or curtailed as the basic skills upon which family problem solving and tension management depend may be overwhelmed, or at least diverted. The authors of PMFF argue that the family's capacity to accommodate to stress and avert potential crises is an excellent indicator of family resilience and health.

Family values and norms will shape every aspect of a family's functioning. The family's values may be either consonant or dissonant from those of society. A family's norms are the sum total of what is or is not considered acceptable within the family. While the PMFF identifies which characteristics are conducive to health or pathological family functioning, it is not possible to take such a position with values and norms. Nevertheless, understanding a family's values and norms is crucial for understanding that family's functioning.

To accomplish these tasks family members are called upon to achieve a high level of role performance. Roles are prescribed and repetitive behaviors involving a set of reciprocal activities with other family members. Collectively, these roles and their performance either facilitate or interfere with successful task accomplishment. The authors classify roles as either traditional or idiosyncratic. Traditional roles contribute to the accomplishment of essential family tasks, but the definition of a traditional role (i.e., father, wife, teenager, etc.) may vary depending on the values and norms of the society and those subcultures in which the individuals in the family are involved. There is no best or correct definition of traditional roles; each family arrives at a definition that works for it. Idiosyncratic roles do not contribute directly to task accomplishment, and are often the expression of individual and/or family pathology. Some families, for example, delegate one member to the role of family scapegoat, sacrificing his or her development to allow the family as a unit to exist in relative comfort.

Effective role performance and definition and task accomplishment in the family unit necessarily involve family communication and affective expression. It is through communication that the information required for effective role performance and task accomplishment is exchanged. The goal of communication—the achievement of mutual understanding—will be met if messages sent are clear, direct, and sufficient, and if receivers are psychologically available and open to receiving them with minimal distortion. In content, a communication can be affective (expression of feeling), instrumental (related to the ongoing task of everyday life), or neutral (neither instrumental nor affective). The more disturbed the family system, the greater the disturbance in affective communication.

Concomitantly, the family members' affective (emotional) involvement with each other and family control, or their way of influencing one another, play a critical role in helping or hindering role performance and definition, communication, and ultimately task accomplishment. The term *affective involvement* refers to the degree and quality of family members' interest and concern for one another. Optimally, the family will meet all members' emotional needs, thus providing the cohesion, security, and sense of being valued that contribute to the development of self-esteem and independence—while at the same time valuing and protecting each member's right to independent thought and behavior.

The quality of involvement will determine whether the relationships are nurturant and supportive, or destructive and self-serving. In contrast to the Circumplex Model of family behavior that implies that optimal affective involvement lies on the midpoint of a continuum between extreme cohesiveness and extreme disengagement, the process model postulates that these two dimensions taken together will determine whether the family environment provides continuing security and autonomy or whether it is exploitative and beneficial only to those who hold power and influence in the family system. There are five types of family affective involvement: (1) uninvolved; (2) interested but devoid of feelings; (3) narcissistic; (4) empathic; and (5) enmeshed. In the uninvolved family both degree and quality of involvement are low. In the case of family systems that show interest but are devoid of feelings, both the intensity and quality of involvement are only slightly higher than in the uninvolved family. The narcissistic family is characterized by higher intensity of affective involvement, but remains nurturant only as long as its members continue to satisfy each other's needs. The empathic family system maintains a high degree of active involvement while remaining supportive and accepting of each other's autonomy. The enmeshed system traps family members in an intense but stifling relationship that, while temporarily decreasing anxiety, does so by interfering with the continuing maturation of any.

Control is a PMFF concept used to describe a variety of interpersonal strategies or techniques to influence members' behavior. Family members will need to influence each other in two distinct situations, either to sustain ongoing functioning or to allow the family to adapt to changing task demands. There are four basic types of family control: (1) rigid; (2) flexible; (3) laissez-faire; and (4) chaotic. Both the maintenance and adaptation components of control will be affected by a given family's style, which may vary in its predictability, constructiveness, and responsibility. Ideally, family control should emphasize consistency of style, educational and nurturing techniques, and achievement and internalization of a sense of personal responsibility. A rigid family style is high on predictability, but low on constructiveness and adaptability. A flexible family system is high on predictability and high on constructiveness. A laissez-faire style combines moderate predictability and low constructiveness. Since almost anything goes, inertia and indecision take the place of organization and action. The chaotic style is extremely low in both predictability and constructiveness.

The Process Model of Family Functioning focuses upon family function rather than structure and thus defines six universal criteria of family functioning. A self-report test—The Family Assessment Measures (FAM III)—developed from the model (Family Assessment Measure III) is being widely used both as a research tool and as a clinical adjunct. The family systems model of the Family Assessment Measure is presented in Figure 11.4.

THE FAMILY ASSESSMENT MEASURE-III

The Family Assessment Measure (FAM-III) was aimed at providing an operational definition of the constructs in the Process Model. The present version of the Family Assessment Measure (III) assesses the family from three different perspectives. (1) The General scale (50 items, nine subscales) focuses on the level of health or pathology in the family from a system perspective. This scale provides an overall rating of family functioning, seven measures relating to the Process Model, plus

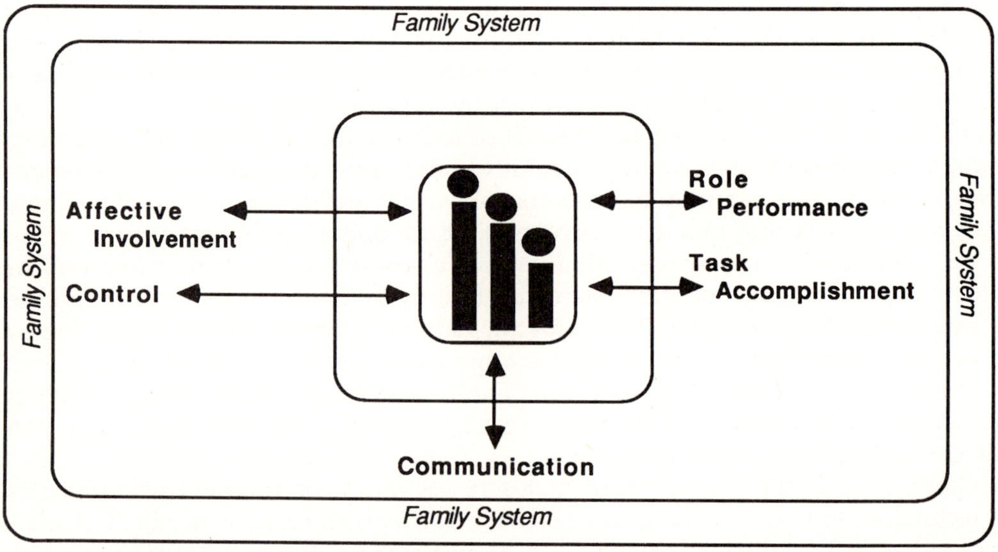

FIGURE 11.4. Family Systems Model of the Family Assessment Measures.

two response style subscales (Social Desirability and Denial). (2) The Dyadic Relationship scale (42 items, seven subscales) focuses on relationships among specific pairs (dyads) in the family. For each dyad, an overall rating of functioning is provided along with an index (subscale) for each construct of the Process Model. (3) The Self-Rating scale (42 items, seven subscales) focuses on the individual's perception of his or her functioning in the family. An overall index is provided along with seven measures relating to the Process Model.

Psychometric Properties

Preliminary analyses have been conducted on FAM-III using a heterogeneous sample of 475 families that were tested at various health and social service settings in the Toronto area. The reliability estimates are provided for the overall rating and various subscales. The estimates for the overall ratings are substantial. For adults—General scale, .93, Dyadic Relationships, .95, and Self-Rating, .89; for children—General scale, .94, Dyadic Relationships, .94, and Self-Rating, .86.

A multivariate comparison of problem and nonproblem families was conducted to provide evidence on the diagnostic power of the FAM-III General scale. "Problem" families were defined as currently having one or more family members receiving professional help for psychiatric or emotional problems, alcohol or drug problems, school-related problems, or major legal problems. These groups were contrasted with nonproblem families. A multiple discriminant analysis was conducted to identify linear combinations of the nine General scale measures that significantly differentiated among the six groups. The two discriminant functions differentiated children from adults and the problem from nonproblem families. Problem families in general are likely to report family dysfunction in roles and affective involvement. Nonproblem families have a tendency to be somewhat higher in social desirability and denial, although these differences appear to be minor. The discriminatory power of FAM-III has not been established for the Dyadic and Self-Rating scales.

THE FAMILY ADAPTABILITY AND COHESION EVALUATION SCALES (FACES)

The Circumplex Model of family behavior provided the basic foundation and overriding framework in the development of the three versions (FACES I, II, and III) of the Family Adaptability and Cohesion Evaluation Scales (FACES). Olson and associates (Olson & H. McCubbin, 1982; Olson, H. McCubbin, et al., 1983; Olson & Barnes, 1982; Olson, Sprenkle, & Russell, 1979; Russell, 1979; Sprenkle & Olson, 1978) have advanced the development of one of the major conceptual frameworks in family therapy and family research. Family Cohesion, Adaptability, and Communication are three dimensions of family behavior that emerged from a conceptual clustering of more than 50 concepts developed to describe marital and family dynamics.

Family Cohesion is defined as the emotional bonding that family members have toward one another. There are four levels: disengaged, separated, connected, and enmeshed. The developers of this framework hypothesized that the central levels separated and connected) are the most viable for family functioning. The extremes (disengaged or enmeshed) are generally seen as problematic.

Family Adaptability is defined as the ability of a marital or family system to change its power structure, role relationships, and relationship rules in response to situational and developmental stress. The four levels are rigid, structured, flexible, and chaotic. It is hypothesized that central levels (structured and flexible) are more conducive to marital and family functioning, while the extremes (rigid and chaotic) are the most problematic for families as they move through the family life cycle.

Communication, the third dimension in the Circumplex Model, is the facilitating dimension of family functioning. Communication is considered critical to movement on the other two dimensions. Positive communication skills (i.e., empathy, reflective listening, supportive comments) enable couples and families to share with each other their changing needs and preferences as they relate to Cohesion and Adaptability. Negative communication skills (i.e., double messages, double binds, criticism) minimize the ability of a couple or family members to share their feelings and thereby restrict their movement on these dimensions.

The Family Cohesion and Adaptability dimensions were integrated into the Circumplex Model as formulated by David H. Olson, Candyce Russell, and Douglas Sprenkle (1980, 1983; Olson, Sprenkle, & Russell, 1979). When Cohesion and Adaptability are placed orthogonally to each other 16 distinct types of marital and family systems are identified by combining the four levels of the Cohesion and four levels of the Adaptability dimensions. Four of the 16 family types are moderate (balanced types) on both the Cohesion and the Adaptability dimensions. Eight types are extreme on one dimension and moderate on the other (mid-range types), and four types are extreme on both dimensions (extreme types).

The Family Adaptability and Cohesion Evaluation Scales (FACES) were initially developed and tested as part of a doctoral dissertation research. Sprenkle focused on the Adaptability dimension and examined the interaction processes of 25 couples in marriage counseling and 25 nonclinical married couples. Russell (1979) studied both the Cohesion and the Adaptability dimensions, testing 31 nonclinical families with adolescent girls. As hypothesized, high-functioning families were moderate on Cohesion and Adaptability, while low functioning families scored at extremes of Cohesion and Adaptability. The family systems model of the Family Adaptability and Cohesion Evaluation Scales is presented in Figure 11.5.

The Family Adaptability and Cohesion Evaluation Scales (FACES, FACES II, FACES III) were designed to enable the researcher or clinician to place individual families or groups of families within the Circumplex Model. This assists in further understanding the dynamics of particular kinds of families and in setting treatment goals and program objectives. The three versions of FACES were designed so that individual family members could describe how they perceived their family. The reading level for the instruments was about seventh grade so that children as young as 12 could understand and respond to the items.

FACES I

FACES I (Olson, Portner, & Bell, 1978) was developed to provide an assessment of Cohesion and Adaptability as perceived by each family member. FACES I items were developed to tap each of nine concepts (emotional bonding, independence, boundaries, coalitions, time, space, friends, decision making and interests/recreation) related to Cohesion and six concepts (assertiveness, control, discipline, negotiation,

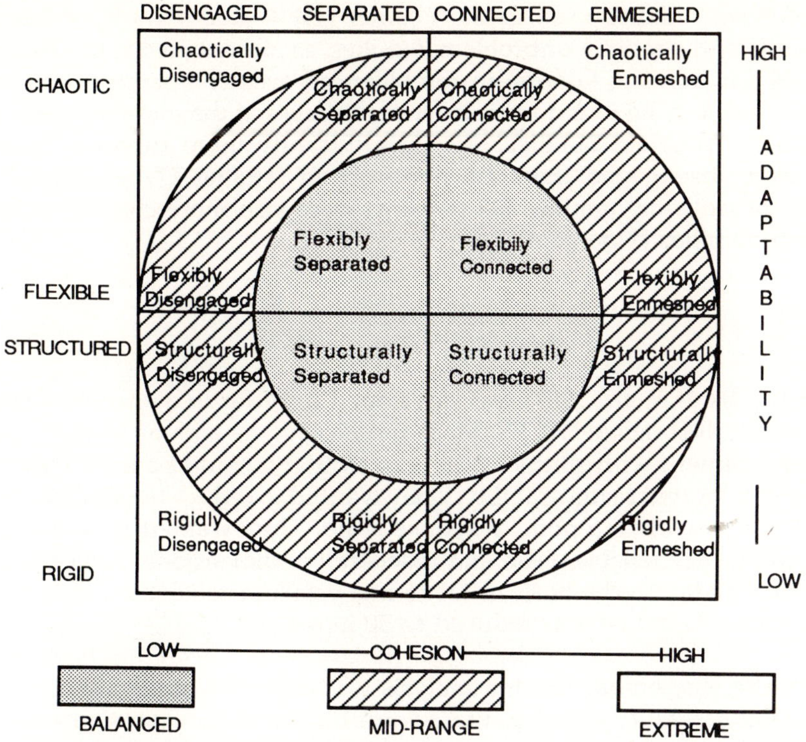

FIGURE 11.5. Family Systems Model of the Family Adaptability and Cohesion Evaluation Scales.

roles, rules) related to Adaptability. Additionally, two items were selected for the high, moderate, and low levels of each concept related to Cohesion and Adaptability. There are 54 items for Cohesion and 42 items for Adaptability, making a total of 96 items in FACES I. In addition, 15 items from the Edmonds' Social Desirability Scale (Edmonds, 1967) were included, making a total of 111 items in FACES I.

Psychometric Properties. A factor analysis of the Adaptability and Cohesion scales was done using data from 201 families with a father, mother, and adolescent, making a total of 603 family members. The factor analysis replicated the initial formulation of the scales where items were written for high, moderate, and low levels of Cohesion and Adaptability. The internal consistency (alpha) reliability for Adaptability was .75 and for Cohesion .83.

Portner (1980), who was involved in the development of all versions of FACES, compared 55 families (parent and one adolescent) in family therapy with a matched control group of 117 nonproblem families. As hypothesized, nonclinic families were more likely to fall in the balanced areas of the Circumplex Model on Cohesion and Adaptability than the clinic families (58 and 42 percent, respectively). Clinic families tended to be more toward the chaotic disengaged extreme (30 percent), with fewer nonclinic families at that extreme (12 percent). Bell (1982), also one of the codevelopers of FACES, studied 33 families with runaways and compared them with the same

117 nonproblem families used in the Portner (1980) study. As hypothesized, he found significantly more nonproblem families as described by the mother and adolescents (but not the fathers) in the balanced area compared to the runaway families. Conversely, he found more runaway families at the mid-range and extreme levels than nonproblem families. Also, significantly more runaway families (29 percent) were disengaged than the nonproblem families (7 percent). A higher percentage of runaway families (23 percent) were also more chaotic compared to nonproblem families (7 percent).

FACES II

FACES II (Olson et al., 1982) was developed in order to overcome some of the limitations with the original FACES. More specifically, the authors wanted to develop a shorter instrument with simple sentences so that it could be used with children and those with limited reading ability. They wanted to reduce the number of double negatives and provide a 5-point response scale. They wanted to develop a scale with two empirically reliable, valid and independent dimensions. After initial testing with 464 adults and on the basis of factor analysis and reliability (alpha) analysis, the initial scale (90 items) was reduced to 50 items.

Psychometric Properties. Factor analysis was done separately for the Cohesion and Adaptability items. Although there were 13 factors for Cohesion and 9 factors for Adaptability, the first 4 factors for each dimension accounted for about 75 percent of the variance. For the reduced scale of 50 items, the Cronbach alpha reliability figure for Cohesion was .91 and for Adaptability was .80.

The 50 items of the initial FACES II were administered to 2412 individuals in a national survey (Olson, H. McCubbin, et al., 1983). On the basis of the factor analysis and reliability checks, the 50-item scale was reduced to 30 items with 2 or 3 items for each of the content areas. The final 30-item scale contains 16 Cohesion items and 14 Adaptability items. There are 2 items for the following eight concepts related to the Cohesion dimension: emotional bonding, family boundaries, coalitions, time, space, friends, decision making, and interest/recreation. There are 2 or 3 items for the six concepts related to the Adaptability dimension: assertiveness, leadership, discipline, negotiation, roles, and rules.

The total sample of 2412 respondents was divided into two equal subgroups. Cronbach alpha figures for each of these groups and the total scale were as follows: (1) total sample—Cohesion, .87, Adaptability, .78; (2) subsample 1—Cohesion, .88, Adaptability, .78; and (3) subsample 2—Cohesion, .86, Adaptability, .79. The test–retest reliability study was conducted in fall 1981, using the 50-item version. The time lapse between the first and second administration of FACES II was 4 to 5 weeks. Respondents were 124 university and high school students who were not currently enrolled in a family studies course. They were asked to describe their "family of origin." The Pearson Product moment correlation for the 50-item FACES II scale was .83 for Cohesion and .80 for Adaptability. The norms on FACES II were based on the parents and adolescents participating in the national survey. Using only cases where there were complete data for all 30 items, a total of 2082 parents and 416 adolescents were used as the normative sample.

FACES III

The new version, FACES III (Olson et al., 1985), is now being developed and tested along with the development of national norms in response to the recognition that the two scales, Cohesion and Adaptability, as measured by FACES I and II, are highly intercorrelated. Because measures of family functioning in the Circumplex Model call for orthogonal dimensions—Cohesion and Adaptability—the developers of FACES III have been able to isolate these two dimensions, which meet this important criteria. The intercorrelation between Cohesion and Adaptability was a low of .05.

The authors recommend the use of "family satisfaction" in the application of and interpretation of FACES information in clinic settings. The alternative hypothesis states that families classified at the extreme on both dimensions will function "well" as long as all individuals indicate satisfaction with the family situation. Therefore the perceived versus ideal discrepancy on the family satisfaction scale, which is recommended to be used along with FACES, is an additional strategy for assessing how individuals feel about their current family system.

THE T-DOUBLE ABCX MEASURES OF FAMILY ADJUSTMENT AND ADAPTATION

The T-Double ABCX Model of Family Adjustment and Adaptation framework (H. McCubbin & M. McCubbin, 1987) emerges as part of a long tradition of theorizing and systematic research linking the family system to the psychological and physical well-being of its members. Dating back to the work of Adolph Meyer (cited in Leif, 1948), who used life charts with his patients to establish the association between the occurrence of particular or multiple life events and onset of illness, scientists (e.g., Holmes & Rahe, 1967; Jenkins, 1979; Patterson & McCubbin, 1983) have continued to pursue this line of inquiry in an effort to provide an individual and family-based explanation for the variability in individual susceptibility to illness and disease.

The T-Double ABCX framework which is also referred to as the Typology Model of Family Adjustment and Adaptation focuses on family efforts to manage the demands it faces (from stressors and strains) with its capability for meeting demands (resources and coping), mediated by the family's appraisal (situational and schema) so as to achieve a balance in family functioning (called adjustment and adaptation). There are two distinct and important phases in the model, adjustment and adaptation phases, separated by a period of family crisis when the family's homeostasis is upset. In contrast to the traditional models of family functioning, which focus upon the internal dynamics and workings of the family, three levels of the family functioning are considered—the individual, the family unit, and the community, each characterized by both demands and capabilities. This is not a static model; rather, there are dynamic interactions (inside the family) and transactions (outside the family) extended over time, as families attempt to maintain or arrive at a balance by using capabilities from one level of the family system to meet demands at another level.

To highlight the important aspects of family functioning, particularly as they apply to self-report measures of functioning, we turn our attention to the critical dimensions of the T-Double ABCX framework as they apply to health and illness research, namely: (1) pile-up of demands—stressors and strains; (2) family typologies; (3) family capabilities—resources; (4) family coping; and (5) family appraisals.

Pile-up of demands is a condition that produces or calls for change in the family system. Because change is implied, a demand can be viewed as a collection of threats or challenges to the family's existing homeostatic functioning. These demands may come from individual family members (i.e., psychological problems, developmental needs, etc.), the community (i.e., work pressures, etc.), or the family (i.e., marital conflicts, etc.) and may take the form of discrete stressors (i.e., events that occur at a discernible point in time) or strains (i.e., condition of tension associated with a residual unresolved problem from the past or need to desire to change something). These demands for change produce tension in the family system, and if this tension is not mediated by the family's own capabilities a state of stress arises. Because demands accumulate and interact with each other, a major event is not necessarily required to push the family demand load beyond the family's threshold to manage it. What is implied in this concept of pile-up is the dynamic nature of family demands; stressors and strains are constantly changing over the course of time.

A family's typology is defined as a set of basic attributes about the family system that characterize and explain how a family system typically appraises, operates, and/or behaves. These predictable and discernible patterns of family behavior, which are reinforced by rules and routines, play an important role in explaining family behavior in the face of stressful life events and transitions. In the face of a severe chronic illness situation, balanced families indicate more positive health outcomes for the chronically ill child (M. McCubbin, 1986). In the face of normative transitions, regenerative families, that is, those with strengths of family hardiness and coherence, are better able to manage hardships and promote other family strengths of bonding, flexibility, predictability, as well as marital and family satisfaction (H. McCubbin, Thompson, & Pirner, 1986). The family typologies utilized in the Family Stress, Coping, and Health Project and described more fully elsewhere (H. McCubbin & Thompson, 1987) are regenerative families, rhythmic families, and traditionalistic families (see Lavee, 1985; M. McCubbin, 1986; McCubbin et al., 1986).

Family capabilities are defined as the potentiality the family has available to it for meeting demands. Family resources, the first of three types of capabilities, are defined as characteristics, traits, competencies, or tangible items that may be brought into play in eliminating or mediating the impact of demands. Resources may be tangible, such as money, or intangible, such as self-esteem, and may come from individual members (i.e., innate intelligence, personality characteristics, esteem, etc.), from the family unit (i.e., cohesiveness, flexibility, communication, etc.), or from the community (i.e., esteem support, network support, medical care, etc.).

Coping is another type of capability that serves to eliminate or mediate the impact of demands. Coping is defined as a specific effort (covert or overt) that an individual member or the family unit uses to eliminate, reduce, or manage a set of demands. Although coping most often has been conceptualized at the individual level, we can also consider family- and even community-level coping if we think of collective group action to eliminate or manage demands. Because the family is a system, coping may be conceptualized as the simultaneous management of competing demands and, therefore, may include a combination of the following strategies: (1) direct action to reduce the number and/or intensity of demands (i.e., doing home treatments for the cerebral palsy child, etc.); (2) direct action to acquire additional resources not already available to the family (i.e., medical assistance and diagnosis, respite care, etc.); (3) maintaining or strengthening existing resources so they can be allocated and reallocated to meet demands (i.e., doing things together as a family to maintain cohesiveness, etc.); (4) managing tension associated with ongoing strains (i.e., exercising, using humor, engaging in enjoyable activities, etc.); and (5) reframing the situation to make it more tolerable or manageable (i.e., lowering expectations in the home while caring for an ill member, emphasizing spiritual beliefs to build hope, etc.).

Family appraisals, specifically situational perceptions and family schemata, have also received additional and appropriate emphasis in the T-Double ABCX framework as important factors in the management of demands. Situational appraisals are assessments done by individual family members or collectively by the family unit of the interactional relationship between (1) the family pile-up of demands—their intensity, controllability, resulting expectations, and potential short- and long-term consequences—and (2) the family's capabilities—their availability, utility, potential mediating or buffering impact, the family's costs in the use of their resources, and the resulting short- and long-term consequences when these capabilities are utilized to meet the demands. Understandably, situational appraisals play a central role in shaping the family members' and the family unit's response(s) to the total stressful and possibly distressful situation. The family systems model of family measures in the T-Double ABCX Model of Family Adjustment and Adaptation is presented in Figure 11.6. followed by two family typologies used in family systems–oriented investigations in Figure 11.7.

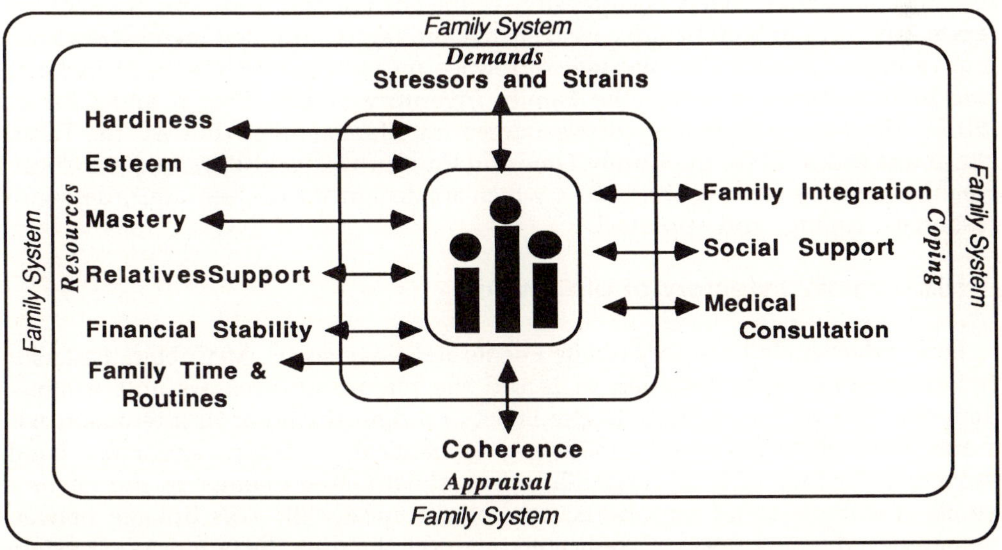

FIGURE 11.6. Family Systems Model of measures in the T-Double ABCX Model of Family Adjustment and Adaptation.

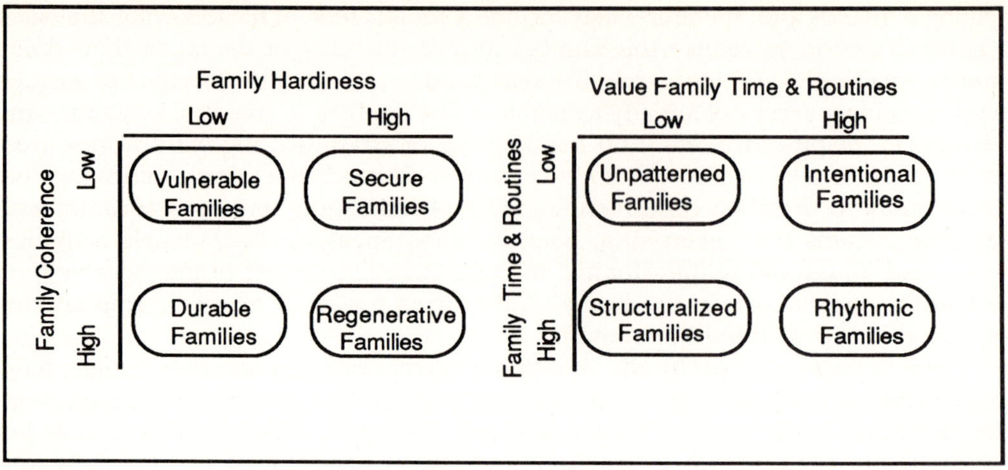

FIGURE 11.7. Family typology of regenerative families and rhythmic families created by the use of family system measures.

FAMILY ADJUSTMENT AND ADAPTATION MEASURES

The T-Double ABCX Framework calls for a constellation of family measures designed to assess the complex relationship between the family's demands and the mediating influences of the family's capabilities—resources, coping, and appraisals. In this chapter we will limit our presentation to four select indices of family functioning that have already been utilized in health care professionals' research. This brief review is suggestive of the current and future potential of self-report measures in both health care research and family-oriented medical or clinical interventions. Specifically, we will introduce measures currently used in health care investigations, namely, the Family Inventory of Life Events and Changes (FILE), the Family Inventory of Resources for Management (FIRM), the Family Hardiness Index (FHI), the Family Time and Routines Index (FTRI), and the Coping Health Inventory for Parents (CHIP), which are designed to assess family demands, resources, coping, and appraisal.

FILE—Family Inventory of Life Events

FILE—the Family Inventory of Life Events and Changes (H. McCubbin, Patterson, & Wilson, 1987) was designed to record the pile-up of stressors and strains—demands that may contribute to the onset of a disease and/or in interaction with a specific medical diagnosis, treatment, or medical condition render the family vulnerable or incapable of responding in a constructive manner to the needs of family member(s) who may be acutely or chronically ill. This linkage between demands and family stress is predicated on understanding the family as a "system" in terms of the interconnectedness of its members. What affects one person in the family affects the others to some degree. Change in any one part of the system requires some readjustment by the whole family system and by its members. Life events and strains, which are experienced by the family as a whole or by any one member, when added together, will have a negative impact upon the stability of the family unit, the health of its members, and the family's response to concurrent or future medical situations.

FILE is a 71-item self-report instrument designed to record normative and nonnormative family demands—stressors, hardships, prior strains—a family unit may experience within a year. Families usually are dealing with several stressors and strains simultaneously, and FILE provides an index of this pile-up, which in turn is an index of a family's vulnerability to crisis. The questionnaire is to be completed by adult family members (together or separately), a single parent, or a cohabiting couple (together or separately). The selection of family stressor and strain items was guided, in part, by those life changes appearing on other individual life change inventories (Coddington, 1972; Dohrenwend, Krasnoff, Askenasy, & Dohrenwend, 1978; Holmes & Rahe, 1967). In addition, situational and developmental changes experienced by families at different stages of the life cycle were included. These items were derived from clinical and research experience of the investigators, and from a careful review of family stress research from the previous decade (H. McCubbin et al., 1980). Each item was worded to reflect a change in a family member or a change in family relationships. This inventory has been used in a wide range of studies including rural farm and nonfarm families and families faced with childhood chronic illness such as cystic fibrosis, myelomeningocele, or cerebral palsy.

The first version of FILE consisted of 171 items, but in our efforts to adapt this inventory for use in prevention-oriented settings (family practice clinics, pediatric clinics, family life education centers, and the like), and in other medical and family counseling clinics, we reduce FILE (Form C) to 71 items grouped into nine subscales: Intra-Family Strains, Marital Strains, Pregnancy and Childbearing Strains, Finance and Business Strains, Work–Family Strains, Illness and Family Care Strains, Family Transitions In and Out, Family Losses, and Family Legal Strains.

Psychometric Properties. The total index of family pile-up of demands (71 items) is reliable with a Cronbach alpha of .81. Select subscales of FILE have respectable reliabilities—Intra-Family Strains, Finance and Business Strains, and Family Legal Strains. Additionally, test–retest reliabilities (4 to 5 weeks apart) ranged from a low of .64 to a high of .84 for the various subscales. The overall test-retest reliability for FILE was .80. Factor analyses were completed on data obtained on two independent samples of husbands and wives (N = 1330 and N = 1410, respectively) representing families from all stages of the family life cycle. The results (H. McCubbin & Patterson, 1983a, 1983b) revealed the same factor structure of nine subscales reported in the initial publication of FILE. Several additional indices of validity have been reported. Specifically, total pile-up of family life stressors and strains was significantly and inversely correlated with measures of changes in the health status of children (for example, pulmonary functioning of children with cystic fibrosis) (H. McCubbin & Patterson, 1983a, 1983b). A greater number of family stressors and strains in a 12-month period was associated with a subsequent decline in the children's pulmonary functioning as recorded during two clinic visits that occurred 3 to 6 months later. Additionally, the pile-up of demands was correlated significantly with measures of family functioning: (1) family cohesion, −.24; (2) independence of family members, −.16; (3) family organization, −.14; and (4) family conflict, +.23.

Family research on development, transitions, and stress has pointed to the obvious fact that stressful life events and strains are, in part, a function of the stage of the family life cycle in which a family may be found. For example, the probability of a family's experiencing the death of a member increases as the family moves into the later stages of the family life cycle. Therefore, it would be advantageous if the norms for family demands were established by stage of the family cycle, rather than developed for all families in a total group. Through the use of data obtained on 1140 couples, or 2280 married individuals, who were representative of seven stages of the family life cycle, we were able to obtain normative data so that families completing FILE could be compared with other families at their respective stages of development (H. McCubbin & Patterson, 1983a, 1983b). The normative data are separated into three levels—low demand, moderate demand, and high demand—on the basis of cutoff scores determined by the mean and one standard deviation.

FIRM—Family Inventory of Resources for Management

In an attempt to assess the family's basic repertoire of resources, FIRM, Family Inventory of Resources for Management (McCubbin, Comeau, & Harkins, 1987), was developed. In order to describe or predict how a family adapts to stressful events and strains, the T-Double ABCX framework calls for information about which resources a family has, does not have, or has depleted. It is hypothesized that families possessing a larger portfolio of resources will manage more effectively and will be better able to adapt to stressful situations.

The selection of items for FIRM was influenced by literature and theory in three major areas: (1) personal resources; (2) the family system internal resources; and (3) community support. Personal resources are resources, qualities, and aids characteristic of individual family members that are available to any family member in need. They include financial (economic well-being), education (contributing to cognitive ability, facilitating realistic perceptions and problem-solving ability), health, and psychological (personality characteristics) attributes (George, 1980; Pearlin & Schooler, 1978).

Family system resources encompass primarily the original concepts identified by Hill (1958), and those in Burr's (1973) synthesis of the literature—family communication and family cohesiveness. Managerial ability (resource management) has been emphasized by proponents of family management frameworks (Deacon & Firebaugh, 1975; Paolucci, Hall, & Axinn, 1977) along with ability to identify resources (Paolucci et al., 1977). Problem-solving ability has been examined as a key family system resource (Aldous, Condon, Hill, Straus, & Tallman, 1971; Hill & Joy, 1979; Reiss, 1971).

Community support, often referred to as social support as defined by Cobb (1976), is information exchanged between people that provides emotional support, resulting in the individual's feeling loved and cared for; esteem support, resulting in the individual's feeling esteemed and valued, and network support, resulting in the individual's feeling he or she is part of a network of mutual obligation and understanding.

FIRM consists of 98 self-report items, and the respondent is asked to evaluate on a scale of 0 to 3 how well the items "describe our family." The four major resources (subscales) identified in FIRM are:

Family Strengths I: Esteem and Communication. This family resource reflects the presence of a combination of personal, family system, and community resources in six areas: (1) family esteem (respect from friends, relatives, co-workers, and among family members); (2) communication (sharing feelings, discussing decisions); (3) mutual assistance (helping each other and relatives); (4) optimism (maintaining a positive outlook on matters); (5) problem-solving ability; and (6) encouragement of autonomy among family members. (Cronbach alpha = .85)

Family Strengths II: Mastery and Health. This family resource includes items that reflect personal, family system, and community support resources along three dimensions: (1) sense of mastery over family events and outcomes (fate control, flexibility, managerial abilities); (2) family mutuality (emotional support, togetherness, cooperation); and (3) physical and emotional health of family members. (Cronbach alpha = .85)

Extended Family Support. This family resource index contains items that indicate the mutual help and support given to and received from relatives. (Cronbach alpha = .62)

Financial Well-Being. This family resource reflects the family's perceived financial efficacy along the dimensions of: (1) ability to meet financial commitments; (2) adequacy of financial reserves; (3) ability to help others (relatives, the needy); (4) optimism about the family's financial future (adequacy of insurance, employment benefits, retirement income, earning power, and the family's financial progress). (Cronbach alpha = .85)

Psychometric Properties. FIRM has been subjected to factor analyses involving a sample of 322 families responding to having a child with either cerebral palsy or myelomeningocele. Additionally, FIRM has been utilized in the study of a normative sample of 2000 midwest families (Light, 1985; H. McCubbin & Patterson, 1981). The findings reported to date indicate the stability of the four resources just described. Additionally, the alpha reliabilities for the four major resources ranged from a low of .62 for Extended Family Social Support to a high of .85 for the three remaining resources. The authors report low to moderate intercorrelations among the four major resources and only a modest association with social desirability.

FHI—The Family Hardiness Index

The Family Hardiness Index (FHI) was developed to measure the characteristic of hardiness as a stress resistance and adaptation resource in families that would function as a buffer or mediating factor in mitigating the effects of stressors and demands, and a facilitation of family adjustment and adaptation over time. Family hardiness specifically refers to the internal strengths and durability of the family unit and is characterized by a sense of control over the outcomes of life events and hardships, a view of change as beneficial and growth producing, and an active rather than passive orientation in adjusting to and managing stressful situations. The Family Hardiness Index (FHI; M. McCubbin, H. McCubbin, & Thompson, 1987) was initially used in an investigation of family traditions, celebrations, and routines in 304 nonclinical families (H. McCubbin et al., 1986) as part of the ongoing research of the Family Stress, Coping and Health Project at the University of Wisconsin-Madison.

The Family Hardiness Index (FHI) was developed to adapt the concept of individual hardiness to the *family unit*. Items were constructed to fit the three components of commitment, challenge, and control and reflect a *we* rather than an *I* orientation. Family hardiness, in the context of the research done by the Family Stress, Coping and Health Project, focuses upon the family's patterned approach to life's hardships and its typical pattern of appraising the impact of life events and changes on family functioning. When applied to the family, hardiness was found to encompass four interrelated components.

Specifically, family hardiness involves the family's co-oriented commitment or its working together to manage difficulties; its confidence in being able to handle problems; its emphasis on viewing hardships as challenges and the seeking of new life experiences as challenges; and its sense of internal control rather than being the victim of circumstances.

Psychometric Properties. The Family Hardiness Index (alpha = .82) is a 20-item instrument consisting of four subscales (Co-oriented Commitment, Confidence, Challenge, and Control) that calls for the respondent to assess the degree to which (false, mostly false, mostly true, true) each statement describes his or her current family situation. The Co-oriented Commitment subscale measures the family's sense of internal strengths, dependability, and ability to work together. The Confidence subscale measures the family's sense of being able to plan ahead, being appreciated for efforts, their ability to endure hardships and experience life with interest and meaningfulness. The Challenge subscale measures the family's efforts to be innovative and active and to experience new things and to learn. The Control subscale measures the family's sense of being in control of family life rather than being shaped by outside events and circumstances.

FTRI—The Family Time and Routines Index

Family routines are a relatively reliable index of family integration, which includes effective ways of meeting common problems and the ability to handle major crises. The Family Time and Routines Index was developed by the Family Stress, Coping and Health Project at the University of Wisconsin-Madison (H. McCubbin, M. McCubbin, & Thompson, 1987) to assess the types of routines used in families and the value placed upon them. This instrument was based upon the Family Routines Inventory (Boyce, Jensen, James, & Peacock, 1983; Jensen, James, Boyce, Hartnett, 1983) and includes 16 additional items with greater emphasis on including teenage members, and the elimination of 10 items from the original Family Routines Inventory.

The Family Time and Routines Index is a 34-item scale (alpha = .88) consisting of eight subscales, Parent–Child Togetherness Routines, Couple Togetherness Routines, Child Routines, Family Meals Routines, Family Togetherness Routines,

Family Chores Routines, Relatives Connection Routines, and Family Management Routines. The index calls for a respondent's assessment of the degree to which (false, mostly false, mostly true, true) each statement describes his or her family behavior. Additionally, the index calls for an assessment of the degree to which the respondent values (views as important) the routine listed.

The Parent–Child Togetherness Routines subscale measures the family's emphasis on establishing predictable communications between parent and child. The Couple Togetherness Routines subscale measures the family's emphasis on establishing predictable routines to promote communication between couples. The Child Routines subscale measures the family's emphasis on establishing predictable routines to promote children's (or teens') sense of autonomy and order. The Family Togetherness Routines subscale measures the family's emphasis on family togetherness to include special events, caring, quiet time, and family time. The Child Chores subscale measures the family's emphasis upon establishing predictable routines to promote child and adolescent responsibilities in the home. The Family Meal Routines subscale measures the family's efforts to establish predictable routines to promote togetherness through family meals together. The Relatives Connection Routines subscale measures the family's effort to establish predictable routines to promote a meaningful connection with relatives. The Family Management Routines subscale measures the family's efforts to establish predictable routines to promote a sense of family organization and accountability needed to maintain family order in the home.

Psychometric Properties. A reasonable set of tests to validate the measure of Family Time and Routines includes the systematic examination of the association between Family Time and Routines and other criterion indices of family strengths hypothesized to be associated with this index of family stability and continuity. Specifically, in a recent investigation (H. McCubbin, et al., 1986), we hypothesized that Family Time and Routines consisting of subscales of Parent-Child Togetherness, Family Meal Routines, Couple Togetherness, Child Routines, Family Togetherness, Family Chores Routines, Family Management Routines, and Relatives Connection Routines would be positively correlated with criterion indices of family bonding (i.e., family cohesiveness), family coherence (i.e., family sense of order and trust), and family celebrations (i.e., family effort to acknowledge special family events and transitions), as well as with indices of family satisfaction, marital satisfaction, and community satisfaction. The hypotheses were confirmed and are presented in Table 11.3.

CHIP—Coping Health Inventory for Parents

One of the major mediating factors and buffering influences to the impact of demands on the family system and their potentially adverse consequences is the coping strategies parents employ to manage tensions and strains. Parental coping takes on added importance as a critical aspect of family functioning in the case of families struggling with a member with chronic illness. Managing the long-term treatment of a member with a chronic illness usually involves a complementary relationship between the health care team and the family unit. The successful care of chronically ill member depends upon the family's willingness to modify family

TABLE 11.3. FAMILY TIME AND ROUTINES INDEX IN RELATIONSHIP TO CRITERION INDICES OF FAMILY FUNCTIONING

Criterion Indices	Correlation with the Family Time and Routines Index*
Family Bonding (FACES II—Olson et al., 1982)	.24
Family Coherence (FCOPES—McCubbin et al., 1982)	.34
Family Celebrations (FCI—H. McCubbin & Thompson, 1987)	.30
Quality of Family Life (Olson & Barnes, 1982), an adaptation of this measure—	
Family Satisfaction	.25
Marital Satisfaction	.26
Community Satisfaction	.19

* $p < .05$

life in response to a complex and usually time-consuming regimen of continuous therapy. Therefore, how the parents cope with the situation could make a difference in health status of chronically ill children over time.

CHIP—Coping Health Inventory for Parents (H. McCubbin, M. McCubbin, Nevin, & Cauble, 1987) is an 80-item questionnaire checklist developed to provide information about how parents individually perceive their overall response to the management of a chronically ill child in the family. The coping behaviors, such as "believing that my child(ren) will get better" or "talking with the medical staff (nurses, social worker, etc.) when we visit the medical center," are listed and parents are asked to record how "helpful" (0 to 3) the coping behavior items were to them in managing the home illness situation.

Following the methodology outlined in prior family coping studies (Boss, H. McCubbin, & Lester, 1979; H. McCubbin, Dahl, Lester, Benson, & Robertson, 1976), the construction of CHIP was guided by the inclusion of important behavior items used in prior studies of family response to stress. The development of additional items focused on: (1) network and social support theory (Caplan, 1976; Cobb, 1976), that is, the family's relationship to the community and family members for emotional, esteem, and network support; (2) individual psychology of coping (Lazarus, 1966; Pearlin & Schooler, 1978), that is, the personal, active, and passive psychological adjustments needed to manage anxieties and emotional tensions; and (3) family medical support, that is, the parents' efforts to communicate with the medical staff and other parents, as well as their attempts to master medical illness and home care issues in order to understand and manage the chronically ill child in the home.

The development of CHIP was influenced by a hierarchical approach to the organization of behavior. In the application of this approach, two general levels of abstraction were defined: (1) coping behaviors (operationally defined through 80 specific items), and (2) coping patterns (combination of coping behaviors into specific patterns). After careful analysis of the items, the initial list was reduced to 45 items, which were grouped by factor analysis into three subscales or three distinct parental coping patterns.

Coping I: Maintaining Family Integration, Cooperation, and an Optimistic Definition of the Situation. This subscale is composed of 19 behaviors that center on the family and the parents' outlook on life and illness, keeping the family together, encouraging cooperation, investing in the children, and encouraging independence in the family.

Coping II: Maintaining Social Support, Self-Esteem, and Psychological Stability. The second subscale involves 18 coping behaviors that focus upon the parents' efforts to maintain a personal sense of well-being through obtaining social support, maintaining self-esteem, and managing psychological tensions and strains.

Coping III: Understanding the Medical Situation through Communication with Other Parents and Consultation with Medical Staff. This subscale involves eight coping behaviors and focuses on the interface between the parent, other parents in a similar situation, and the medical staff and its program, as well as parental effort to understand and master the medical information needed to cope with the illness.

Psychometric Properties. The psychometric details of CHIP are presented elsewhere (H. McCubbin & Patterson, 1981; H. McCubbin, M. McCubbin, et al., 1983; M. McCubbin, 1984; M. McCubbin, 1986). Briefly, three coping patterns derived from factor analysis represented 71 percent of the variance of the original correlation matrix. Cronbach's alphas, computed for one item each coping pattern, indicated respectable reliabilities of .79 (Coping I), .79 (Coping II), and .71 (Coping III).

Additionally, the CHIP subscales were correlated with independent assessments of family functioning and changes in the health status of children with cystic fibrosis. When used by mothers, all three coping patterns were significantly correlated with the family interpersonal relationship dimensions of family life. Specifically, mothers' coping efforts directed at family integration, cooperation, and optimism (Coping I) were positively associated with family cohesiveness ($r = .21$); their efforts at maintaining social support, esteem, and emotional stability (Coping II) were significantly correlated with family expressiveness ($r = .19$); and their efforts at medical consultation (Coping III) were positively associated with family cohesiveness ($r = .19$). In contrast, two coping patterns used by fathers were associated with system maintenance dimensions of family life. Specifically, fathers' coping efforts directed at integration, cooperation, and optimism (Coping I) were associated with family organization ($r = .32$), and their efforts at medical communication and consultation (Coping III) were associated with both family organization ($r = .22$) and family control ($r = .19$). Similar to mothers' Coping I, their efforts at family integration, cooperation, and optimism (Coping I) were also significantly correlated with family cohesiveness ($r = .36$) and in addition, inversely correlated with family conflict ($r = -.21$). In summary, mothers' three coping patterns were validated by their positive association with family cohesiveness and expressiveness. Fathers' coping patterns were validated by their association with family cohesiveness, conflict, organization, and control.

Parental coping, as measured by CHIP, was also validated against health status indices. Specifically, mothers' efforts to maintain family integration, cooperation, and an optimistic definition of the situation (Coping I) were validated against the criterion index of positive gains in the child's height and weight ($r = .20$). Additionally, mothers' Coping II efforts were significantly correlated ($r = .23$) with positive changes in the child's pulmonary functioning. Fathers' coping pattern of maintaining social support, self-esteem, and psychological stability was significantly correlated with positive gains in children's height–weight index ($r = .22$) and pulmonary functioning index ($r = .31$).

SUMMARY AND CONCLUSIONS

Child health assessment has much to gain from investing in systematic assessments of family system functioning. Self-report measures of family system functioning are but one among many strategies used to make these important assessments. By introducing, discussing, and to some degree appraising extant self-report measures, we hope to shed light upon this developing but very complex arena of family measurement, and more importantly to encourage further research in this area.

We have much to gain from the continued use of self-report measures of family system functioning, and over time we will be able to advance the development of these measures, improve their reliabilities and validities, and further substantiate the linkage between the family environment and the psychological and physical health of family members. With this in mind, we can anticipate major developments and constructive findings in the immediate future.

While each instrument or set of instruments discussed here is in need of continued refinement and rigorous assessments, there appears to be a growing commitment to advance the development of instruments grounded in theory, supported by empirical tests of reliability and validity, and with a direct link to the psychological and physical health status and physiological changes in family members. It may be premature to express excitement at the prospect of uncovering or discovering the pathways between the family and the human body, but it is reassuring to note the emergence of efforts at least to examine the linkage.

Family systems research has much to gain from this line of scientific inquiry. It is possible that self-report measures can play a central role in understanding the family's role in fostering or undermining children's emotional and social development; in understanding why some families fall apart in the face of childhood chronic illnesses; in understanding the role of the family in supporting or undermining psychological and psychiatric interventions; and in understanding the role of the family system in promoting rehabilitation and recovery of children and adolescents afflicted with an illness or who have received medical treatment requiring home care. Surely, family systems self-report measures, even with all their psychometric limitations, have and will continue to serve an important function in the advancement of research and practice linking the family environment to the present and future health status of family members, particularly children.

References

Ackerman, N. (1958). *The psychodynamics of family life*. New York: Basic.

Aldous, J., Condon, R., Hill, R., Straus, M., & Tallman, I. (1971). *Family problem-solving*. Hinsdale, IL: Dryden.

Bell, R. (1982). *Parent-adolescent interaction in runaway families*. Unpublished doctoral dissertation, University of Minnesota, St. Paul.

Bishop, D. S., & Epstein, N. B. (1979). *Research on teaching methods*. Paper presented at the International Forum for Trainers and Family Therapists. Tavistock Clinic, London.

Boss, P., McCubbin, H., & Lester, G. (1979). The corporate executive wife's coping patterns in response to routine husband-father absence. *Family Process, 18*, 79–86.

Boyce, W., Jensen, E., James, S., & Peacock, J. (1983). The Family Routines Inventory: Theoretical origins. *Social Science & Medicine, 17*(4), 193–200.

Burr, W. (1973). *Theory construction and the sociology of the family*. New York: Wiley.

Caplan, G. (1976). The family as a support system. In G. Caplan & M. Killilea (Eds.), *Support systems and mutual help*. New York: Grune & Stratton.

Cobb, S. (1976). Social support as a moderator of life stress. *Psychosomatic Medicine, 38*, 300–314.

Coddington, R. D. (1972). The significance of life events as an etiologic factor in the diseases of children II: A study of the normal population. *Journal of Psychosomatic Research, 16*, 205–213.

Comley, A. (1973). Family therapy and the family physician. *Canadian Family Physician, 16*, 78–81.

Deacon, R., & Firebaugh, F. (1975). *Home management context and concepts*. Boston: Houghton Mifflin.

Dohrenwend, B. S., Krasnoff, L., Askenasy, A. R., & Dohrenwend, B. P. (1978). Exemplification of a method of scaling life events: The PERI life events scale. *Journal of Health & Social Behavior, 19*, 205–229.

Edmonds, V. (1967). Marital conventionalization: definition and measurement. *Journal of Marriage and the Family, 29*, 681–688.

Eichel, E. (1978). Assessment with a family focus. *Journal of Psychiatric Nursing & Mental Health Services, 16*, 11–15.

Epstein, N. B., & Bishop, D. S. (1973). State of the art-1973. *Canadian Psychiatric Association Journal, 18*, 175–183.

Epstein, N. B., Bishop, D., & Baldwin, L. (1982). McMaster Model of Family Functioning: A view of the normal family. In F. Walsh (Ed.), *Normal family processes*. New York: Guilford.

Epstein, N. B., Levin, S., & Bishop, D. (1976). The family as a social unit. *Canadian Family Physician, 22*, 1411–1413.

Fuhr, R. A., Moos, R. H., & Dishotsky, N. (1981). The use of family assessment and feedback in ongoing family therapy. *American Journal of Family Therapy, 9*, 24–36.

Garmezy, N., & Rutter, M. (Eds.) (1983). *Stress coping and development in children*. New York: McGraw-Hill.

George, L. (1980). *Transitions in later life*. Belmont, CA: Brooks/Cole.

Hill, R. (1958). Generic features of families under stress. *Social Casework, 49*, 139–150.

Hill, R., & Joy, C. (1979). *Conceptualizing and operationalizing category systems for phasing of family development*. Unpublished manuscript, University of Minnesota.

Holmes, T. H., & Rahe, R. (1967). The social readjustment rating scale. *Journal of Psychosomatic Research, 11*, 213–218.

Jenkins, C. D. (1979). Psychosocial modifiers of response to stress. *Journal of Human Stress, 5*, 3–15.

Jensen, E. W., James, S. H., Boyce, W. T., & Hartnett, S. A. (1983). The Family Routines Inventory: Development and validation. *Social Science & Medicine, 17*, 4, 201–211.

Lavee, Y. (1985). *Family types and family adaptation to stress: integrating the circumplex model of family systems and the family adjustment and adaptation response model*. Unpublished doctoral dissertation, University of Minnesota, St. Paul.

Lazarus, R. S. (1966). *Psychological stress and the coping process*. New York: McGraw-Hill.

Leif, A. (Ed.) (1948). *The commonsense psychiatry of Dr. Adolf Meyer*. New York: McGraw-Hill.

Light, H. K. (1985, June). *How strong is your family?: Perceptions of farm men and farm women*. Paper presented at the American Home Economics Association Annual Meeting and Exposition, Fargo, ND.

McCubbin, H., Comeau, J., & Harkins, J. (1987). Family Inventory of Resources for Management (FIRM). In H. McCubbin & A. Thompson (Eds.), *Family assessment inventories for research and practice*. Madison: University of Wisconsin, Madison.

McCubbin, H., Dahl, B., Lester, G., Benson, D., & Robertson, M. (1976). Coping repertoires of families adapting to prolonged war-induced separations. *Journal of Marriage & the Family, 38*, 461–471.

McCubbin, H., Joy, C., Cauble, A., Comeau, J., Patterson, J., & Needle, R. (1980). Family stress, coping, and social support: A decade review. *Journal of Marriage & the Family, 42*, 855–871.

McCubbin, H., Larson, A., & Olson, D. (1987). F-COPES Family Crisis Oriented Personal Scales. In H. McCubbin & A. Thompson (Eds.), *Family assessment inventories for research and practice*. Madison: University of Wisconsin, Madison.

McCubbin, H., & McCubbin, M. (1987). Family stress theory and assessment: The T-Double ABCX Model of Family Adjustment and Adaptation. In H. McCubbin & A. Thompson (Eds.), *Family assessment inventories for research and practice*. Madison: University of Wisconsin, Madison.

McCubbin, H., McCubbin, M., Nevin, R., & Cauble, A. E. (1987). Coping Health Inventory for Parents (CHIP). In H. McCubbin & A. Thompson (Eds.), *Family assessment inventories for research and practice*. Madison: University of Wisconsin, Madison.

McCubbin, H., McCubbin, M., Patterson, J., Cauble, A. E., Wilson, L., & Warwick, W. (1979). CHIP—Coping Health Inventory for Parents: An assessment of parental coping patterns in the care of the chronically ill child. In H. McCubbin, A. E. Cauble, & J. M. Patterson (Eds.), *Family stress, coping and social support*. New York: Springer.

McCubbin, H., McCubbin, M., Patterson, J., Cauble, A. E., Wilson, L., & Warwick, W. (1983). CHIP—Coping Health Inventory for Parents: An assessment of parental coping patterns in the care of the chronically ill child. *Journal of Marriage & the Family, 45*, 359–370.

McCubbin, H., McCubbin, M., & Thompson, A. (1987). Family Time and Routines Scale. In H. McCubbin & A. Thompson (Eds.), *Family assessment inventories for research and practice*. Madison: University of Wisconsin, Madison.

McCubbin, H., & Patterson, J. (1981). *Systematic assessment of family stress, resources and coping: Tools for research, education and clinical intervention*. St. Paul, MN: Department of Family Social Science.

McCubbin, H. I., & Patterson, J. (1983a). The family stress process: The Double ABCX Model of Adjustment and Adaptation. In M. Sussman, H. McCubbin, & J. Patterson (Ed.), Social Stress and the Family: Advances and Developments in Family Stress Theory and Research. *Marriage & Family Review* (Vol. 6). Binghamton, NY: Haworth.

McCubbin, H. I., & Patterson, J. M. (1983b). The family stress process: The Double ABCX Model of Adjustment and Adaptation. In H. McCubbin, M. Sussman, & J. Patterson (Eds.), *Advances and developments in family stress theory and research*. New York: Haworth.

McCubbin, H. I., Patterson, J. M., & Wilson, L. (1987). Family Inventory of Life Events and Changes (FILE). Form A. In H. McCubbin & A. Thompson (Eds.), *Family assessment inventories for research and practice*. Madison: University of Wisconsin, Madison.

McCubbin, H., & Thompson, A. (1987). Family Celebrations Index. In H. McCubbin & A. Thompson (Eds.), *Family assessment inventories for research and practice*. Madison: University of Wisconsin, Madison.

McCubbin, H. I., & Thompson, A. I. (1987). *Family assessment inventories for research and practice*. Madison: University of Wisconsin, Madison.

McCubbin, H., Thompson, A., & Pirner, P. (1986). *Family rituals, typologies, and family strengths*. Madison: Family Stress Coping and Health Project, University of Wisconsin, Madison.

McCubbin, M. (1986). *Family stress and family types: Chronic illness in children*. Doctoral dissertation, University of Minnesota.

McCubbin, M. (1984). Nursing assessment of parental coping with cystic fibrosis. *Western Journal of Nursing Research, 6*, 4.

McCubbin, M., McCubbin, H., & Thompson, A. (1987). Family Hardiness Index. In H. McCubbin & A. Thompson (Eds.), *Family assessment inventories for research and practice*. Madison: University of Wisconsin, Madison.

Moos, R. (1974). *Family Environment Scales*. Palo Alto: Consulting Psychologists Press.

Moos, R. (1979). Evaluating family and work settings. In P. Ahmed & G. Coelho, (Eds.), *New directions in health*. New York: Plenum.

Moos, R., Bromet, E., Tsu, V., & Moos, B. (1979). Family characteristics and the outcome of treatment for alcoholism. *Journal of studies in alcohol, 40*, 78–88.

Moos, R., & Fuhr, R. (1982). The clinical use of social ecological concepts: The case of an adolescent girl. *American Journal of Orthopsychiatry, 52*, 111–122.

Moos, R., & Moos, B. (in press). *Family Environment Scales Manual*. Palo Alto: Consulting Psychology Press.

Murdock, G. P. (1960). The universality of the nuclear family. In N. W. Bell & E. F. Vogel (Eds.), *A modern introduction to the family*. Glencoe, IL: Free Press.

Olson, D. H., & Barnes, H. L. (1982). *Quality of life*. Family Social Science, University of Minnesota, St. Paul.

Olson, D. H., & McCubbin, H. (1982). Circumplex model of marital and family systems V: Application to family stress and crisis intervention. In H. I. McCubbin, A. E. Cauble, & J. M. Patterson (Eds.), *Family Stress, coping and social support*. Springfield, IL: Charles C. Thomas.

Olson, D., McCubbin, H., Barnes, H., Larsen, A., Muxem, A., & Wilson, M. (1983). *Families: What makes them work*. Beverly Hills: Sage.

Olson, D. H., Portner, J., & Bell, R. (1978). *Family Adaptability and Cohesion Evaluation Scales*. St. Paul, MN: Family Social Science, University of Minnesota, St. Paul.

Olson, D. H., Portner, J., & Bell, R. Q. (1982). *FACES II: Family Adaptability and Cohesion Evaluation Scales*. Family Social Science, University of Minnesota, St. Paul.

Olson, D. H., Portner, J., & Lavee, Y. (1985). *FACES III*. Family Social Science, University of Minnesota, St. Paul.

Olson, D. H., Russell, C. S., & Sprenkle, D. H. (1980). Marital and family therapy: A decade review. *Journal of Marriage & Family, 42*, 973–993.

Olson, D. H., Russell, C. S., & Sprenkle, D. H. (1983). Circumplex Model VI: Theoretical update. *Family Process, 22*, 69–83.

Olson, D., Sprenkle, D., & Russell, C. (1979). Circumplex Model of Marital and Family Systems I: Cohesion and Adaptability dimensions, family types and clinical applications. *Family Process, 18*, 3–28.

Paolucci, B., Hall, O., & Axinn, N. (1977). *Family decision making: An ecosystem approach*. New York: Wiley.

Parsons, T., & Bales, R. B. (1955). *Family: Socialization and interaction process*. Glencoe, IL: Free Press.

Patterson, J. & McCubbin, H. (1983). *A-COPE—Adolescent Coping Orientation for Problem Experiences* (Research Instrument). Madison, WI: University of Wisconsin.

Pearlin, L., & Schooler, C. (1978). The structure of coping. *Journal of Health & Social Behavior, 19*, 2–21.

Portner, J. (1980). *Parent-adolescent interaction of families in treatment*. Unpublished doctoral dissertation, University of Minnesota, St. Paul.

Rado, S. (1961). Towards the construction of an organized foundation for clinical psychiatry. *Comprehensive Psychiatry, 2*, 67–73.

Reiss, D. (1971). Varieties of consensual experience III: Contrast between families of normals, delinquents, and schizophrenics. *Journal of Nervous & Mental Disease, 152*, 73–95.

Russell, C. S. (1979). Circumplex Model of Marital and Family Systems III: Empirical evaluation with families. *Family Process, 18*, 29–45.

Sigal, J. J., Rakoff, V., & Epstein, N. B. (1967). Indicators of therapeutic outcome in conjoint family therapy. *Family Process, 6*, 215–226.

Skynner, A. C. (1969). A group-analytic approach to conjoint family therapy. *Journal of Child Psychology & Psychiatry, 10*, 81–106.

Smilkstein, G. (1978). The family APGAR: A proposal for a family function test and its use by physicians. *Journal of Family Practice, 6*, 1231–1239.

Smilkstein, G. (1984). The physician and family function assessment. *Family Systems Medicine, 2*, 263–278.

Sprenkle, D. H., & Olson, D. H. (1978). Circumplex Model of Marital Systems IV: Empirical study of clinic and non-clinic couples. *Journal of Marriage & Family Counseling, 4*, 59–74.

Steinhauer, P. S., Santa-Barbara, J., & Skinner, H. A. (1984). The Process Model of Family Functioning. *Canadian Journal of Psychiatry, 29*, 77–88.

Tallman, I. (1970). The family as a small problem group. *Journal of Marriage & the Family, 32*, 94–104.

Westley, W. A., & Epstein, N. B. (1960). *The silent majority*. San Francisco: Jossey-Bass.

PART III

SPECIALIZED FOCI OF ASSESSMENT

12

Measuring Children's Adjustment to Hospitalization and to Medical Procedures

LAWRENCE J. SIEGEL

One certainty in modern life is a visit to a physician and dentist, beginning in childhood. Each day, thousands of children undergo numerous medical and dental procedures. Children are typically introduced to the health care system early in life for immunizations that are required prior to school attendance, for periodic well-child examinations, and for dental examinations and/or treatment.

Despite significant advances in preventive dental health, almost all children require some type of dental treatment. Most of this involves restorative dental work for the treatment of dental caries or tooth extraction. Modern dental equipment is designed to enable the dentist to complete prophylaxis or treatment in the shortest possible time with minimal discomfort. Furthermore, pharmacology has given the dentist various analgesic agents for the alleviation of pain. Despite these developments in current dental practice, invasive dental procedures can be highly distressing to many children (Melamed, 1979; Siegel, in press).

Approximately four million children are hospitalized during a given year, representing 6 percent of all children under 18 years of age. The average number of days that a child remains in the hospital is 6 (McCerthy & Kozak, 1985). About one-third of all children are hospitalized at least once before they reach adulthood (Prugh, 1983). While many children remain in the hospital for a brief period of time, often for only a day, they are likely to encounter numerous aversive experiences and invasive medical procedures that pose a significant psychological threat. Among the various invasive and painful medical procedures that are likely to be distressing to the hospitalized child are venipunctures, injections, cardiac catheterizations, lumbar punctures, and bone marrow aspirations. Even noninvasive and nonpainful procedures such as X rays or physical examinations can be anxiety provoking, particularly for young children.

In addition to the actual medical procedures, there are a number of potential sources of stress for the hospitalized child, whether he or she is undergoing diagnostic tests, medical treatment, or surgery. Among those factors that have been suggested as contributing to a child's emotional distress in the hospital are: separation from family members, unfamiliarity with the hospital environment and its personnel, immobility, disruption of typical routines and loss of control over daily events, concerns about bodily harm and embarrassment, and distortions and misconceptions about the purpose of the hospitalization and medical procedures (Siegel, 1983).

The nature of the child's hospitalization may be elective, episodic, or chronic (Barowsky, 1978). Most admissions to the hospital are for elective diagnostic medical procedures and surgery. Typically, these situations are planned hospitalizations in which there is an opportunity to prepare the child in advance for the events that he or she will experience. Episodic hospitalizations represent admissions on an emergency basis, and because they are usually unpredictable, they do not typically permit the child to be prepared in advance for the experience. Finally, there are some children who enter the hospital on a repeated basis, often for prolonged time periods. This last group of children most often are diagnosed as having a chronic illness or medical condition such as kidney disease, cystic fibrosis, or leukemia. In addition, some chronic diseases in children are highly life threatening, and as a result, admission to the hospital may have a considerably different meaning for these children and their families. Therefore, while all children may encounter many similar experiences while in the hospital, the nature of their medical problems and the purpose of the admission can present different challenges to the child's adaptation to the experience. While it is recognized that the child's illness certainly will have an impact on his or her adjustment, this chapter considers adjustment primarily as it pertains to the child's response to medical procedures and the hospital experience regardless of the medical or health-related condition of the child.

An ecological approach to the study of children's adjustment to their medical and dental treatment is possible because of naturally occurring stressful experiences in these health care settings. Children cannot readily avoid medical and dental treatment when it is necessary, because adults typically determine when treatment and contact with health care professionals occur. As a result, escape or avoidance behaviors are impractical and the child must, therefore, confront the potentially stressful procedures and events. Although the severity of the illness or physical condition can enhance the stressfulness of the situation for the child, at least some portion of children's reactions can be attributed to the aversive properties of the setting itself. These situations represent relatively controlled environments in which stressful stimuli that elicit distress-related behaviors can be easily identified. Furthermore, because children typically have repeated contacts with medical and dental procedures, there is a unique opportunity to study the effects of repeated experiences and long-term adaptability to these health care settings (Melamed, Klingman, & Siegel, 1983; Melamed & Siegel, in press).

The purpose of this chapter is to familiarize the reader with a number of issues pertaining to the assessment of children's adjustment to hospitalization and to the medical and dental procedures that children experience while in various health care settings. Interest in this area has been multidisciplinary, and has been addressed primarily in the medical, dental, nursing, and psychological literature. Children's adjustment to hospitalization and medical and dental procedures has been investigated in the context of: (1) factors influencing children's responses to health care settings and procedures; and (2) children's responses to various preparation programs designed to reduce the distress of hospitalization and medical and dental procedures.

Following a discussion of the parameters of adjustment in children undergoing medical and dental procedures and/or hospitalization, an overview of the major approaches to the clinical and research assessment of children in this area will be presented. Factors associated with children's adjustment to health care settings and events that should be considered in a comprehensive assessment of children's reactions to hospitalization and medical procedures will also be reviewed. It is recognized that pain from disease and injury and as a result of painful medical and dental procedures is an important determinant of children's overall adjustment to health care settings and treatment. This factor will be discussed only briefly, however, since a detailed review of pain assessment is presented elsewhere in this volume. In addition, this chapter describes the methodology for assessing children's responses to special hospital environments such as intensive care units, recovery rooms, and isolation facilities. Finally, directions for future research and clinical practice will be discussed.

AN OPERATIONAL DEFINITION OF ADJUSTMENT TO HOSPITALIZATION AND HEALTH CARE PROCEDURES

The concept of adjustment is defined in the broadest sense in this chapter as children's *responses* to the procedures and settings in which health care is delivered. These responses are often subsumed in the literature under the global label of *psychological upset* (other similar constructs include *anxiety*, *fear*, *distress*) manifested by the child while undergoing medical or dental procedures (Thompson, 1985; Vernon, Foley, Sipowicz, & Schulman, 1965). Therefore, whether or not a child adequately adjusts to these health care experiences is judged against the extent to which the child exhibits some level of psychological upset.

A number of authors have noted that concepts such as anxiety, fear, and pain are closely linked in children (Jeans, 1983; Poznanski, 1976) and are difficult to distinguish behaviorally (Shacham & Daut, 1981; Sternbach, 1968). Similarly, LeBaron and Zeltzer (1984) found that many children had difficulty distinguishing between the concepts of *scared* and *hurt*. They suggest that the difficulty in assessing these variables in children is due largely to their reciprocal relationship, rather than the cognitive inability of children to make appropriate distinctions between the two concepts.

In acute pain experiences such as those involved in many invasive medical and dental procedures, anxiety and pain basically represent different sides of the same coin. They relate to each other in a cyclical manner. Anxiety potentiates pain, and pain promotes anxiety (Katz, Varni, & Jay, 1984; Siegel, in press).

Given this difficulty in distinguishing between anxiety and pain in children experiencing acute, noxious stimulation, Katz, Kellerman, and Siegel (1980, 1981) have proposed the more general concept of *behavioral distress* to encompass both of these concepts. This chapter therefore adopts the use of the term *behavioral distress* when referring to the combined manifestations of pain, anxiety, and general emotional upset in children undergoing health care procedures.

A major difficulty in assessing children's adjustment to hospitalization and medical and dental procedures pertains to the relative incidence or "base rate" of children's distress-related responses in health care settings. In order adequately to evaluate the degree of children's adjustment to these experiences, it is important to have some idea of the *typical* responses and the *extent of variation* of these responses in given clinical populations.

Even a cursory review of the literature on the psychological adjustment of children to health care procedures and settings indicates that there are few methodologically sound studies in this area (Siegel, 1976). Much of the early work on the effects of hospitalization and medical treatment on children was in case study form or presented descriptive or anecdotal evidence with few objective data (e.g., Chapman, Loeb, & Gibbons, 1956; Jackson, Winkley, Faust, Cermak, & Brutt, 1953; Jessner, Blom, & Waldfogel, 1952, Prugh, Staub, Sands, Kirschbaum, & Lenihan, 1953). Evidence from these early reports suggested that the incidence of children's stress-related reactions during and following hospitalization for diagnostic procedures, medical treatment, and surgery varied from 10 to 30 percent for "severe" untoward responses to as much as 90 percent for "mild" reactions. These emotional responses have been reported to manifest themselves as a variety of behavior problems, including sleep and appetite disturbances, regressive and compulsive behaviors, anger and aggression, enuresis and encopresis, and phobias and social withdrawal (Prugh & Eckhardt, 1980).

Among the methodological problems with much of the literature in this area are the failure of investigators clearly to operationalize and describe the psychological variables that they are attempting to measure during and after the health care experience, the failure to demonstrate acceptable reliability and validity of the measures used, the failure to use raters or observers who are "blind" to the purpose of the study or the child's experimental condition, and the failure to use multiple observers to obtain data on observer reliability (Melamed & Siegel, 1980; Vernon et al., 1965). In addition, differences between studies on a number of important dimensions, such as the measures used to assess the child's response to the hospitalization or procedures and the time at which the child's behavior was measured, variability in the health care procedures, and differences in a number of patient variables prohibit a comparison of results from one study to the next (Siegel, 1983). Given these methodological problems, there is a relative absence of appropriate norms for the incidence of distress-related responses in hospitalized children and in children undergoing health care procedures in general.

A MULTIDIMENSIONAL ASSESSMENT OF CHILDREN'S RESPONSES TO HOSPITALIZATION AND HEALTH CARE PROCEDURES

The early literature on the assessment of children's reactions to health care experiences primarily involved the anecdotal descriptions of children's distress-related behaviors and/or unidimensional global measures. For example, in a study by Prugh and colleagues (1953), the hospitalized child was rated as adequate, difficult, or inadequate in the ability to "relate successfully to peer and adult members of the ward group, together with his capacity for reality testing and his ability to master anxiety successfully in accordance with his age level, through verbalization and play" (p. 81). Similarly, Vaughan (1957) used reports from nurses to determine the incidence of "disturbance on the ward" following surgery in young hospitalized children. Jessner and colleagues (1952) compared the posthospital reactions of children undergoing tonsillectomies with ratings of prehospital adjustment on the basis of the mother's retrospective reports and psychiatric observations of the child. Prehospital adjustment was rated as adequate, neurotic trends, or disturbed. Posthospital reactions were rated as severe upset, mild upset, or improved. Children rated as severe upset were those who exhibited marked or persisting disturbances in any of the following areas: sleep, speech, tics and mannerisms, fears, and regressive behaviors.

Many of these early studies, which represent the preponderance of literature on children's adjustment to hospitalization and health care, used inadequate methodology for measuring children's responses to the hospital experience. Among the problems with these studies is the use of a single, global measure of adjustment based on multiple sources of information. In addition, few of these studies used multiple observers who were blind to the child's experimental condition. Finally, many of the studies fail adequately to describe the bases by which they classify children regarding their degree of adjustment or emotional upset.

Children's emotional responses to health care have traditionally been assessed during two basic time periods. The majority of studies have measured children's *immediate responses*, assessing their reactions during the actual health care procedures or during the period of hospitalization. In addition, some investigations have assessed children's *posthospital* or *postprocedural responses*, evaluating the child's reaction at some period following his or her experience with the health care setting or procedure. This post–health care assessment has ranged from a period immediately following the medical or dental procedure to a period of from 2 days to more than a decade following the child's discharge from the hospital (Thompson, 1985).

The current *zeitgeist* in this area is to regard children's emotional distress as a complex, multidimensional phenomenon that necessitates a multidimensional assessment approach (Melamed & Siegel, 1980). Anxiety and/or emotional distress is a complex array of responses, rather than a single, clearly defined response. That is, anxiety may manifest itself as one or more of three basic classes of responses, including behavioral (overt motor behavior), cognitive–affective, and physiological (changes mediated by the autonomic nervous system) (Lang, 1968, 1977; Melamed & Siegel, 1980).

There is an impressive body of research that suggests that measures of anxiety or distress do not correlate very highly with one another (Lang, Melamed, & Hart, 1970). Because these low correlations are particularly prevalent in measures of childhood anxiety (Melamed & Siegel, 1980; Siegel & Ridley-Johnson, 1985), it is important to assess concurrently all three response systems that may reflect a child's emotional response to medical and dental settings and procedures. For example, a child's self-report of distress may not be congruent with how he or she actually behaves during a stressful procedure. Similarly, the child's physiological responses to potentially anxiety-provoking events may indicate visceral arousal, yet the child may exhibit few disruptive motor responses or avoidance behaviors. Given these potential differences in responding across the three systems, which modality do we select? At present, there are not sufficient data to suggest that any one of these three response systems deserves primary consideration. Furthermore, different measures of stress-related behaviors within a single response system may vary. For instance, heart rate, muscle tension, and skin conductance may not equally reflect physiological arousal. Therefore, where feasible, emotional distress should *not* be inferred on the basis of a single indicator of autonomic arousal. Instead, it is the *pattern* of relationships between responses that is important when assessing children's reactions to health care procedures. Individuals may differ in their tendency to exhibit certain patterns of responses in different systems or in the same system at different times (Lacey, 1967). Therefore, when group data are being evaluated, it is important to be aware of these individual differences when reporting mean group effects. It has also been noted that desynchrony or discordance between systems may appear because of differential rates or change in the target behaviors (Hodgson & Rachman, 1974). This suggests that it is important to sample the behaviors at different time periods within the same setting. It is only by doing a profile analysis of concordance and desynchrony between the three response systems that the process of change in emotional distress can be understood. One would expect, for example, that techniques directed at arousal reduction would have more specific effects on the physiological system, whereas the behavior change methods would induce cooperative behavior while still leaving the child aroused in the visceral system. In sum, the potency of treatment effects should be evaluated by assessing changes in particular dependent measures and by observing interrelationships between measures.

In addition, it has been suggested that the three response systems reflecting emotional distress may be differentially important depending on the medical or dental procedure being studied (Melamed et al., 1983). For example, with health care procedures that require that the child exhibit few motor responses and that necessitate considerable cooperative behaviors (i.e., cardiac catheterizations, restorative dental treatment), measures of observable behaviors would be particularly important. Similarly, with procedures in which excessive physiological arousal might be problematic, physiological indices such as heart rate or muscle tension specifically should be evaluated.

Numerous assessment methods have been used for evaluating the behavioral, cognitive, and physiological components of anxiety and distress in children undergoing diagnostic and treatment procedures in various health care settings. Techniques for assessing each of these response systems are discussed in detail.

Behavioral Observations

Measures of children's motor or overt responses are the most frequently used instruments for assessing children's distress-related behaviors in medical and dental settings. Observational measures involve observers or raters who document the occurrence of specified behaviors during specific time intervals. Trained, independent observers may be used to obtain a sample of the child's behavior, or parents and/or various health care providers may be used to assess overt manifestation of distress through rating scales or checklists. Two basic approaches to the assessment of overt behavioral distress have been used with children in health care settings: (1) recording the occurrence and/or frequency of specific behaviors; and (2) rating a particular dimension of children's behavior in specific situations using a Likert-type scale (Thompson, 1985).

A variety of observation scales have been developed specifically for measuring distress-related behaviors in children undergoing medical and dental procedures. One of the earliest such scales, the Observer Rating Scale of Anxiety (ORSA), was developed by Melamed and Siegel (1975). This behavioral observation scale consists of 29 categories of verbal and motor behavioral manifestations of children's anxiety in medical settings. Among the responses rated by an observer include such anxiety-related behaviors as crying, stiff body posture, and verbalizations pertaining to being separated from mother or to being anxious. A time-sampling procedure is used in which an observer indicates the presence or absence of each response category during consecutive 3-minute intervals throughout the period of observation. The frequency of responses observed during the total period of observation represents the child's score on this measure. Data on the reliability and validity of this instrument have been reported in several studies (Ferguson, 1979; Melamed, Dearborn, & Hermecz, 1983; Melamed, Meyer, Gee, & Soule, 1976).

Melamed and her colleagues (Melamed, Hawes, Heiby, & Glick, 1975; Melamed, Weinstein, Hawes, & Katin-Borland, 1975) developed the Behavior Profile Rating Scale (BRPS). This instrument has been employed frequently in dental settings to measure the frequency of distress-related disruptive behaviors in children undergoing dental treatment. The BPRS measures 27 different responses that relate to problematic behaviors in separating from the mother, or disruptive responses during the dental procedures. Behaviors are recorded across successive 3-minute intervals. This scale is presented in Table 12.1. As can be seen from the table, each category is weighed by a factor that indicates the degree of disruptiveness as determined by dentists' ratings. The total score is obtained by multiplying the frequency at which the behavior in each category occurred by its weighted factor, and adding across all categories. The score is then divided by the number of 3-minute intervals to yield a score representing the frequency of disruptive behaviors per 3-minute interval. This measure has been used in a number of studies with children undergoing dental treatment and has been shown to have good reliability and validity (Klorman, Hilpert, Michael, LaGana, & Sveen, 1980; Klorman, Michael, Hilpert, & Sveen, 1979; Melamed, Yurcheson, Fleece, Hutcherson, & Hawes, 1978; Siegel & Peterson, 1980, 1981).

The Procedure Behavior Rating Scale (PBRS) was developed by Katz and colleagues (1980) to measure children's behavioral distress while undergoing invasive and highly stressful medical procedures such as bone marrow aspirations and lumbar punctures. The PBRS consists of 25 items indicative of distress in children such as crying, clinging, verbal expressions of fear, and behaviors necessitating that the child be physically restrained. Each behavior is coded by observers for occurrence during discrete phases of the medical procedure.

TABLE 12.1. BEHAVIOR PROFILE RATING SCALE

	Successive 3-Minute Observation Periods									
	1	2	3	4	5	6	7	8	9	10
Separation from mother										
(3) Cries										
(4) Clings to mother										
(4) Refuses to leave mother										
(5) Bodily carried in										
Office behavior										
(1) Inappropriate mouth closing										
(1) Choking										
(2) Won't sit back										
(2) Attempts to dislodge instruments										
(2) Verbal complaints										
(2) Overreaction to pain										
(2) White knuckles										
(2) Negativism										
(2) Eyes closed										
(3) Cries at injection										
(3) Verbal message to terminate										
(3) Refuses to open mouth										
(3) Rigid posture										
(3) Crying										
(3) Dentist uses loud voice										
(4) Restraints used										
(4) Kicks										
(4) Stands up										
(4) Rolls over										
(5) Dislodges instruments										
(5) Refuses to sit in chair										
(5) Faints										
(5) Leaves chair										

Source: From "Reduction of Fear-Related Dental Management Problems with Use of Filmed Modeling" by B. G. Melamed, D. Weinstein, R. Hawes, and M. Katin-Borland, 1975, *Journal of the American Dental Association, 90,* pp. 822–826. Reprinted by permission.

A significant revision of the PBRS by Katz and colleagues (1980) was developed by Jay and Elliott (1980). This revision, the Observation Scale of Behavioral Distress (OSBD), uses 11 operationally defined distress-related behaviors weighed on a scale of 1 to 4 according to their intensity. The behaviors and their respective intensity weights are: cry (1.5), scream (4.0), physical restraint (4.0), verbal resistance (2.5), request emotional support (2.0), muscular rigidity (2.5), verbal pain (2.5), flail (4.0), nervous behavior (1), and information seeking (1.5). Behaviors are recorded during consecutive 15-minute intervals during each of four phases of the medical procedures. Jay and her colleagues have reported reliability and validity data on the OSBD in several investigations (Jay, Elliott, Ozolins, Olson, & Pruitt, 1985; Jay, Ozolins, Elliott, & Caldwell, 1983).

LeBaron and Zeltzer (1984) developed the *Procedure Behavior Checklist* PBCL), based on Katz and colleagues' (1980) PBRS. The PBCL comprises eight behaviors reflecting anxiety and pain. In addition, the observer rates the intensity of behavior on a scale of 1 to 5 (1 = very mild, 5 = extremely intense). LeBaron and Zeltzer interestingly found that scores on the PBCL were more consistently associated with self-report and behavioral ratings of anxiety than of pain. In addition, the use of intensity ratings appeared to contribute little to differentiating the behavior of children and adolescents undergoing bone marrow aspirations.

Additional observation scales have been reported in the literature. Because there are limited data regarding their reliability and validity, they will be noted briefly. One observational scale has been employed specifically with very young children. Chambers, Fields, and Machen (1981) and Fields, Machen, Chambers, and Pfefferle (1981) developed a measure for obtaining continuous data on anxiety-related behaviors in children 36 to 60 months old undergoing dental procedures. Gross, Stern, Levin, Dale, and Wojnilower (1983) used a four-category observational scale to measure children's responses to venipuncture. A time-sampling procedure was used to record the following behaviors: crying, escape, resistance, and aggression. Vocal, verbal, facial, and motor responses reflecting general distress were recorded in an observational study by Hester (1979), who assessed the reactions of young children receiving immunization injections.

Using an observation scale to measure children's behaviors during cast removal, Johnson, Kirchoff, and Endress (1975) recorded "minor signs of distress" (e.g., body tension) and "major signs of distress" (e.g., pulling away, kicking, screaming). Naylor, Coates, and Kan (1984) developed a measure to assess children's behavior during cardiac catheterization involving nine categories of child and staff behaviors.

Ballard, Gipson, and Pratt (1981) developed an 11-item Child Medical Distress Scale to record children's behavior while undergoing allergy immunization injections. A factor analysis, based on the observational ratings of 850 children receiving injections, suggested four basic components of children's expressions of distress during invasive medical procedures: (1) physical struggling; (2) crying; (3) respondent behaviors such as flinching; and (4) distressed appearance.

An elaborate observational measure for assessing children's general adjustment to the hospital was developed by Cormier (1979). Each child was observed with a 45-item scale using a time-sampling procedure. The major categories that are coded with this instrument are child behaviors, the location of the child, the child's activities at the time of observation, the adults involved, and the nature of the adult–child interactions. A factor analysis of the observational data yielded three factors that corresponded to different typologies of adjustment to the hospitalization. Factor I was characterized by friendliness, cooperative behavior, smiling, playing, and verbalizing. A second factor assessed children who were withdrawn and passive, exhibiting limited verbalizations and frequent self-stimulation behavior. Factor III characterized children who were irritable, complaining, aggressive, and prone to excessive periods of crying.

The second basic approach to measuring children's behavioral responses to health care procedures is the use of rating scales. Typically this assessment technique has involved a behaviorally anchored, Likert-type scale in which some dimension of behavior is rated along a numerical continuum. In the majority of studies in which these scales have been used, a single rating is obtained based on an overall judgment of the child's behavior during specific medical or dental procedures.

An early example of such a rating scale is the Global Mood Scale developed by Vernon, Foley, and Schulman (1967). This 7-point scale, which is presented in Table 12.2, has been used to assess hospitalized children during various activities on a pediatric ward (Schulman, Kaspar, & Child, 1970), while undergoing anesthesia induction (Vernon, 1973; Vernon & Bailey, 1974), and during an injection for preoperative medication (Vernon, 1974). Interrater reliabilities with this measure generally have been reported in the moderate range. There are few data on the relationship of the Global Mood Scale to other measures of distress in children.

Another rating scale of behavioral distress that has received widespread use with children was developed by Frankl, Shiere, and Fogels (1962). The Frankl Scale consists of four categories of behavior (ranging from definitely positive to definitely negative) that pertain to varying degrees of distress and cooperation with the procedures. This scale and variations of this instrument have been used primarily in dental settings (Klorman et al., 1979; Klorman, Ratner, Arata, King, & Sveen, 1978; Machen & Johnson, 1974; Wright & Alpern, 1971). In addition, the Frankl Scale has been used to assess young children undergoing a physical examination and injections (Broome, 1986; Shaw & Routh, 1982). Interrater reliabilities with this

TABLE 12.2. GLOBAL MOOD SCALE

1. Attentive and active in happy or contented way and/or interested in play or other constructive activity
2. Attentive to surroundings but not especially happy appearing and/or unconstructive play and activities
3. Passive, vacant expression, generally quiet and no play, dozing or sleeping
4. Unhappy, worried, or anxious appearance without crying
5. Marked unhappiness—whining, whimpering, moaning, or soft crying, isolated indicators of distress
6. Moderate crying or intermittent but fairly constant sobbing, several noncrying reactions suggesting distress
7. Screaming full blast, intense and constant crying without paying attention to anything

Source: From "Effects of Mother–Child Separation and Birth Order on Young Children's Responses to Potentially Stressful Experiences" by D. T. A. Vernon, J. M. Foley, and J. L. Schulman, 1967, *Journal of Personality and Social Psychology, 5*, pp. 162–174. Copyright 1967 by the American Psychological Association. Reprinted by permission of the publisher and author.

scale generally have been reported to be quite high. Systematic data on the correlations of the Frankl Scale with other measures of anxiety and distress, however, are lacking.

A number of investigators have used separate ratings of anxiety and cooperation when assessing children's responses to health care procedures (Katz et al., 1981; Klorman et al., 1980; LeBaron & Zeltzer, 1984; Peterson & Shigetomi, 1981; Schwartz, Albino, & Tedesco, 1983; Siegel & Peterson, 1980). It has been suggested that separate ratings of these dimensions are necessary since distress may manifest itself as inhibited motor behavior (i.e., freezing or white knuckles) rather than as overt motor responses. Thus a highly cooperative or compliant child is not necessarily a nonanxious one.

Wolfer and Visintainer (1975) constructed two such scales, which they call the Manifest Upset Scale and the Cooperation Scale. The scales range from 1 (little or no fear or anxiety including calm appearance, no crying or verbal protest; complete cooperation including active participation in and assistance with the procedure) to 5 (extreme emotional distress including agitated hard crying or screaming and/or strong verbal protest; extreme resistance, strong avoidance, and the necessity to restrain the child). These scales have been used to rate hospitalized children's behavior during several "stress points" including a physical examination, blood test, preoperative injection, transportation to the operating room, and anesthesia induction. Similar measures of anxiety and cooperation using a 6-point Likert scale were developed by Venham, Bengston, and Cipes (1978) for use with children undergoing dental treatment. Ratings were made during three separate phases of the dental treatment session.

Research indicates that separate ratings of distress and cooperation tend to correlate highly with each other, suggesting that both measures may be tapping a similar factor (Siegel & Peterson, 1980; Venham, Gaulin-Kremer, Munster, Bengston-Audia, & Cohan, 1980; Visintainer & Wolfer, 1975). In addition, several studies have indicated high correlations between ratings of children's distress during medical and dental procedures and scores of behavioral distress from observational measures (Jay et al., 1983; Katz et al., 1980; Siegel & Peterson, 1980).

A final method used to rate children's responses to health care relies on parental report. These measures have been used almost exclusively to obtain data regarding the child's behavior during the posthospital period.

The parent report instrument that has been employed the most in the research literature is the Posthospital Behavior Questionnaire (Vernon, Schulman, & Foley, 1966). This measure consists of 28 items considered to be behavioral indicators of stress in children. Examples of several questions that parents are asked on this scale include: "Does your child seem to be afraid of leaving the house with you?" and "Does your child spend time just sitting or lying and doing nothing?" Each item is rated on a 5-point scale ranging from 1 (much less than before) to 5 (much more than before). Thus parents are asked to compare their child's current (i.e., posthospital) behavior with their recall of their child's behavior before entering the hospital. A test–retest coefficient of .65 was reported for a 1-month retest interval. The validity of this scale was established by comparing total scores with independent ratings by a psychiatrist following interviews with the child and parents. The correlation between total scores and ratings of behavior change following hospitalization was in the moderate range ($r = .47$). A factor analysis of this questionnaire yielded six factors: (1) general anxiety and regression; (2) separation anxiety; (3) anxiety about sleep; (4) eating disturbance; (5) aggression toward authority; and (6) apathy–withdrawal. Additional data regarding the validity of this measure are provided in a number of studies (Cassell, 1965; Ferguson, 1979; Sipowicz & Vernon, 1965; Tarnow & Gutstein, 1983; Vernon, 1973; Wolfer & Visintainer, 1979). Other approaches to parental reports of children's posthospital behavior are illustrated in studies by Melamed and Siegel (1975), Naylor and colleagues (1984), and Skipper and Leonard (1968).

Measures that assess behavioral indicators of emotional distress offer several advantages over measures of the other response systems, particularly with young children undergoing health care procedures. Unlike physiological measures, observations of the child's behavior can be made in a relatively unobtrusive manner. In addition, obtaining data regarding various aspects of a child's overt behaviors is not dependent on the child's abilities or attitudes, as is the case when assessing cognitive–affective components of distress.

Behavioral ratings of children in health care settings that are based on specific, concrete behaviors are an improvement over global ratings of distress that rely to a greater extent on the subjective judgment of the raters. In addition to providing more objective criteria, the former type of observational measure allows for parametric evaluations of its internal properties. The latter, however, may be more practical for use in applied clinical as opposed to experimental situations. Furthermore, the reliability and validity of these more global rating scales can be improved considerably by limiting the period of observation to shorter time intervals and to specific time-limited events rather than by rating the child in a more general manner over extended time periods (e.g., the child's overall response to 3 days in an intensive care unit).

Several observation scales have used weighted factors or intensity ratings of degree of distress or disruptiveness in addition to recording the frequency of occurrence of the child's behavior. While it might appear that using such scales would provide greater sensitivity than observations resulting from scales that use only frequency recordings, there are currently few data regarding the superiority of either type of scale for measuring children's distress-related behaviors.

Behavioral ratings based on parent report can provide useful data regarding the child's response to health care settings and procedures, particularly during the posthospital period when observation of the child's behavior is limited to the parents. It is important to recognize, however, that reporting errors are inherent in retrospective recall and that reliability of these data is significantly reduced when the measures are obtained at long time intervals following the child's discharge from the hospital.

Given the scope of this chapter, it is not possible to review the literature regarding specific findings of children's overt behaviors in health care settings. However, there are some data that merit a brief note because of the remarkably consistent findings across studies. Basically, the literature indicates that younger children exhibit substantially more overt indices of behavioral distress than do older children and adolescents during actual medical and dental procedures (Ballard et al., 1981; Gross et al., 1983; Katz et al., 1980; LeBaron & Zeltzer, 1984). It would appear that the older age groups, on the other hand, show more behavioral withdrawal.

Self-Report Measures

A number of self-report measures have been used to assess children's subjective experience of distress associated with medical and dental procedures. Other self-report instruments have been used to obtain information about cognitions pertaining to children's feelings, attitudes, and overall emotional reactions to the health care experience.

Self-report measures of children's anxiety and distress typically ask the child to rate the extent to which specific symptoms or events are experienced in particular settings or situations. In addition, children may be asked to rate the intensity of their subjective feelings of distress based on their general experience or before, during, and/or immediately following exposure to the health care procedure.

Some investigators have made a distinction between measures of trait and state or situational anxiety and distress (Spielberger, 1966). Trait measures are presumed to assess more stable or generalized characteristics of the child, while situational measures tend to assess a transitory state that presumably varies over time and across situations and occurs in response to specific events.

The most frequently used self-report instruments for assessing children's responses to medical and dental procedures are "fear thermometer" ratings of distress or "faces" rating scales. Fear thermometers are pictorial representations of a thermometer with a numerical scale (i.e., 0 to 10, or 0 to 100), 0 indicating no fear and the highest number reflecting the most fear. The child is instructed to point to the place on the thermometer that shows how anxious or afraid he or she is at a particular moment or in response to specific medical or dental events or procedures (Katz et al., 1980; Melamed et al., 1978; Melamed & Siegel, 1975).

Faces scales consist of a series of faces varying in the degree to which they depict anxiety or unhappiness. For example, the first face in the series would be a smiling face indicating no anxiety or distress, while the last face would be a very negative one representing high levels of anxiety or distress. The faces in between are graded from positive to very negative. Several studies have used the faces scales to assess children's self-reported distress in medical and dental settings (e.g., Katz et al., 1980; LeBaron & Zeltzer, 1984).

A variation of the faces scale was developed by Venham, Bengston, and Cipes (1977). In the Picture Test (see Fig. 12.1), the child is presented with eight pairs of pictures indicating various emotional reactions. The child is asked to select the little boy in each picture who feels the most like the way he or she feels. The total score is the number of times that the more "anxious" member of each pair is chosen. This measure has been used primarily with young children undergoing dental treatment (Klorman et al., 1978; Siegel & Peterson, 1980; Venham & Gaulin-Kremer, 1979; Venham & Quatrocelli, 1977).

Several self-report measures have been developed that assess fears in children that are specific to the medical or dental setting. The Hospital Fears Rating Scale (Melamed & Siegel, 1975) is a self-report scale comprising 8 items from the subscale Medical Fears that was factor-analyzed from the Fear Survey Schedule for Children (Scherer & Nakamura, 1968). Another 8 items having face validity for assessing hospital fears and 9 nonrelated "filler" items were also included. The child is instructed to rate the degree of his or her fear for each item on a fear thermometer.

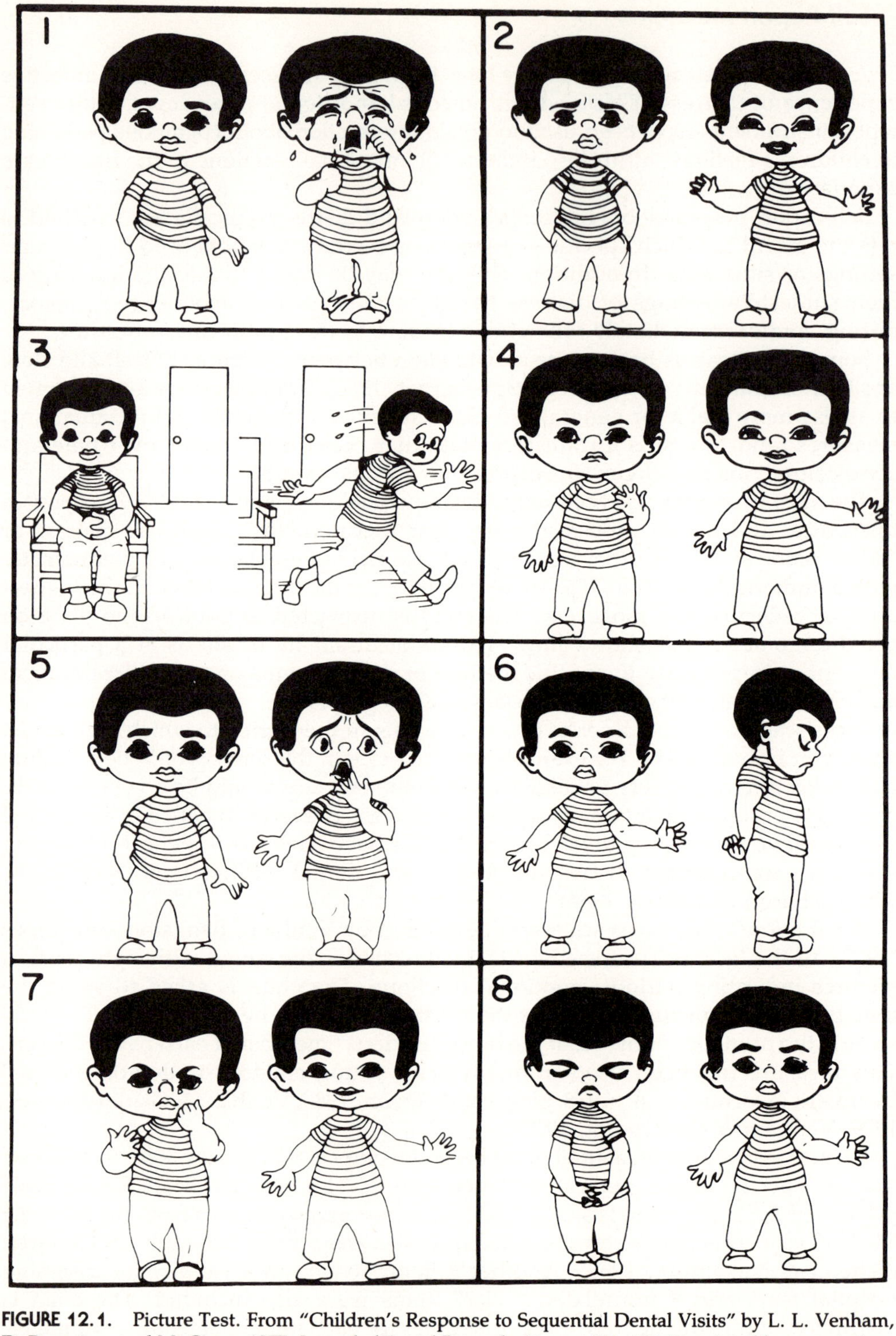

FIGURE 12.1. Picture Test. From "Children's Response to Sequential Dental Visits" by L. L. Venham, D. Bengston, and M. Cipes, 1977, *Journal of Dental Research*, *56*, pp. 454–459. Reprinted by permission.

The sum of the child's ratings on the 16 medical fear items is the total score for this measure. This measure is presented in Table 12.3 and has been used in a number of studies with hospitalized children (Faust & Melamed, 1984, 1979; Melamed, Dearborn, & Hermecz, 1983; Peterson & Shigetomi, 1981; Tarnow & Gutstein, 1983). A similar 12-item scale, the Medical Fear Questionnaire, is reported by Broome (1986). In this measure, the child is asked to rate how fearful he or she is for each event on a 3-point scale (1 = not at all; 3 = a lot).

Melamed and colleagues (Melamed, Hawes, Heiby, & Glick, 1975; Melamed, Weinstein, Hawes, & Katin-Borland, 1975) have also modified the Children's Fear Survey Schedule to include items that are relevant specifically to the dental setting. Examples of some of the items that the child rates using a fear thermometer include the dentist's drill, having your mouth checked, and getting an injection.

A number of self-report anxiety inventories have also been used to measure children's responses to health care settings. Among the most frequently used anxiety inventories include the Children's Manifest Anxiety Scale (Castaneda, McCandless, & Palermo, 1956) and the State-Trait Anxiety Inventory for Children (Spielberger, Edward, Lushene, Montouri, & Platzek, 1970). These instruments tend to provide more global measures of distress that are nonspecific to medical or dental settings and procedures.

Finally, a number of investigators have assessed children's cognitions that pertain to their conceptions and understanding of hospitalization, illness, and medical

TABLE 12.3. CHILDREN'S HOSPITAL FEARS RATING SCALE

Instructions: I want to find out how afraid you are of some different things. Listen, and when I name something I want you to tell me how afraid you are of it by putting a mark on this thermometer. If you feel very afraid of the thing I say, put a mark on top (point). If you don't feel afraid at all, put a mark on the bottom (point to the bottom). And if you feel somewhere in between, put a mark somewhere in between the top and the bottom. (Run your finger up and down scale between top and bottom.)

Here's the first one: Elevators. How afraid are you of elevators?

Ex.: Elevators

How afraid are you of:

_____ sharp objects
_____ having to go to the hospital
_____ getting a shot from the nurse or doctor
_____ making mistakes
_____ spiders
_____ going to bed in the dark
_____ going to the dentist
_____ strange or mean looking dogs
_____ going to the doctor
_____ flying in an airplane
_____ getting punished
_____ getting a haircut
_____ thunderstorms
_____ germs or getting a serious illness
_____ the sight of blood
_____ deep water or the ocean
_____ being alone without your parents
_____ having an operation
_____ ghosts or spooky things
_____ getting carsick
_____ people wearing masks
_____ getting sick at school
_____ not being able to breathe
_____ getting a cut or injury
_____ falling from high places

care. Children's health care concepts and knowledge can influence the manner in which they respond to health care experiences. The major focus of this literature has been the investigation of developmental changes that occur in children's health care conceptualizations.

Campbell (1975), for example, asked hospitalized children 6 to 12 years old for their definition of illness. The children's responses were placed by two independent raters into 11 categories pertaining to somatic feeling states, objective detectable indicators, and psychosocial indicators. Consistent development trends were observed in the children's definitions of illness ranging from undifferentiated feeling states (e.g., feeling sick) to specified and localized somatic states (e.g., stomach aches), visible external signs (e.g., swollen arm), objective signs not clearly visible (e.g., hot forehead), and, finally, specific disease concepts (e.g., diabetes, appendicitis). Thus the children's developmental level of cognitive sophistication was consistent with their progression in sophistication of their definitional concepts of illness.

Three stages in the development of a concept of illness were identified in hospitalized children 5 to 9 years of age by Simeonson, Buckley, and Monson (1979). In the first stage, the child's thought process involved magical thinking and circular logic, with illness being viewed as the result of some specific human action (e.g., becoming ill after eating someone else's food). In the second stage, children viewed illness as caused by one specific external factor related to illness or health (e.g., illness caused by germs or a cut finger). Finally, illness in the third stage was viewed in terms of generalized or abstract notions of physical susceptibility (e.g., illness caused by getting a virus from another person or because the pancreas is not producing sufficient insulin to use the sugar in the blood).

Bibace and Walsh (1980) interviewed children 4, 7, and 11 years old, asking them 12 questions pertaining to the causes and cures of illness. The children's responses were classified according to Piaget's three broad stages of cognitive development. Each of these stages was further subdivided into two subcategories as follows: (1) preoperational stage—phenomenism and contagion; (2) concrete operational stage—contamination and internalization; and (3) formal operational stage—physiological and psychophysiological. Approximately 70 percent of 4-year-olds have phenomenistic explanations, 75 percent of 7-year-olds provided contaministic explanations, and 70 percent of 11-year-olds gave physiological explanations.

Similarly, Brewster (1982) studied chronically ill hospitalized children's concepts of their illness, their understanding of the purpose of medical procedures, and the role of the medical staff. The results indicated that children 5 to 12 years old proceed through a predictable, maturational cognitive sequence of three stages in the conceptual development of the understanding of the causes of illness and three stages in the understanding of the intent of medical procedures.

Several investigators have measured children's knowledge about hospitalization and medical and dental procedures following exposure to various preparation programs (Faust & Melamed, 1984; Klingman, Melamed, Cuthbert, & Hermecz, 1984; Roberts, Wurtele, Boone, Ginther, & Elkins, 1981). Information acquired by the child through the preparation procedure is typically assessed by means of multiple-choice questionnaires.

Self-report measures of children's responses to health care experiences present a challenge to the clinician and researcher. These measures rely on the ability and willingness of children accurately to describe their own feelings and thoughts. The use of self-report instruments of distress is particularly problematic with young children who are limited in their conceptual abilities and have difficulty discriminating and translating internal states such as anxiety or fear into ratings on a fear thermometer or making qualitative judgments such as "a little bit" or "a lot" of fear.

Generally, self-report measures of children's distress in health care settings do not correlate highly with measures of distress-related behaviors (Melamed & Siegel, 1980; Winer, 1982). Certainly, one possible reason for these findings is the unreliability of self-report instruments with young children. For example, Ferguson (1979) found no relationship between scores on the Hospital Fears Rating Scale and several observational and physiological measures. These results are not unexpected, considering that this self-report instrument was administered to children as young as 3 years old. LeBaron and Zeltzer (1984) have also suggested that the low correlations between self-report and observational data may result from the fact that self-report reflects the private experiences of distress and discomfort while overt behaviors may largely reflect an interpersonal dimension of distress. Some evidence for this view comes from the study by Katz and colleagues (1980), who found that children and adolescents did not differ significantly in their *experience* of distress (as measured through self-report) during a stressful medical procedure, but they did differ in the types of overt behaviors exhibited during the observations. These findings further suggest that self-report measures may be particularly important to use with older children and adolescents. Yet as noted earlier, while this age group may be highly distressed or anxious, they tend not to show behavioral indicators of distress as overtly as young children.

One method for increasing confidence in the reliability of children's self-report data regarding concepts such as *afraid* or *scared* has been suggested by LeBaron and Zeltzer (1984). They asked children to describe how they felt during a painful medical procedure in order to determine whether their numerical ratings on a faces scale were consistent with their verbal descriptions.

An area that has received almost no attention in the literature pertains to a possible social desirability response set with children. Studies are needed to assess the extent to which socially desirable responding is a factor in children's responses on self-report instruments of distress. This response set may present a particular problem with older males who might be reluctant to acknowledge fear or anxiety regarding specific medical and dental procedures.

Physiological Measures

Numerous indices of autonomic nervous system activity reflecting physiological arousal have been used to assess children's emotional reactions to medical and dental procedures and settings. Physiological responses may be monitored by highly sophisticated psychophysiological equipment or through less complex procedures such as radial pulse rate. Indirect measures of physiological activity have been assessed in hospitalized children through various indices of physical recovery from surgery. In addition, several investigators have reported the use of biochemical markers of distress-related responses in children undergoing hospitalization or specific health care procedures.

There is considerable research evidence that marked desynchrony often occurs between different physiological responses in the same person. Thus each individual has his or her own idiosyncratic pattern of responses such that some persons may be primarily heart responders, while others may primarily respond on measures of electrodermal activity (Lacey & Lacey, 1968). As a result, it is suggested that more than one physiological measure of distress and anxiety be used in order to evaluate the different patterns of responses within each individual.

A variety of physiological measures presumed to reflect distress have been used in the literature with children. The measures employed in medical and dental settings include heart rate or pulse rate (e.g., Faust & Melamed, 1984; Johnson et al., 1975; Klingman et al., 1984; Melamed et al., 1983; Siegel & Peterson, 1980; Venham et al., 1978), respiration rate (e.g., Klingman et al., 1984; Simpson, Ruzicka, & Thomas, 1974), muscle tension (e.g., Ferguson, 1979; Simpson et al., 1974), blood pressure (e.g., Skipper & Leonard, 1968), and digital blood volume (e.g., Klorman et al., 1980). Measures of electrodermal activity such as basal skin response, galvanic skin response, and skin resistance have also been used in a number of investigations (e.g., Klingman et al., 1984; Klorman et al., 1979; Venham et al., 1978).

The most frequently used physiological indices of distress in children have been measures of cardiovascular activity, such as heart rate and pulse rate. Most studies have recorded radial pulse rate by means of manual palpation for a period of 30 to 60 seconds. Other investigators have used electrocardiogram recordings from psychophysiological equipment.

An interesting method for measuring heart rate responses in hospitalized children is described by Burling and Collipp (1969). In a study designed to assess the most stressful experiences for children hospitalized for nonsurgical reasons, the emotional responses of children 15 months to 10 years of age were measured using a portable ECG pulse monitor. Heart rate was monitored during the first several days of the child's hospitalization for consecutive 12-hour time periods each day. In addition, an observer followed each child throughout the day noting the events that the child experienced. A summary of the data record from one of the children is presented in Figure 12.2. The results from this study clearly indicated that the single most distressing event for the children is the venipuncture.

Another commonly used measure of anxiety and distress for children undergoing medical and dental procedures is the Palmar Sweat Index (PSI) (Dabbs, Johnson, & Leventhal, 1968; Johnson & Dabbs, 1967; Thompson & Sutarman, 1953). The PSI is a plastic impression method that permits the investigator to quantify sweat gland activity from the child's finger. The number of active sweat glands provides a measure of transitory physiological arousal. Melamed and her colleagues have found the PSI to be a reliable and valid measure of children's distress-related reactions in medical and dental settings (Faust & Melamed, 1984; Melamed & Siegel, 1975; Melamed et al., 1976; Melamed et al., 1978).

Investigations of children's response to hospitalization for surgery frequently have utilized a number of physiological and physical indicators of postoperative recovery (Melamed & Siegel, 1975; Peterson & Shigetomi, 1981; Skipper & Leonard, 1968; Wolfer & Visintainer, 1979). It is presumed that these measures are sensitive to the child's overall emotional reactions to the experience. Typically, measures of recovery are assessed while the child is in the hospital, although several investigators have used parental report to obtain these data following the child's discharge from the hospital. Table 12.4 lists the various physical and physiological measures of

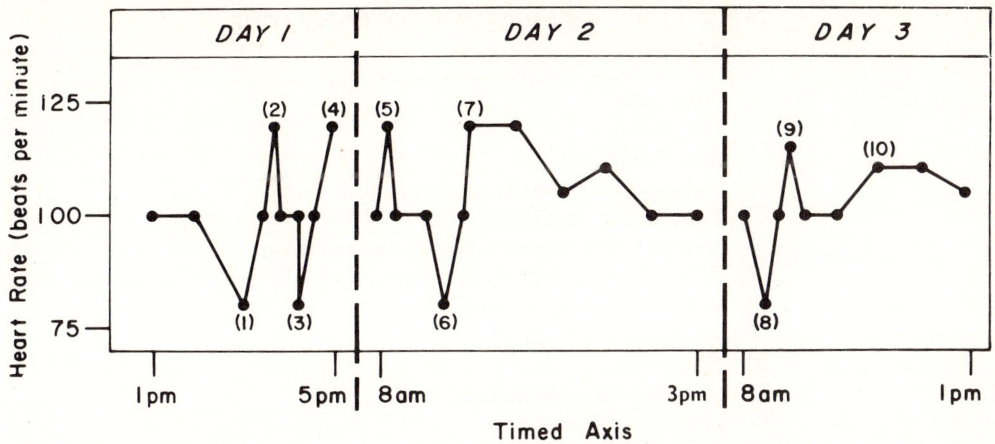

FIGURE 12.2. Timed axis. Observation of this 5-year-old African girl was begun in the emergency room. Increases in heart rate were noted: needle (2, 5, 9), eating (4), recreation (7, 10). Decreases in heart rate were noted: doctor's visit (1, 3, 6, 8). It is difficult to explain the decreases in heart rate during each visit of the doctor. (From "Emotional Responses of Hospitalized Children: Results of Pulse-Monitor Study" by K. A. Burling and P. J. Collipp, 1969, *Clinical Pediatrics, 8,* pp. 641–646. Reprinted by permission.)

postoperative recovery reported in the literature. As can be seen from the table, most of the measures assess either vital signs or medical complications.

Another physiological parameter that has been used is various biochemical markers presumed to be associated with stress-related reactions. Barnes, Kenney, Call, and Reinhart (1972) studied the neuroendocrine responses of children undergoing open heart surgery. Twenty-four-hour urine samples were collected at several time periods including before and after surgery, before and after suture removal, the day before discharge from the hospital, and at 1- and 3-month clinic visits following discharge. The urine was analyzed using a measure of corticosteroids (17-hydroxycorticosteroids). For all children, corticosteroid levels were highest the day before surgery and just prior to suture removal. In addition, urinary cortisol levels were higher during the hospitalization than at the outpatient clinic assessments. Ratings of anxiety by a nurse and psychiatrist were not significantly correlated with the corticosteroid measure.

Cortisol production was also an index of psychological distress in a study by Knight and colleagues (1979). Children hospitalized for elective surgery were evaluated three times including 2 weeks prior to hospital admission, the day after admission, and the day after surgery. Urinary cortisol levels were found to be related to several coping patterns and adjustment ratings on the hospital ward.

Katz and colleagues (1982) measured endorphin levels from spinal fluid in children undergoing lumbar punctures. The findings indicated that there was an inverse relationship between observational and self-report measures of anxiety and distress assessed during the medical procedure and endorphin levels in the spinal fluid.

Physiological measures of anxiety and distress offer similar advantages to observational measures in that they do not depend on the child's verbal and cognitive

TABLE 12.4. MEASURES OF POSTOPERATIVE RECOVERY

1. Pulse rate
2. Temperature
3. Blood pressure
4. Frequency of nausea or vomiting
5. Time to first voiding
6. Number of analgesics and sedatives used
7. Ease of emergence from anesthesia
8. Volume of fluid intake
9. Solid food consumed
10. Infections
11. Length of hospitalization
12. Time to ambulation

abilities as do self-report instruments. As is not the case with self-report and observational measures, the assessment of physiological indicators of distress can necessitate the use of highly sophisticated equipment and require considerable technical expertise. Some methods for obtaining physiological measures may require the child to be cooperative with the procedure. Furthermore, these measures may be difficult to assess in naturalistic settings where the child is mobile.

One of the primary methodological problems in the use of physiological measures of distress in children is the interpretation of the pattern of relationships between different physiological variables. It is unclear, for example, what the findings mean when a child undergoing a medical procedure shows an increase in heart rate, a decrease in skin conductance, and no change in muscle tension when compared to a resting baseline assessment. Additional research is needed to clarify the significance of this variability in responding both within an individual and between different individuals.

The literature demonstrates rather consistently that heart rate is a sensitive measure of physiological distress in children in health care settings. It appears to be useful as a measure of children's response to medical and dental procedures and as a measure of change in intervention programs designed to reduce the distress associated with these procedures. Heart rate also has been shown to have moderate correlations with observational measures of distress.

While measures of physical recovery can be relatively cost-efficient to obtain, there are several factors that make interpretation of the findings difficult. Few studies have standardized the time at which various postoperative recovery measures are assessed. For example, various measures might be obtained 2 hours following surgery for one child, while the same measures with another child might be assessed 6 hours after surgery. Different postsurgery time intervals can introduce a variety of variables that may affect findings such as level of emergence from anesthesia and need for pain medications. Similarly, the amount and type of medications that the child is receiving as well as the type and seriousness of the child's surgery can influence the physical and physiological variables that are measured. These factors have not typically been considered when the data are reported in the literature.

The particular method of physiological assessment used depends largely on the goals of the investigator. Measures such as pulse rate obtained through manual palpation or the Palmar Sweat Index might be used where the investigator is interested in assessing a single event that is reflected in a very brief time period (such as the period immediately before and after a venipuncture). If the investigator is interested in measuring *continuous* changes in physiological indices over longer time intervals, then the use of psychophysiological equipment would be an appropriate consideration. Finally, when the goal is to assess physiological reactivity as a global response reflecting a period as long as 24 hours, biochemical measures of distress might be useful.

ASSESSING CHILDREN'S RESPONSES TO SPECIAL HOSPITAL ENVIRONMENTS

Some children require medical care that is inherently more traumatic than that encountered during routine elective admission to the hospital. Several investigators have assessed the adjustment problems encountered by children who are exposed to unusually stressful environments within the hospital, including the emergency room, intensive care units, and isolated or protected environments.

An emergency admission to the hospital represents a crisis situation for the child and his or her family (Axlerod, 1976). The child's illness or injury may be life threatening and necessitate immediate diagnosis, treatment, or surgery. This situation requires that efforts be directed toward a rapid adjustment of the child and family to a frightening series of events. The emergency room staff is also under considerable pressure to attend quickly to the medical needs of the child, making it difficult to attend concurrently to the child's emotional reactions.

Despite the inherent stresses of an emergency admission, there has been little research on children's behavior under these conditions. An interesting study by Roskies, Bedard, Gauvreau-Guilbaut, and LaFortune (1975) compared extensive observations of the behavior of eight children admitted on an emergency basis with observations of the behavior of eight children having elective admissions. They were also interested in the effects that the parents' and staff's behavior had on the children's reaction to the hospital. Subjects were included in the study if they were 4 to 8 years old, accompanied by at least one parent, conscious (so that they could be observed), had come directly to the hospital, and were eventually admitted to the pediatric ward. At least 6 hours of observations of the natural sequence of events in the admissions process were obtained for each child, including at least 1 hour of observation on the ward. The number and type of people present during the emergency and elective admission and the nature of the interactions that occurred with the parents and child were also recorded. The observations were later categorized into the number of painful events that the child experienced and the number of positive, negative, and neutral interactions that occurred between the parent and child. The results indicated that, on all the dimensions that were measured, the emergency admission was considerably more stressful for the parents and children than were elective admissions. For example, children in the emergency group experienced an average of eight painful procedures during the first 6 hours in the hospital, compared to an average of three for the elective group, and they were separated from their parents much earlier than were children in the elective group. While parent–child interactions in the elective group were characterized by an equal number of positive and neutral interactions, the majority of the interactions in the emergency group were either neutral or negative.

Another particularly stressful environment for the hospitalized child is the intensive care unit, where children with a life-threatening condition must receive medical care. The child is typically immobilized, subjected to numerous painful medical procedures, and exposed to an unfamiliar and highly threatening setting. A child in a pediatric intensive care unit (PICU) is confronted with periods of overstimulation alternating with periods of sensory deprivation (Rothstein, 1980). In a study by Cataldo, Bessman, Parker, Pearson, and Rogers (1979), behavioral observations were conducted on 99 children on the PICU during a 2-month period. These children were admitted for injuries, surgery, or illness. The average length of stay in the PICU was approximately 5 days. Six categories of child behavior were observed: waking state, position, verbalization, eye contact, activity, and affective state. The behavior of caregivers was also observed, including verbalizations to the child and number and type of persons at his or her bedside. The observations indicated that approximately one-third of the children were conscious and alert in the PICU but were not responsive to their environment, frequently staring into space and not attending to anything specific. In addition, there was a low rate of verbalizations by the children and a high level of neutral or unresponsive affective behaviors.

Barnes (1975) examined children's responses to a PICU following heart surgery. The children's levels of consciousness as indicated by their responses to various PICU experiences and events were evaluated by behavioral observations and interviews. Observations during routine activities in the unit averaged 4 hours each day for the first 3 days following surgery. Units of behavior were coded for the types of phenomena that the children referred to in their verbalizations, such as treatments and procedures, persons, events, and furnishings. In addition, each behavioral response was rated as to its level of consciousness including alertness (accurate understanding of phenomena), distortion (exaggeration or misunderstanding of the phenomena), fantasy (imagined responses), affective memory (responses referring to an emotional experience prior to hospitalization), and dreams. Analysis of the data revealed a high degree of accuracy in children's perceptions, with approximately 60 percent of all responses classified as alert. As many as 35 percent of the children's responses reflected some type of distortion.

Kellerman and his colleagues (Kellerman et al., 1976; Kellerman, Rigler, & Siegel, 1979) have discussed the effects of protected environments, or reverse isolation, on pediatric patients. Where the risk of infections must be minimized, some children need to be confined, often for extended periods of time, to a room where the air is continually cleaned. The use of such environments is particularly common with children undergoing chemotherapy for cancer in which the medication significantly increases the risk of infection by affecting the child's immunological system. Prolonged isolation can have a potentially deleterious effect on the child's psychological adjustment because of potential sensory deprivation as a result of confinement to a limited area and to a limited number of persons.

Kellerman and his colleagues studied 14 children with cancer who were hospitalized in a protected environmental unit while undergoing chemotherapy. The children ranged in age from 3 to 17 years old and had an average stay in the isolation unit of 92 days. Ratings of the children were conducted three times each day using 36 behavioral categories related to physical discomfort, affect, perceptual–motor functioning, activity level, management problems, appetite and sleep patterns, and social–interpersonal functioning. Based on these data, no significant or prolonged psychological effects were noted in the children. While some children evidenced transitory periods of depression, this problem was effectively reduced by providing the children with stimulating activities. The authors stress that these positive findings can be attributed to the comprehensive psychosocial program that is provided on a daily basis, including recreational and stimulating activities, and a daily routine. Similar investigations of children undergoing cancer chemotherapy in protected hospital environments are reported by Powazek, Goff, Schyving, and Paulson (1978) and Hollenbeck and colleagues (1980).

ASSESSING COPING RESPONSES IN HEALTH CARE SETTINGS

In recent years, the study of coping processes in children has received greater emphasis. Because of their potential importance in the prevention and early intervention in stress-related adjustment problems, researchers have begun to identify self-generated cognitive and behavioral coping strategies that children use in response to stressful experiences such as medical and dental procedures (Siegel, 1979). The majority of investigations have taken a process rather than a trait approach to measuring children's characteristic methods of coping with health care experiences. Instead of using inventories or questionnaires to assess coping as in the adult literature, most of the studies with children have used interview procedures and/or behavioral observations to identify children's coping strategies in specific health care settings.

Siegel (1981a, 1981b) conducted an ecological assessment of self-generated coping strategies used by hospitalized children to determine whether children who make an optimal adjustment to hospitalization for illness or surgery use coping strategies different from those of children who make a less satisfactory adjustment to the experience. This investigation was particularly interested in assessing the cognitive and behavioral coping responses in which children engaged during stressful and painful medical procedures. A multidimensional assessment approach was used to evaluate the anxiety level and response to pain of 80 children, 8 to 14 years old, who were hospitalized for minor elective surgery. In addition, the evening before surgery and following several stress points (e.g., blood test, diagnostic procedures, preoperative injection), a structured interview was conducted with the children to evaluate, among other things, their typical coping responses to painful and anxiety-provoking experiences both in and out of the hospital. An example of one of the interview questions was: "Pretend your best friend has to go to the doctor for a blood test like the one you just had. What advice would you give so that your friend wouldn't be worried about it or so it wouldn't bother her [or him]? Did you do any of those things or think about any of those things when you had your blood test?"

Children were classified as successful copers if they were consistently rated by a nurse and physician as being cooperative with the procedures, showing low anxiety, and manifesting high thresholds for physical discomfort. On the other hand, unsuccessful copers were defined as being uncooperative, showing high anxiety, and manifesting low tolerance for discomfort. The results indicated that successful copers had more accurate information about why they were in the hospital and asked more questions about the hospital than unsuccessful copers. Successful copers also reported using a greater number of different strategies for managing stressful and painful experiences than unsuccessful copers, such as imagery-based rehearsal in which they planned how they might confront a stressful or painful event prior to its occurrence. Unsuccessful copers, on the other hand, reported using significantly more negative self-statements regarding their ability to tolerate discomfort, such as thinking about how much the needle was hurting, and reported thinking more often about past experiences where they were unable effectively to tolerate painful procedures similar to those encountered in the hospital. A multiple regression analysis revealed that the number of different coping strategies used by the children accounted for most of the variance of successful coping, followed by the extent of accuracy of their knowledge regarding the reason for their hospitalization, with 23 percent and 18 percent of the variance, respectively. Table 12.5 lists the coping categories used to classify the children's responses to the coping interview.

Information-seeking versus information-avoiding coping methods used by children undergoing stressful medical procedures during hospitalization for surgery were assessed by Peterson and Toler (1986). The child's cognitive coping style reflecting an information-seeking disposition was measured by the interview developed by Siegel (1981a, 1981b). A Coping Behaviors Scale was used to measure observable coping strategies used by the child during a blood test, during anesthesia induction, and in the recovery room following surgery. The behaviors assessed by this scale included positive assertion with the medical staff, level of activity during a medical procedure, verbal discussion of the procedure, watching the procedure, and asking questions concerning the procedure. In addition, the child's behavioral distress during the medical procedures was measured using the observational scale developed by Katz and colleagues (1980).

The interview measure of coping was found to be associated with a number of general and specific coping behaviors measured by parents and observers. Furthermore, the child's response to medical procedures was influenced by the child's coping style as assessed by the interview. High information-seeking scores predicted lower rates of distress-related behaviors during various medical procedures and were associated with children who were better informed about hospital procedures and surgery prior to admission to the hospital.

The coping strategies used by children undergoing routine dental treatment were investigated by Curry and Russ (1985). A Behavioral Coping Observation Scale was developed to assess children's coping behaviors during dental treatment. The BCOS consists of three basic behavioral categories including information seeking, support seeking, and direct efforts to maintain control. In addition, a Cognitive Coping Interview was developed to assess the children's cognitions (i.e., thoughts, self-statements, wishes) during four major procedures of dental treatment (explorer exam, injection of anesthetic, placement of rubber dam, and cavity preparation). The child is interviewed and his or her responses are coded according to six possible cognitive coping categories.

These two measures were used to identify the cognitive and behavioral coping strategies employed by 30 children, 8 to 10 years old, who were undergoing restorative dental treatment. The results indicated that the coping responses used by the

TABLE 12.5. CATEGORIES OF COPING STRATEGIES

Category	Definition of Coping Strategy
Distraction—external	Indicates that he or she does something to divert his or her attention away from the procedure by focusing on some aspect of the immediate environment (e.g., looking at a picture on the wall, counting floor tiles)
Distraction—internal	Indicates that he or she does something to divert his or her attention away from the procedure by focusing on some part of the body or sensation unrelated to the procedure (e.g., concentrates on heart beating)
Distraction—imagery	Indicates that he or she thinks about or imagines some pleasant event, activity, or situation to divert attention away from the procedure (e.g., thinks about playing an electronic game, imagines self at school, thinks about being at a party)
Reinterprets sensations	Indicates an attempt to reinterpret or alter by some cognitive process (other than by distraction) the *sensory stimulation* produced by the procedure (e.g., thinks about it as being cool or as pressure rather than as hurting, burning, or stinging)
Fantasy	Imagines he or she is some imaginary character who does not feel pain (e.g., Superman) or pretends that some magical event is happening (e.g., waving a magic wand) to make the pain disappear
Mental rehearsal	Indicates some attempt to prepare for the experience by mentally planning how he or she will confront it
Information seeking—relevant	Indicates an attempt to ask questions or gather information relevant to the medical procedure
Information seeking—irrelevant	Indicates an attempt to ask questions or gather information that is unrelated to the medical procedure
Positive self-statements	Indicates thinking about positive aspects of the procedure; reassures self that he or she can tolerate the procedure; thinks about handling previous procedures successfully; makes self-reinforcing statements for doing well during the procedure; thinks about the experience (e.g., "The doctor is doing this to help me," "It doesn't hurt so bad, I can get through this okay")
Negative self-statements	Indicates thinking about distressing aspects of the *current* procedure and problems in tolerating it (e.g., thinks about how much it was hurting and wanting it to stop)

(*Table continues on p. 290.*)

TABLE 12.5. *(Continued)*

Category	Definition of Coping Strategy
Catastrophizing thoughts	Indicates thinking about distressing or bad things that *might* happen or have occurred in the past (e.g., thinks about the last time it really hurt)
Affective expression	Indicates that he or she thought about or actually displayed some affective response (e.g., cried, yelled, got angry) as a means of tension or stress reduction
Affective inhibition	Indicates an attempt to reduce emotional distress by specifically controlling or inhibiting feelings such as trying not to cry or yell
Relaxation	Indicates that he or she engaged in some activity or thought about something with the specific intent of relaxing or making self feel calm
Seeking help or emotional support	Indicates that he or she thought about asking or actually asked someone for help, comfort, sympathy, or emotional support such as asking the nurse to hold his or her hand or thought about mother being in the room to call for help or comfort if needed
Physical activity	Indicates that he or she attempts to place a part of the body in a certain position (e.g., holds arm rigid) or that he or she engages in a particular physical activity (e.g., holds breath, massages arm) for the specific purpose of reducing discomfort
Seeks active termination of procedure	Engages in any activity or thinks about engaging in an activity with the specific purpose of *immediately* terminating the procedure (e.g., escaping from the room, pushing the doctor away, verbalizing that he or she wants the procedure stopped)
Passive acceptance	Indicates some decision that presumes that nothing could be done to change the situation or to make it better or less stressful in some way
No strategy reported	After sufficient prompting from the examiner, indicates that he or she did not engage in any activity or did not think about anything

children were distributed across all of the categories assessed. Every subject reported employing at least two cognitive coping responses and was observed using at least one behavioral coping response. Older children used a greater number and variety of cognitive coping responses than the younger children. The scores from the behavioral and cognitive measures were not significantly correlated with each other, suggesting that there may be a differential use of these strategies across children.

Burstein and Meichenbaum (1979) assessed the defensive disposition (coping style) of children 4 to 9 years of age who were scheduled for minor surgery. Defensive style was measured by observing the child's preference for play materials and recording the amount of time each child spent playing with hospital-relevant or hospital-nonrelevant toys. Observations were obtained a week before surgery, the night before surgery, and a week after surgery. An interview also was conducted 7 months following hospitalization in which the child was asked to recall various hospital experiences. Children who selected hospital-relevant toys a week prior to surgery (low-defensive children) had lower self-reported anxiety scores after surgery than children who chose toys not related to the hospital (high-defensive children). At the 7-month follow-up assessment, low-defensive children recalled more stressful events from their hospitalization than did high-defensive children.

Play behavior was also used as a measure of children's attempts to cope with impending hospitalization for elective surgery in a study by Tarnow and Gutstein (1983). The purpose of this study was to assess children's naturalistic attempts at preparatory behavior before surgery through information seeking and rehearsal of events. Children were observed during three different 5-minute time periods. During the first period, the child was left alone to paly in a room with two boxes, one containing hospital-related materials and the other having a variety of age-appropriate toys. During the second observation period, an experimenter asked the child to demonstrate what would happen in the hospital using the medically related equipment. Finally, parents were instructed to use the hospital play materials to prepare their children for surgery.

Children's level of active preparatory behavior was rated using a 4-point scale ranging from 0 (complete lack of involvement) to 3 (active involvement in an integrated fashion). Self-report and observational measures of distress also were assessed during the three observation periods. No significant relationships were found between the children's preparatory play behavior and the measures of their distress. Higher levels of active preparatory play were associated with fewer post-hospital behavior problems.

Knight and colleagues (1979) used a structured interview and Rorschach responses to categorize coping styles (defensive styles) in children hospitalized for elective surgery. Urinary cortisol levels were used as a measure of physiological distress. Children who were rated as using the defensive styles of intellectualization or a mixed pattern of defenses had significantly lower cortisol production rates than children who were rated as using denial, displacement, or projection.

Hyson (1983) examined coping behaviors in children ranging in age from 6 to 60 months while undergoing a routine physical examination. Coping responses were operationalized using White's (1974) strategies of adaptation, which include information seeking (looking, asking questions), comfort seeking (contact with mother, familiar objects), and autonomy (attempts to control, structure, or protest). In addition, the child's facial expressions of emotion were classified according to a system developed by Izard (1977) and Ekman, Freisen, and Ellsworth (1972). Behavioral observations were obtained using an elaborate procedure reported by Caldwell and Honig (1971) that results in a sequential and continuous record of behavior. The results indicated that information-seeking behaviors were the most common among children of all ages in the period just before the examination. Autonomy behaviors were the predominant coping responses during the actual physical examination although age differences were noted in the specific type of autonomy responses that were exhibited.

Pidgeon (1981) studied the coping functions of the questions asked by young hospitalized children. Question asking was viewed as a means of helping children to manage novelty and incongruity in their environment, to establish supportive social contacts with adults in a stressful situation, to influence the actions of others, and to achieve cognitive clarity or reality testing. The spontaneous questions of children 3 to 5 years old were sampled in structured and unstructured situations during the first 2 days after admission to the hospital. Using Piaget's functional classification system, the largest number of children's questions (53 percent) were about the actions and intentions of hospital personnel regarding therapeutic activities, play and social activities, and routine care. The second largest category of children's questions were about the names of objects and persons in the hospital environment. These findings suggest that the preschool-age child maintains a vigilant orientation in the hospital and that preparation procedures should include information about the actions and intentions of hospital personnel and the identification of familiar and unfamiliar objects.

Using Lazarus's stress and coping paradigm, Caty, Ellerton, and Ritchie (1984) did a content analysis of the coping strategies reported in 39 case studies of hospitalized children 20 months to 10 years of age. The majority of behaviors reported in the case studies were classified in the Action/Inaction dimension (64.3 percent). The Information Exchange dimension accounted for 31.1 percent of the behaviors while 4.6 percent of the behaviors were categorized in the Intrapsychic dimension. Younger children displayed greater numbers of behaviors in the Action/Inaction dimension while older children showed a greater tendency to exhibit behaviors that were information focused, reflecting their greater cognitive and verbal abilities.

ASSESSMENT OF PARENTAL FACTORS

Several areas of research have examined the effects of parental (usually maternal) behaviors on children's responses to health care procedures. There is a considerable literature that emphasizes the importance of assessing parental attitudes, expectations, and child management techniques as determinants of children's reactions to medical and dental experiences. One such area of research concerns the relationship between maternal anxiety and the child's anxiety and cooperation during medical and dental procedures. This factor has been of concern to investigators, not only because of the effect of the anxiety on the parents, but also because of the possibility that the parents' anxiety might be communicated to the child. Maternal anxiety typically has been evaluated by self-report inventories. A significant, positive relationship between parental anxiety and children's distress-related responses in health care settings has been reported in several studies (Jay et al., 1983; Johnson & Baldwin,

1968, 1969; Koenigsberg & Johnson, 1972). Other investigators, however, have found no relationship between parental anxiety and the child's behavior during medical and dental procedures (Klorman et al., 1978; Klorman et al., 1979; Schulman et al., 1970). As Winer (1982) has noted, the tendency for more anxious mothers to have more distressed children has been shown primarily with younger children. He suggests that as children increase with age they generally develop greater independence from their mothers, thereby reducing the influence of the mother's anxiety on the child.

A second area of research that has addressed parental factors in health care settings with children is the study of the effect of the mother's presence versus absence during medical and dental procedures on the child's behavior. There is a lack of consensus in the literature regarding the effect of a parent's presence during medical and dental treatment on the child. Those who advocate the presence of a parent suggest that the parent has a positive influence primarily by inhibiting anxiety in the young child. On the other hand, those who suggest that parents should not be present during procedures argue that parents have a negative influence on the child's behavior by interfering with the dental procedures and communicating their own anxiety to the child.

Venham and his colleagues (Venham, 1979; Venham et al., 1978) have systematically evaluated the effects of the mother's presence on the child's response to dental stress. In one study, they varied whether the mother was present or absent over two dental sessions. A number of physiological, self-report, and behavioral measures failed to reveal a significant effect. However, the mother's presence during the first session and absence during the second session tended to result in lower anxiety and greater cooperation in the child than the reverse order. Younger children generally were more anxious on the second visit regardless of the mother's presence.

A second study in which the decision regarding the parent–child separation was left to the mother and child indicated that the presence or absence of the mother did not produce any significant differences in the child's behavior. In general, the mother's influence on the child depended on the manner in which she responded during the dental treatment. If she was calm and responded with confidence when her child was moderately anxious, no adverse reactions occurred from the child. Thus it would appear that the quality of the mother–child relationship and her specific behavior in the dental operatory (and not merely her presence or absence) are the critical variables (Venham, 1979).

Shaw and Routh (1982) investigated the effects of mothers' presence on the behavior of 18-month-old and 5-year-old children receiving routine immunization injections. Children in both age groups whose mothers were present during the injection were rated as exhibiting significantly more negative behaviors than children whose mothers were absent. The investigators suggest that the findings indicate that under the conditions of a minor anxiety-provoking experience, young children may inhibit their distress if the mother is absent. These findings do not necessarily imply that the children were less fearful.

In a similar study, Gross and colleagues (1983) observed the behavior of children 4 to 10 years of age who were undergoing a venipuncture. One-half of the children had their mothers present while half of the children's mothers remained in the waiting room. Regardless of age, children whose mothers were present displayed significantly more crying before the blood test than children whose mothers were absent. No differences in behavior were observed during the blood test. The authors concluded that mothers may serve as a discriminative stimulus for crying behavior in the presence of an aversive event.

Another parent variable that has been examined is child-rearing attitudes and practices. These investigations assume that disciplinary techniques and other parental practices pertaining to child management can influence the manner in which a child copes with stressful events such as medical and dental procedures. The relationship between child-rearing practices and young children's responses to a dental examination and prophylaxis was investigated by Venham and colleagues (1979). Child-rearing practices were measured by home observations and a self-report questionnaire. The findings indicated that children's heart rate and observer-rated anxiety were significantly correlated with a number of child-rearing techniques. Children who were less anxious during dental treatment tended to come from home environments with greater structure and had mothers who provided sufficient limits on their behavior, including rewards and punishment.

Zabin and Melamed (1980) examined the relationship between parents' disciplinary style and children's anxiety during hospitalization for surgery. Disciplinary methods were measured by a questionnaire assessing how parents respond to their children in stressful situations such as having an injection, being afraid of thunder and lightning, and falling off a bicycle. Parents who reported using positive reinforcement, modeling, and persuasion as techniques for encouraging their children to manage stressful situations tended to have children who exhibited low anxiety during the hospitalization. On the other hand, children with high anxiety scores were more likely to have parents who used punishment, force, and the reinforcement of dependent behaviors.

In an interesting study by Bush, Melamed, Sheras, and Greenbaum (1986), the influence of actual maternal behaviors on children's reactions to a medical examination was investigated in an outpatient clinic. Fifty children from 4 to 10 years of age were observed interacting with their mothers immediately prior to the examination. Observations were obtained using the Dyadic Prestressor Interaction Scale developed by the investigators. This instrument measures four categories of child behaviors (attachment, distress, exploration, and prosocial) and six categories of parent behaviors (informing, distracting, reassuring, ignoring, restraining, and agitation). Maternal use of informing and distracting was associated with children's exploration of the treatment room, prosocial behavior, and fewer distress-related behaviors. The relationships between these parent–child variables were particularly stronger with younger children (less than 5 years, 9 months). Self-reported maternal anxiety was not associated with either the mother's or their children's behavior in the examining room.

ASSESSING THE BEHAVIOR OF HEALTH CARE PROVIDERS

The nature of the child's interaction with health care providers such as physicians, dentists, and nurses can influence the child's response to hospitalization and medical and dental procedures. It is generally acknowledged that the doctor's or dentist's behavior can affect the extent to which a child is calm and cooperative or anxious and highly disruptive during various procedures. This issue is of particular importance considering that the degree of cooperation of the child can influence the quality and speed with which the procedures are performed. Several investigators have attempted to assess the relationship between the communication style or behavior management strategies of health care providers and children's behavior during medical and dental procedures.

Hyson, Snyder, and Andujar (1982) examined the relationship between the doctor's style of interaction and the child's behavior during a routine physical examination. Three characteristics of the physician's interactions were assessed, including warmth (proximity to the child and expressions of empathy), child involvement (extent to which the doctor talked with the child and permitted the child to handle medical instruments), and mother involvement (extent to which the doctor spoke with the mother and encouraged the mother to hold the child on her lap). The physician's warmth was found to be associated with positive responses by the child. Neutral and passive behaviors exhibited by children were associated with a pattern of interaction characterized by low warmth and limited child involvement.

Melamed, Bennett, and colleagues (1983) investigated the effects of dentists' use of instructions alone; instructions plus praise for cooperative behavior (positive reinforcement); instructions plus criticism, restraint, or loud voice for inappropriate behavior (punishment); and instructions with both contingent reward and punishment. Observations with children 4 to 12 years old revealed that instructions alone facilitated cooperation over subsequent sessions. The use of contingent praise and punishment also reduced disruptive behavior. Increased disruptiveness was observed with the use of praise or punishment alone. The punishment-only condition was associated with higher levels of self-reported anxiety.

When level of previous experience and degree of fear regarding dental treatment were taken into account, differential treatment effects occurred for the different management strategies. Children with previous dental experience or a high degree of initial disruptiveness became calm and cooperative when treated with both positive reinforcement for compliance and punishment for inappropriate behavior. They reported more anxiety and feelings of being less in control with a neutral dentist who did not provide direct feedback about the appropriateness of their responses. On the other hand, children who were new to the dental setting or low in reported dental fears reported heightened anxiety if treated by a dentist using punishment in response to noncompliant behavior.

Naturally occurring interactions between 25 dentists and preschool-age children undergoing dental treatment were analyzed using a lag sequential technique by Weinstein, Getz, Ratener, and Domoto (1982). A lag sequential analysis is a statistical procedure by which one can assess the probability that a particular behavior will be followed by other types of behaviors. The categories of dentist communication observed included directive guidance (provided statement of instruction, expectation, or feedback concerning child's behavior), permissive behavior (allowed problem behavior to continue or tried to persuade child to cooperate), and coercive behavior (attempted to overcome problems by verbal or nonverbal force). Child behaviors were classified into fear- and non–fear-related categories. Dentist direction and reinforcement were followed by the least fear-related behaviors. Coercive behaviors (i.e., dentist found fault, threatened, acted gruff) provided the greatest probability of fear-related behavior. Fear-related responses were most likely to occur when the dentist held or restrained the child. The investigators concluded that dentists were less likely to use direction or reinforcement after the child's fear-related behavior. Dentists were more likely to use rules, coercion, and coaxing after the child's fear-related behaviors. Thus the data suggest that dentists more frequently respond to the fearful child with behaviors that are counterproductive or ineffective in reducing distress.

SUMMARY AND CONCLUSIONS

Numerous methodological improvements in assessment of children's adjustment to hospitalization and medical procedures have occurred during the past several decades. Assessment procedures have progressed from unidimensional, global measures with unsatisfactory reliability and validity to empirically validated measurement procedures reflecting a multidimensional approach to children's responses to medical events. These advances in assessment procedures, however, have introduced a number of complex issues which remain to be resolved through additional research. One important area that remains to be clarified, for example, is the clinical significance of discordant relationships among measures of the different systems of emotional distress in children undergoing medical procedures. While each response system is uniquely important to the assessment of children's distress-related behaviors, further research is needed to evaluate how each target response is differentially affected by such factors as cognitive-developmental level, the nature of the medical event, and type of intervention program used.

Research has yet to determine what constitutes optimal levels of adjustment and adaptive levels of anxiety for hospitalized children. It is yet unclear, for example, whether high levels of anxiety prior to medical procedures or surgery are detrimental to the subsequent adjustment of the child.

Longitudinal studies are needed to assess the extent to which a child's response to medical procedures varies across time. What factors influence whether a child habituates or becomes sensitized to medical procedures? Are measures of the various response systems of distress in children differentially influenced by a child's repeated exposure to particular medical procedures? Research needs to provide data regarding these issues.

One area that has received virtually no attention in the literature is the assessment of the *positive* effects of the hospital experience on children's behavior. Vernon and Schulman (1964), for example, found that a number of children showed reductions in behavior problems following their hospitalization. Vernon et al. (1965) note that hospitalization, particularly where the child has received psychological preparation, may be beneficial to some children by fostering a sense of accomplishment and maturity through mastering the stress of various experiences in the hospital. Similarly, Guerin (1977) has proposed that hospitalization can be a positive life experience, particularly for children from multi-problem, low-income families. She indicates that the hospital can provide a temporary respite for a child from a chaotic home situation by providing the child with a structured environment in an atmosphere of supportive and caring adults who are concerned with the child's physical and emotional well-being. Future research is needed which addresses the possible short-term and long-term benefits of hospitalization on the child's development.

Children's typical modes of responding to stressful situations influence their ability to manage hospitalization and painful and anxiety-provoking medical procedures and likely affect their ability to benefit from preparation programs. Investigators are beginning to make progress in assessing the cognitive and behavioral coping strategies that children use when undergoing medical and dental procedures. Further work is needed to develop empirically validated measures of children's cognitions and behaviors that they actually use when confronted with stressful situations. Such information will be useful in developing effective interventions for reducing the distress associated with medical and dental procedures.

References

Axlerod, B. H. (1967). Mental health considerations in the pediatric emergency room. *Journal of Pediatric Psychology, 1,* 14–17.

Ballard, B. D., Gipson, M., & Pratt, A. C. (1981, April). *Behavioral treatment of children's distress caused by painful allergy treatment injections.* Paper presented at the meeting of the Rocky Mountain Psychological Association, Denver.

Barnes, C. M. (1975). Levels of consciousness indicated by responses of children to phenomena in the intensive care unit. *Maternal–Child Nursing Journal, 4,* 215–285.

Barnes, C. M., Kenney, F. M., Call, T., & Reinhart, J. B. (1972). Measurement in management of anxiety in children for open heart surgery. *Pediatrics, 49,* 250–259.

Barowsky, E. I. (1978). Young children's perceptions and reactions to hospitalization. In E. Gellert (Ed.), *Psychosocial aspects of pediatric care.* New York: Grune & Stratton.

Bibace, R., & Walsh, M. (1980). Development of children's concepts of illness. *Pediatrics, 66,* 912–917.

Brewster, A. B. (1982). Chronically ill hospitalized children's concepts of their illness. *Pediatrics, 69,* 355–362.

Broome, M. E. (1986). The relationship between children's fears and behavior during a painful event. *Children's Health Care, 14,* 142–145.

Burling, K. A., & Collipp, P. J. (1969). Emotional responses of hospitalized children: Results of a pulse-monitor study. *Clinical Pediatrics, 8,* 641–646.

Burstein, S., & Meichenbaum, D. (1979). The work of worrying in children undergoing surgery. *Journal of Abnormal Child Psychology, 7,* 121–132.

Bush, J. P., Mèlamed, B. G., Sheras, P. L., & Greenbaum, P. E. (1986). Mother–child patterns of coping with anticipatory medical stress. *Health Psychology, 5,* 137–157.

Caldwell, B. M., & Honig, A. S. (1971). APPROACH: A procedure for patterning responses of adults and children (coding manual). Abstracted in *Catalog of Selected Documents in Psychology, 1,* 1.

Campbell, J. D. (1975). Illness is a point of view: The development of children's concepts of illness. *Child Development, 46,* 92–100.

Cassell, S. (1965). Effects of brief puppet therapy upon the emotional responses of children undergoing cardiac catheterization. *Journal of Consulting and Clinical Psychology, 29,* 1–8.

Castaneda, A., McCandless, B. R., & Palermo, D. S. (1956). The children's form of the Manifest Anxiety Scale. *Child Development, 27,* 317–326.

Cataldo, M. F., Bessman, C. A., Parker, L. H., Pearson, J. E. R., & Rogers, M. C. (1979). Behavioral assessment for pediatric intensive care units. *Journal of Applied Behavior Analysis, 12,* 83–97.

Caty, S., Ellerton, M. L., & Ritchie, J. A. (1984). Coping in hospitalized children: An analysis of published case studies. *Nursing Research, 33,* 277–282.

Chambers, W. L., Fields, H. W., & Machen, J. B. (1981). Measuring selected disruptive behaviors of the 36-to-60 month-old patient, I. Development and assessment of a rating scale. *Pediatric Dentistry, 3,* 251–256.

Chapman, A. H., Loeb, D. G., & Gibbons, M. J. (1956). Psychiatric aspects of hospitalizing children. *Archives of Pediatrics, 73,* 77–78.

Cormier, P. P. (1979). Identification of typologies derived from child behaviors in the hospital as predictors of psychological upset. *Journal of Psychiatric Nursing & Mental Health Services, 17,* 28–31.

Curry, S. L., & Russ, S. W. (1985). Identifying coping strategies in children. *Journal of Clinical Child Psychology, 14,* 61–69.

Dabbs, J. M., Johnson, J. E., & Leventhal, H. (1968). Palmar sweating: A quick and simple measure. *Journal of Experimental Psychology, 78,* 347–350.

Ekman, P., Friesen, W. V., & Ellsworth, P. C. (1972). *Emotion in the human face: Guidelines for research and an integration of findings.* New York: Pergamon.

Faust, J., & Melamed, B. G. (1984). Influence of arousal, previous experience, and age on surgery preparation of same day of surgery and inhospital pediatric patients. *Journal of Consulting & Clinical Psychology, 54,* 359–365.

Ferguson, B. F. (1979). Preparing young children for hospitalization: A comparison of two methods. *Pediatrics, 64,* 656–664.

Fields, H. W., Machen, J. B., Chambers, W. L., & Pfefferle, J. C. (1981). Measuring selected disruptive behavior of the 36 to 60 month-old dental patient. II: Quantification of observed behavior. *Pediatric Dentistry, 3,* 257–261.

Frankl, S. N., Shiere, F. R., & Fogels, H. R. (1962). Should the parent remain with the child in the dental operatory? *Journal of Dentistry for Children, 29,* 150–163.

Gross, A. M., Stern, R. M., Levin, R. B., Dale, J., & Wojnilower, D. A. (1983). The effect of mother–child separation on the behavior of children experiencing a diagnostic medical procedure. *Journal of Consulting & Clinical Psychology, 51,* 783–785.

Hester, N. K. (1979). The preoperational child's reaction to immunization. *Nursing Research, 28,* 250–255.

Hodgson, R., & Rachman, S. (1974). Desynchrony in measures of fear. *Behaviour Research & Therapy, 12,* 319–326.

Hollenbeck, A. R., Sussman, E. J., Nannis, E. D., Strope, B. E., Hersh, S. P., Levine, A. S., & Pizzo, P. A. (1980). Children with serious illness: Behavioral correlates of separation and isolation. *Child Psychiatry & Human Development, 11,* 3–11.

Hyson, M. C. (1983). Going to the doctor: A developmental study of stress and coping. *Journal of Child Psychology & Psychiatry, 24,* 247–259.

Hyson, M. C., Snyder, S. S., & Andujar, E. M. (1982). Helping children cope with checkups: How good is the "good patient"? *Children's Health Care, 10,* 139–144.

Izard, C. E. (1972). *Human emotions.* New York: Plenum.

Jackson, K., Winkley, R., Faust, O. A., Cemack, E., & Brutt, M. M. (1953). The problem of emotional trauma in the hospital treatment of children. *Journal of the American Medical Association, 149,* 1536–1538.

Jay, S. M., Elliott, C. H., Ozolins, M., Olson, R. A., & Pruitt, S. D. (1985). Behavioral management of children's distress during painful medical procedures. *Behaviour Research & Therapy, 23,* 513–520.

Jay, S. M., Ozolins, M., Elliott, C., & Caldwell, S. (1983). Assessment of children's distress during painful medical procedures. *Health Psychology, 2,* 133–147.

Jeans, M. E. (1983). The measurement of pain in children. In R. Melzack (Ed.), *Pain measurement and assessment.* New York: Raven.

Jessner, L., Blom, G. E., & Waldfogel, S. (1952). Emotional implications of tonsillectomy and adenoidectomy in children. In R. S. Eissler (Ed.), *The psychoanalytic study of the child* (Vol. 7). New York: International University Press.

Johnson, R., & Baldwin, D. C., Jr. (1968). Relationship of maternal anxiety to the behavior of young children undergoing dental extraction. *Journal of Dental Research, 47,* 801–805.

Johnson, R., & Baldwin, D. C., Jr. (1969). Maternal anxiety and child behavior. *Journal of Dentistry for Children, 36,* 87–92.

Johnson, J. E., & Dabbs, J. M. (1967). Enumeration of active sweat glands: A simple physiological indicator of psychological changes. *Nursing Research, 16,* 273–275.

Johnson, J. E., Kirchoff, K. T., & Endress, M. P. (1975). Altering children's distress behavior during orthopedic cast removal. *Nursing Research, 24,* 404–410.

Johnson, J. E., Leventhal, H., & Dabbs, J. M. (1971). Contributions of emotional and instrumental response processes in adaptation to surgery. *Journal of Personality & Social Psychology, 20,* 55–64.

Katz, E. R., Kellerman, J., & Siegel, S. E. (1980). Behavioral distress in children with cancer undergoing medical procedures: Developmental considerations. *Journal of Consulting & Clinical Psychology, 48,* 356–365.

Katz, E. R., Kellerman, J., & Siegel, S. E. (1981). Anxiety as an affective focus in the clinical study of acute behavioral stress: A reply to Shacham and Daut. *Journal of Consulting & Clinical Psychology, 49,* 470–471.

Katz, E., Sharp, B., Kellerman, J., Marston, A., Hershman, J., & Siegel, S. (1982). Beta-endorphin immunoreactivity and acute behavioral distress in children with leukemia. *Journal of Nervous & Mental Disease, 170,* 72–77.

Katz, E. R., Varni, J., & Jay, S. M. (1984). Behavioral assessment and management of pediatric pain. In M. Hersen, R. M. Eisler, & P. M. Miller (Eds.), *Progress in behavior modification.* New York: Academic.

Kellerman, J., Rigler, D., & Siegel, S. E. (1979). Psychological responses of children to isolation in a protected environment. *Journal of Behavioral Medicine, 2,* 263–274.

Kellerman, J., Rigler, D., Siegel, S. E., McCue, K., Pospisil, J., & Uno, R. (1976). Pediatric cancer patients in reverse isolation utilizing protected environments. *Journal of Pediatric Psychology, 1,* 21–25.

Klingman, A., Melamed, B. G., Cuthbert, M. I., & Hermecz, D. A. (1984). Effects of participant modeling on information acquisition and skill utilization. *Journal of Consulting & Clinical Psychology, 52,* 414–422.

Klorman, R., Hilpert, P. L., Michael, R., LaGana, C., & Sveen, O. B. (1980). Effects of coping and mastery modeling on experienced and inexperienced pedodontic patients' disruptiveness. *Behavior Therapy, 11,* 156–168.

Klorman, R., Michael, R., Hilpert, P. L., & Sveen, O. B. (1979). A further assessment of predictors of the child behavior in dental treatment. *Journal of Dental Research, 58,* 2338–2343.

Klorman, R., Ratner, J., Arata, C. L. G., King, L. B., & Sveen, O. B. (1978). Predicting the child's uncooperativeness in dental treatment from maternal trait, state, and dental anxiety. *Journal of Dentistry for Children, 45,* 62–67.

Knight, R. B., Atkins, A., Eagle, C., Evans, N., Finklestein, J. W., Fukushima, D., Katz, J., & Weiner, H. (1979). Psychological stress, ego defenses, and cortisol production in children hospitalized for elective surgery. *Psychosomatic Medicine, 41,* 40–49.

Koenigsberg, S. R., & Johnson, R. (1972). Child behavior during sequential dental visits. *Journal of the American Dental Association, 85,* 128–132.

Lacey, J. I. (1967). Somatic response patterning and stress: Some revisions of activation theory. In M. H. Appley & R. Trumbull (Eds.), *Psychological stress: Issues in research.* New York: Appleton-Century-Crofts.

Lacey, J. I., & Lacey, B. B. (1968). Verification and extension of the principle of autonomic response stereotypy. *American Journal of Psychology, 71,* 50–73.

Lang, P. J. (1968). Fear reduction and fear behavior: Problems in treating a construct. In J. M. Shlier (Ed.), *Research in psychotherapy* (Vol. 3). Washington, DC: American Psychological Association.

Lang, P. J. (1977). Physiological assessment of anxiety and fear. In J. D. Cone & R. P. Hawkins (Ed.), *Behavioral assessment: New directions in clinical psychology.* New York: Brunner/Mazel.

Lang, P. J., Melamed, B. G., & Hart, J. (1970). Automating the desensitization procedure: A psychophysiological analysis of fear modification. *Journal of Abnormal & Social Psychology, 76,* 220–234.

LeBaron, S., & Zeltzer, L. (1984). Assessment of acute pain and anxiety in children and adolescents by self-reports, observer reports, and a behavior checklist. *Journal of Consulting & Clinical Psychology, 52,* 729–738.

Machen, J. B., & Johnson, R. (1974). Desensitization, model learning, and the dental behavior of children. *Journal of Dental Research, 53,* 83–87.

McCerthy, E., & Kozak, L. (1985). *Hospital use by children: United States, 1983.* Washington, DC: National Center for Health Statistics.

Melamed, B. G. (1979). Behavioral approaches to fear in dental settings. In M. Hersen, R. M. Eisler,

& P. M. Miller (Eds.), *Progress in behavior modification* (Vol. 7). New York: Academic.

Melamed, B. G., Bennett, C. G., Jerrill, G., Ross, S. L., Bush, J. P., Hill, C., Courts, F., & Ronk, S. (1983). Dentists' behavior management as it affects compliance and fear in pediatric patients. *Journal of the American Dental Association, 106*, 324–330.

Melamed, B. G., Dearborn, M., & Hermecz, D. A. (1983). Necessary considerations for surgery preparation: Age and previous experience. *Psychosomatic Medicine, 45*, 517–525.

Melamed, B. G., Hawes, R. R., Heiby, E., & Glick, J. (1975). Use of filmed modeling to reduce uncooperative behavior of children during dental treatment. *Journal of Dental Research, 54*, 801–979.

Melamed, B. G., Klingman, A., & Siegel, L. J. (1984). Childhood stress and anxiety: Individualizing cognitive behavioral strategies in the reduction of medical and dental stress. In A. W. Meyers & W. E. Craighead (Eds.), *Cognitive behavior therapy with children*. New York: Plenum.

Melamed, B. G., Meyer R., Gee, C., & Soule, L. (1976). The influence of time and type of preparation on children's adjustment to hospitalization. *Journal of Pediatric Psychology, 1*, 31–37.

Melamed, B. G., & Siegel, L. J. (1975). Reduction of anxiety in children facing hospitalization and surgery by use of filmed modeling. *Journal of Consulting & Clinical Psychology, 43*, 511–521.

Melamed, B. G., & Siegel, L. J. (1980). *Behavioral medicine: Practical application in health care*. New York: Springer.

Melamed, B. G., & Siegel, L. J. (in press). Coping behaviors in children facing medical stress. In T. Field, P. McCabe, & N. Schneiderman (Eds.), *Stress and coping* (Vol. 2). Hillsdale, NJ: Erlbaum.

Melamed, B. G., Weinstein, D., Hawes, R., & Katin-Borland, M. (1975). Reduction of fear-related dental management problems with use of filmed modeling. *Journal of the American Dental Association, 90*, 822–826.

Melamed, B. G., Yurcheson, R., Fleece, E. L., Hutcherson, S., & Hawes, R. (1978). Effects of film modeling on the reduction of anxiety-related behaviors in individual varying in level of previous experience in the stress situation. *Journal of Consulting & Clinical Psychology, 46*, 1357–1367.

Naylor, D., Coates, T. J., & Kan, J. (1984). Reducing distress in pediatric cardiac catheterization. *American Journal of Disease of Children, 138*, 726–729.

Peterson, L., & Shigetomi, C. (1981). The use of coping techniques to minimize anxiety in hospitalized children. *Behavior Therapy, 12*, 1–14.

Peterson, L., & Toler, S. M. (1986). An information seeking disposition in child surgery patients. *Health Psychology, 5*, 343–358.

Pidgeon, V. (1981). Functions of preschool children's questions in coping with hospitalization. *Research in Nursing & Health, 4*, 229–235.

Powazek, M., Goff, J. R., Schyving, J., & Paulson, M. A. (1978). Emotional reactions of children to isolation in a cancer hospital. *Journal of Pediatrics, 92*, 834–837.

Poznanski, E. O. (1976). Children's reactions to pain: A psychiatrist's perspective. *Clinical Pediatrics, 15*, 114–119.

Prugh, D. (1983). *The psychosocial aspects of pediatrics*. Philadelphia: Lea Febiger.

Prugh, D. G., & Eckhardt, L. O. (1980). Stages and phases in the responses of children and adolescents to illness and injury. In B. W. Camp (Ed.), *Advances in behavioral pediatrics* (Vol. 1). New York: JAI.

Prugh, D. G., Staub, E. M., Sands, H. H., Kirschbaum, R. M., & Lenihan, E. A. (1953). A study of the emotional reactions of children and families to hospitalization and illness. *American Journal of Orthopsychiatry, 23*, 70–106.

Roberts, M. C., Wurtele, S. K., Boone, R. R., Ginther, C., & Elkins, P. D. (1981). Reduction of medical fears by use of modeling: A preventive application in a general population of children. *Journal of Pediatric Psychology, 6*, 293–300.

Roskies, E., Bedard, P., Gauvreau-Guilbaut, H., & LaFortune, D. (1975). Emergency hospitalization of young children: Some neglected psychological considerations. *Medical Care, 13*, 570–581.

Rothstein, R. (1980). Psychological stress in families of children in a pediatric intensive care unit. *Pediatric Clinics of North America, 27*, 613–620.

Scherer, M. W., & Nakamura, C. Y. (1968). A fear survey schedule for children (FSS-FC): A factor-analytic comparison with manifest anxiety (CMAS). *Behavior Research & Therapy*, 173–182.

Schulman, J. L., Kaspar, J. C., & Child, D. (1970). Videotape sampling of the child's day in the hospital. *Journal of Pediatrics, 76*, 728–731.

Schwartz, B. H., Albino, J. E., & Tedesco, L. A. (1983). Effects of psychological preparation on children hospitalized for dental operations. *Journal of Pediatrics, 102*, 634–638.

Select Panel for the Promotion of Child Health (1981). *Better health for our children*. DHHS Publication Number (PHS) 79-55071.

Shacham, S., & Daut, R. (1981). Anxiety or pain: What does the scale measure? *Journal of Consulting & Clinical Psychology, 49*, 468–469.

Shaw, E. G., & Routh, D. K. (1982). Effect of mother presence on children's reaction to aversive procedures. *Journal of Pediatric Psychology, 7*, 33–42.

Siegel, L. J. (1976). Preparation of children for hospitalization: A selected review of the research literature. *Journal of Pediatric Psychology, 1* 26–30.

Siegel, L. J. (1981a, April). *Naturalistic study of coping strategies in children facing medical procedures*. Paper presented at the meeting of the Southeastern Psychological Association, Atlanta.

Siegel, L. J. (1981b, August). *An ecological assessment of children coping in the hospital*. Paper presented at the meeting of the American Psychological Association, Los Angeles.

Siegel, L. J. (1983). Hospitalization and medical care of children. In C. E. Walker & M. C. Roberts (Eds.), *Handbook of clinical child psychology*. New York: Wiley.

Siegel, L J. (in press). Dental treatment. In D. Routh (Ed.), *Handbook of pediatric psychology*. New York: Guilford.

Siegel, L. J., & Peterson, L. (1980). Stress reduction in young dental patients through coping skills and sensory information. *Journal of Consulting & Clinical Psychology, 48*, 785–787.

Siegel, L. J., & Peterson, L. (1981). Maintenance effects of coping skills and sensory information on young children's response to repeated dental procedures. *Behavior Therapy, 12*, 530–535.

Siegel, L. J., & Ridley-Johnson, R. (1985). Anxiety disorders of childhood and adolescence. In P. H. Bornstein & A. E. Kazdin (Eds.), *Handbook of clinical behavior therapy with children*. Homewood, IL: Dorsey.

Simeonsson, R. J., Buckley, L., & Monson, L. (1979). Conceptions of illness causality in hospitalized children. *Journal of Pediatric Psychology, 4*, 77–84.

Simpson, W. J., Ruzicka, R. L., & Thomas, N. R. (1974). Physiological responses of children to initial dental experience. *Journal of Dentistry for Children, 41*, 465–470.

Sipowicz, R. R., & Vernon, D. T. A. (1965). Psychological responses of children to hospitalization. *American Journal of Diseases of Children, 109*, 228–231.

Skipper, J., & Leonard, R. C. (1968). Children, stress, and hospitalization: A field experiment. *Journal of Health & Social Behavior, 9*, 275–287.

Spielberger, C. D. (1966). Theory and research on anxiety. In C. D. Spielberger (Ed.), *Anxiety and behavior*. New York: Academic.

Spielberger, C. D., Edward, C. D., Lushene, R., Montouri, J., & Platzek, D. (1970). *Manual for the State-Trait Anxiety Inventory for Children*, The How I Feel Questionnaire. Palo Alto, California: Consulting Psychologist Press.

Sternbach, R. A. (1968). *Pain: A psychophysiological analysis*. New York: Academic.

Tarnow, J. D., & Gutstein, S. E. (1983). Children's preparatory behavior for elective surgery. *Journal of the American Academy of Child Psychiatry, 22*, 365–369.

Thompson, M. L., & Sutarman (1953). The identification and enumeration of active sweat glands in man from plastic impressions of the skin. *Transactions of the Royal Society of Topical Medicine & Hygiene, 47*, 412–417.

Thompson, R. H. (1985). *Psychosocial research on pediatric hospitalization and health care: A review of the literature*. Springfield, IL: Charles C. Thomas.

Vaughn, G. F. (1957). Children in hospital. *Lancet, 272*, 1117–1120.

Venham, L. L. (1979). The effects of mother's presence on child's response to sequential dental visits. *Journal of Dental Research, 56*, 454–459.

Venham, L. L., Bengston, D., & Cipes, M. (1977). Children's response to sequential dental visits. *Journal of Dental Research, 56,* 454–459.

Venham, L. L., Bengston, D., & Cipes, M. (1978). Parent's presence and the child's response to dental stress. *Journal of Dentistry for Children, 45,* 213–217.

Venham, L. L., & Gaulin-Kremer, E. A. (1979). A self-report measure of situational anxiety for young children. *Pediatric Dentistry, 1,* 91–96.

Venham, L. L., Gaulin-Kremer, E., Munster, E., Bengston-Audia, D., & Cohan, J. (1980). Interval rating scales for children's dental anxiety and uncooperative behavior. *Pediatric Dentistry, 2,* 195–202.

Venham, L. K., Murray, P., & Gaulin-Kremer, E. (1979). Child-rearing variables affecting the preschool child's response to dental stress. *Journal of Dental Research, 58,* 2042–2045.

Venham, L. L., & Quatrocelli, S. (1977). The young child's response to repeated dental procedures. *Journal of Dental Research, 56,* 734–738.

Vernon, D. T. A. (1973). Use of modeling to modify children's responses to a natural potentially stressful situation. *Journal of Applied Psychology, 58,* 351–356.

Vernon, D. T. A. (1974). Modeling and birth order in response to painful stimuli. *Journal of Personality & Social Psychology, 29,* 794–799.

Vernon, D. T. A., & Bailey, W. C. (1974). The use of motion pictures in the psychological preparation of children for induction of anesthesia. *Anesthesiology, 40,* 68–74.

Vernon, D. T. A., Foley, J. M., & Schulman, J. L. (1967). Effects of mother-child separation and birth order on young children's responses to potentially stressful experiences. *Journal of Personality & Social Psychology, 5,* 162–174.

Vernon, D. T. A., Foley, J. M. Sipowicz, R. R., & Schulman, J. L. (1965). *The psychological responses of children to hospitalization and illness.* Springfield, IL: Charles C. Thomas.

Vernon, D. T. A., Schulman, J. L., & Foley, J. M. (1966). Changes in children's behavior after hospitalization. *American Journal of Disease of Children, 111,* 581–593.

Visintainer, M. A., & Wolfer, J. A. (1975). Psychological preparation for surgical pediatric patients: Effects on children's and parent's stress responses and adjustment. *Pediatrics, 56,* 187–202.

Weinstein, P., Getz, T., Ratener, P., & Domoto, P. (1982). The effect of dentists' behaviors on fear-related behaviors in children. *Journal of the American Dental Association, 104,* 32–38.

White, R. W. (1974). Strategies of adaptation: An attempt at systematic description. In G. V. Costello & J. R. Adams (Eds.), *Coping and adaptation.* New York: Basic.

Winer, G. A. (1982). A review and analysis of children's fearful behavior in dental settings. *Child Development, 53,* 1111–1133.

Wolfer, J. A., & Davis, C. E. (1970). Assessment of surgical patients' preoperative emotional condition and postoperative welfare. *Nursing Research, 19,* 402–414.

Wolfer, J. A., & Visintainer, M. A. (1975). Pediatric surgical patients' and parents' stress responses and adjustment. *Nursing Research, 23,* 244–255.

Wright, G. Z., & Alpern, G. D. (1971). Variables influencing children's cooperative behavior at the first dental visit. *Journal of Dentistry for Children, 38,* 60–64.

Wurster, C. A., Weinstein, P., & Cohen, A. J. (1979). Communication patterns in pedodontics. *Perceptual & Motor Skills, 48,* 159–166.

Zabin, M. A., & Melamed, B. G. (1980). Relationship between parental discipline and children's ability to cope with stress. *Journal of Behavioral Assessment, 2,* 17–38.

13

Assessing Stressful Life Events in Childhood and Adolescence

JAMES H. JOHNSON
ANDREW S. BRADLYN

During their development, children and adolescents experience a variety of events that result in significant changes in their lives. Examples include the birth of a sibling, parental separation, divorce, or death of a family member, all of which may be associated with significant changes in peer and family interactions and lifestyle. Given the potentially disruptive effects of such events, mental health and other child care professionals have become increasingly interested in examining the degree to which stressful events experienced by children may contribute to the development of both physical and mental health problems.

In considering the topic of life stress and life stress assessment, it is useful to note that a variety of definitions of *stress* have been presented over the years. There are, for example, definitions that emphasize a stimulus-oriented perspective, defining it in terms of the experiencing of specific types of noxious or aversive stimuli. Others, such as Selye (1982), have focused on the organism's biological or psychological response to presumably stressful situations. Most recently, Lazarus (see Lazarus & Folkman, 1984) and others have defined *stress* as resulting from an interaction between the person and his or her environment; thus stress results from experiencing events or situations that are appraised by individuals as threatening or as placing demands on them that exceed their ability to cope. It is this last, more cognitively oriented conceptualization that will be utilized here in examining the relationship between life events experienced by both children and adolescents and the extent to which the experiencing of these events is linked to health-related problems. The purpose of this chapter is threefold. First, several frequently used measures for assessing life change in children and adolescents will be described. In the second section, findings regarding the relationship between life stress scores and physical health will be reviewed. Finally, recommendations for future assessment directions will be provided, with particular emphasis being placed on the role of moderator variables in mediating the effects of life stress.

ASSESSING LIFE EVENTS: LIFE CHANGE UNIT MEASURES

Coddington Life Events Record

The Life Events Record, developed by Coddington (1972a, 1972b), is perhaps the most well-known and widely used life stress measure for children.

The measure is a listing of various events judged to be frequently experienced by children and adolescents. Depending upon the age of the child, there are from 30 to 42 items on the scale. The preschool version, for example, lists 30 events, the elementary version 36 events, the junior high version 40 events, and the senior high version 42 events. The parents of very young children are asked to complete the measure for their children, while older children complete the checklist themselves. Respondents are asked to indicate which of the events listed have been experienced during the recent past, and the number of times the event(s) has been experienced. Life change scores are computed by summing values termed "life change units" that have been assigned to the various events. These item weights were initially obtained by asking 243 raters (teachers, pediatricians, mental health workers) to rate a list of events according to the average amount of social readjustment required. To provide a reference value, "birth of a sibling" was assigned an arbitrary value of 500, and raters were asked to assign each of the other events a value greater than or less than 500 to indicate greater or lesser degrees of readjustment. Average readjustment ratings were then calculated, and life change units determined by dividing ratings for each event by the constant 10 and rounding the resulting figure. For example, on the senior high school version divorce of a parent is assigned a value of 77, death of a parent a value of 87, and hospitalization a value of 58. A total life stress score is then obtained by summing change units associated with the specific life events that the child has reportedly experienced. Normative data have been provided by Coddington (1972b), who administered the Life Events Record to a large sample of children and adolescents drawn from the general population in order to obtain developmental data regarding the average amount of social readjustment experienced by those at various ages. The total sample for this study consisted of more than 3500 children ranging in age from preschoolers to senior high school students, and varied in sex, race, and socioeconomic status. Data provided by this investigation yielded means and standard deviations for life stress scores obtained by children of various age groups. Here it may be noted that the data suggest a strong relationship between the age of the child and the amount of life change reported, with older children reporting significantly higher levels of change than younger children. Normative data are useful in providing a means of determining whether a child is reported to have experienced a significantly higher amount of life change than similar-aged peers.

Validity Studies. Data supporting the validity of the Life Events Record have been provided by a large number of studies investigating the relationship between life change obtained from this measure and various indices of child health and adjustment. In general, it has been found that the scores derived from this scale are related to a wide variety of dependent measures. Two of the more methodologically sound health-related investigations are representative of studies that have used this scale.

Padilla, Rohsenow, and Bergman (1976), in a prospective study, examined the relationship between reported life changes and accident frequency in a sample of 103 seventh grade boys. The children completed a modified version of the Life Events Record, with life event scores being obtained by summing life change units associated with events that were reported to have been experienced in the last 12 months. Children who scored in the upper and lower 27 percent of the distribution of these scores were then selected for further study.

The subjects were interviewed weekly over a 5-month period to obtain information about the occurrence and severity of any accidents they might have experienced. All interviewers were blind to the children's initial life event scores. Padilla and colleagues (1976) report that subjects who had initially reported higher levels of life change reported having significantly more accidents than those children who had low (bottom 27 percent of the distribution) life event scores. Although it is potentially problematic to rely on self-reported accident frequency and intensity, this investigation is noteworthy for its prospective nature and the fact that the interviewers were blind to the subjects' initial life stress scores.

An investigation reported by Hodges, Kline, Barbero, and Flanery (1984) examined the reported life events of children with recurrent abdominal pain (RAP) and their parents, and children who were classified as psychiatric referrals and normal controls. Thirty children (11 males, mean age of 10 years; 19 females, mean age of 11 years) who met specific diagnostic criteria for RAP were administered the Coddington Life Events Record. Equal numbers of children referred to a psychiatric clinic, as well as volunteers from the general population with no history of RAP or psychiatric treatment, completed the same measure. The parents of the children completed a modified version of the Schedule of Recent Experiences (Holmes & Rahe, 1967), in addition to several life event items taken from Sarason, Johnson, and Siegel's (1978) Life Experiences Survey. Life events were reported for the previous 12-month period.

Comparisons of the life stress scores for these three groups indicated that children with recurrent abdominal pain reported significantly higher life stress scores than did children in the normal control group (as did children in the psychiatric group). Hodges and colleagues (1984) noted that children in the RAP and psychiatric groups obtained life stress scores that were from one to two standard deviations above the normative mean for 10-year-olds, as reported by Coddington (1972b). No differences were found for the measure of overall life stress reported for the parents, however. In addition to these illustrative studies, Coddington life stress scores have been found to be significantly related to recurrent chest pain (Pantell & Goodman, 1983) and adolescent pregnancy (Coddington, 1979).

Reliability Findings. While there are data such as those just described that support the validity of the Coddington scales, there are presently no data available addressing the question of the reliability of this measure.

Additional Life Change Unit Measures

The Children's Life Events Inventory is a British modification of the Coddington Life Events Record. Developed by Monaghan, Robinson, and Dodge (1979), this is a 40-item instrument that was constructed in much the same fashion as the original scale, with some changes in item content. There have been no validity or reliability data reported.

Yeaworth, York, Hussey, Ingel, and Goodwin (1980) have developed a 31-item instrument comprising events deemed appropriate for adolescents. In contrast to the Coddington scale in which professionals were asked to rate events for life change units, adolescents themselves provided the ratings. Rather than ask how much readjustment would be necessary, Yeaworth and colleagues (1980) asked the adolescents to rate how upsetting each event would be for them. Although mean life change scores are presented for the sample of 207 adolescents, the authors report no validity or reliability data. An investigation reported by Ferguson (1981) utilized an expanded version of this scale (items related to adolescent suicide were included) with a small (N = 25) sample of gifted, White, suburban ninth graders. The reports of these gifted children yielded lower stress scores on this measure than did a sample of 71 nongifted students; additionally, life stress scores were found to be significantly correlated with an index of suicidal ideation.

Finally, the High School Social Readjustment Scale (Tolor, Murphy, Wilson, & Clayton, 1983) has been developed specifically for use with high school students. Psychologists, high school teachers, and high school students themselves provided estimates of the amount of readjustment associated with each of 52 events. Tolor and colleagues (1983) note that these groups were quite similar in their rank ordering of the events. No validity or reliability data have been reported for this instrument.

General Evaluation of Life Change Unit Measures

Although life change unit measures have been the most frequently used methods for assessing life events, with the exception of the Coddington scale, there are few validity data to support their use. Even here, without adequate reliability data one must still be cautious in drawing conclusions from investigations using this instrument.

Other limitations of the Coddington Life Events Record (and similar measures) are apparent. First, the scale yields only an overall measure of life change and, like its adult counterpart, the Schedule of Recent Experiences (Holmes & Rahe, 1967), makes no distinction between positive and negative life events. Implicit in the development of these measures, then, is the assumption that it is *change per se*, and not the desirability of those changes, that is stressful and related to adverse outcomes. Related to this issue, it may be noted that several investigations with adults suggest that it may be more appropriate to conceptualize life stress in terms of negative life change (Johnson & Sarason, 1979a; Mueller, Edwards, & Yarvis, 1977; Sarason et al., 1978; Vinokur & Selzer, 1975). These authors have reported investigations in which only negligible relationships were found between positive change and relevant dependent measures, while indices of negative change were found to be consistently correlated with stress-related measures. To the extent that these findings with adult subjects are generalizable to children (data related to this issue will be presented in a later section), the failure to separate positive and negative life events represents a major limitation of the Coddington scale and its variations.

A second limitation relates to the use of life change units in deriving life stress scores. Life change units are purported to represent the amount of change resulting from or the degree of stressfulness associated with experiencing specific events. If one accepts the assumption that the stressfulness of specific events depends not merely on the occurrence of that event, but also on the child's appraisal of the event, it is appropriate to question whether values derived from the average ratings of others can adequately represent the stressfulness associated with any specific event for any specific child. Indeed, an investigation by Yamamoto and Felsenthal (1982) suggests that adult ratings of life events may not, in some instances, correspond to children's self-ratings of those same events.

A final area of concern with the Coddington-type scales centers on the degree to which the items can be assumed to provide an adequate sampling of life events experienced by children and adolescents. Events included in such measures have typically been derived from the authors' experience, instead of relying on more empirical methods of test construction or the surveying of children and adolescents themselves to determine which events they report as stressful.

In light of these limitations, three areas for improvement are apparent. First, any measure of life events for children and adolescents should contain a broad, representative sample of such events, including those suggested by children and adolescents themselves. Secondly, the measure should allow the separate assessment of positive and negative life changes. Finally, a method to assess the impact of life changes on specific children, rather than relying on group averages, would allow for a more sensitive instrument. It is only recently that measures have been developed that take into account such factors; these measures are the focus of the following section.

ASSESSING LIFE EVENTS: NON–LIFE CHANGE UNIT MEASURES

In contrast to measures such as the Coddington Life Events Record, several instruments have been developed on the assumption that undesirable events may have a different and perhaps more detrimental effect on the individual than desirable events. In this model, then, life stress is conceptualized in terms of events that exert a negative impact on an individual. These measures typically provide for the separate assessment of desirable and undesirable change. Three such measures, the Life Events Checklist (Johnson & McCutcheon, 1980), the Junior High Life

Experiences Survey (Swearingen & Cohen, 1985), and the Adolescent Perceived Events Scale (Compas, Davis, & Forsythe, 1985), can be considered within this category.

Life Events Checklist

Johnson and McCutcheon (1980) have reported an alternative life change measure that is suitable for older children and adolescents. The Life Events Checklist comprises a listing of 46 events, with spaces provided for respondents to report events not specifically listed. Items were selected from the Coddington Life Events Record, adult life stress scales (with those items appropriately modified for use with children and adolescents), and events that the authors judged to be frequently experienced by children and adolescents. Importantly, to provide for a more adequate sampling of events, additional items were obtained by asking 44 Black children and White children and adolescents from varying socioeconomic backgrounds to list the five most stressful events experienced during the previous year. Table 13.1 illustrates the general format of this measure.

The first 18 events on the scale are events over which the child is likely to have little personal control and that are unlikely to be confounded with measures of health and adjustment. Items 19 to 46 are events that are likely to function as stressors when experienced but that are potentially under the control of the individual.

The Life Events Checklist yields two values, a positive life change score and a negative life change score. As discussed in the previous section, this distinction is supported by the results of a number of investigations with adults that have reported that positive and negative changes are differentially associated with relevant dependent variables. As can be seen, rather than taking a life change unit approach,

TABLE 13.1. EXAMPLES OF EVENTS INCLUDED IN THE LIFE EVENTS CHECKLIST

Event	Type of Event		Impact or Effect of Event on Your Life			
1. Moving to a new home	Good	Bad	No effect	Some effect	Moderate effect	Great effect
2. New brother or sister	Good	Bad	No effect	Some effect	Moderate effect	Great effect
3. Changing to a new school	Good	Bad	No effect	Some effect	Moderate effect	Great effect
4. Serious illness or injury of a family member	Good	Bad	No effect	Some effect	Moderate effect	Great effect
8. Death of a family member	Good	Bad	No effect	Some effect	Moderate effect	Great effect
9. Parents separated	Good	Bad	No effect	Some effect	Moderate effect	Great effect

Source: Adapted from Johnson & McCutcheon, 1980.

the analysis of events also takes into account the *individual's subjective appraisal* of each event. Preliminary normative data derived from the positive and negative changes reported by 213 male and female subjects drawn from the general population are also provided.

Validity Studies. Several recent studies have provided preliminary support for the usefulness of the Life Events Checklist. Using a preliminary version of the checklist, Gad and Johnson (1980) reported negative life change scores to correlate significantly with a variety of factors including visits to a physician during the previous year, reports of diagnosed illness, reports of physical health problems, visits to a school counselor, reports of personal problems, difficulty coping with personal problems, and reported drug use. Positive life change scores were found to be correlated with fewer variables, including a negative relationship with visits to a physician. Interestingly, reports of personal problems were also related to the positive life change score, but the correlation was much lower than that obtained for the index of negative change.

Johnson and McCutcheon (1980) investigated the relationship between Life Events Checklist scores and a number of dependent variables, including locus of control orientation, depression, trait anxiety, and emotional maladjustment. Additional measures included self-reports of school days missed because of illness, reports of physical health problems, and self-ratings of present health and health within the previous year. In order to determine the degree to which responses to the checklist might be biased by subjects' attempts to respond in a socially desirable manner, the relationship between life change scores and scores on a measure of social desirability was also examined.

Analyses based on the entire sample yielded significant correlations between negative life change scores and reports of depression, anxiety, emotional maladjustment, and an externally oriented locus of control, with higher levels of reported negative life change being associated with higher levels of reported depression and so forth. High levels of positive life changes were also found to be significantly related to an internal rather than external locus of control orientation. There were no significant correlations between either of the life change scores and the measure of social desirability. No significant correlations between either reported positive or negative life change and physical health were obtained.

When the data were analyzed as a function of the sex of the respondent, several interesting findings were reported. For males, there was a significant relationship between negative life change and school days missed as a result of illness, reports of physical health problems, and ratings of present health status. The authors also reported that higher reported levels of positive life change were associated with lower ratings of maladjustment. For females, there were no significant correlations between life change scores and indices of physical health. However, significant correlations were obtained between negative life change scores and indices of maladjustment and external locus of control. Thus the scores derived from the Life Events Checklist were found to correlate with a variety of relevant dependent variables; additionally, support was provided for the independent assessment of positive and negative life events. The possibility that the correlates of life stress scores for males and females may differ was also suggested.

Wenet (1979) compared the Life Events Checklist scores from 25 male adolescent sex offenders with those obtained from an equal number of male adolescents drawn from the general population who were matched for age. Wenet reported that there were significant differences between the two groups on the measure of reported negative life change. Negative life change scores for the offender group were approximately three times those reported by the control group. No group differences were obtained for reported positive life changes.

Brand, Johnson, and Johnson (1986) provide additional support for the validity of the Life Events Checklist. In their study of 141 children from 10 to 17 years old with juvenile-onset or insulin-dependent diabetes mellitus, measures of negative life change were significantly associated with certain biochemical measures of diabetic control that have previously been demonstrated to be sensitive to the effects of stress. These authors reported no significant relationship between any of the dependent variables and positive life change scores. Finally, other investigators (Greenberg, Siegel, & Leitch, 1983; Smith, Gad, & O'Grady, 1983) have also reported significant correlations between scores on the Life Events Checklist and additional measures of health and adjustment.

Reliability Studies. Two studies bearing on the reliability of the Life Events Checklist have been reported. Brand and Johnson (1982) administered the Life Events Checklist to 50 children and adolescents (10 to 17 years old) drawn from a university laboratory school. In an effort to collect data regarding the test–retest reliability of this measure, the checklist was readministered 2 weeks later. Positive and negative life change scores were computed by summing the impact scores of reported events that were rated as desirable and those that were rated as undesirable (impact rating procedure), and also by simply summing the numbers of positive and negative events reported, giving each a rating of 1 (unit rating procedure). Using the simple unit rating procedure, test–retest correlations for positive and negative life change scores were .69 ($p < .001$) and .72 ($p < .001$), respectively. When scores were derived using the impact of rating procedure, test–retest correlations were .71 ($p < .001$) for positive and .66 ($p < .001$) for negative change scores. Thus these data suggest that the Life Events Checklist demonstrates adequate reliability over a 2-week interval, particularly when one considers that some events may have actually been experienced between the two testings.

Data bearing on the interrater reliability of the LEC have been reported by Gilbert (1985), who administered the LEC to a sample of children and adolescents (N = 45; age range from 11 to 18 years). Collateral information was obtained by asking the mothers of these subjects to complete this measure by reporting events experienced by their children during the past 12 months. While there was a tendency for mothers to underestimate the number of events experienced (and the impact of these events), significant correlations between child or adolescent and parent reports of events were obtained. When weighted indices of positive and negative change were considered separately, the obtained correlations were .48 and .60, respectively. It should be noted, however, that correlations in both of these studies were based on total positive and negative change scores and suggest not necessarily that the same events are being reported each time, but only the degree to which the total magnitude of events is reported consistently across time and respondents.

General Evaluation of the Life Events Checklist. The studies just reviewed suggest that Life Events Checklist scores are reasonably reliable, and that they correlate in the expected direction with a variety of relevant dependent measures. Additionally, scores on the Life Events Checklist have been demonstrated to differentiate between clinic and nonclinic groups. Finally, the fact that positive and negative life change scores were found to be differentially related to dependent measures supports the desirability of separate assessment of positive and negative change events as opposed to the commonly used total score procedure for assessing life change events.

Given the relative newness of this instrument, several areas requiring additional research are evident. Further investigations of the test–retest reliability of the Life Events Checklist over a longer time interval are needed to establish the stability of the resulting scores; it will also be important to establish exact agreement figures in order for researchers to have confidence that respondents are reporting the *same* events from administration to administration. Additional studies involving collateral reports by significant others are also necessary to establish the adequacy of this instrument. Finally, studies comparing the Life Events Checklist with other life change measures in the prediction of health and adjustment problems would be especially useful.

Additional Non–Life Change Unit Instruments

The Junior High Life Experiences Survey (Swearingen & Cohen, 1985) is in many respects similar to the Johnson and McCutcheon (1980) Life Events Checklist. This instrument consists of 39 items similar in content to items included in the child measures previously described, as well as spaces to add events not listed. Respondents are asked to report events occurring within the past 6 months and to rate those experienced events as positive, neutral, or negative. Respondents must then rate the impact of those events on a 7-point Likert scale (from "very good change" to "very bad change"). Thus one can derive positive, negative, and/or total life change scores, which are based on either a simple count of the number of events or the sum of the impact ratings.

Preliminary data regarding this instrument are provided by Swearingen and Cohen in an investigation in which 233 seventh and eighth grade males and females were administered the JHLES. Measures of state–trait anxiety and depression as well as the number of school days missed during the most recent grading period were also collected. The authors report that negative life change scores were associated with higher levels of self-reported anxiety, depression, and school absences. Positive change scores were generally unrelated to these variables; the only significant correlation with positive change scores was for the measure of depression, in which higher levels of reported positive change were associated with lower levels of depression. These findings provide further support for the separate calculation of positive and negative change scores in life stress research, as they suggest that indices of negative change demonstrate a higher association with various dependent measures than does the simple summing of life change unit scores used in the Coddington scale and its modifications.

An additional measure, the Adolescent Perceived Events Scale (APES), has been developed by Compas and colleagues (1985). It is similar to the Life Events Checklist and Junior High Life Experiences Survey described previously in that it allows for the separate assessment of positive and negative life events and for obtaining individualized impact ratings of events. The APES is different from previous scales in that it provides a broader sample of life events, including the assessment of daily stressors (hassles), pleasures, and major life changes.

The scale was developed in a multistage procedure with a large number of adolescents ($N = 654$) first being surveyed to determine major life events experienced within the past 6 months, as well as daily hassles and pleasures experienced within this same time period. The addition of daily hassles was based on investigations with adults (DeLongis, Coyne, Dakof, Folkman, & Lazarus, 1983; Kanner, Coyne, Schaefer, & Lazarus, 1981) that suggested that many daily events can be perceived as stressful and may be more highly correlated with indices of health and adjustment than are major life events. Pleasant events were included because of suggestions by some life stress investigators (Felner, 1984; Felner, Farber, & Primavera, 1983) that the potentially adaptive significance of positive events has been largely ignored in the life stress literature.

Secondly, using multidimensional scaling procedures, the dimensions most commonly used by adolescents in their appraisal of events were identified. In their sample of 36 male and female adolescents (12 to 20 years old), three dimensions emerged as relevant: (1) desirability; (2) impact; and (3) generality of cause, which was relevant in only one age group. Because the relevant dimensions varied as a function of age, three slightly different versions of the APES were constructed. For young adolescents (12 to 14 years old) events are rated on the single dimension of desirability. Adolescents between the ages of 15 and 17 are asked to rate events on the dimensions of desirability, impact, and cause. For respondents in the oldest group (18 to 20 years old) events are rated on two dimensions, desirability and impact.

Preliminary validity data have been reported in a study (Compas et al., 1985) relating APES scores to the Hopkins Symptom Checklist (Derogatis, Lipman, Rickels, Uhlenhuth, & Covi, 1974) as a measure of psychological symptoms. The Hopkins Symptom Checklist is a 58-item self-report measure that yields a total symptom index as well as subscales related to depression, anxiety, obsessive–compulsive characteristics, interpersonal sensitivity, and somatization.

Correlational analyses indicated that weighted negative event scores were significantly associated with each of the Hopkins Symptom Checklist subscales. Consistent with previous investigations that have assessed positive and negative events separately, weighted positive change scores were significantly correlated with fewer variables. Significant relationships were determined between weighted positive change scores and measures of anxiety and obsessive–compulsive characteristics only.

Test–retest reliability for the version of the APES appropriate for older adolescents is also provided by Compas and colleagues (1985). Fifty-one college freshmen, 17 to 20 years old, were asked to report events occurring during the previous 3 months, and the measure was then readministered 2 weeks later. At the second testing, respondents were asked to report events experienced during the same 3-month time period that had been assessed during the first testing.

The overall correlation between the total number of events reported at Time 1 and Time 2 was .77 ($p < .001$), and the percentage of agreement for specific events reported at the two testings was 89. It should be noted that this latter figure is important in establishing the degree to which specific events are reported or not reported consistently over time, and represents an important psychometric advance over the simple total score correlation. These findings suggest that the respondents were quite consistent in their reports at each testing.

Adequate levels of reliability were also determined when positively and negatively reported events were considered separately. Test–retest correlations between weighted positive and negative scores were .84 and .74, respectively. The overall percentage of agreement score for events rated as positive and negative at both Time 1 and Time 2 was 93. These data suggest that, at least for older adolescents reporting events over a 2-week interval, the APES possesses adequate test–retest reliability.

A final study reported by Compas and colleagues (1985) examined the interrater reliability of this measure. The authors asked a small group of adolescent college freshmen ($N = 34$) to complete the APES and then compared their scores with the responses of a roommate or close friend of the subject who served as a collateral informant. In addition to reporting the experiencing of events, the collateral informant was asked to indicate whether the events were perceived by the subject as desirable or undesirable. The resulting percentage of agreement figure for reports of events experienced and not experienced was 82. When the desirability of events was taken into account, percentage of agreement for events reported by both respondents as either positive or negative was 87 percent. These findings suggest that the life events reported by the respondents were likely to have been events actually experienced by the subject, rather than the result of inaccurate or biased reporting.

Although very new, this scale appears to have several advantages for use with adolescents. First, it provides the most extensive listing of life events of any existing adolescent measure. As was not the case with most previous measures, specific attention was also focused on including a larger sample of events that were likely to be perceived as positive by adolescent respondents. It is encouraging that preliminary data suggest that indices of life change derived from the scale are significantly related to measures that might be expected to be associated with stressful life events.

These positive attributes notwithstanding, there are several limitations of the APES that need to be addressed in future research. Although reliability and validity data have been reported, these data are based almost exclusively on administration of the APES to older adolescent and college samples. This heavy reliance on data obtained from older adolescents means that there is a paucity of information regarding the validity of this measure with much younger adolescents. Clearly, more data on younger age groups are necessary.

Finally, while it is apparent that the APES demonstrates adequate reliability for events reported over a 3-month interval (at least for college students), reliability for events assessed over a longer time interval would be desirable. Although it is possible that the recall of events over a longer period of time may be impaired by a variety of factors, such as memory, the fact that many life event investigations ask respondents to report events occurring over a longer time interval (typically 12 months) makes these data especially relevant. Despite these limitations, the Adolescent Perceived Events Scale represents one of the more well-developed measures available for use with older adolescent populations.

ASSESSMENT OF LIFE EVENTS IN FAMILIES

Adolescent–Family Inventory of Life Events and Changes

Rather than focusing exclusively on child or adolescent life events, McCubbin, Patterson, Bauman, and Harris (1982) have developed the Adolescent–Family Inventory of Life Events and Changes (A-FILE) to provide a measure of family-related stressors. This approach evolved from viewing the family as a social system made up of interconnected members and therorizing that all events affecting one member affect other family members as well. Patterson and McCubbin (1983) posit that life changes experienced by the family will be associated with a decline in both family functioning and the functioning of individuals within the family system (see McCubbin & McCubbin, Chapter 11, this volume).

The A-FILE consists of 50 self-report items, designed to assess life events and changes experienced by members of the adolescent's family. Item content reflects family-related events similar to those included in adult and child life event measures. McCubbin and colleagues (1982) also included events that are believed to be experienced by families as a result of moving through different stages of the family life cycle. Both positive and negative events are included, as all are assumed to require at least some readjustment in the regular pattern of interaction among family members. Examles of events included within each of the six categories of events are presented in Table 13.2.

Scoring of the A-FILE involves simply computing the unweighted sum of the total number of life events experienced, with no separation of desirable and undesirable events. An attempt was originally made to use weights similar to those

TABLE 13.2. EXAMPLES OF A-FILE EVENTS

Transitions (14 items)
- Parents separated or divorced
- Family moved to a new home

Losses (7 items)
- Parent died
- Death of a close friend or family member

Responsibilities and strains (19 items)
- Parent(s) and teenager(s) have increased arguments (hassles) over choice of friends and/or social activities
- Increase in parent's time away from family
- Family member ran away

Legal conflict (2 items)
- Family member was robbed or attacked (physically or sexually)
- Family member went to jail, juvenile detention, or was placed on court probation

Sexuality (4 items)
- Unmarried family member became pregnant
- Family member had abortion

Substance abuse (4 items)
- Family member drinks too much alcohol

Source: Adapted from McCubbin, Patterson, Bauman, & Harris (1982)

derived by Coddington (1972a) and Holmes and Rahe (1967). However, these proved to be no more useful than the simpler unit rating procedure.

Validity and Reliability Studies. In addition to providing normative data on 500 male and female junior and senior high school students, the authors have reported preliminary data concerning the validity and reliability of the A-FILE. In a test–retest reliability study, A-FILE scores were obtained for 74 junior and senior high school students after a 2-week interval. McCubbin, Needle, and Wilson (1985) report a test–retest correlation coefficient of .84, suggesting adequate test–retest reliability. The authors also note that overall scores derived from the A-FILE have been found to correlate with variables such as health locus of control, with higher A-FILE life event scores being associated with lowered perceptions of control over health-related behaviors. McCubbin and colleagues (1985) have found A-FILE scores to be significantly correlated with reports of adolescent substance abuse, such as cigarette, marijuana, and alcohol consumption. It should be noted that scores on a companion measure, the Family Inventory of Life Events (FILE; Patterson & McCubbin, 1983), developed for use with other family members, have also been determined to correlate significantly with child health status when administered to families having a chronically ill child (cystic fibrosis). Scores on this measure have also been shown to correlate significantly with general measures of family functioning, such as assessed by the Moos (1976) Family Environment Scale.

Thus despite the limited data currently available regarding the validity of the A-FILE, findings related specifically to this measure, when considered along with those obtained from the FILE, appear to provide tentative support for the usefulness of family-based life event measures; however, additional research is clearly required.

METHODOLOGICAL CONCERNS IN LIFE STRESS ASSESSMENT

Having considered the nature and adequacy of several child, adolescent, or family life event measures, it would seem important to comment at least briefly on a range of more general methodological issues relevant to life event assessment. These questions have to do with issues such as the importance of assessing event desirability, the method of weighting specific events, the best source of life event data, as well as the sampling of life events.

While the results of several studies with adults (cf. Sarason et al., 1978; Vinokur & Selzer, 1975) and children (cf. Compas et al., 1985; Gad & Johnson, 1980; Johnson & McCutcheon, 1980; Swearingen & Cohen, 1985) have found negative life event scores to be more highly correlated with measures of psychological adjustment than global scores (positive and negative events combined), there is less information available regarding the relationship between positive and negative life events and physical health outcomes. At this time, there are only three investigations that have considered health-related variables (Brand et al., 1985; Greene, Walker, Hickson, & Thompson, 1985; Smith et al., 1983). Each of these investigations found that negative life change scores were more highly correlated with the dependent measures than were positive change scores. Given the positive findings in investigations of psychological adjustment, and the promising findings of health-related investigations, it would seem prudent to assess positive and negative life events separately. Failure to do so may result in lowered correlations and a loss of important data.

The actual determination of the valence of a particular event can be accomplished either by asking judges to categorize an event as desirable or undesirable or by having each subject make that determination. The available research does not provide a strong argument for or against either method. Results from studies with adult subjects (e.g., Mueller et al., 1977; Vinokur & Selzer, 1975) indicate that positive and negative change scores determined either way were equally predictive of measures of adjustment; similar findings with adolescents have been reported by Swearingen and Cohen (1985).

In addition to the issue of assessing event desirability, there is that of how experienced events should be weighted. As has been indicated, several approaches have been used. Most notable in this regard is the use of life change units to weight events, as is advocated by Coddington (1972), and the use of individualized impact ratings as provided for in the Life Events Checklist (Johnson & McCutcheon, 1980). Other approaches have involved simple counts of the number of events experienced. At present, there seem to be few data supporting the superiority of any of these approaches over others. While intuitively it seems that some events have a much greater impact on the person than other events, and should thus be weighted differently, research to date has failed to show any method of weighting to be superior to a simple count of the number of positive and negative events experienced. Thus while the separate assessment of positive and negative events appears to have received considerable support, the importance of the differential weighting of events is unclear (Johnson, 1982; Johnson & McCutcheon, 1980). Further research on this issue seems warranted.

Another question has to do with *who* should report the life events. Although it might be argued that the child or adolescent is the ideal respondent, there are instances where the child is either too young to provide accurate recall of events or unavailable, and the parent is placed in this role. While both parents and children have been utilized as respondents in the investigations previously described, only the Gilbert (1985) study provides data addressing the agreement of parent and child or adolescent report.

In the Gilbert (1985) investigation, children and adolescents (11 to 19 years old) and their parents were asked to complete the Life Events Checklist. Results of this study yielded only moderate correlations between life stress scores provided by parent and child, and depending upon the method used to compute the scores, ranged from .35 to .60. Gilbert (1985) reports that children and adolescents reported significantly more events than did their parent.

Although this study does not provide information regarding the relative accuracy of parent and child reports of life events, it does suggest that the reports obtained are not identical. As noted previously, this study does not provide any data regarding the occurrence or nonoccurrence of specific events. Future research to determine the degree to which the two respondents agree on particular events is necessary.

A final issue has to do with the sampling of life events and the adequacy with which life event measures provide a representative sampling of such events. With the exception of that of Compas and colleagues (1985), child and adolescent life change measures fail to assess many of the day-to-day stressors referred to by other investigators as hassles (Kanner et al., 1981; Lazarus, DeLongis, Folkman,

& Gruen, 1985). Lazarus and his colleagues (e.g., DeLongis et al., 1982; Kanner et al., 1981; Lazarus et al., 1985) report findings with adults that suggest that measures of daily small events or hassles may be more highly correlated with health-related measures than are measures of major life change. It is conceivable that the reliance on only one class of events (major life events) reduces the probability of determining significant relationships between life events or daily hassles and health-related outcomes. Compas and colleagues' (1985) inclusion of a broader range of items represents an appropriate and significant modification of life event measures.

THE RELATIONSHIP BETWEEN LIFE CHANGE AND PHYSICAL ILLNESS

While research into the effects of life stress has become popular only within the past 10 to 15 years, there are now more than 1000 published studies in this area, and the number of such investigations is increasing each year. One reason for the increasing popularity of this area relates to the fact that life stress measures have been found to relate to a host of physical health problems.

Studies with adults, for example, have suggested significant relationships between measures of life change and problems such as cardiac death and myocardial infarction (Edwards, 1971; Lundberg, Theorell, & Lind, 1975; Rahe & Lind, 1971; Rahe & Paasikivi, 1971; Theorell & Rahe, 1971), hypertension (Lal, Ahuja, & Madhukar, 1982), pregnancy and birth complications (Gorsuch & Key, 1974; Nuckolls, Cassell, & Kaplan, 1972), and menstrual discomfort (Siegel, Johnson, & Sarason, 1979). Reported life stress has also been found to relate to symptom severity, degree of control over illness, or recurrent symptoms in individuals with chronic illnesses such as asthma (De Araujo, Van Arsdel, Holmes, & Dudley, 1973), diabetes (Bradley, 1977), and genital herpes (Watson, 1983). Wyler, Masuda, and Holmes (1971) have also found a significant relationship between life stress and illness severity, with higher life stress scores being associated with more serious types of illness. Finally, other investigators have reported relationships between life stress scores and athletic injuries (Bramwell, Wagner, Masuda, & Holmes, 1975) and work-related accidents (Levenson, Hirschfeld, Hirschfeld, & Dzubay, 1983).

While it is necessary to interpret these findings with caution (as few studies allow one to infer the existence of a causal relationship), these findings taken together support the hypothesis that reports of adult life stress are significantly associated with a variety of physical health problems. This conclusion is generally consistent with the views of Holmes and Masuda (1974), who have suggested that, rather than being associated just with stress-related disorders, life stress may contribute to the development of a range of physical problems by increasing one's susceptibility to illness. Despite the intuitive appeal of this hypothesis, we actually know very little regarding the mechanism(s) by which life stress may increase the probability of physical health problems, although there are studies that suggest that stress can adversely influence immunocompetence, thus making the person more susceptible to a range of health problems (Jemmott & Locke, 1984).

While the large majority of life stress investigations have been with adults, investigators have recently turned their attention to the correlates of reported life stress in younger individuals. Here, life stress, assessed via measures such as those described earlier, has been found to be related to a broad range of children's health problems. In the sections to follow we will examine life change as it relates to general health status, including accidental injury, the onset of specific health problems, and the exacerbation of chronic illness.

Life Stress and General Health Status

Accidents account for more than 100,000 deaths in the United States each year. In 1980, accidental injury was responsible for 46 percent of all deaths in children between the ages of 1 and 4 years; this is three times the number of deaths resulting from congenital anomalies, which represent the second leading cause of death. For children between the ages of 5 and 14 years, accidents account for 55 percent of all deaths (Baker, O'Neill, & Karpf, 1984). It has been suggested that the ratio of nonlethal accidents to lethal accidents may be as high as 200 to 1 (Barnett & Einhorn, 1972); thus accidents represent a serious health problem for children and adolescents and are a growing public concern. Because of this, researchers have begun to investigate a variety of factors, including stress, that may contribute to accidental injuries in children. Padilla and colleagues' (1976) investigation, which was reviewed previously, represents one such attempt to examine this relationship. Two additional studies merit consideration (see also Wright, Flagler, & Friedman, Chapter 20, this volume).

Beautrais, Fergusson, and Shannon (1982) investigated the relationship between family life changes and childhood morbidity in 1265 children between the ages of 1 and 4 years. Major life changes during the child's first 4 years of life were obtained by having the parents complete a modified version of the Holmes and Rahe (1967) scale. Information pertaining to a variety of factors was obtained: visits to a general practitioner, hospital attendance, and hospital admissions for several types of illness, hospital admissions for accidental poisoning, burns, and scalds, hospital admissions for other types of accidents (lacerations, bruising, fractures), and suspect home conditions. Beautrais and colleagues (1982) reported increased levels of family stress to be associated with an increased incidence of various types of accidents, as well as with suspect home conditions and the development of various types of physical illness (respiratory and gastrointestinal problems). The authors note that there was a general trend for morbidity rates to increase in direct proportion to the amount of stress reported. In fact, children from families that reported 12 or more major life events were found to be, on the average, six times more likely to have been hospitalized than were children from families reporting 3 or fewer life events. Children whose families reported high levels of stress were also more likely to have been seen by a private practitioner or to have had contact with a hospital as an outpatient. Importantly, the significant relationships between reported stress and child morbidity were obtained even after controlling for such variables as maternal age, ethnic status, educational level, and family size, thereby decreasing the probability that these findings were the result of an extraneous uncontrolled-for variable(s).

A final study relevant to this topic was reported by Coddington and Troxell (1980), who obtained life stress scores for 114 high school football players and then monitored these students to determine the frequency of athletic injuries during the subsequent football season. Those students who reported events such as parental illness, separations, divorces, and deaths in the family were found to be significantly more likely to sustain significant athletic injury than those who did not report such events. These findings are similar to those reported by Bramwell and colleagues (1975), who found that major injuries to college football players were related to the level of life events reported. Taken together, these findings suggest a general relationship between the amount of life stress experienced by the child, adolescent, and/or family and accidental injuries of various types.

Aagaard, Husfeldt, and Husfeldt (1983) reported the results of a prospective investigation of children seen within a general practice in Denmark. The authors collected information concerning sociodemographic factors, diseases, and reported life events (using a modified version of the Coddington scale) for 386 children and families contacting their general practitioner. One year later, information regarding the children's current health status was obtained; specifically, Aagaard and colleagues (1983) were interested in admissions to the hospital, number of contacts with the physician, and the parents' perceptions of the children's health status. This information was supplemented with data from the medical records at the hospital and general practitioner. The authors report that higher levels of reported life events were associated with an increased probability of visits to the physician, but did not appear to be related to hospitalizations within the year-long period of the investigation.

Several other investigations already reviewed in this chapter have examined the relationship between life change and more general measures of child health and illness. For example, Gad and Johnson (1980) found that measures of negative life change were significantly correlated with the number of visits to the physician, reports of diagnosed illness, and self-reports of physical health problems. Johnson and McCutcheon (1980) also found that, for male subjects, reported life event scores were significantly correlated with the number of school days missed because of illness, reports of physical health problems, and self-ratings of physical health. Finally, Hotaling, Atwell, and Linsky (1970) examined the relationship between life stress (as reported on the senior high version of the Coddington Life Events Record) and the number of illnesses over the last 12 months and ratings of physical health during the study (based on number of illnesses and degree of incapacitation). Life stress scores were found to be significantly related to seriousness of illness, although no relationship was found when number of illnesses was taken as the dependent measure. Further examination of the data by assessing the differential relationship between measures of positive and negative life change and seriousness of illness suggested that the previously obtained relationship was primarily attributable to the effects of negative change, since only the negative change measure was found to relate significantly to the seriousness of illness index.

Life Change and Specific Health Problems

Perhaps the earliest investigation to examine the relationship between life events and the occurrence of illness was that reported by Meyer and Haggerty (1962). Although these authors did not use any of the previously described instruments, they followed 100 children prospectively for a period of 12 months; throat cultures for streptococcal infections were taken from each child every 2 weeks. For a measure of life events, family members were also asked to keep a diary of "upsetting" events experienced during this time and to record any illnesses. The results of this study suggested that the 2 weeks prior to the emergence of a streptococcal infection were typically marked by an increased level of upsetting events, and that these were correlated with clinical manifestations of upper respiratory tract illness. While not all infections were preceded by upsetting events, the authors found that the probability of infection significantly increased when stressful events were experienced. This is cautiously interpreted as suggesting that stressful events may contribute to the development of this particular variety of illness.

Some studies have dealt with life events in relation to several specific illnesses. For example, Heisel, Ream, Raitz, Rappaport, and Coddington (1973) obtained life stress scores on children with a variety of health problems including 34 children with juvenile rheumatoid arthritis (JRA), 31 children hospitalized for appendectomies or herniorrhaphies, 32 children seen on a general pediatric inpatient service for a variety of physical complaints, and 35 children diagnosed with hemophilia. Subjects in each of the first three groups were assessed with regard to the degree of life stress experienced during the year preceding the current admission, using the Coddington Life Events Record. For hemophilic children, the relationship between the number of hemorrhages and life events that occurred during each year of a 2-year period was examined. When life stress scores for children in the JRA, general pediatric, and surgery groups were individually compared to life stress scores reported by a normative sample of healthy children (Coddington, 1972b), each of these groups reported significantly higher life stress scores. Among children with hemophilia, a general relationship between life stress scores and hemorrhagic episodes was also obtained. Coddington (1979) notes, however, that the strength of this relationship was attentuated when the frequent hospitalizations experienced by these children were taken into account. Heisel and colleagues (1973) interpret their findings as evidence for a general relationship between stressful life change and the development of childhood illness, or in the case of hemophilia, the exacerbation of an already existing illness.

Cardiovascular Risk Factors. An investigation reported by Gillum, Prineas, Gomez-Marin, Chang, and Finn (1984) presents data on the relationship between life events and cardiovascular risk factors. As part of a large-scale investigation of children's blood pressure, Recent Life Events questionnaires were completed by the parents of 1505 school children between the ages of 6 and 9 years (mean age was 8.9 years). Blood pressure, pulse rate, height, weight, and skin fold thickness were collected biannually during the 1977–1978 school year. Gillum and colleagues (1984) report that the frequency of reported life events was not significantly related to blood pressure at either baseline or follow-up; similarly, no relationship was obtained between reported life events and any of the other risk factor measures. The frequency of reported events was found to be related to measures of socioeconomic status, with higher life event scores being associated with children from lower socioeconomic status households. Race was also determined to be a significant variable in the relationship, as Black and American Indian children were reported to have experienced significantly more life events in the past 12 months than other children.

Pregnancy. Although not properly considered an illness, pregnancy in adolescence is recognized as a high-risk condition for both the mother and fetus. In

1980, there were more than 3,600,000 live births in the United States. Girls less than 15 years of age delivered 10,169 live births, while 552,151 children were born to mothers between the ages of 15 and 19 years. Significantly, pregnant girls less than 15 years of age have a 60 percent higher maternal mortality rate than older mothers (Carey, McCann-Sanford, & Davidson, 1981). Additionally, young mothers, particularly those less than 20 years of age, are more likely to give birth to premature infants and infants with a variety of perinatal and neonatal difficulties (Placek, 1977). Given the increase in the frequency of teenage pregnancies in recent years, many investigators have sought to identify factors that may contribute to pregnancy in this age group.

For example, Coddington (1979) obtained information regarding the amount of life stress experienced over a 12-month period (which covered events occurring up to 7 to 10 months prior to conception) from 121 pregnant adolescents between the ages of 14 and 19 years. A control group of 261 adolescent girls who were not pregnant provided similar information. Comparisons of these groups in terms of overall level of life stress suggested that pregnant adolescents reported significantly higher levels of prior life change than did subjects in the control group. Particularly noteworthly were the differences reported regarding family life events, over which the adolescent had little or no control. Pregnant subjects reported death or illness of a parent, death of a grandparent, and separation of parents more often than did the adolescents who were not pregnant. There was also a nonsignificant trend for pregnant subjects to report the death of a sibling more often than nonpregnant subjects.

Coddington (1979) also examined the relationship between reported life stress and obstetric complications. Information for 55 of the cases just mentioned was obtained through record review; no relationship between life stress scores and complications was found. Coddington (1979) notes that this was not unexpected; previous research (Nuckolls et al., 1972) suggested that the relationship between life stress scores and obstetric complications for adult subjects may be mediated by other variables, such as social support or the degree of psychosocial assets displayed by the expectant mother. In Nuckolls and colleagues' (1972) study, women reporting high life stress and low levels of support were at greater risk. Given that potential moderators of this relationship were not assessed in the Coddington (1979) study, it is possible that life stress scores may have been related to complications in some undetermined subset of the sample, even in the absence of a significant overall correlation. The role of moderator variables will be examined in more depth in a later section of this chapter.

As a final point in the discussion of this study, it should be noted that the differences between pregnant and nonpregnant adolescents may be at least partially accounted for by sociodemographic differences between the two groups, as the groups differed in terms of both race and socioeconomic status. That is, Black females were overly represented among pregnant adolescents, as were those from lower socioeconomic groups. Given research findings that suggest that Black adolescents as a group are more likely to report higher levels of life stress (negative change events) and that life stress appears to be negatively correlated with socioeconomic variables (Gad & Johnson, 1980), the failure to control for such factors represents a significant limitation of this study. Further research, designed to clarify the relationship between life stress and adolescent pregnancy and control for such confounding factors, is needed.

Recurrent Pain. In addition to Hodges and colleagues' (1984) study described earlier, several recent investigations have examined the relationship between life events and recurrent pain in children and adolescents. In one such investigation (Pantell & Goodman, 1983), 100 adolescents presenting to a medical school adolescent clinic with symptoms of recurrent chest pain were studied. Using items from the Coddington Life Events Record as a semistructured interview, these authors report that 31 percent of the subjects reported the occurrence of significant negative events within 6 months of the onset of their pain. Unfortunately, a control group was not similarly studied, and the authors did not report specific life change scores for the recurrent pain subjects.

Greene and colleagues (1985) also examined the relationship between life stress scores and recurrent abdominal or chest pain. One hundred and seventy-two children and adolescents (11 to 19 years old) seen in a medical center adolescent clinic were routinely administered Johnson and McCutcheon's Life Events Checklist. On the basis of a complete medical history, physical examination, and laboratory findings, patients were placed into one of six diagnostic groups: (1) those who simply received a routine checkup; (2) those who had acute minor illnesses (without abdominal or chest pain); (3) those with abdominal pain, chest pain, or headache that had a clinically diagnosed physical origin; (4) those who had recurrent abdominal pain, chest pain, or headache without an identifiable physical basis; (5) those with behavioral problems; and (6) those displaying chronic illnesses of various types.

There were no differences between any of the groups in terms of positive change scores on the LEC. However, those patients reporting recurrent pain without an identifiable physical origin and those presenting with behavioral problems as primary concerns were found to differ from all other groups with regard to the amount of negative change reported. These findings are consistent with those reported by Hodges and colleagues (1984) in suggesting a significant relationship between life stress scores and recurrent pain (without physical basis) displayed by children and adolescents. In considering the results of their investigation, Greene and colleagues (1985) suggest that life stress measures may be useful additions to the armamentarium of the practitioner in assessing adolescent problems, and that they may facilitate the exploration of psychosocial factors associated with physical problems.

Respiratory Illness. Boyce and colleagues (1973) examined the relationship between life stress and respiratory illness in 58 children (mean age 4.3 years). Subjects in this study attended a day-care–elementary school center. As part of a larger study, each of these children was assessed 5 days per week over a 1-year time period to obtain clinical and laboratory data concerning the presence and severity of respiratory tract illness. Specifically, four dependent measures were examined: number of illnesses; average duration of illness; average severity of illness; and a composite sickness score. At the end of the 1-year study period, the parents of these children were interviewed retrospectively to assess the degree of life stress experienced during the time period (life stress was assessed via the Coddington Life Events Record).

Life change scores were found to be positively correlated with average duration and severity of illness, but not with the number of illnesses. Additional multiple regression analyses, which focused on the relationship between life stress scores and dependent measures while controlling for several potentially confounding variables (sex, race, age, family size), also provided support for an association between reported life stress and these variables.

Children in the study were also classified as coming from families characterized by high or low attention to routine. Analyses of the joint relationships among life stress scores, adherence to family routine, and illness were found to provide support for the combined effects of the predictor variables (life stress scores and family routine) when the illness severity index was considered. The results suggested that children who were reported to have experienced high levels of life stress and who resided in a highly routinized family were most likely to have increased severity of illness scores. Thus these data support the hypothesis that reported life stress is a predictor of respiratory illness duration, whereas severity of illness can best be predicted by considering the joint effects of life change and adherence to family routines. In addition to providing a measure of support for the association between child life stress and respiratory illness, this investigation highlights an issue raised earlier regarding the potentially important contribution of moderator variables to this association. Although the authors initially hypothesized that the relationship between life stress and illness would be attenuated by a high level of family routinization, the role of family routine in the life stress–respiratory illness relationship was not in that direction. Boyce and colleagues (1973) reported that high life stress scores in a highly routinized family were associated with an increased severity of respiratory difficulties. While the reasons for this interaction are unclear, the role of the family in coping with life stress merits further investigation.

Childhood Cancer. An additional illustration of studies examining the relationship between measures of life change and the onset of specific types of childhood illness is provided by Jacob and Charles (1980), who extended the work of earlier studies by Green and his colleagues (Green, 1952, 1954; Green, Young, Swisher, & Miller, 1955). In this series of studies, these investigators reported that 31 of 33 pediatric leukemic patients had experienced major losses or separations in the 2 years preceding the onset of their illness. One-half of these losses were reported to have occurred in the 6-month interval immediately prior to the onset of the disease.

Jacob and Charles (1980) compared the life stress scores of 25 children with leukemia, lymphoma, or other malignancy to a well-matched group (matched for age, sex, and socioeconomic status) of control children. The children in the control group were recruited from a general pediatric clinic and presented with a range of less serious physical complaints such as sore throat and respiratory infection. Life events experienced by the family (and thus presumably influencing the child) were assessed by having the parents retrospectively complete the Schedule of Recent Experiences (Holmes & Rahe, 1967) with regard to events experienced by the child or family during the year prior to the onset of illness.

In terms of the total life change unit scores, mean scores of 197 and 91.8 were determined for the childhood cancer group and the control group, respectively; this difference was statistically significant. A comparison of the number of events experienced indicated that the childhood cancer group was reported to have experienced approximately twice the number of events as control subjects (5.7 vs. 2.8).

Jacobs and Charles (1980) also examined the extent to which specific events were reported more frequently for the childhood cancer group than for the general pediatric clinic subjects. Among these events were marital separation, death of a close family member (52 percent of children in the cancer group had experienced parental separation or loss of a family member other than the parent during the past year, as opposed to 16 percent of the control group), change in residence (72 percent vs. 24 percent), change in schools (56 percent vs. 32 percent), change in the health of a family member (60 percent vs. 24 percent), change in the number of arguments among family members (20 percent vs. 4 percent), and others. These findings suggest, then, that children with cancer differ from controls not only in terms of reported levels of overall stress, but also to some extent in terms of the specific events reported. Appropriately, the authors caution against construing these results as evidence of a causal relationship between family life stress and childhood cancer; however, these findings are suggestive, and further studies in this area are in order.

Juvenile-Onset Diabetes. Leaverton, White, McCormick, Smith, and Sheikholislam (1980) examined the relationship between parental loss and the onset of diabetes in children. They compared a group of 121 insulin-dependent diabetic children less than 18 years of age with a control group of 37 children drawn from the general population who were matched for age, sex, race, and socioeconomic status. Parent reports of life events were used to obtain data on parental loss as well as other stressors. When diabetic and control children were compared for the occurrence of parental loss (by separation, divorce, or death) before the onset of diabetes, a significant relationship was obtained. Parental loss was reported in 42 percent of the families of diabetic children, and in only 19 percent of the families of control children. These findings were interpreted as support of parental loss as an antecedent factor in the development of diabetes, although it is clear that a causal relationship cannot be assumed. Stein and Charles (1971) also reported a higher frequency of parental loss and serious family disturbance in a group of diabetic children than in a comparison group of children with other chronic illnesses.

Life Events and the Exacerbation of Chronic Illness

In contrast to the investigations just described that examined the relationship between reported life events and the onset of various illnesses, several authors have investigated the relationship between reported life events and changing health status in children and adolescents with chronic illnesses. Research addressing this relationship will be the focus of this section.

Bedell, Giordani, Amour, Tavormina, and Boll (1977) examined the relationship between reported life events and physical health problems in children attending a 3-week summer camp for the chronically ill. Forty-five children with a range of illnesses including diabetes, asthma, and cystic fibrosis were administered the Coddington Life Events Record in addition to certain personality instruments. The camp counselors, who were blind to the children's life events scores, were then asked to record the frequency of any physical health problem related to their illness while at camp.

The results of this study indicated that children with high levels of reported life events demonstrated significantly more illness-related episodes than did those children with low life events scores. During the 3-week camp, children with high life events scores experienced 69 illness-related episodes, as compared to only 19 episodes by children with low life events scores. The authors do not indicate whether any specific illness was more highly related to illness episodes while at camp, nor do they provide data supporting the reliability with which the illness-related episodes were observed, suggesting that these results must be cautiously interpreted.

A number of studies have examined the relationship between reported life events and juvenile-onset diabetes in children. For example, Chase and Jackson (1981) administered the Coddington Life Events Record to 84 children and adolescents with insulin-dependent diabetes mellitus during routine clinic visits. Life events were reported retrospectively over the past 3 months, which generally covered the time elapsed since the last clinic appointment. A variety of biochemical and clinical measures, reflecting the degree to which the child's diabetes was under control, were obtained within this same 3-month period. Life stress scores were found to be associated with a number of dependent measures including triglyceride and serum glocose concentrations, and cholesterol values. Children with elevated hemoglobin A1 values (a measure considered to be a cumulative index of blood sugar levels over the past 3 months) were also found to have higher life stress scores than those children with more clinically normal values. Finally, Chase and Jackson (1981) report that the life stress scores for children who had one or more hospitalizations during the previous 3 months for ketoacidosis were significantly higher than those for children who had not been hospitalized (mean life stress scores of 208 and 122, respectively). It is important to note that, while this investigation does provide support for the relationship between life events and diabetic control, the relationship held only for older subjects in the sample (15 to 19 years old).

Brand and colleagues (1986) examined the relationship between life stress scores and diabetic control in a group of 141 children and adolescents between the ages of 10 and 17 years attending a 2-week diabetes camp. The Johnson and McCutcheon (1980) Life Events Checklist was administered to determine life events reports during the past 1-year period. Additionally, blood and urine sugar levels, hemoglobin A1, and an index of urine ketone levels were obtained as measures of diabetic control while the children were at camp. Each camper also completed a locus of control measure, to assess the degree to which the relationship between reported life events and diabetic control might vary as a function of the child's perception of control over his or her environment.

Brand and colleagues (1986) report no significant relationship between positive change scores and any of the measures of diabetic control. Negative life change scores, however, were found to be significantly related to urine ketone levels. This relationship was determined primarily for younger males whose locus of control was internally oriented. It is noteworthy that the strongest relationship between negative change scores and ketone levels was found for the internally oriented rather than the externally oriented children. Brand and colleagues (1985) speculate that, given the belief that one is capable of exerting a degree of control over one's environment (internal locus of control), experiencing life changes that are outside of one's control (e.g., parental loss) may actually be more stressful than if one sees such events as clearly uncontrollable (external locus of control). No significant correlations between life change scores and blood and/or urine sugar measures were obtained.

The results of Brand and colleagues' (1986) and Chase and Jackson's (1981) investigations do provide some measure of support for a relationship between reported life changes and some aspects of diabetic control. Brand and colleagues' study, however, suggests that primarily negative changes are related to measures of control, and that this relationship does vary as a function of age, sex, and locus of control.

The health status of adolescents with cystic fibrosis was the focus of a recent investigation by Smith and colleagues (1983). These authors administered the Johnson and McCutcheon (1980) Life Events Checklist to a sample of 26 adolescents (mean age 15 years) and compared their scores to the scores of subjects from the general population. No significant differences were found for life events scores between the two groups. The authors also categorized each patient with regard to the degree of impairment exhibited (based on measures of pulmonary function, X ray, and a rating of the patient's overall condition). When patients were categorized along the severity of impairment dimension, it was found that patients with more severe impairment reported life events scores that were significantly higher than those patients with milder impairment. These differences were obtained only for measures of negative life events, and were found regardless of whether negative change scores were based on a simple count of negative events reported or on a sum of the impact ratings associated with those events. Somewhat similar findings have been reported by Patterson and McCubbin (1983), who found increased levels of reported life stress experienced by the family (as reported on the Family Inventory of Life Events) to be related to pulmonary function in children with cystic fibrosis.

Child Life Stress and Health Status: An Overview and Summary

The investigations reviewed here provide tentative support for a relationship between life changes and the health status of children and adolescents. Scores on measures of life events were found to be associated with the frequency of childhood accidents and adolescent pregnancy. Data examining the relationship between these measures and self-report indices of general health status support such a relationship in regard to variables such as the number of visits to a physician, reports of physical health problems, reports of diagnosed illness, and number of school days missed because of illness. In studies examining the onset of illness, life events were found to be associated with the occurrence of juvenile rheumatoid arthritis, recurrent abdominal pain, childhood cancer, and the duration and severity of childhood illness. The results of other investigations suggest that reported life events may be related to changes in the health status of children and adolescents with chronic diseases such as diabetes and cystic fibrosis. Let us now consider some of the issues that have implications for future research, specifically the implication of causality and the potential role of moderator variables, and examine the effects of these problems on the interpretation of the relationship between life events and physical health status.

While the data presented in this chapter have tended to support the relationship between cumulative life changes and child health status, the exact nature of that relationship remains unclear; there are not yet sufficient data to conclude that it is life change that exerts a causal effect on child health and not vice versa. Because the majority of these studies are correlational in nature, any assumptions regarding causality must be made with a great deal of caution. Clearly, a prospective longitudinal assessment strategy is necessary to deal adequately with this issue (Kobasa, 1985). Only by collecting data in a prospective manner can researchers begin to address questions regarding biased recall (Brown, 1974) and the temporal relationship between the occurrence of life events and health-related problems.

In examining the relationship between life change and physical health status, it also becomes apparent that the correlations, while statistically significant, are generally small and thus account for a relatively minimal proportion of the variance in the dependent measures. For example, few studies report correlations greater than .30 or .40. The small percentage of variance accounted for is directly related to our ability to make predictions. While the exact nature of the measure of life stress employed may have an effect on producing small correlation coefficients, the adult literature would suggest that the failure to consider the important role of moderator variables may also be a major contributing factor (Sarason et al., 1979). Many life stress investigations have addressed the relationship between physical health and life change without considering other important variables that may mediate an individual's response to life change(s). For example, variables such as social support (Wilcox, 1981), perceived control (Lefcourt, Miller, Ware, & Sherk, 1981), sensation seeking (Smith, Johnson, & Sarason, 1978), and hardiness (Kobasa, Maddi, & Kahn, 1982) are among those reported to influence a person's response to life events. While most of these studies have been with adults, studies with children and adolescents have also provided support for the moderating role of variables such as locus of control (Brand et al., 1986), family structure (Boyce et al., 1973), and social support (Sandler, 1980). Although not examined extensively due to a lack of adequate measures, it is likely that other variables such as coping style might also be found to serve as moderators of the effects of life stress on children and adolescents. It is clear from the research conducted thus far that one should not assume a direct relationship between life events and health outcomes. Greater attention to the role of moderator variables in future research will most likely lead to the identification of stronger and more meaningful relationships between life events and child health status.

In conclusion, the focus of this chapter has been on describing the various life event measures currently available, reviewing research regarding their adequacy, and examining research findings regarding the relationship between cumulative life changes and child health status. While there are presently fewer studies investigating this relationship than there are investigating the association between life change and psychological adjustment, existing studies do suggest a link between life change and child health. Prospective investigations that examine the role of moderator variables in mediating the response to these events are now needed to help us gain a better understanding of the exact nature of this relationship.

References

Aagaard, J., Husfeldt, P., & Husfeldt, V. (1983). Social factors and life events as predictors for children's health: A one year prospective study. *Acta Paediatrica Scandinavia*, 72, 275–281.

Baker, S. P., O'Neill, B., & Karpf, R. (1984). *The injury fact book*. Lexington, MA: Lexington Books.

Barnett, H. L., & Einhorn, A. H. (1972). *Pediatrics*. New York: Appleton-Century-Crofts.

Beautrais, A. L., Fergusson, D. M., & Shannon, F. T. (1982). Life events and childhood morbidity: A prospective study. *Pediatrics, 70,* 935–940.

Bedell, J. R., Giordani, B., Amour, J. L., Tavormina, J., & Boll, T. (1977). Life stress and the psychological and medical adjustment of chronically ill children. *Journal of Psychosomatic Research, 21,* 237–242.

Boyce, T. W., Jensen, E. W., Cassell, J. C., Collier, A. M., Smith, A. H., & Raimey, C. T. (1973). Influence of life events and family routines on childhood respiratory tract illness. *Pediatrics, 60,* 609–615.

Bradley, C. (1979). Life events and the control of diabetes mellitus. *Journal of Psychosomatic Research, 23,* 159–162.

Bramwell, S. T., Wagner, N. N., Masuda, M., & Holmes, T. H. (1975). Psychosocial factors in athletic injuries. *Journal of Human Stress, 1,* 6–20.

Brand, A. H., & Johnson, J. H. (1982). Note on the reliability of the Life Events Checklist. *Psychological Reports, 50,* 1274.

Brand, A. H., Johnson, J. H., & Johnson, S. B. (1986). *Life stress and diabetic control in insulin-dependent diabetic children and adolescents. Journal of Pediatric Psychology, 11,* 481–495.

Brown, G. (1974). Meaning, measurement and stress of life events. In B. S. Dohrenwend & B. P. Dohrenwend (Eds.), *Stressful life events: Their nature and effects.* New York: Wiley.

Carey, W. B., McCann-Sanford, T., & Davidson, E. C. (1981). Adolescent age and obstetric risk. *Seminars in Perinatology, 5,* 9–17.

Chase, H. P., & Jackson, G. G. (1981). Stress and sugar control in children with insulin-dependent diabetes mellitus. *The Journal of Pediatrics, 98,* 1011–1013.

Coddington, R. D. (1972a). The significance of life events as etiologic factors in the diseases of children: A survey of professional workers. *Journal of Psychosomatic Research, 16,* 7–18.

Coddington, R. D. (1972b). The significance of life events as etiologic factors in the disease of children: A study of a normal population. *Journal of Psychosomatic Research, 16,* 205–213.

Coddington, R. D. (1979). Life events associated with adolescent pregnancies. *Journal of Clinical Psychiatry, 40,* 180–185.

Coddington, R. D., & Troxell, J. R. (1980). The effect of emotional factors on football injury rates: A pilot study. *Journal of Human Stress, 6,* 3–5.

Compas, B. E., Davis, G. E., & Forsythe, C. J. (1985). *Assessment of major and daily life events during adolescence: The Adolescent Perceived Events Scale.* Unpublished manuscript, University of Vermont.

Compas, B. E., & Wagner, B. M. (1985). *Reciprocal relationships of life events and daily hassles with psychological symptoms: A prospective study.* Paper presented at the annual convention of the American Psychological Association, Los Angeles.

De Araujo, G., Van Arsdel, P. P., Holmes, T. H., & Dudley, D. L. (1973). Life change, coping ability and chronic intrinsic asthma. *Journal of Psychosomatic Research, 17,* 359–363.

DeLongis, A., Coyne, J. C., Dakof, G., Folkman, S., & Lazarus, R. S. (1983). Relationship of daily hassles, uplifts, and major life events to health status. *Health Psychology, 1,* 119–136.

Derogatis, L. R., Lipman, R. S., Rickels, K., Uhlenhuth, E. H., & Covi, L. (1974). The Hopkins Symptom Checklist. *Pharmacopsychiatry, 7,* 79–110.

Edwards, M. K. (1971). *Life crises and myocardial infarction.* Unpublished master's thesis, University of Washington, Seattle.

Felner, R. D. (1984). Vulnerability in childhood: A preventative framework for understanding children's efforts to cope with life stress and transitions. In M. C. Roberts & L. Peterson (Eds.), *Prevention of problems in childhood.* New York: Wiley.

Felner, R. D., Farber, S. S., & Primavera, J. (1983). Transitions and stressful life events: A model for primary prevention. In R. D. Felner, L. A. Jason, J. N. Moritsugu, & S. S. Farber (Eds.), *Preventative psychology: Theory, research, and practice.* New York: Pergamon.

Ferguson, W. (1981). Gifted adolescents, stress and life changes. *Adolescence, 16,* 973–985.

Gad, M. T., & Johnson, J. H. (1980). Correlates of adolescent life stress as related to race, SES, and levels of perceived social support. *Journal of Clinical Child Psychology, 9,* 13–16.

Gilbert, B. (1985). *Physiological responsivity to venipuncture and speech giving in insulin-dependent diabetic adolescents at two levels of diabetic control and their nondiabetic peers.* Unpublished doctoral dissertation, University of Florida.

Gillum, R., Prineas, R., Gomez-Marin, O., Chang, P., & Finn, S. (1984). Recent life events in school children: Race, socioeconomic status and cardiovascular risk factors. *Journal of Chronic Diseases, 37,* 839–851.

Gorsuch, R. L., & Key, M. K. (1974). Abnormalities of pregnancy as a function of anxiety and life stress. *Psychosomatic Medicine, 36,* 352–361.

Green, W. A. (1952, March). *Psychological factors and reticuloendothelial disease.* Paper presented at the annual meeting of the American Psychosomatic Society, Chicago.

Green, W. A. (1954). Psychological factors and reticuloendothelial disease: Preliminary observations on a group of males with lymphomas and leukemias. *Psychosomatic Medicine, 16,* 220–230.

Green, W. A., Young, L. E., Swisher, S. N., & Miller, G. (1955). Psychological factors and reticuloendothelial disease: Observations on a group of females with lymphomas and leukemias. *Psychosomatic Medicine, 18,* 284–303.

Greenberg, M. T., Siegel, J. M., & Leitch, C. J. (1983). The nature and importance of attachment relationships to parents and peers during adolescence. *Journal of Youth & Adolescence, 12,* 373–386.

Greene, J. W., Walker, L. S., Hickson, G., & Thompson, J. (1985). Stressful life events and somatic complaints in adolescents. *Pediatrics, 75,* 19–22.

Heisel, J. S., Ream, S., Raitz, R., Rappaport, M., & Coddington, R. D. (1973). The significance of life events as contributing factors in the diseases of children. *Behavioral Pediatrics, 83,* 119–123.

Hodges, K., Kline, J. J., Barbero, G., & Flanery, R. (1984). Life events occurring in families of children with recurrent abdominal pain. *Journal of Psychosomatic Research, 28,* 185–188.

Holmes, T. H., & Masuda, M. (1974). Life change and illness susceptibility. In B. S. Dohrenwend & B. P. Dohrenwend (Eds.), *Stressful life events: Their nature and effects.* New York: Wiley.

Holmes, T. H., & Rahe, R. H. (1967). The social readjustment rating scale. *Journal of Psychosomatic Research, 11,* 213–218.

Hotaling, G. T., Atwell, S. G., & Linsky, A. S. (1978). Adolescent life change and illness: A comparison of three models. *Journal of Youth & Adolescence, 7,* 393–403.

Jacobs, T. J., & Charles, E. (1980). Life events and the occurrence of cancer in children. *Psychosomatic Medicine, 42,* 11–24.

Jemmott, J. B., & Locke, S. E. (1984). Psychosocial factors, immunologic mediation, and human susceptibility to infectious diseases: How much do we know? *Psychological Bulletin, 95,* 78–108.

Johnson, J. H. (1982). Life events as stressors in childhood and adolescence. In B. Lahey & A. Kazdin (Eds.), *Advances in clinical child psychology.* New York: Plenum.

Johnson, J. H., & McCutcheon, S. M. (1980). Assessing life stress in older children and adolescents: Preliminary findings with the Life Events Checklist. In I. G. Sarason & C. D. Spielberger (Eds.), *Stress and anxiety.* Washington, DC: Hemisphere.

Johnson, J. H., & Sarason, I. G. (1979). Moderator variables in life stress research. In I. G. Sarason & C. D. Spielberger (Eds.), *Stress and anxiety,* Washington, DC: Hemisphere.

Kanner, A. D., Coyne, J. C., Schaefer, C., & Lazarus, R. S. (1981). Comparison of two modes of stress measurement: Daily hassles and uplifts versus major life events. *Journal of Behavioral Medicine, 4,* 1–19.

Kobasa, S. (1985). Longitudinal and prospective methods in health psychology. In P. Karoly (Ed.), *Measurement strategies in health psychology.* New York: Wiley.

Kobasa, S. C., Maddi, S. R., & Kahn, S. (1982). Hardiness and health: A prospective study. *Journal of Personality and Social Psychology, 42,* 168–177.

Lal, N., Ahuja, R. C., & Madhukar, A. (1982). Life events in hypertensive patients. *Journal of Psychosomatic Research, 26,* 441–445.

Lazarus, R. S., DeLongis, A., Folkman, S., & Gruen, R. (1985). Stress and adaptational outcomes: The problem of confounded measures. *American Psychologist, 40,* 770–779.

Lazarus, R. S., & Folkman, S. (1984). *Stress, appraisal, and coping.* New York: Springer.

Leaverton, D. R., White, C. A., McCormick, C. R., Smith, P., & Sheikholislam, B. (1980). Paternal loss antecedent to childhood diabetes mellitis. *Journal of the American Academy of Child Psychiatry, 19,* 678–689.

Lefcourt, H. M., Miller, R. S., Warc, E., & Sherk, D. (1981). Locus of control as a modifier at the relationship between stressors and moods. *Journal of Personality and Social Psychology, 41*, 357–369.

Levenson, H., Hirschfeld, M. L., Hirschfeld, A., & Dzubay, B. (1983). Recent life events and accidents: The role of sex differences. *Journal of Human Stress, 9*, 4–8.

Lundberg, V., Theorell, T., & Lind, E. (1975). Life changes and myocardial infarction: Individual differences in life change scaling. *Journal of Psychosomatic Research, 19*, 27–32.

McCubbin, H. I., Needle, R. H., & Wilson, M. (1985). Adolescent health risk behaviors: Family stress and adolescent coping as critical factors. *Family Relations, 34*, 51–62.

McCubbin, H. I., Patterson, J. M., Bauman, E., & Harris, L. (1982). Adolescent—Family Inventory of Life Events. In D. Olson, H. McCubbin, H. Barnes, & A. Larsen (Eds.), *Family Inventories*. St. Paul, MN: Author.

McCubbin, H. I., Patterson, J. M., & Wilson, L. R. (1982). Family inventory of life events and changes. In D. Olson, H. I. McCubbin, H. Barnes, & A. Larsen (Eds.), *Family inventories*. St. Paul, MN: Author.

Meyer, R. J., & Haggerty, R. J. (1962). Streptococcal infections in families. *Pediatrics, 29*, 539–549.

Monaghan, J. H., Robinson, J. O., & Dodge, J. A. (1979). The Children's Life Events Inventory. *Journal of Psychosomatic Research, 23*, 63–68.

Moos, R. (1974). *Preliminary manual for the Family Environment Scale*. Palo Alto, CA: Consulting Psychologists Press.

Mueller, D. P., Edwards, D. W., & Yarvis, R. M. (1977). Stressful life events and psychiatric symptomatology: Change or undesirability. *Journal of Health & Social Behavior, 18*, 307–317.

Nuckolls, K. B., Cassell, J., & Kaplan, B. H. (1972). Psychosocial assets, life crisis and the prognosis of pregnancy. *American Journal of Epidemiology, 95*, 431–441.

Padilla, E. R., Rohsenow, D. J., & Bergman, A. B. (1976). Predicting accident frequency in children. *Pediatrics, 58*, 223–226.

Pantell, R. H., & Goodman, B. W. (1983). Adolescent chest pain: A prospective study. *Pediatrics, 71*, 881–886.

Patterson, J. M., & McCubbin, H. I. (1983). The impact of family life events and changes on the health of a chronically ill child. *Family Relations: Journal of Applied Family & Child Studies, 32*, 255–264.

Placek, P. (1977). Maternal and infant health factors associated with low infant birth weight. In P. Reed and F. Stanley (Eds.), *The Epidemiology of Prematurity*. Baltimore: Urban and Schwarzenberg.

Rahe, R. H., & Lind, E. (1971). Psychosocial factors and sudden cardiac death: A pilot study. *Journal of Psychosomatic Research, 15*, 19–24.

Rahe, R. H., Mahan, J. L., & Arthur, R. J. (1970). Prediction of near-future health changes from subject's preceding life changes. *Journal of Psychosomatic Research, 14*, 401–406.

Rahe, R. H., & Paasikivi, J. (1971). Psychosocial factors and myocardial infarction—II: An outpatient study in Sweden. *Journal of Psychosomatic Research, 15*, 33–39.

Rubin, R. T., Gunderson, E. K. E., & Arthur, R. J. (1971). Life stress and illness patterns in the U.S. Navy—V: Prior life changes and illness onset in a battleship crew. *Journal of Psychosomatic Research, 15*, 89–94.

Sandler, I. N. (1980). Social support resources, stress and maladjustment of poor children. *American Journal of Community Psychology, 8*, 41–52.

Sarason, I. G., Johnson, J. H., & Siegel, J. M. (1978). Assessing the impact of life changes: Development of the Life Experiences Survey. *Journal of Consulting & Clinical Psychology, 46*, 932–946.

Selye, H. (1982). History and present status of the stress concept. In L. Goldberger & S. Breznitz (Eds.), *Handbook of stress: Theoretical and clinical aspects*. New York: Free Press.

Siegel, J. M., Johnson, J. H., & Sarason, I. G. (1979). Life stress and menstrual discomfort. *Journal of Human Stress, 5*, 41–46.

Smith, M. S., Gad, M. T., & O'Grady, L. (1983). Psychosocial functioning, life change, and clinical status in adolescents with cystic fibrosis. *Journal of Adolescent Health Care, 4*, 230–234.

Smith, R. E., Johnson, J. H., & Sarason, I. G. (1978). Life change, the sensation seeking motive, and psychological distress. *Journal of Consulting and Clinical Psychology, 46*, 348–349.

Stein, S. P., & Charles, E. (1971). Emotional factors in juvenile diabetes mellitus: A study of early life experiences of adolescent diabetics. *American Journal of Psychiatry, 128,* 56–60.

Swearingen, E. M., & Cohen, L. H. (1985). Measurement of adolescents' life events: The Junior High Life Experiences Survey. *American Journal of Community Psychology, 13,* 69–85.

Theorell, T., & Rahe, R. H. (1971). Psychosocial factors and myocardial infarction: 1. An inpatient study in Sweden. *Journal of Psychosomatic Research, 15,* 25–31.

Tolor, A., Murphy, V., Wilson, L. T., & Clayton, J. (1983). The High School Social Readjustment Scale: An attempt to quantify stressful events in young people. *Research Communications in Psychology, Psychiatry & Behavior, 8,* 85–111.

Tolor, A., & Murphy, V. M. (1985). Stress and depression in high school students. *Psychological Reports, 57,* 535–541.

Vinokur, A., & Selzer, M. L. (1975). Desirable versus undesirable life events: Their relationship to stress and mental distress. *Journal of Personality & Social Psychology, 32,* 329–337.

Watson, D. B. (1983). The relationship between genital herpes and life stress as moderated by locus of control and social support. *Dissertation Abstracts International, 43,* 12.

Wenet, G. (1979). *Life stress and the adolescent sexual offender: A comparative study.* Unpublished manuscript, University of Washington.

Wilcox, B. L. (1981). Social support, life stress, and psychological adjustment: A test of the buffering hypothesis. *American Journal of Community Psychology, 9,* 371–379.

Wyler, A. R., Masuda, M., & Holmes, T. H. (1971). Magnitude of life events and seriousness of illness. *Psychosomatic Medicine, 33,* 115–122.

Yamamoto, K., & Felsenthal, H. M. (1982). Stressful experiences of children: Professional judgments. *Psychological Reports, 50,* 1087–1093.

Yeaworth, R. C., York, J., Hussey, M. A., Ingle, M. E., & Goodwin, T. (1980). The development of an adolescent life change event scale. *Adolescence, 15,* 91–98.

14

Assessing Children's Health Concepts

DAVID S. GOCHMAN

A research literature is slowly but steadily emerging in the area of youngsters' health-related concepts. Blos's benchmark review (1978) identified major research dealing with beliefs about illness causality, concepts of health, concepts of death and dying, beliefs about mental illness, concepts of treatment, and concepts of hospitalization. Kalnins and Love's more recent review (1982) summarized an appreciable amount of research and organized it conceptually. The most current evaluations of children's health concepts (Bruhn & Parcel, 1982; Gochman, 1985) make it clear, however, that more systematic research is needed in this largely unexplored area, and that more attention must be paid to problems of assessment.

This chapter begins with some pertinent definitions and then presents a broad range of assessments of health-related concepts. It continues with a discussion of

This chapter contains selected passages from "Family Determinants of Children's Concepts of Health and Illness" by D. S. Gochman, 1985, in *Health, Illness, and Families: A Life-Span Perspective*, edited by D. C. Turk and R. D. Kern. These passages have been reprinted with permission of John Wiley & Sons, Inc. © 1985. This chapter also contains passages from *Youngsters' health cognitions: Cross-sectional and longitudinal analyses*, by D. S. Gochman, 1986, reprinted with the permission of Health Behavior Systems, © 1986.

major lines of inquiry and an examination of research and methodological issues, and concludes with speculation about future research directions.

DEFINITIONS

Health Concepts

In this new and emerging area, there are few clear-cut, consensual definitions. The domain of health concepts can be defined either narrowly or broadly. A narrow definition is limited to how youngsters define health and illness, and to what they believe the terms *health* and *illness* mean. A broad definition embraces a variety of health-related concepts including—but not restricted to—beliefs about causes of illness, conceptions about parts of the body, expectations about encountering health problems, beliefs about how much control persons have over their health, assessments of health status, perceptions of and attitudes about hospitalization, health professionals, and medical interventions, and the value or priority attached to health. This broader construction is more appropriate for this chapter. It widens the limited range of research available for discussion and increases its representativeness. However, all possible health-related concepts *cannot* be considered in this chapter.

Assessment

A second definitional issue surrounds the term *assessment*. In the area of children's health concepts there are few established assessment techniques. There are no widely accepted instruments with clearly demonstrated psychometric properties—such as reliability and validity—based on rigorous standardization procedures involving large, heterogeneous populations. Instead, *assessment*, as it is considered in this chapter, involves *describing* the range of diverse procedures used to collect research data rather than analyzing them critically and comparatively. This meaning is congruent with Graham and Lilly's (1984, p. 2) current usage. Moreover, the function of such assessments is to increase knowledge and understanding of behavior in general, rather than to increase clinical understanding of—and ultimately improve predictions about—single individuals (e.g., Lanyon & Goodstein, 1982, p. 23).

RANGE OF HEALTH CONCEPTS ASSESSSED

The consideration of the assessment of children's health-related concepts proceeds topically rather than in terms of theoretical models, major concepts, or specific assessment procedures and instruments. This organizational scheme reflects the reality of the field. Although a number of investigations have been linked to specific theoretical models, particularly to that of Piaget, and observations are often interpreted through particular theoretical concepts, these are exceptions. Assessment of children's health-related concepts does not appear to unfold as the logical and natural outgrowth of either theoretical or conceptual development, or of instrumental sophistication and precision. Rather, it has developed in an ad hoc fashion, made up of a number of diverse investigations, few of which were conceptually related to one another in a rigorous way, or employed the same assessment techniques. In this sense the assessment of children's health-related concepts parallels the assessment of personality in general. For example, Lanyon and Goodstein (1982) assert: "The typical *measures* of personality in use today . . . tend to be atheoretical" (p. 35); few personality assessment techniques can be considered to be rationally derived from theory.

The major topics discussed in this section are beliefs about the causality of illness, beliefs about hospitalization and treatment, beliefs about body parts, definitions of health and illness, and health motivation.

Beliefs About Causality of Illness

Nagy's studies (e.g., 1951, 1953) provide some of the earliest assessments of children's health concepts. Nagy assessed beliefs about germs, contagion, and the causes of illness in samples of Hungarian, British, and American youngsters. These beliefs were assessed in several ways. There were individual interviews, in which each child was asked, "What illnesses have you had?" and "What makes us ill?"; children's drawings of germs, followed by "What is a germ?" and "Please explain what you have drawn"; essays written in school classrooms on the subject "What makes us ill?"; replies to written test questions such as "In what way do germs enter our bodies?" "What do germs do in our bodies?" and "In what way do germs leave our bodies?"; and interview questions: "Have you ever heard the word 'germ'?" "What does it mean?" "Through what ways do germs go into our body?" "What are they doing inside?" "When we are not ill any more, what happens to the germs?" The several samples consisted of children between the ages of 3 and 12, representing varied socioeconomic and cultural backgrounds. A different combination of methods and questions was used with each sample.

From these diverse assessments, Nagy observed developmental changes in beliefs about the causes of illness: Very young respondents, those younger than 5, seemed incapable of grasping the real origins of illness; those 6 and older appeared to be able to apply the concepts of infection with a precision that increased with age. Nagy's conclusions were based on percentile distributions rather than on statistical analyses.

Piagetian Concepts of Cognitive Development. Several investigators have examined beliefs about causality from a Piagetian perspective. Simeonsson, Buckley, and Monson's assessments (1979), which were added to some standardized measures of Piagetian conservation, egocentrism, and causality, consisted of six questions: (1) "How can children keep from getting sick?" (2) "What does medicine do?" (3) How do children get sick?" (4) "How do children get stomachaches?" (5) "How do children get bumps or spots?" (6) "When children are sick, how do they get better again?" The sample was made up of 60 hospitalized youngsters ranging in age from 4 to 11. For half of the sample these verbal questions were supplemented with appropriate illustrations (e.g., a child in a hospital bed, medicine, etc.).

On the basis of these assessments, Simeonsson, Buckley, and Monson (1979) concluded that "conceptions of illness causality follow a developmental progression of stages similar to that reported for other domains" (p. 82). They progress from global, undifferentiated beliefs, sometimes involving magical thinking and superstition, to attributions about specific events, sometimes involving violation of rules, to generalized abstractions, involving such basic concepts as infection and differentiated bases for treatment.

Myers-Vando, Steward, Folkins, and Hines (1979) provide another assessment of beliefs about the causality of illness from a Piagetian framework. To a standardized assessment of Piagetian "conservation," they added a projective-type task in which the respondent was asked to tell a story about a picture of a child lying in bed, and to speculate on how the child became ill and might become better, and an interview about the respondent's own illness experiences, including causes and recovery. Interjudge ratings of responses to both tasks, taken as a whole, demonstrated reliability of .87. Respondents were 12 youngsters ranging in age from 8 to 16 who had congenital heart disease and 12 others matched on age, sex, and social class who had no physical, emotional, or intellectual problems. On the basis of their assessments, Myers-Vando and colleagues concluded that, while the children with chronic cardiac disease tended to attain lower levels of general conceptual functioning on the conservation tasks than did the controls, contrary to the study's predictions that the emotional distress resulting from having to cope with chronic disease would result in lower levels of understanding of illness causality, the two groups did *not* differ in their responses to the measures of illness causality.

In a related study, Carandang, Folkins, Hines, and Steward (1979) assessed beliefs about illness causality in siblings of youngsters with diabetes. On the basis of these assessments, the authors concluded that the stresses of dealing with a sibling's illness were reflected in decreased ability to conceptualize the causes and treatment of illness at the same level of cognitive maturity demonstrated by controls who were presumably not faced with such stress.

Neuhauser, Amsterdam, Hines, and Steward (1978) assessed youngsters' concepts of healing in terms of Piagetian developmental stages. In an orally administered questionnaire, they asked 24 White, middle-class children, 12 of whom were 4 and 5 years old and 12 of whom were 8 and 9 years old, questions such as: "How did you know when you were hurt [sick]?" "When you were hurt, how did you heal [get better]?" "How did that work to help you heal [get better]?" "What was going on inside your body that helped you heal [get well]?" "How does that work? Can you show me?" A Piagetian conservation task was used to determine the level of cognitive functioning. Among other findings, Neuhauser and colleagues observed that youngsters who were functioning at the concrete operational level more frequently used internal cues in the more abstract situation of an illness than did the preoperational children.

Piagetian Concepts of Moral Development. In research derived from Piagetian concepts of moral development, Kister and Patterson (1980) assessed the degree to which youngsters employed concepts of contagion and immanent justice in their explanations of the causes of illness and accidents. To assess the use of contagion concepts, respondents were asked: "If a boy your age went to school one day, and the girl sitting next to him had [the ailment], would he have to be careful so he wouldn't catch [the ailment] from her?" This forced-choice question was followed by "How come?" or "Why not?" If the ailment was labeled as contagious, the respondent was asked: "Let's say the boy really didn't want to get [the ailment]. Would it be better for him to sit next to the girl with [the ailment], across the room from her, or does it make a difference where he sits?" The stories and questions dealt with a contagious illness (cold), a noncontagious illness (toothache), and an accident (scraped knee).

In the assessments of immanent justice, respondents were told a story wherein a youngster had committed a "minor transgression" and had subsequently experienced an illness: "Once a boy your age disobeyed his mother. Was that a nice thing to do? Well, that afternoon, he got a cold. Do you think he got a cold because he disobeyed his mother? What made him get a cold? Let's pretend he didn't disobey his mother. Do you think he would get a cold anyway? Why [not]?" In addition, similar stories were related for a noncontagious illness (toothache), an accident (scraped knee), and a nonhealth event (a bridge breaking as the boy was crossing it).

These formats included both forced-choice and open-ended responses. Interrater agreement for the forced-choice responses was reported to be .93. Respondents were 60 middle-class children of both sexes, 15 each from preschool, kindergarten, and second and fourth grades. They were all interviewed by a female.

On the basis of their assessments, Kister and Patterson concluded that as children grow older, they are less likely to overgeneralize the concept of contagion, and less likely to employ concepts of immanent justice.

Concerned about possible differences in perceptions between sick, hospitalized children and healthy ones, Brodie investigated anxiety about illness and included assessments of beliefs about causality (1974), particularly about illness as punishment. Brodie asked a sample of 408 students in first, third, and fifth grades questions such as "Do you think boys and girls who misbehave get sick more often than those who are good?" "If you play more than you should can you get sick?" "If you fight with other children can you get sick?" and "Can children get sick because they tell lies?" Brodie concluded "that the majority of the children, regardless of age, do not perceive illness as do sick children. Instead of viewing illness as possible punishment, or [believing] that their parents may be displeased with them when they become ill . . . healthy children simply reject these ideas" (p. 1157).

Beliefs About Hospitalization and Treatment

Psychoanalytically oriented observations of hospitalized children comprise another line of research with early beginnings. Deutsch's clinical insights based on "long years of psychoanalytic experience and collecting and reconstructing observations which originally were not intended to answer the questions included here" (1942, p. 105) provided assessments of the meaning that surgical procedures had for hospitalized youngsters. Deutsch noted the potential that such procedures have for being interpreted by the child as punishment and for evoking fears of separation and death.

Similar case history approaches to assessment confirm Deutsch's conclusions that children often view hospitalization very differently than do adults, and that they perceive it as rejection, abandonment, and/or punishment (e.g., Barowsky, 1978; Chapman, Loeb, & Gibbons, 1956; Jessner, Blom, & Waldfogel, 1952; Vernon, Foley, Sipowicz, & Schulman, 1965, chap. 8). Steuart's case history assessments (1952) also noted the impact of hospitalization on dependency behaviors in youngsters.

Matus, Kinsman, and Jones (1978) have developed a standardized, rigorous way of assessing youngsters' beliefs about hospitalization and treatment for asthma. Seventy-two pediatric hospitalized patients with chronic respiratory disease, ranging in age from 7 to 15 years, responded to a 79-item questionnaire dealing with stigma associated with asthma, perceptions of the patient's role and the role of others in the treatment of the condition, and attitudes toward the personnel involved in the treatment, as well as other relevant attitudes. Items included: "This hospital is usually just a step on the way to something worse," "The nurses are very nice to their patients," and "Coming to a hospital is good insurance against having to have more hospitalization." Respondents indicated their level of agreement with each item on a 5-point scale. Factor analyses revealed seven clusters: minimization of severity; passive observance of illness; bravado; expectation of staff rejection; moralistic authoritarianism; stigma; and external control. Additional analyses indicated that the cluster scores themselves had sufficient internal consistency (coefficients ranged from .76 to .89) and stability between successive administrations (coefficients, with a single exception, ranged from .69 to .79).

From their assessments, Matus and colleagues concluded that "stable attitude structures in regard to chronic asthma and treating agents are already present during childhood" (p. 617).

Beliefs About Body Parts

Gellert, noting the lack of research on how young persons view their bodies (1962, 1978), and observing the need "for developing further the methods used in gathering, organizing, and reporting relevant data" (1962, p. 297), devised a standardized questionnaire technique, the Gellert Index of Body Knowledge, to assess this area rigorously and systematically. This index required youngsters to respond, in individual interviews, to questions such as: "What do you have inside you?" "Tell me as many things as you can think of that are inside you." "Show me the head." "What is in the head?" (Probe: "Tell me all the things that are in the head.") "Make a circle where, and about how big the heart is." "What does the heart do?" (Probe: "What is it for?") "What would happen if we didn't have a heart?"

Other questions probed specifically about bones, the stomach, ribs, the liver, skin, lungs, nerves, the bladder, and bowel movements to assess how well children could locate them and what functions they served. (Appropriate probes were used as necessary.) Data were obtained from a pilot sample of 96 youngsters ranging in age from 4 years and 7 months to 16 years and 11 months—all but 4 of whom were hospitalized. Gellert devised a system of response categories and, with the independent judgments of a collaborator, was able to demonstrate interjudge reliabilities of between .69 and .91 for a range of organ functions (1962, p. 403). On the basis of this assessment process and from this sample, Gellert concluded that as children grow older their reality orientation predictably increases and they acquire more valid and accurate notions of how the body and its component organs function. In addition, from a theoretical perspective, Gellert's assessments suggested that egocentrism and concreteness are more characteristic of the way in which younger children—in contrast to older ones—view their bodies. Older children demonstrated greater degrees of articulation of parts of the various body systems, and increased conceptions of permanent as opposed to fluid structures (e.g., materials ingested or egested) than did younger ones.

Gellert further noted the congruence between these observations and a Piagetian conception of development. Moreover, her data suggested that the modal age for "correct" or adult-type responses was either 9 to 10, or 11 to 12. Such data are considered "strong evidence that knowledge about the body increases sharply around the age of 9 years" (1962, p. 388). Gellert's thorough presentation of data (1962) did not, however, include systematic statistical analyses of these developmental changes. The trends are inferred from tabular presentation of percentages. Nonetheless, the work remains an important pioneer effort at standardizing an assessment procedure relevant to children's health concepts, and at codifying and quantifying results.

Johnson and Wellman (1982), building in part on the work of Nagy and Gellert, assessed children's conceptions of the brain and of the mind in a series of four interrelated studies. Respondents ranged in age from 3 to 15 (with some adults as controls). In two studies the assessment procedures consisted of asking two general questions: "Where is your brain?" and "What does your brain do?" In the first of these, respondents were also asked whether the brain was needed for each of a list of tasks, including mental acts such as thinking, knowing, and remembering; feelings; school and motor tasks; involuntary acts such as coughing and blinking; and sensory activities. In the second study, they were asked instead whether each of these acts could be performed without the brain, as well as whether the brain and mind were in the same or different places, whether each could exist without the other, and whether the brain helps a variety of body parts.

The third and fourth study each consisted of a sample aged 3 to 5 years. In one, respondents were shown pictures of a variety of activities, analogous to those dealt with in the first two studies, and were asked: "Do you need your brain to think . . . tell a story . . . wiggle your toes?" In the final study, respondents were asked if the brain was inside or outside.

On the basis of these assessments, Johnson and Wellman conclude that by 4 years of age children are aware that the brain is internal and that it is associated with a variety of mental acts. Young children do not, as a rule, confound the brain with the head.

> During the school years, concepts of mind and brain become increasingly differentiated: the mind as a nonmaterial entity, more closely associated with mental acts. . . . Only older subjects . . . exhibited a more technical understanding that the brain is as essential for all behavior, including noncognitive involuntary responses. (p. 232)

The use of variations in the questions and tasks provided Johnson and Wellman with evidence of convergent validity. For example, the failure of very young children in the first study to regard the brain as necessary for more than a limited set of strictly mental–intellectual actions is observed again in the second study where the questions were asked in a different way.

Definitions of Health and Illness

Rashkis's work on children's conceptions of health (1965) complements these studies of children's conceptions of the disease process and of their body parts. Rashkis's assessments consisted of play-period interviews that began with respondents interacting with toys and other play materials, including plastic dolls. When the respondents became involved with the dolls and began to fantasize about them, interviewers asked them, "How are they?" referring to the dolls, and upon the child's response, 16 questions about health were asked in conversational fashion. These questions dealt with the meaning of health ("What is it like to be well?" "How do we feel when we are well?"); responsibility for health ("Can we keep ourselves well?" "Can others keep us well?" "Who can keep us well?" "What do we do to be well?" "What do others do to keep us well?"); health and ideas of reference ("Do grownups [children] like us to be well?"); and prevalence of health ("Are grownups [children] well?" "How many grownups [children] are well?" "All or most grownups [children] *or* some or few grownups [children]?" "Do some grownups [children] stay well more than other grownups [children] stay well?" "Are there some grownups [children] who always stay well?"). On the basis of responses of 54 elementary school children, ranging in age from 4 years and 9 months to 8 years and 9 months and representing a wide range of socioeconomic backgrounds, Rashkis observed that, while the modal response to the question "What is it like to be well?" was "not sick," there were no statistically significant differences between this and other responses for the total sample. However, there were statistically significant grade-related differences in the frequency of *pleasant* responses: Older youngsters more often than younger ones equated being well with positive, pleasant states. Younger ones more than older ones tended to respond either that they didn't know or in terms of not being sick. Rashkis interprets these and other observations as reflecting the inability of younger children, that is, those below age 7, to integrate their health-related feelings and experiences into a clear, conscious conception of health as a positive state.

Furthermore, these assessments revealed that physicians—more so than family members—are likely to be perceived as the persons responsible for health. The data support the view that youngsters have a protective image of adults, and Rashkis interprets this as a generalized expectancy arising from the young person's continued positive contact with parents.

Natapoff's assessments of concepts of health and illness (1978) were conducted within a Piagetian framework. The three main questions Natapoff asked were "What does the word *health* mean?" "How do you feel when you are healthy?" "Can you be part healthy and part not healthy at the same time?" The respondents in Natapoff's study were first, fourth, and seventh graders in a suburban community, representing blue-collar, white-collar, and professional families.

On the basis of these assessments, Natapoff observed that youngsters were most likely to equate being healthy with—in order of preference—feeling good, their ability to do things they wanted to do, and not being sick. They were least likely to equate being healthy with being happy or having a strong body. They equated not being healthy with being sick and not being able to do things. Natapoff interprets age group data as suggesting that older children demonstrate greater analytic processes, greater levels of abstraction in their thinking, and greater ability to see part–whole relationships than do younger ones. Following the Piagetian model, Natapoff suggests that children's concepts of health and illness move from preoperational, eogcentric, syncretistic functioning (those younger than 7 or 8), through concrete operational functioning (from 8 to 10 years old), to the formal operational functioning of those older than 10.

Campbell's investigations of how children's concepts of illness evolve and change (e.g., 1975a, 1975b, 1978) provide another set of assessments of definitions of illness. Campbell's assessments involved interviews with 264 youngsters 6 through 12 years old, from intact White families, who had been hospitalized as short-term patients, and who had led normal, active lives prior to their entering the hospital. Youngsters were asked, "Now, I'm wondering about how you know when you're sick. When you say you are sick, what do you mean? On one day you know you are well; on another you know you are sick. Okay, what's the difference?" Campbell devised a coding scheme (1975b) to determine whether or not 11 "themes," such as nonspecific feeling states or disease-specific concepts, were present in the responses. The median intercoder agreement coefficient for these themes was .89; for no theme was it lower than .70. On the basis of these assessments, Campbell concluded that youngsters show both age-specific and developmental consensus in their use of these themes, and that their "conceptual sophistication" increases with age.

Closely related to issues of definitions of health and illness are Mechanic's assessments of youngsters' willingness to report symptoms when feeling ill, risk-taking attitudes, denial of pain attitudes, and perceptions of when a doctor is necessary (1964). Mechanic's assessments required youngsters to compare themselves with descriptions of other children their age, as follows: "Larry and Linda usually *tell* others when they don't feel well while Bob and Betty usually *do not tell* others when they don't feel well." The respondents then had to indicate whether they were more like the first two children or more like the last two.

Finally, Marshall, Hassanein, Hassanein, and Paul (1970) demonstrated that Osgood's semantic differential technique could be used to assess the concept of *sick*, as well as the concepts of *doctor*, *nurse*, and *hospital*, in a sample of 180 youngsters 9 years old.

Health Motivation

Few assessments exist of health motivation in young populations. The Health Ideation Pictures (HIP) were an early attempt at assessing the degree to which health is valued by youngsters (Gochman, 1970). This projective-type task consisted of eleven 5-by-7-inch black-and-white drawings in which youngsters were depicted in a variety of activities, each of which had the potential for eliciting health content. Respondents were asked to tell a story about each picture, but were not specifically probed for health content. Responses from a sample of 31 Cub Scouts, 8 through 10 years old, drawn from a middle-class population, were either tape-recorded or written down verbatim during interviews. A coding system was devised to measure the presence of health ideation, that is, degree to which health content was freely mentioned, and adaptive health behavior, that is, degree to which preventive or corrective health behavior was mentioned. Interjudge reliability, measured by Kendall's *tau beta* coefficients, ranged from .695 to 1.00 for the different pictures. Furthermore, analyses of scores for all pairs of pictures revealed that, for health ideation, there were 43 significant correlations out of 55. Actual values of the correlation coefficients were attenuated because of the lack of variability in the responses themselves.

Although the HIP were used briefly in subsequent research, they were cumbersome to administer and to score. Moreover, their failure to elicit much health content readily suggested that health was not especially important or generally motivating among the youngsters sampled. This finding may have been due in part to a task effect: In the free-response atmosphere of the HIP, youngsters are not asked specifically about health.

As an alternative, the Mouth Appearance Pictures were developed (Gochman, 1975). In contrast to the Health Ideation Pictures, these were a forced-choice assessment procedure in which youngsters were presented with nine pairs of mouths and were required to choose between a more attractive but less healthy mouth and a less attractive but healthier mouth. Respondents circled the one mouth in each pair that they would like to have. There were three degrees of attractiveness (straight, moderately crooked, and severely crooked teeth) and three degrees of health (two, five, and eight cavities). Considerable care was taken in the drafting of the pictures to eliminate any apparent racial characteristics. As an additional precaution, the pictures were printed on buff-toned paper to minimize cues for racial identification.

In a sample of 774 youngsters in grades 3 through 9, taken from schools in both inner-city and suburban areas, interitem analyses revealed that the MAP are an internally consistent measure. The coefficients ranged from .56 to .76 (Gochman, 1975).

MAJOR LINES OF CURRENT RESEARCH

Recent overviews of current research on the assessment of children's health beliefs (e.g., Bruhn & Parcel, 1982) suggest that two major conceptual models predominate: (1) the health-belief model; and (2) the concept of locus of control derived from social learning theory.

The Health-Belief Model

The health-belief model (e.g., Rosenstock, 1974) is an essentially cognitive paradigm for predicting the likelihood of persons taking health actions. In its original form, the model postulated that perceptions of being susceptible to some condition, the perceived severity or seriousness of that condition, and perceptions of the benefits or actions that prevent or treat that condition are all positively related to the likelihood that a person will engage in some specific preventive health behavior. According to Green (1974), reference is made to this model in "virtually every dissertation related to health behavior" (p. 324). The model has since been extended to deal with sick-role, illness behaviors and responses to chronic conditions (e.g., Janz & Becker, 1984).

A series of interrelated studies, begun in 1967, marked one of the first assessments of a cluster of these beliefs and related concepts in young populations (e.g., Gochman, 1969, 1971a, 1971b, 1972, 1977, 1986).

Perceived Vulnerability. In the original formulation of the health-belief model, perceived susceptibility was defined with reference to a single health problem. Gochman conceptually defined it as the degree to which youngsters believe they are susceptible to—or might encounter—a variety of health problems or conditions, and termed this generalized expectancy *perceived vulnerability*.

Perceived vulnerability was assessed through responses to a series of expectancy-type questions. The assessment tool went through several revisions before emerging in a final 15-item form. The general question format (e.g., Gochman, 1972) is: "What chance is there of your getting the flu during this next year?" The other specific health problems are: a bad accident, like breaking an arm; a rash; a fever; having a tooth pulled; a sore throat; a toothache; a cold; bleeding gums; an upset stomach; being sick enough to miss a week of school; a cavity; a bad headache; breaking or cracking a tooth; and cutting a finger accidentally.

For each question subjects selected the one response from seven alternatives that best expressed their own expectancy. These alternatives were: "no chance," "almost no chance," "a small chance," "a medium chance," "a good chance," "almost certain," and "certain"; were scored respectively from 1 to 7, and treated as a quasi-interval scale (e.g., Cureton, 1968). Pilot work demonstrated the suitability of this format for the target populations.

Special instructions ensure that the questions and response alternatives are clearly understood. (Details of instructions and suitability are provided in Gochman, 1986.) The measure was revealed to be reliable in terms of internal consistency. In a sample of 774 respondents in grades 3 through 9, interitem correlation coefficients were significant in 101 of 105 pairs (Gochman, Bagramian, & Sheiham, 1972). In other large samples odd–even correlation coefficients of .66 and .68 were obtained; a smaller subsample revealed the measure to be reliable in terms of stability as well, with a test–retest correlation coefficient of .82 (Gochman, 1986).

Alternative instruments to assess perceived vulnerability have also been developed. Urberg and Robbins (1984, p. 370), for example, expanded the Gochman measure to 22 items, to provide greater variety and to increase the severity of the health problems. In addition, they devised a 12-item scale dealing with perceptions of vulnerability to the negative consequences of smoking. They report internal consistency, using Cronbach's alpha, of at least .80 for their assessment procedures.

Perceived Benefits. In the original model *perceived benefits* were broadly conceived as the set of "beliefs regarding the relative effectiveness of the known available alternatives in reducing the disease threat to which the individual feels subjected" (Rosenstock, 1974, p. 331). Because Gochman's research dealt with populations that were not identified as being at risk, and because earlier research suggested that health may not be salient in young populations (Gochman, 1971b), a corollary conception was proposed for perceived benefits: beliefs about the health outcomes or the health impact of specific actions *in relation to other outcomes or impacts*.

Gochman's assessments of perceived benefits thus consisted of two forced-choice-type questions. In each, the respondent had to select *two* out of four responses. One question asked: "If you go to the dentist, finish the sentence by circling the *two* answers that best tell why *you* go. If you don't go, circle only "I don't go." "The sentence began: "I go to the dentist because . . . " and the four responses were: "I want to keep my teeth for a long time," "I don't want my teeth to look crooked," "I don't want to have toothaches," and "I want my teeth to look clean."

A similar question asked why respondents brushed their teeth. In each question, two of the four answers reflected perceived health benefits (e.g., "I don't want to have toothaches") and two reflected perceived appearance (nonhealth) benefits (e.g., "I want to have a nice smile").

For each question, respondents choosing two nonhealth responses were given a score of 1; those choosing one health and one nonhealth response were given a score of 2; and those selecting two health responses were given a score of 3. The magnitude of these scores reflected the degree to which youngsters perceived health benefits accruing to their actions. (Additional details about this assessment procedure are provided in Gochman, 1986.)

Eisen and his colleagues (e.g., Eisen, Zellman, & McAlister, 1985) elaborate on alternative ways of assessing perceptions of benefits of health actions.

Intentions to Take Health Actions. *Intentions to take health actions* refer to those beliefs about the likelihood of engaging in some specific health-promoting behavior at some future time. Such intentions include *preventive attitudes,* the degree to which young persons see themselves as preventively oriented in the future. This was assessed through a series of nine expectancy-type questions, such as "What chance is there that when you are grown up you would visit a doctor even if you don't feel sick?" The other preventive behaviors were: ". . . probably find yourself smoking some cigarettes every day"; ". . . eat some vegetables and fruits every day"; ". . . forget to use safety belts when you ride in a car"; ". . . get some exercise every day"; ". . . use a lot of your spending money to buy tasty snacks like candy, cake, and potato chips"; ". . . want to have a fever thermometer in your home"; "first go to the drugstore if you felt sick and needed help"; and ". . . get a flu shot if it were given free."

For each question the youngsters selected one of seven response alternatives: "no chance," "almost no chance," "a small chance," "a medium chance," "a good chance," "almost certain," and "certain." Responses were scored as follows: 1 for the "no chance" alternative through 7 for the "certain" alternative, with appropriate scoring reversals, so that the highest preventive score would be 7. (Details on instructions, reliability, and suitability are found in Gochman, 1986.)

Related Health Concepts. Other cognitions assessed in Gochman's studies include: intentions of making dental visits, general evaluative beliefs about teeth, and beliefs about tooth-brushing frequency. (These are described in detail in Gochman, 1986.)

Perceived Seriousness. Although the concept of perceived seriousness—or perceived severity—has not been examined as systematically in young populations as other derivatives of the health-belief model, Eisen and his colleagues (e.g., Eisen et al., 1985) have developed an assessment of *perceived seriousness* in the context of a young female's perceptions of what she would suffer if she were to become pregnant. Their assessment consists of items such as "If a teenage girl has an unplanned pregnancy, it's not a big problem since she can raise her baby alone."

Beliefs About Specific Illnesses. Michielutte and Diseker (1982), guided by the health-belief model, assessed children's perceptions of selected diseases through a series of semantic differential-type questions. Respondents were asked to evaluate cancer, heart disease, diabetes, and mental illness in terms of whether: "most people never recover / most people recover completely"; "I have a big chance of getting it / I have no chance of getting it"; "scares most people / scares hardly anybody"; "a very mild disease / a very poweful disease"; "very well understood by doctors / hardly anything is known about it"; "many people get it / almost nobody gets it." From their sample of 295 seventh graders in an urban county in North Carolina, they were able to conclude that youngsters perceive cancer differently than they do other diseases. Cancer is perceived negatively in relation to other diseases in terms of perceived susceptibility and severity; that is youngsters believe that it is more severe and that persons have more of a chance of getting it, and it is "the least understood" and holds "the least promise for recovery" (p. 848).

Locus of Control

The second major conceptual framework underlying research on the assessment of health beliefs is locus of control. Stemming from social learning theory, models of locus of control suggest that the degree to which persons perceive themselves as being in control of events in their lives has important implications for their behavior. The implications of locus of control for health-relevant behavior are systematically identified by Wallston and Wallston (1978). The prototype of locus of control scales for children was developed by Bialer (1961). The principal extension of locus of control to the assessment of children's health-related concepts was developed by Parcel and his associates (e.g., Parcel & Meyer, 1978). Recognizing the importance of creating "specific scales for specific categories of behavior" (Parcel & Meyer, 1978, p. 150), Parcel initially developed a preliminary instrument of 30 items consisting of statements that were derived "from adaptations of some items from the [Wallston, Wallston, & Kaplan] adult locus of control scale and from statements contained in elementary-grade health education textbooks" (Parcel & Meyer, 1978, p. 150). These questions were administered in both written and oral form to an initial sample of 168 youngsters, in second through sixth grades, in two parochial elementary schools. Children responded to these items in a "yes" or "no" manner.

On the basis of analyses of internal consistency and differences between grades, sexes, and schools, a revised 20-item instrument was developed. This revised assessment tool, the Children's Health Locus of Control (CHLC) Scale, consisted of items such as: "There is nothing I can do to keep from getting sick"; "I can do many things to fight illness"; "It is the teacher's job to keep me from having accidents at school." This was administered to 140 third, fourth, and fifth graders in a single elementary school, along with the Nowicki-Strickland Children's Locus of Control Scale.

Kuder-Richardson analyses indicated that the CHLC had an internal reliability coefficient of at least .72. A test–retest intraclass reliability coefficient of .62 indicated that the instrument was acceptably stable. Moreover, a correlation coefficient of .501 between the CHLC and the Nowicki-Strickland scale led Parcel and Meyer to suggest that the CHLC had "construct" validity.

Parcel and Meyer's factor analysis of the Children's Health Locus of Control Scale (1978) indicates that locus of internal control is multidimensional in young populations. Three major factors emerged: general beliefs about the degree that youngsters control their own health; beliefs about the degree that health and illness are determined by chance or luck; and beliefs about the degree to which powerful agents such as physicians and nurses determine health and illness outcomes. Such findings increase understanding of what the assessment of locus of control means in young populations. They also have the potential to increase the precision with which the concept is used, and offer opportunities to develop differential predictions and assessments for the three subscales.

RESEARCH AND METHODOLOGICAL ISSUES

For the purposes of this chapter, research and methodological issues are organized (somewhat arbitrarily) as follows: research issues are those related to theories, concepts, and general frames of reference that underlie the assessment of children's health concepts; methodological issues are those related to specific assessment procedures or techniques, and/or their external validity or generalizability.

Research Issues

Two major issues that confront the assessment of children's health-related concepts are conceptual clarity and theroetical alternatives.

Conceptual Clarity. There is great need for increased conceptual clarity in the area of children's health-related concepts. What, for example, is meant by beliefs about health and illness? A task force on children's health concepts (Bruhn & Parcel, 1982) reports: "In the entire area of cognitive systems, concepts need to be sharper and clearer and they need to be integrated with theory" (p. 151).

With few exceptions (e.g., Campbell, 1975a; Gochman, 1972; Neuhauser et al., 1978; Simeonsson et al., 1979), as Bibace and Walsh (1981) and Crider (1981) note, research on children's health concepts has not been derived systematically from theoretical models of development. The potential breadth of this area must be acknowledged, and its challenge accepted. Children's concepts about health and illness represent the varied ways in which youngsters relate themselves to the many dimensions of health (and/or illness) that impinge upon them. Abstracting additionally from Bruhn and Parcel (1982), concepts of health and illness can be seen to embrace *what* children know, as well as *how* they organize this knowledge; how they evaluate health, that is, their attitudes, values, and feelings about health; their health-related beliefs—whether or not these are veridical—together with the organizational structure of these beliefs, that is, how these beliefs are related to one another. Concepts of health and illness can embrace children's body images, and how children process health-relevant stimuli or data (Bruhn & Parcel, 1982, pp. 149–153).

Within this potentially broad range, specific variables should be clearly defined conceptually, and systematically related to a specifiable theory, model, or paradigm. Assessments would be more meaningful and have greater value if they were based on more clearly defined concepts. Furthermore, there would be hope for meaningful comparisons between, and replications of, findings. Currently, it is not unusual for different researchers to use a single term such as *perceived vulnerability* to refer to entirely different dimensions of beliefs (e.g., Gochman, 1977; Lewis & Lewis, 1982).

Increased conceptual clarity would also reduce the likelihood of confounding key concepts. Within the original health-belief model, for example, motivational characteristics were imputed to high levels of perceived susceptibility and perceived severity, together with perceptions of available actions or benefits (e.g., Rosenstock,

1974). Motivation was thus equated with expectations, beliefs, and perceptions. Motivation has a well-defined place in psychological theory (e.g., Birney, 1968; O'Kelly, 1968) that implies priorities that energize and organize behaviors. Separate assessment of health motivation and perceived vulnerability (e.g., Gochman, 1977) has shown them to be empirically independent. Such data support the position that motivation is not to be inferred or imputed from other cognitions. Confounding such characteristics presents problems for the development of assessment research, as well as for health professionals who inappropriately assume that some target group possesses selected psychological characteristics.

Factor analysis may prove to be valuable in developing such clarification. Dielman, Leech, Becker, Rosenstock, and Horvath's factor analysis (1980) of several health beliefs demonstrates that items that assess perceived susceptibility (vulnerability) to specific conditions (e.g., "How much of a chance do you think there is—in the next few months—that you might have a pain in your stomach?") are factorially distinct from those assessing general and specific health concerns (e.g., "When you are sick, how much do you worry about it?"). Such findings strengthen the position that perceived susceptibility (vulnerability) is distinct from worry about health or appraisal of health status, assessments of which have at times been used as indices of perceived susceptibility (e.g., Lewis & Lewis, 1982).

While Dielman and colleagues (1980) also suggest that perceived susceptibility may not be unidimensional, the final factor structure they present does not, by itself, argue this unequivocally. While the susceptibility items appear to load on three factors (perceived susceptibility / specific conditions; perceived seriousness of and susceptibility to disease; and perceived susceptibility / general), several of the items load nearly equally well on two of the three, diminishing the clarity of the distinctiveness of the proposed three factors. Other careful analyses of larger amounts of conceptually derived assessments should facilitate the clarification process.

Theoretical Development and Theoretical Alternatives. Although the health-belief model has continued to be a highly productive theoretical research formulation, it is not in itself a theory of psychological development. The assessment of children's health concepts requires the continued elaboration of alternative developmental paradigms to the area of health beliefs and health behaviors. Piagetian and Lewinian models of cognitive development, together with social learning theory, offer promise for future progress in the field. In addition, the derivatives of Heider's balance theory (Heider, 1958) that emerge periodically, such as attribution theory (e.g., Kelley, 1967) or behavioral intention theory (Fishbein & Ajzen, 1975), might prove to be productive.

Attribution theory "refers to the process of inferring or perceiving the dispositional properties of entities in the environment" (Kelley, 1967, p. 193). In allowing for "the allocation of causality between the environment and the self" (p. 196), the theory relates attribution of validity to information received from other persons to perceptions of these sources. In the area of children's health concepts, attribution theory points to potential targets of assessment procedures: the acceptability of health education programs and health-related messages from health professionals and significant others, and the changes in—or acquisitions of—health concepts that result from these messages.

Behavioral intention theory indicates that the intention to engage in a specified behavior is the best predictor of a person's behavior (Fishbein & Ajzen, 1975, pp.

381–382). Accordingly, a child's intentions of engaging in selected health and safety behaviors are another target for assessment procedures. Chassin and colleagues (1981) investigated adolescents' smoking behaviors by assessing selected cognitions derived from Fishbein and Ajzen's model—attitudes toward the act of smoking, their normative beliefs about smoking, and intentions to smoke—along with a selection of other variables. Attitudes toward the act of smoking were assessed through semantic–differential-type questions about smoking being fun, pleasant, and nice; and by responses to items about the consequences of smoking such as "If I smoke, I will be relaxed" multiplied by "Being relaxed is good." Normative beliefs were assessed by items such as "My friends think that I should smoke cigarettes." Behavioral intentions were assessed by items such as "I plan to smoke cigarettes a month from now."

Chassin and colleagues observed that beliefs derived from behavioral intention theory, that is, beliefs about the act of smoking and normative beliefs, were the best predictors of intentions to smoke of the range of cognitions they explored.

Duryea and Martin's (1981) assessments of the degree of distortion present in young persons' perceptions of the smoking behavior of their peers is relevant to the normative-beliefs component of behavioral intention theory.

Methodological Issues

Three major methodological concerns are apparent in the assessment of children's health-related concepts: psychometric analyses, data bases, and procedures.

Psychometric Analyses. The overview of the major areas of children's health-related concepts demonstrates that these have been assessed in a variety of ways. They have ranged from single, global questions asked in face-to-face interviews, such as "What makes us ill?" (e.g., Nagy, 1951) to multiitem questionnaire scales derived from specific concepts in specific theoretical models with specific multiple response alternatives, such as measures of perceived vulnerability / perceived susceptibility (e.g., Dielman et al., 1980; Gochman, 1977). They have employed self-reports; responses to figures and pictures; and open-ended, projected, forced-choice, and closed-ended formats. There is always advantage and protection in such diversity. It widens the range of available information, increases the degree to which certain kinds of data emerge, and to some degree ensures against measurement error. But, against the background of such diversity, serious psychometric problems can be observed.

At the outset are some critical questions about the very nature of the phenomena being observed. To what degree are children's health-related concepts essential aspects of personality? Some health-related concepts do seem to resemble personality characteristics, for example, health locus of control (Parcel & Meyers, 1978) and perceived vulnerability (Gochman & Saucier, 1982). But scant attention has been paid to how to conceptualize them as dimensions of personality. Are these and similar health-related concepts to be considered traits, that is, relatively enduring dispositions that transcend situations, or states, that is, situationally dependent, or reflections of person–environment interactions (Lanyon & Goodstein, 1982).

Are they to be considered to be "achievements?" Can they be compared to skills and abilities? Prior to developing appropriate psychometric guidelines or models for assessing them, there must be some consensus about what they are—or at least what specific health concepts are.

To the degree that some of them are considered as dimensions of personality, or skills, or "achievements," then it becomes imperative to explore and improve their psychometric properties. For the most part, little attention has been paid to reliability and validity.

In some instances reliability has been considered in terms of interjudge or interrater reliability (e.g., Campbell, 1975b; Gellert, 1962; Kister & Patterson, 1980; Myers-Vando et al., 1979). In other instances, it has been considered in terms of internal consistency (e.g., Gochman, 1975; Parcel & Meyers, 1978). But generally, questions about reliability have not been predominant in developing instruments to assess children's health-related concepts. Evidence exists that some scales are reliable in terms of stability over time (Gochman, 1986; Parcel & Meyer, 1978), but stability has not been a major concern in most assessments of children's health concepts. To the degree that a specific concept is supposed to reflect a relatively enduring characteristic, then concern with stability must be increased. If, instead, a concept is considered to reflect a less permanent dimension in the child's life, then concern with stability need not be as great. However, if developmental aspects of health concepts are at issue, then some evidence of stability is necessary in order to distinguish developmental changes from measurement error.

Nor have questions of validity been systematically addressed. While virtually all of the assessments discussed would seem to have some degree of "face" validity (i.e., they seem to be measuring whatever it is they're purported to be measuring), there have been few attempts to determine the degree to which the measures demonstrate validity in other ways. Do the assessment procedures have "test" validity? Can they be validated by using other measures assessing the same concepts? As is not the case in such as intelligence, aptitude, ability, or achievement testing, in which there is an abundance of assessment tools available (a numerical abundance, not necessarily a qualitative one), in the area of children's health-related concepts, in which there is no consensus on what to measure, there are as yet no established "benchmarks." One notable exception is Parcel's Health Locus of Control Scale (Parcel & Meyer, 1978), which was compared with the Nowicki-Strickland Children's Locus of Control Scale and demonstrated its "concurrent" or "test" validity with a correlation of .501. Moreover, a 9-item short form of the Parcel scale was satisfactorily validated against the factor structure of the long form (Bush, Parcel, & Davidson, 1982). Furthermore, Parcel and Meyer straightforwardly equated internal locus of control with "an achievement" and introduced the concept of item difficulty, found in achievement testing, as a way of analyzing individual items.

In addition, assessments of adolescents' perceptions of vulnerability to health problems in the present (within the next year) were observed to be related to their perceptions of being vulnerable to more serious health problems in later adulthood (Gochman & Saucier, 1982).

Validity can also be addressed through the ability of an assessment procedure to "predict" some behavior or performance in the future. Currently there is little clear-cut evidence that assessments of children's health-related concepts can be used to predict either concurrent or future health-related behaviors. But, unlike other forms of assessment, such as ability, aptitude, or intelligence testing, assessments of health-related concepts in youngsters have not, for the most part, been undertaken in order to make such predictions. Nor, as is not the case with clinical assessments, have they been undertaken to classify youngsters for diagnosis and treatment.

Finally, although a few attempts have been made (e.g., Gochman, 1977) to demonstrate construct validity for some concepts and their assessment techniques, by and large, the atheoretical nature of the concepts and their assessments has not led to systematic construct validation. Briefly (it is impossible in this context to be more detailed about what is meant by *construct validity*), to demonstrate construct validity in an appropraite, systematic way, it would first be necessary to develop a theoretical model in which a health-related concept is seen to be a consequence of one or more antecedent variables, such as socialization experiences, health status, family characteristics, or peer characteristics. Next, it would be necessary to make specific predictions differentially linking these antecedent variables with the health-related concept. Then the theroetical model would predict specific linkages between the concept and other concepts (both health and non–health related), as well as linkages between the concept and current and future observable behaviors. For each of the specified variables, multiple assessment procedures would have to be developed, each assessment logically derived from the theoretical variable it is intended to measure. This highly complex formula has not yet been followed, even in a limited way, in the domain of the assessment of children's health-related concepts.

Data Bases. Evidence that expectations of health problems are relatively stable and organized by age 8 or so (Gochman, 1971a, 1986) points to the critical importance of studying younger, preschool populations to increase understanding of the way in which such concepts emerge. While some work with younger populations has already been done (e.g., Johnson & Wellman, 1982), innovative, creative measures to assess health-related concepts in children as young as 2 or 3 are particularly needed. The development of an array of pictorial, play, and other assessment techniques that minimize oral and verbal skills is an especially important methodological challenge.

In addition, assessments of children's health-related concepts must be conducted on populations other than those that are readily available (and sometimes captive), since such limited data bases restrict the generalizability of what is made known through the assessment process.

Assessments of children's health-related concepts must be conducted systematically on heterogeneous populations, and the assessment instruments must be appropriate for socioeconomically, ethnically, racially, and culturally diverse groups. Although some evidence exists that socioeconomic status itself is not a significant determinant of selected health-related concepts in older children (e.g., Gochman, 1972, 1975, 1986), there is a need to ensure that the effects of it and other social factors have been fully investigated.

There is also a need to control for health status and health history in the assessment process. Although Brodie's work (1974) suggests that healthy children view illness differently than do ill, hospitalized children, very little assessment research has attempted to compare beliefs about health and illness, in some controlled, systematic way, in healthy and nonhealthy youngsters. Questions can be raised about whether health history and health status have any appreciable influence on youngsters' health-related concepts (e.g., Gochman, 1971b), but definitive answers have not been provided.

Procedural Issues. Decisive investigations of children's health-related concepts will require integrated cross-sectional and longitudinal assessments. Careful longitudinal study will reveal the degree to which observed changes are attributable to cognitive development or to instrument effects. However, longitudinal research is fraught with problems. It is difficult to follow large numbers of children for a period of years, particularly in a transient, mobile society. Even where evidence exists that a target population has been stable, the closing of industries or the construction and opening of new schools may present unforeseen problems in any systematic follow-ups. Moreover, funding sources are increasingly reluctant to make the long-term commitment required for longitudinal study.

FUTURE DIRECTIONS

Three frames of reference might lead to more fruitful and meaningful assessment research in the future: a commitment to *health behavior* research, systemic models, and demedicalization and wellness.

Health Behavior Research

A Working Definition. The codifying and increased visibility of behavioral medicine (Schwartz & Weiss, 1978) have been exceptionally important steps in addressing health problems, and in reinforcing the ties between medicine and medical technology on the one hand, and knowledge and research methods from the social and behavioral sciences on the other. Although it is clear that the findings emanating from behavioral medicine are being translated in important ways into newer approaches to alleviate disorders, behavioral medicine by itself is only one frame of reference relevant to the assessment of health concepts.

A definition more relevant to research in the area of children's health concepts is that proposed for *health behavior*. As a working definition, the term substantively denotes

> those personal attributes such as beliefs, expectations, motives, values, and other cognitive elements; personality characteristics, including affective and emotional states and traits; and overt behavior patterns, actions, and habits that relate to health maintenance and wellness, to health restoration and to health improvement. (Gochman, 1982b, p. 169)

This working definition further states "that these personal attributes are influenced by, and otherwise reflect family structure and processes, peer group and social factors, and societal, institutional, and cultural determinants" (p. 169). Such a working definition stands independently of pathology, of specific disorders, and of the medical model. It embraces issues of health maintenance in general, as well as behaviors related to specific disorders. The definition embraces both mental and somatic health and recognizes their linkages, in contrast to behavioral medicine, which excludes, with some few exceptions, nonphysical problems.

There is an important directional aspect to the working definition of health behavior: Health behavior research is the interdisciplinary study of the phenomena included in the substantive definition. Health behavior research does not belong to any one discipline or profession, but would involve anthropologists, sociologists, psychologists, social workers, health educators and planners, physicians, nurses, and other health and human service professionals working together to increase rigorous, *basic* research on those personal attributes that relate to maintaining, restoring, and improving health (Gochman, 1982b, p. 170). It seems far more likely that progress in assessing children's health-related concepts will stem from such basic research efforts than that it will stem from the illness-focused, clinically oriented research fostered by behavioral medicine.

Health-Germane Motivation. An important future task for health behavior researchers is the identification of those motives that are germane to health-related behaviors. While health as a motive is not generally salient in young populations (e.g., Gochman, 1971b, 1975, 1982a), other motives may be both potent and relevant in generating health behaviors. Clearly, it is important to distinguish the wish to possess good health from other motives that might be at least as potent in fostering health behaviors. Such motives might include youngsters' wishes to be active physically and socially, to advance academically, and to succeed occupationally and vocationally. Very little systematic research has been done to date on the assessment of such motives in young populations. Such assessments will require diligence and creativity and pose an important challenge to health behavior researchers and to those interested in developing better linkages between health behavior research and the area of child development.

Beliefs and Behaviors. A second important task for future health behavior research is the systematic investigation of the relationships between children's health-related concepts and their overt health actions and behaviors. Although presumptions have been made that behaviors are based on beliefs, and although the major models or paradigms in this area are cognitive, there is yet little evidence that health beliefs and health behaviors are clearly related in young populations. Weisenberg, Kegeles, and Lund (1980) and Kegeles and Lund (1982) raise serious questions about these presumed relationships. It remains for future investigations to assess health-related beliefs and behaviors in a rigorous, systematic fashion, and thus help to clarify their relationships.

Taxonomy of Health Concepts. A third task facing health behavior researchers is compiling a taxonomy of health-related concepts. Success in such a task hinges on increasing the clarity of the concepts involved and on the accumulation of larger amounts of rigorously derived data. There is a need for a complete catalog of health-related beliefs, expectations, perceptions, motives, values, understandings, and other cognitions, along with their definitions, theoretical derivations, empirical measurements, and relationships—both theoretical and empirical—with other variables. Such a compendium would help define a universe of target variables for assessment instruments and processes.

Systemic Models

Systemic models are a second frame of reference that might facilitate the future assessments of youngsters' health concepts. Health-related beliefs, attitudes and perceptions must be examined as systems, that is, as wholes in themselves, and as parts—or subsystems—of other systems. The observation that beliefs about vulnerability, for example, behave as systems (e.g., Gochman, 1973; Gochman & Sheiham, 1978) suggests that future investigations might assess the systemic attributes of other groups of beliefs, such as perceived locus of control, preventive attitudes, and perceptions of causality. Assessment instruments might explore the degree to which such cognitive clusters demonstrate general systemic properties of differentiation, openness to information, and interdependence (e.g., Bertalanffy, 1950; Harvey, Hunt, & Schroder, 1961; Rokeach, 1960; Weiss, 1939). Furthermore, future investigations might assess how particular systems of health-related beliefs relate to other such systems, and the degree to which attributes such as differentiation and interdependence vary in consistent ways in individuals.

Demedicalization and Wellness

A third frame of reference for the future assessment of health concepts in youngsters emerges from critical examinations of the overmedicalization of contemporary American society. Fox (1977) has cogently argued for a thoughtful reconsideration of the overuse of the health–illness metaphor. Bruhn, Williams, and Fitzsimmons (1980) urge increased demedicalization and personal assumption of responsibility in the area of health. Harris and Guten (1979), noting that research on health behavior selects medically approved behaviors such as direct contact with health professionals or compliance with medical regimens, propose instead the inclusion of any behavior believed by an individual to protect, promote, or maintain health regardless of whether the behavior is medically defined as effective. The term *wellness*, itself increasingly overused in inappropriate ways, has been rigorously defined by Bruhn and Cordova (1977) to denote the development of abilities to seek actively to change life situations so that persons can function at their capacity, including the development of competence to deal responsibly with their health.

The concepts of demedicalization and wellness thus have the potential for directing assessments away from dealing strictly with illnesses and professionally defined health issues, and toward the skills, coping mechanisms, and adaptive and proactive capacities of persons. Such thinking can generate different health-related concepts as targets for assessment than are currently typically identified. For example, in the future assessments might be made of youngsters' beliefs about how well they generally cope with demands and challenges, including the challenge of remaining healthy and safe. Assessments might also be made of the priority that youngsters attach to adept personal and social functioning; their ability to distinguish between what might be identified as behavior problems and what might be more justifiably termed illnesses; and their overuse of the illness metaphor. These would all comprise "health-related" concepts.

Herold's analysis (1983) of how the health-belief model can be extended to the area of contraception and Eisen and colleagues' (1985) assessments of beliefs related to pregnancy and contraception reflect this nonmedical, "social functioning" view of health. Other existing examples of such demedicalized assessments are Wellman and Johnson's investigations of children's development of concepts of how the body functions nutritionally (1982); Harris and Guten's moving away from physician-defined health-protective behaviors (1979); and Lau and Hartman's nonmedicalized approach to research on common sense, subjective experiences, and representations of the causes, courses, and consequences of diseases (1983).

References

Barowsky, E. I. (1978). Young children's perceptions and reactions to hospitalization. In E. Gellert (Ed.), *Psychological aspects of pediatric care*. New York: Grune & Stratton.

Bertalanffy, L. von (1950). The theory of open systems in physics and biology. *Science, 111*, 23–29.

Bialer, I. (1961). Conceptualization of success and failure in mentally retarded and normal children. *Journal of Personality, 29*, 303–320.

Bibace, R., & Walsh, M. E. (1981). Children's conceptions of illness. In R. Bibace & M. E. Walsh (Eds.), Children's conceptions of health, illness, and bodily functions. *New directions in developmental psychology* (Vol. 14). San Francisco: Jossey-Bass.

Birney, R. C. (1968). Motivation: Human motivation. In D. L. Sills (Ed.), *International encyclopedia of the social sciences* (Vol. 10). New York: Macmillan and Free Press.

Blos, P., Jr. (1978). Children think about illness: Their concepts and beliefs. In E. Gellert (Ed.), *Psychological aspects of pediatric care*. New York: Grune & Stratton.

Brodie, B. (1974). Views of healthy children toward illness. *American Journal of Public Health, 64*, 1156–1159.

Bruhn, J. G., & Cordova, F. D. (1977). A developmental approach to learning wellness behavior: Part I. Infancy to early adolescence. *Health Values, 1*, 246–254.

Bruhn, J. G., & Parcel, G. S. (1982). Current knowledge about the health behavior of young children: A conference summary. In D. S. Gochman & G. S. Parcel (Eds.), Children's health beliefs and health behavior. *Health Education Quarterly, 9*, 167–174.

Bruhn, J. G., Williams, J. A., & Fitzsimmons, E. L. (1980). *Self-responsibility for health: Focus on the child and the family. Final report of a conference*. Galveston: University of Texas Medical Branch.

Bush, P. J., Parcel, G. S., & Davidson, F. R. (1982, August). *Reliability of a shortened children's health locus of control scale*. Paper presented at the meeting of the American Psychological Association, Washington.

Campbell, J. D. (1975a). Attribution of illness: Another double standard. *Journal of Health & Social Behavior, 16*, 114–126.

Campbell, J. D. (1975b). Illness is a point of view: The development of children's concepts of illness. *Child Development, 46*, 92–100.

Campbell, J. D. (1978). The child in the sick role: Contributions of age, sex, parental status, and parental values. *Journal of Health & Social Behavior, 19*, 35–51.

Carandang, M. L. A., Folkins, C. H., Hines, P. A., & Steward, M. S. (1979). The role of cognitive level and sibling illness in children's conceptualization of illness. *American Journal of Orthopsychiatry, 49*, 474–481.

Chapman, A. H., Loeb, D. G., & Gibbons, M. J. (1956). Psychiatric aspects of hospitalizing children. *Archives of Pediatrics, 73*, 77–88.

Chassin, L., Presson, C. C., Bensenberg, M., Corty, E., Olshavsky, R. W., & Sherman, S. J. (1981). Predicting adolescents' intentions to smoke cigarettes. *Journal of Health & Social Behavior, 22*, 445–455.

Crider, C. (1981). Children's conceptions of the body interior. In R. Bibace & M. E. Walsh (Eds.), Children's conceptions of health, illness, and bodily functions. *New directions in developmental psychology* (Vol. 14). San Francisco: Jossey-Bass.

Cureton, E. E. (1968). Psychometrics. In D. L. Sills (Ed.), *International encyclopedia of the social sciences* (Vol. 13). New York: Macmillan and Free Press.

Deutsch, H. (1942). Some psychoanalytic observations in surgery. *Psychosomatic Medicine, 4*, 105–115.

Dielman, T. E., Leech, S. L., Becker, M. H., Rosenstock, I. M., & Horvath, W. J. (1980). Dimensions of children's health beliefs. *Health Education Quarterly, 7,* 219–238.

Duryea, E. J., & Martin, G. L. (1981). The distortion effect in student perceptions of smoking prevalence. *Journal of School Health, 51,* 115–118.

Eisen, M., Zellman, G. L., & McAlister, A. L. (1985). A health belief model approach to adolescents' fertility control: Some pilot program findings. *Health Education Quarterly, 12,* 185–210.

Fishbein, M., & Ajzen, I. (1975). *Belief, attitude, intention, and behavior: An introduction to theory and research.* Reading, MA: Addison-Wesley.

Fox, R. (1977). The medicalization and demedicalization of American society. In J. H. Knowles (Ed.), *Doing better and feeling worse: Health in the United States.* New York; Norton.

Gellert, E. (1962). Children's conceptions of the content and functions of the human body. *Genetic Psychology Monographs, 61,* 293–405.

Gellert, E. (1978). What do I have inside me? How children view their bodies. In E. Gellert (Ed.), *Psychosocial aspects of pediatric care.* New York: Grune & Stratton.

Gochman, D. S. (1969) Measuring health-relevant expectancies. *Psychological Reports, 24,* 880.

Gochman, D. S. (1970). The Health Ideation Pictures (HIP): Reliability and internal consistency. *Perceptual & Motor Skills, 30,* 271–278.

Gochman, D. S. (1971a). Children's perceptions of vulnerability to illness and accidents: A replication, extension and refinement. *HSMHA Health Reports, 86,* 247–252.

Gochman, D. S. (1971b). Some correlates of children's health beliefs and potential health behavior. *Journal of Health & Social Behavior, 12,* 148–154.

Gochman, D. S. (1972). The development of health beliefs. *Psychological Reports, 31,* 259–266.

Gochman, D. S. (1973). A context for dental health education. *International Journal of Health Education, 16* (Suppl.), 3–8.

Gochman, D. S. (1975). The measurement and development of dentally relevant motives. *Journal of Public Health Dentistry, 35,* 160–164.

Gochman, D. S. (1977). Perceived vulnerability and its psychosocial context. *Social Science & Medicine, 11,* 115–120.

Gochman, D. S. (1982a, August). *Health motivation in youngsters: A longitudinal replication.* Paper presented at the meeting of the American Psychological Association, Washington.

Gochman, D. S. (1982b). Labels, systems and motives: Some perspectives for future research and programs. In D. S. Gochman & G. S. Parcel (Eds.), Children's health beliefs and health behavior. *Health Education Quarterly, 9,* 167–174.

Gochman, D. S. (1985). Family determinants of children's concepts of health and illness. In D. C. Turk & R. D. Kerns (Eds.), *Health, illness, and families: A life-span perspective.* New York: Wiley.

Gochman, D. S. (1986). *Youngsters' health cognitions: Cross-sectional and longitudinal analyses.* Louisville: Health Behavior Systems.

Gochman, D. S., Bagramian, R. A., & Sheiham, A. (1972). Consistency in children's perceptions of vulnerability to health problems. *HSMHA Health Service Reports, 87,* 282–288.

Gochman, D. S., & Saucier, J. F. (1982). Perceived vulnerability in children and adolescents. In D. S. Gochman & G. S. Parcel (Eds.), Children's health beliefs and behaviors. *Health Education Quarterly, 9,* 46–59.

Gochman, D. S., & Sheiham, A. (1978). Cross-national consistency in children's beliefs about vulnerability. *International Journal of Health Education, 21,* 188–193.

Graham, J. R., & Lilly, R. S. (1984). *Psychological testing.* Englewood Cliffs, NJ: Prentice-Hall.

Green, L. W. (1974). Editorial. In M. H. Becker (Ed.), The health belief model and personal health behavior. *Health Education Monographs, 2,* 324.

Harris, D. M., & Guten, S. (1979). Health-protective behavior: An exploratory study. *Journal of Health & Social Behavior, 20,* 17–29.

Harvey, O. J., Hunt, D. E., & Schroder, H. M. (1961). *Conceptual systems and personality organization.* New York: Wiley.

Heider, F. (1958). *The psychology of interpersonal relations.* New York: Wiley.

Herold, E. S. (1983). The health belief model: Can it help us to understand contraceptive use among adolescents? *The Journal of School Health, 53,* 19–21.

Janz, N. K., & Becker, M. H. (1984). The health-belief model: A decade later. *Health Education Quarterly, 11,* 1–47.

Jessner, L., Blom, G. E., & Waldfogel, S. (1952). Emotional implications of tonsillectomy and adenoidectomy on children. *The Psychoanalytical Study of the Child, 7,* 126–169.

Johnson, C. N., & Wellman, H. M. (1982). Children's developing conceptions of the mind and brain. *Child Development, 53,* 222–234.

Kalnins, I., & Love, R. (1982). Children's concepts of health and illness and implications for health education: An overview. In D. S. Gochman & G. S. Parcel (Eds.), Children's health beliefs and health behaviors. *Health Education Quarterly, 9,* 8–19.

Kegeles, S. S., & Lund, A. K. (1982). Adolescents' health beliefs and acceptance of a novel preventive dental activity: Replication and extension. In D. S. Gochman & G. S. Parcel (Eds.), Children's health beliefs and health behaviors. *Health Education Quarterly, 9,* 96–112.

Kelley, H. H. (1967). Attribution theory in social psychology. In D. Levin (Ed.), Current theory and research in motivation. *Nebraska symposium on motivation* (Vol. 15). Lincoln: University of Nebraska Press.

Kister, M. C., & Patterson, C. J. (1980). Children's conceptions of the causes of illness: Understanding of contagion and use of immanent justice. *Child Development, 51,* 839–846.

Lanyon, R. I., & Goodstein, L. D. (1982). *Personality assessment.* New York: Wiley.

Lau, R. R., & Hartman, K. A. (1983). Common sense representations of common illness. *Health Psychology, 2,* 167–185.

Lewis, C. E., & Lewis, M. A. (1982). Children's health related decision making. In D. S. Gochman & G. S. Parcel (Eds.), Health beliefs and health behaviors. *Health Education Quarterly, 9,* 129–141.

Marshall, C. L., Hassanein, K. M., Hassanein, R. S., & Paul, C. L. (1970). Attitudes toward health among children of different races and socioeconomic status. *Pediatrics, 46,* 422–426.

Matus, I., Kinsman, R. A., & Jones, N. F. (1978). Pediatric patient attitudes toward chronic asthma and hospitalization. *Journal of Chronic Diseases, 31,* 611–618.

Mechanic, D. (1964). The influence of mothers on their children's health attitudes and behavior. *Pediatrics, 33,* 444–453.

Michielutte, R., & Diseker, R. A. (1982). Children's perceptions of cancer in comparison to other chronic illnesses. *Journal of Chronic Diseases, 35,* 843–852.

Myers-Vando, R., Steward, M. S., Folkins, C. H., & Hines, P. (1979). The effects of congenital heart disease on cognitive development, illness causality concepts, and vulnerability. *American Journal of Orthopsychiatry, 49,* 617–625.

Nagy, M. H. (1951). Children's ideas on the origin of illness. *Health Education Journal, 9,* 6–12.

Nagy, M. H. (1953). The representation of "germs" by children. *Journal of Genetic Psychology, 83,* 227–240.

Natapoff, J. N. (1982). A developmental analysis of children's ideas of health. In D. S. Gochman & G. S. Parcel (Eds.), Children's health beliefs and health behaviors. *Health Education Quarterly, 9,* 34–45.

Neuhauser, C., Amsterdam, B., Hines, P., & Steward, M. (1978). Children's concepts of healing: Cognitive development and locus of control factors. *American Journal of Orthopsychiatry, 48,* 335–341.

O'Kelly, L. I. (1968). Motivation: The concept. In D. L. Sills (Ed.), *International encyclopedia of the social sciences* (Vol. 10). New York: Macmillan and Free Press.

Parcel, G. S., & Meyer, M. P. (1978). Development of an instrument to measure children's locus of control. In B. A. Wallston & K. A. Wallston (Eds.), Health locus of control. *Health Education Monographs, 6,* 149–159.

Rashkis, S. R. (1965). Children's understanding of health. *Archives of General Psychiatry, 12,* 10–17.

Rokeach, M. (1960). *The open and closed mind: Investigations into the nature of belief systems and personality systems.* New York: Basic.

Rosenstock, I. M. (1974). Historical origins of the health-belief model. In M. H. Becker (Ed.), The health belief model and personal health behavior. *Health Education Monographs, 2,* 328–335.

Schwartz, G. E., & Weiss, S. M. (Eds.) (1978). *Proceedings of the Yale Conference on Behavioral Medicine.* DHEW Publication No. NIH 78-1424.

Simeonsson, R. J., Buckley, L., & Monson, L. (1979). Conceptions of illness causality in hospitalized children. *Journal of Pediatric Psychology, 4,* 77–84.

Steuart, G. W. (1952). Emergency hospitalization of young children: The psychological effects. *South African Medical Journal, 7,* 472–476.

Urberg, K., & Robbins, R. (1984). Perceived vulnerability in adolescents to the health consequences of cigarette smoking. *Preventive Medicine, 13,* 367–376.

Vernon, D. T. A., Foley, J. H., Sipowicz, R. P., & Schulman, J. L. (1965). *The psychological responses of children to hospitalization and illness: A review of the literature.* Springfield, IL: Charles C. Thomas.

Wallston, B. S., & Wallston, K. A. (1978). Locus of control and health: A review of the literature. In B. S. Wallston & K. A. Wallston (Eds.), Health locus of control. *Health Education Monographs, 6,* 107–117.

Weisenberg, M., Kegeles, S. S., & Lund, A. K. (1980). Children's health beliefs and acceptance of a precentive activity. *Journal of Health & Social Behavior, 21,* 59–74.

Weiss, P. (1939). *Principles of development.* New York: Holt, Rinehart & Winston.

Wellman, H. M., & Johnson, C. N. (1982). Children's understanding of food and its functions: A preliminary study of the development of concepts of nutrition. *Journal of Applied Developmental Psychology, 3,* 135–148.

15

Pain Assessment in Children I: Concepts and Measurement Strategies

PAUL KAROLY

Beginning at birth, the human organism is confronted with pain. The normal stresses of living and/or the burdens of a chronic or acute medical condition bring pain into even sharper relief. Pediatricians, health psychologists, nurses, and other health professionals are therefore likely to encounter, at various levels, the pain problems of infants, children, and adolescents; it is not unreasonable to expect that these practitioners should be able to draw upon a fundamental store of knowledge, constructed on a valid empirical and clinical data base. As this chapter will illustrate, the conceptual and technical basis of pediatric pain assessment is an emerging enterprise rather than a fully formed science. Current limitations in measurement stem from both active misconception and passive neglect, and the future of pain treatment for children rests squarely upon the ability of researchers and practitioners to systematize their theories and assessment methodologies and to organize their energies on behalf of a woefully understudied population.

The preparation of this chapter was supported in part by grant #PMH 39246-03, establishing the Preventive Intervention Research Center (PIRC) at Arizona State University.

An editorial in the *New England Journal of Medicine* (Angell, 1982) noted: "Pain is soul-destroying. No patient should have to endure pain unnecessarily." Unfortunately, it would appear from the tenor of recent surveys that this humanitarian sentiment is being applied somewhat selectively—namely, to *adult* pain sufferers. A perusal of contemporary research journals will, for example, reveal that, relative to the study of pain in adults, pediatric pain has attracted little attention (cf. Eland & Anderson, 1977; Schechter, 1984; Varni & Thompson, 1986). The day-to-day practice of medicine, in diagnostic, interventive, and postoperative settings, has likewise handled pediatric pain rather unceremoniously and often naively.

Swafford and Allen (1968) found that, over a 4-month period, only 26 of 180 children admitted to their intensive care unit received narcotic medication, under the assumption that children didn't require pain relief. Schechter, Allen, and Hanson (1986), after reviewing the charts of 90 children and 90 adults (matched for sex and diagnosis), found that, overall, adults received twice the dosage of narcotics that children did, with the discrepancy growing as increased time in hospital was required. Further, narcotics were less likely to be ordered for younger than for older children. In addition to suffering postoperative neglect, it has been shown that children undergoing lumbar punctures, bone marrow aspirations, neonatal circumcisions, and burn debridement procedures, among others, tend to receive little or no analgesic preparation, especially when medication level is left to the discretion of the staff (Eland & Anderson, 1977; Mennie, 1974; Schechter, 1984).

The narrow scope of extant conceptual models and the technical difficulties associated with obtaining reliable self-descriptions from children will occupy the bulk of our attention in this chapter. It is also worth noting that inattentiveness to the needs of children in pain can in part be attributed to medical and/or nursing "myths" concerning the nature of nociception. Among the misconceptions noted are the following:

Children's "immature nervous systems" (slow degree of cortical development) prevent them from feeling pain as adults do—particularly along the *intensity* dimension.

Children are more susceptible than adults to the addictive potential of narcotic analgesics.

Sleeping children are not in pain.

Children cannot localize their pain.

Children recover more quickly from painful experiences (and will not remember them for very long).

These and other beliefs have been found to be either unverifiable or incorrect; yet portions of the clinical community continue to espouse them (cf. Eland & Anderson, 1977; Hawley, 1984; Jacox, 1981).

Despite the availability of technological and data-analytic tools for debunking some of the folklore in pediatric pain, many basic concepts remain fuzzy and many core issues remain as yet ill defined. Lavigne, Schulein, and Hahn (1986), for example, have articulated three fundamental problems. First, the generally accepted definition of pain tends to blend both subjective ("an unpleasant sensory and emotional experience") and objective ("associated with actual or potential tissue damage") elements; and different assessment methods are often used to tap the distinct facets. Second, pain and emotionality (particularly anxiety) have to date proven to be "inextricably confounded." And, third, the developmental aspects of pain have remained largely unresearched, with undue reliance still placed upon adult-oriented measurement strategies in clinical work with children.

The definition of pain (as an unpleasant sensory and emotional experience associated with damage to bodily tissue) issued by the International Association for the Study of Pain (IASP) in 1979 is consistent with the most widely accepted theoretical perspective, the *gate-control model* of Melzack and Wall (1965, 1983). The view that pain is multidimensional and that its modulation is a complex process involving afferent (sensory transmission), central (cortical), and motor networks has served to liberate the study and treatment of pain from the confining influence of the traditional linear, reductionist, input–output model, thereby undergirding the multidisciplinary study of nociception. Nonetheless, the role of cognitive organizational and control processes in pain and the potential contribution of situational variables to the perception and self-modification of nociceptive signals have not been systematically investigated in youngsters with painful medical conditions or in physically healthy children. Despite its obvious utility, then, the IASP definition of pain remains strongly medical (or body centered) and focuses perhaps too much on the short-term aspects of adaptation (cf. Karoly, 1985). From a developmental standpoint also, the current conceptualization offers little guidance—except that age-related changes in sensory detection and emotionality might be important in differentiating the adult from the child pain experience.

As this brief commentary has shown, the field of pediatric pain assessment is fairly rudimentary as a clinical undertaking, as a domain of experimental investigation, and as a breeding ground for theory. In the interest of incremental advancement, the objectives in this chapter include: (1) a presentation of an expanded conceptual model of the psychosocial dimensions of pain, touching upon several sources of mediation; and (2) a review of both current and promising methods of pediatric pain assessment. A detailed illustrative analysis of a common childhood disorder—recurrent abdominal pain—is presented in the next chapter of this volume.

RECURRENT PAIN AS AN INFORMATION CONTROL–ACTION SYSTEM

Pain is commonly referred to as a sensory event, an affective response, a symptom of disease or injury (trauma), a complaint not clearly attributable to a known medical condition, and an unpleasant sensory by-product of medical and dental procedures (cf. Lavigne et al., 1986; Varni, 1984). To index pain as described, researchers often rely upon biochemical, psychophysiological (e.g., heart rate, skin conductance), or behavioral measures. Because of the real and presumed difficulties in assessing pain in children at the experiential level—necessitating self-report—the tendency toward molecular levels of analysis has been especially prevalent in pediatric settings. It is almost as if the assumption is being made that *there is very little information contained in a pain display aside from the fact that the child is experiencing hurt or discomfort beyond normal*. While this assumption seems quite valid as applied to acute (short-term, stimulus-induced) pain, it may be misleading and counterproductive in the case of chronic pain.

If children are forced to live with the unpleasant sensation called pain for a protracted period of time, they *think* about it (where it comes from, why they are stricken, what can be done to reduce or eliminate it), they *talk* about it (to fellow patients on hospital wards, or to parents and siblings at home), they try to *prepare* for it, they develop *styles of communicating their pain nonverbally*, and if the pain persists long enough, they develop *ways of using pain to control others* as well as *ways of controlling the pain*. Children on a burn unit have been observed to engage in discussions with one another about the nature of their treatment, often communicating exaggerated accounts of their suffering at the hands of the staff (Beales, 1982). Children with recurrent headaches have been known to report an increase in pain when school examinations draw nearer (Varni, Katz, & Dash, 1982). Children with chest pain are sometimes accompanied to the physician's office by parents who expect their child to die prematurely (Coleman, 1984). Countless examples exist that illustrate the limitations of a categorical approach to the assessment of pain (particularly as an event that either occurs or doesn't occur) and of a mechanistic and unidimensional (single cause, single effect) model of pain causality (cf. Karoly & Jensen, 1987; Schwartz, 1984). In place of these, a multilayered *contextual model* of assessment is suggested, along with an information processing–action control perspective on understanding the processes inherent in the extended pain experience. This section will focus upon the latter (followed by a discussion of the multiple-contexts assessment model).

First, it is suggested that a useful way to talk and think about chronic pain is as a *verb*—to pain (or to be in pain)—rather than as a noun (a state, a thing, an end product). By this it is *not* meant that pain is nothing more than pain behavior (e.g., grimacing, crying, rubbing, etc.). Instead, it is asserted that pain is an activity that permits an affective, behavioral, cognitive, and environmental *level of analysis*, depending upon one's domain of interest. Pain is a process that unfolds over time and in context, like familiar constructs that we are used to thinking about in such terms—for example, *eating*. Eating is an activity that can be looked upon purely at the motoric level, as a series of hand-to-mouth movements and their biochemical correlates and consequences. Similarly, eating is associated with affect—from deprivation to satiety. Eating is also something we think about, plan, and evaluate—an activity that has *symbolic meaning* to us. In addition, eating is situationally cued and constrained (that is, we typically eat in restaurants rather than in restrooms). There is more to eating than just being hungry, or chewing, or digesting. Whether a given eating episode is adaptive is dependent upon other factors—it possesses no absolute value. Eating varies in terms of being perceptually *figural* versus being *unattended* (background); and whether it is relevant to current pursuits depends upon how closely proprioceptive signals are monitored. Finally, one can choose to control (exhibit or inhibit via conscious means) the act of eating, depending upon either personal judgment or environmental pressures calling for increased or decreased food consumption. Each of these facets of eating holds in the case of "paining" (and the reader is strongly urged to construct his or her own comparisons).

Could we ever hope to understand and/or treat obese children if all we knew about them was how much they eat when they are at their hungriest? Of course not. To understand fully the processes involved in overeating, we would want to know about its long- and short-term antecedents, the child's beliefs about food, the role of situational cues, family models, peer group norms, reinforcement contingencies, self-reactions, the workings of the digestive organs, fat cell count, and a host of *biopsychosocial* variables that provide the context for overeating. No single factor would be relied upon to capture the "essence" of a complex process. Yet, interestingly, the most common assessment of children's pain (sometimes the only measure taken) is intensity level (cf., Varni, Jay, Masek, & Thompson, 1986). The traditional interest in indexing children's perceptions of pain intensity is doubtless linked to the medical community's desire to coordinate analgesic drug dosage with bodily need. While this practice may make sense in the treatment of acute pain, it loses much of its relevance when applied to prolonged, chronic pain conditions.

Continuing with the surprisingly apt analogy between pain processes and eating processes, we note that a heuristically and clinically productive approach to the study of appetite derives from the field of cybernetics or control theory. It is an approach that is compatible with both a molecular (biochemical) emphasis and a higher-order, cognitive emphasis.

Control theory, information theory, and *cybernetics* are terms that refer broadly to a model of regulatory activity within any system (biological or mechanical) that: (1) interacts with its environment in order to maintain a sensed state close or equal to a predetermined standard; and (2) does so by means of a negative feedback process. *Negative feedback* implies that the system perceives an existing state of affairs, compares the input against a reference (preferred or preset) value, and, if a discrepancy is detected, acts to reduce the discrepancy (the effects being opposite, or *negative,* to the initial state). Guyton (1982) describes the human body as consisting of thousands of control systems, typified by the respiratory system, which regulates the concentration of carbon dioxide in extracellular fluid, or the baroreceptor system, which regulates arterial pressure. The overall biologic goal is homeostasis, and, as Rodin (1982) has noted; "most of our life-maintaining biological processes depend upon autoregulatory, homeostatic processes. . . . In some ways this precise reflex system may serve as a metaphor and conceptual model for self-regulation at the behavioral level as well" (p. 63). That is, many self-regulatory processes depend upon learned, instrumental, consciously mediated activities as well as upon innate, biologically programmed responses (as are involved in breathing or blood pressure maintenance).

A frequently cited exemplar of a negative feedback–based self-regulating mechanical system is the thermostatically controlled air-conditioning system in the home. Indeed, because cybernetics (or control theory) originated in the engineering and communication sciences, many mechanical analogies are applied to the description of people—as in likening homeostasis to the operation of a thermostat. In recent years, it has become popular also to view the nervous system as a cybernetic, internal regulatory system, which, instead of merely reacting in a linear (input–output) fashion to environmental stimulation, operates in the service of higher-order reference standards (cf. Powers, 1972). Eating, for example, has been linked to an organismic set point, such that individuals who successfully diet may be prone to eat and regain their lost pounds because of the body's desire to achieve a genetically preset weight level. The question before us, of course, is whether a cybernetic perspective can assist us in penetrating the complexities of the chronic pain experience; an experience that we have suggested is more closely analogous to the contextually embedded, multicausal, yet centrally modulated process of eating than it is to the peripheral, "bottom-up" process of sensory signal detection.

To understand chronic pain in control theory terms we should perhaps begin by pointing out that what is controlled in any human self-regulating system is *information*. The brain, the executive of the system and the arbiter of its hierarchically ordered reference standards, deals only with middlemen, not directly with the changing energy patterns of the external (nonbodily) environment. Direct contact with heat and cold, mechanical or tactile pressure, and the like occur at the level of the sense receptor, which then changes, or *transduces*, the original signal into patterns of neural firing decoded within higher cortical centers.

Information in any system is indexed (its value is fixed) by the amount of uncertainty that is reduced by its receipt. Of course no system (including the human information processing system) could be called adaptive if all input were the same (if there were no alternative possibilities) and uncertainty were reduced to zero. The nervous system operates against a background of "noise" from which a signal is abstracted by virtue of the signal's redundancy or information value. In the domain of nociception, it is commonly asserted that *only acute pain possesses significant information value*. For example, Melzack and Wall (1983) note that acute pain provides a signal of injury and an impetus to action in the interest of promoting relief or recovery. Chronic pain, by contrast, is a signal that "persists after all possible healing has occurred or, at least, long after pain can serve any useful function, and is no longer simply a symptom of injury or disease" (p. 55).

It is more in keeping with contemporary cognitive psychology to view chronic pain as involving a *potentially dysfunctional information system* than to view it as possessing minimal information value. To articulate the difference between acute and chronic pain signals, I shall make use of the model of depth (or levels) of processing that was popularized by Craik and his colleagues (Craik & Lockhart, 1972; Craik & Tulving, 1975) and is consistent with other hierarchical conceptions of information processing (e.g., Gallistel, 1980; John, 1976; Konorski, 1967; Martindale, 1981; Powers, 1972; Rasmussen, 1986). Basically, it is assumed that stimuli can be analyzed to varying degrees of complexity or "depth," and that the more extensive (deeper) the analysis, the greater the degree of understanding, recall, and interpretation. It has been argued that the analysis of raw sensations occurs at a shallow level of processing (localized in the sensory cortex), and that a sensory signal takes on meaning only when it is analyzed semantically (at a later stage) (cf. Martindale, 1981). Another important characteristic of self-regulating, multilevel cognitive systems is their close connection to arousal, activation, or action. Recall that in cybernetics any sensed deviation from a reference level will call forth a behavior designed to reduce the deviation. Or, as Powers (1972) put it: "The only reason for which any higher organism acts is to counteract the effects of disturbances (constant or varying) on controlled quantities" (p. 47). The action system component provides the warrant for our thinking about pain as a verb, reminding us that pain involves *doing* as well as *feeling*. Thus the pain system can be conceptualized in terms of: (1) shallow (sensory) processing; (2) meaning analysis (at deeper levels); and (3) an associated action system, the most obvious elements of which consist of pain exhibition (communication) or pain control. Such a system is depicted in Figure 15.1, wherein the arrows indicate connection (and direction of influence is two way).

Thus from our cybernetic, levels-of-processing view, it may be asserted that acute pain does not need to be processed very deeply because it is time limited and open to few alternative interpretations (e.g., it possesses a high degree of certainty). It calls forth a limited repertoire of responses (actions) as well. It is clear, therefore, why it carries high information value. On the other hand, chronic pain,

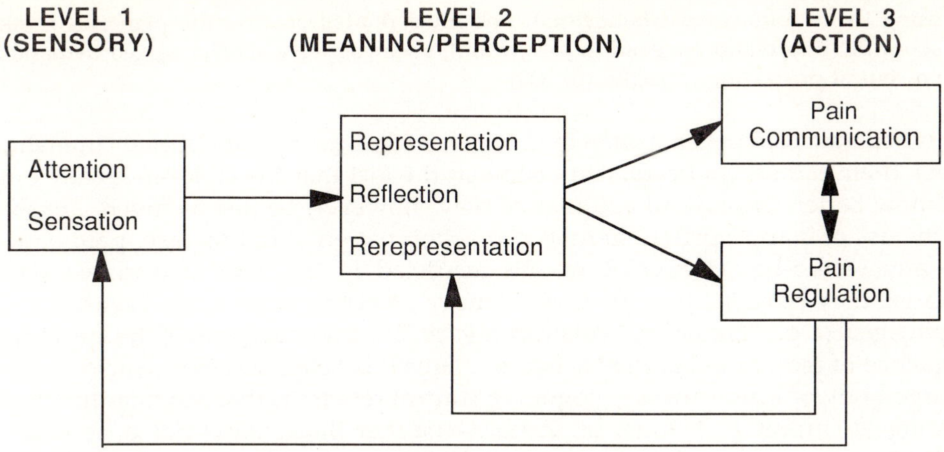

FIGURE 15.1. A model of recurrent pain as an information control–action system.

being more ambiguous, is subject to deeper levels of processing—and it is here that the potential for dysfunctional regulation enters the picture. That is, while acute pain is largely stimulus activated, chronic pain experience is influenced mainly by subjectively held reference values that can be organized around representational models (schemata) of *pain events* and *pain goals*. These event and goal representations are capable of influencing lower-level sensory encoding as well as the action system (cf. also Karoly & Jensen, 1987; Leventhal & Everhart, 1979).

Recurrent sensory experiences of pain contribute to the internal representation (model or schema). Similarly, the model of internal events helps determine what stimuli are attended to and labeled as pain. The process is thus a dialectical one. It is hypothesized that one factor potentially limiting the quality of representation-driven processing in chronic pain will be the structural organization of the internal model, varying along a simplicity (rigidity) versus complexity (flexibility) dimension. That is, a simple model ("that particular sensation I feel is either pain or it isn't" or "any sensation coming from my stomach is either hunger or pain") is efficient, but it also carries the likelihood of confirmatory bias and resistance to experiential modification (cf. Winfrey & Goldfried, 1986).

A second potential source of dysfunctionality has to do with the operation of the action system, which can be activated by environmental or sensory cues or by the pain schema. Pain patients (adults as well as children) may tend either to communicate their pain experiences or to seek to cope with (regulate) their felt pain by means of self-defeating, inefficient action patterns. Specifically, automatized (or overlearned) behaviors that were once effective in communication or control may be emitted inappropriately by pain patients, particularly when stressed by too much affect (fear, anxiety) or too much information (conflicting goals). As Semmer and Frese (1985) pointed out:

> When an action has been automatized, its starting point may not be consciously controlled, and it is, therefore, resistant to change once begun. Further it is difficult to stop using an automatized behavior and to replace it with another one. . . . To stop

> using them (automatized behaviors), one must reintellectualize the plan and think about the information needed to carry it out; such cognitive activity placed demands on central processing capacity. (p. 303)

Thus pediatric pain patients often tend to behave in ways that are labeled "immature," while their parents and caretakers bemoan the fact that the children "really ought to know better." Failure to automatize may, however, be just as much a problem as the use of inappropriate, stereotyped action patterns. In this case, pain patients (or any would-be self-regulators) are restricted in the flow of effective actions because they have *not* learned how to move smoothly from a representation of a coping goal (e.g., "I must try to distract myself") to the enactment of the appropriate sequence of motor or cognitive activities. Thus it is being asserted (consistent with a large body of action theory–cognitive control research) that schema-driven processing in chronic pain must be flexible—neither thoughtless nor obsessive—in order to serve as a guide to long-term adaptation.

MEDIATORS AND MECHANISMS

The foregoing discussion of information–control theory in pain has left a great deal of room for consideration of dynamic elements, those individual difference factors, developmental parameters, ecological constraints, and other structural or functional features that allow the model to be applied to specific patients under specific conditions. While space limitations prohibit a systematic appraisal of theoretically derived or empirically verified mediators of the chronic pain process in children, a brief analysis shall be undertaken concerning both the contents and processes of pain "cognizing," which tend to vary as a function of age and experience. Such contents and processes are the key anchoring points for a relational (noncategorical) understanding of chronic pain (and should be the foci of a comprehensive, relational *assessment* of chronic pain as well).

To assist in this analysis, Table 15.1 and Table 15.2 present summaries of the hypothesized pain information processing constructs along with their constituent parts (Table 15.1) and the processes or functions that presumably act upon these elements (Table 15.2). It is considered heuristically useful, for example, to distinguish between, say, a pain memory (at the meaning level, Table 15.1) and the processes involved in retrieving it, evaluating it, or verbalizing it (Table 15.2).

Cognitive Developmental Factors

The frequently cited recognition that pain experience (particularly the sensory–perceptual and evaluative components) may vary with age and/or cognitive maturation has not yet precipitated broad-based longitudinal investigations. Instead, interest has tended to focus upon cross-sectional (or age-specific) differences in children's language use and comprehension and their conceptual handling of health- and illness-related concepts, usually (but not exclusively) orchestrated around a Piagetian framework (cf., Bibace & Walsh, 1981; Thompson & Varni, 1986). While such work is extremely important, allowing clinicians to gauge the degree of effective communication between themselves and their young patients, it has tended to be

TABLE 15.1. CONTENT DIMENSIONS ASSOCIATED WITH CHRONIC PAIN AS AN INFORMATION CONTROL–ACTION SYSTEM

The Sensory Level

Attentional foci
Pain threshold
Pain tolerance limit

The Relational Meaning (Schematic) Level

Perception of intensity
Pain-related memories
Pain-related self-appraisals
General self-appraisals (self-knowledge)
Body consciousness
Orientation toward past
Orientation toward future
Attitudes toward medicine and medical interventions
Treatment preferences
Health values
Affective reactions (depression, anxiety, etc.)
Attributions of suffering
Pain-related goals, values and standards
Self-efficacy attributions
Personal theory(ies): pain causation; pain modification (external); pain modification (self); rational and irrational beliefs about pain; pain locus of control-responsibility
Knowledge base (pain specific and general)

The Action Level

Problem-solving attitudes and skills
Behavioral enactment skills (e.g., relaxation, assertiveness)
Cognitive coping skills (e.g., distraction, self-instruction, meditation)
Sick-role behaviors (e.g., help-seeking patterns, medical compliance patterns)
Pain behaviors (e.g., crying, bracing, wincing, etc.)

highly symptom centered. As Varni and colleagues (1986) note, "developmentally appropriate assessment instruments that measure more than just pain intensity are noticeably lacking" (p. 170).

The present framework offers a number of directions for future assessment research. Referring to Table 15.1, for example, we see that children's schemata about pain can provide an intricate yet potentially informative context within which to understand the significance of a pain intensity report or a behavioral (overt) pain response. Would not a child's request for medication be less ambiguous if we also possessed data on that child's beliefs about pain causation and about the role of medicine in treatment? Similarly, the singular fact that a child evidences an excellent grasp of the subtle nuances among pain labels could be interpreted more

TABLE 15.2. PROCESSING MECHANISMS ASSOCIATED WITH CHRONIC PAIN AS AN INFORMATION CONTROL–ACTION SYSTEM

Attentional scanning and perceptual signal detection
Arousability, habituation, central inhibitory mechanisms, temperament, peripheral fiber sensitization
Patterns of self-monitoring, field dependence–independence
Activation of pain-related images by environmental stimuli
Activation of pain-related concepts by environmental stimuli
Cognitive style differences in:
Encoding
Retrieval
Organization and storage (configuration and retention in memory)
Transformation (e.g., feature extraction, perspective shift)
Evaluative processing (judgment, attribution, matching, rules formulation)
Propositional logic (condition–action rule use) and causal reasoning
Operant and respondent thought
Goal (standard) setting and resetting
Learning:
Associative processing (verbal and nonverbal)
Overlearning
Vicarious learning and modeling
Operant conditioning
Symbol manipulation
Nonconscious (automatic) processing
Action identification
Social (Interactional) processes:
Modeling
Recognition and evaluation of "place rules"
Contingent and noncontingent social reward–social punishment
Stimulus overload–underload
Language
Self-directed, inner speech and imagery manipulation

fully if one also knew the degree to which that child accurately monitors proprioceptive signals or engages in verbal and/or nonverbal elaboration of past experiences (see Table 15.2).

A potentially salient (though unstudied) dimension in children's pain experience may be the relation between sensory encoding and *self-knowledge*. The present emphasis on the processes of representation, reflection, and rerepresentation (or schema construction) is consistent with recent developmental studies of children's emergent sense of identity and competence (cf. Harter, 1987; Ruble, 1987). It has been postulated that children develop a sense of uniqueness, continuity across time and settings, and self-worth as a function of organismic and social constraints and cognitive appraisals. If children are, indeed, "motivated to construct rules or theories about themselves and their social environments" (Ruble, 1987, p. 244), then it would stand to reason that chronic illness, injury, or other pain-related experiences could have an important impact upon self-definition(s) and that self-definition(s) would, in turn, influence the interpretation and memory of pain or illness experiences (cf. also Breakwell, 1986). Of course, age-related differences in reasoning ability, motive structure, family norms and expectations, self-monitoring propensity, and the like would set further limits on the relationship between pain expression and self-knowledge.

Individual differences and/or age-related differences in information-seeking style may affect not only pain schemata but action strategies as well. The work of Suzanne Miller (e.g., Miller & Green, 1985) suggests that preferences (learned or innate) for avoidance or approach (blunting vs. monitoring) under conditions of stress may interact with situational parameters in determining the effectiveness of children's coping efforts.

Temperament

Although thus far only cognitive–developmental or behavioral concepts have been afforded much attention, the control theory view discussed here recognizes the role of sensory–biologic parameters. To borrow Varni's (1983) term, our model is *cognitive–biobehavioral* in nature. Recognition of biological constraints has typically meant an analysis of the "medical" dimensions of pain (e.g., the child's vital signs, medication use, physical mobility, history of hospitalizations, and any specific disease markers associated with the pain symptomatology); it has not led to a careful or systematic examination of an organismic facet likely to influence such things as attentional style, threshold, pain tolerance, body awareness, affectivity, or coping strategies (among others)—namely, the child's temperament. Although quite familiar in developmental pediatrics in general, the concept of temperament has been given little, if any, empirical attention in pediatric pain assessment. *Temperament* is usually understood to refer to a stylistic aspect of behavior emerging out of innate constitution in interaction with parental socialization and resulting in differences in behavioral tempo, rhythmicity, energy level, distractibility, mood, arousability, and the like (Carey, 1982; Chess & Thomas, 1984; Seifer, Chapter 7, this volume). Admittedly oversimplified, the temperament clusters most often discussed are the "easy child" (characterized by adaptability to change), the "difficult child" (biologically irregular, nonadaptable, given to intense affective reactions), and the "slow-to-warm-up child" (who combines negative responses to novelty with slow adaptability over time). Temperament factors may play a significant role in types of pediatric pain not clearly attributable to disease (e.g., recurrent abdominal pain or migraine headache), predisposing the susceptible youngster to the potentially damaging effects of prolonged stress. Similarly, highly reactive and physically active youngsters are said to be at risk for pain due to injury (Carey, 1986).

An important concept growing out of temperament studies such as Chess and Thomas's New York Longitudinal Study is that of *goodness of fit*, postulating that healthy functioning depends upon a compatibility between the child's characteristics and the demands and expectations of his or her encountered environment. Strictly speaking, then, it is the interaction of a child's behavioral style and family attributes that best represents the potential *risk factor* for pathological outcomes among the chronically ill, including but not limited to youngsters with pain complaints.

Sociocultural Factors

A fundamental assumption of action-theoretic models is that actions and cognitions are partly created and controlled by social forces. Members of social communities (including subunits, such as families and peer groups) share functionally important representations called social conventions, which affect an individual's perceptions, conscious representations, and interpretative styles (cf. Von Cranach, Mächler, & Steiner, 1985). While it has long been recognized that a child with a chronic pain problem can influence family dynamics, it is less common for investigators to search out the mechanisms whereby family dynamics influence pain onset and maintenance (Flor & Turk, 1985). However, since family-centered tuition and modeling are crucial determinants of reference values (standards, set points, etc.) for pain tolerance, pain display, pain labeling, and pain-related goals and incentives, it is clear that the child–family transaction must be characterized by a bidirectional flow of information and action.

Any complex system (setting) makes "demands" upon its members, even when those members are children with pain complaints and/or painful medical conditions. Settings activate different styles of information processing and often provide markers denoting which features (inputs) are relevant and which can be ignored. The precise nature of the dialectical interchange between the pediatric pain patient and his or her social world, while not easily understood, is clarified by the concept of goodness of fit noted previously. That is, the adaptive processing of pain-relevant information can be facilitated or hindered by one's social environment—facilitated if parents, siblings, friends, relatives, and teachers match their demands or expectancies to the child's resource capacities, and disrupted if there is a distinct mismatch (overload or underutilization). In applying the information control–action system model to individual children it will be necessary, therefore, to assess the family, peer, and school environments with respect to their facilitative or disruptive role in the young patient's life. The data deriving from self-report methods or task simulations (two methods that are justifiably popular) can be quite misleading if one ignores the transactional nature of child adaptation and the real-world goodness of fit between the patient and his or her context.

A FRAMEWORK FOR PEDIATRIC PAIN ASSESSMENT

The translation of the conceptual model just outlined into practical assessment procedures should be fostered by means of a compatible measurement model. The tendency to avoid or sidestep measurement models or to build models around existing instruments has been the norm in adult pain assessment, and clearly poses a danger to the pediatric domain as well. However, the information–action control perspective would appear capable of addressing the problems of subjectivity, emotionality, variability, and developmental relevance that have for so long plagued the field of child pain assessment.

Elsewhere, the author and his associates have outlined a *pain context* model (Karoly, 1985; Karoly & Jensen, 1987), the characteristics of which are consistent with a biopsychosocial perspective on children's pain. The context model, as its name suggests, advocates a nonreductionistic, multivariable, transactional approach to pain as a product and as a process. Unlike some assessment frameworks, however, the context approach does not uniformly recommend the use of multiple response modes as a means of triangulating upon the "essence" of pain. Instead, the assessor's major purpose in seeking to gauge an individual's pain experience serves as the starting point in the selection of an assessment battery. Among the system's guiding principles are the following:

Pain must be addressed *relationally*. No single index is sufficient to reflect the experience of pain nor to capture the meaning pain holds for the individual. Both the *social* and *temporal* embeddedness of pain need to be included in any relational assessment.

The three major interpretive contexts of pain are its biomedical (psychophysiologic) aspects, its experiential dimensions, and its relational meaning (see Table 15.3).

Any assessment enterprise should include a competency-based rather than strictly a deficiency-based perspective on the patient.

The so-called objective or behavioral aspects of pain are critical primarily because they are outputs that are fed back to the actor and observed and interpreted by significant others in the patient's life (communicative products). Behaviors are not more real than other dimensions.

The elements of the three major facets of the context model are presented in Table 15.3. A fourth facet is the theoretical or interpretive context within which medical and allied health professionals operate. It will not be discussed in this chapter (but see Karoly & Jensen, 1987, chap. 1).

TABLE 15.3. THE THREE PRIMARY CONTEXTS OF PAIN AND THEIR FACETS

Context I:	*Biomedical Aspects*
	a. Medical and surgical history
	b. Physical diagnosis related to pain complaints
	c. Medication use (present and past)
	d. Family health history and current practices
	e. Neurophysiological status
	f. Doctor–patient relationships
Context II:	*Focal–Experiential Dimensions*
	a. Sensory–perceptual
	b. Affective
	c. Performance (functional, motoric)
	d. Interpersonal
	e. Verbal
	f. Cognitive–representational
Context III:	*Meaning–Relational Dimensions*
	a. Developmental–temporal
	b. Motivational (rehabilitative)
	c. Normative adjustmental
	d. Situational
	e. Vocational–academic
	f. Familial
	g. Self-understanding–self-regulatory

The Three Contexts of Pain

The archetypical interpretative context for pain is the biomedical (Context I). Here, physicians and nurses seek to uncover the pathophysiology of pain disorders and, secondarily, the psychological contributors to adjustment. Where there is evidence of tissue damage or organic involvement (circulatory or neurological problems), the assessment of pain—particularly acute pain—appears to serve a *tracking* function. Pain location and intensity provide clues as to the organic "source" of pain (diagnosis) and the efficacy of surgical or pharmacologic interventions. Noninvasive treatments (e.g., hypnosis) can also be tracked by changes in symptom report. The medical community seems to favor modes of pain assessment that can be applied under conditions of minimal patient cooperation—for it is under stressful circumstances that most pediatric cases are seen (cf. Schechter, 1985). Thus observational methods, simple self-report indices (e.g., fear thermometers), and physiologic methods (e.g., GSR, spectrographic analyses of infant vocalizations) are most often chosen.

When children's pain persists (for at least 6 months) after "healing" has ostensibly taken place or when no clear organic pathology can be identified, the assessment process takes on a different, often controversial, complexion. Wide variation in children's responses to known injury, painful medical procedures, or disease also implicates such elusive factors as personality, emotionality, hypochondriasis, pain proneness, defense mechanisms, and a host of similar constructs that over the years have been thrown into the diagnostic stew called *psychogenic pain*. Abdominal pain, limb pain, and headache are among the pediatric "medical" problems most often labeled psychiatric, calling forth vague causal accounts, "buttressed" typically by nonstandardized assessment devices (cf. Beales, 1982; Poznanski, 1976). Data of a fundamental, biomedical sort can be extremely valuable; but they should be limited to the facets noted in Table 15.3. Family history, a thorough medical examination including appropriate ancillary tests, and any other standard medical procedures represent the range of applicability of Context I measurement. Limiting pediatric pain assessment to within-the-body modes of analysis, however, does not accord with contemporary conceptual models (such as the gate-control theory), and can severely handicap rehabilitative efforts, especially in "chronic" cases.

Context II assessment focuses upon the experience and expression of hurt and suffering, tapping the *what* of pain in contrast to the *why* or *where* (facets included in Context I). A major assumption of Context II is that pain is a multiply determined amalgam of sensory, cognitive, and action elements that cannot be reduced to any single facet without sacrificing the emergent quality of the experience (cf. Melzack & Wall, 1983). To date, the sensory intensity aspect of children's pain has received the most attention from assessors, typically via visual analogue scales, pain thermometers, and color spectrum ratings (Varni et al., 1986). Observational indices (performance measures) and physiological methods are also used—typically in research studies rather than in clinical protocols—but are labor intensive compared to self-report measures (cf. Katz, Kellerman, & Siegel, 1980; Melamed & Siegel, 1975). Unfortunately, contemporary methods of experiential analysis have been selected more often on the basis of convenience than on the basis of their ability reliably to address a specific assessment question. (Sometimes the costlier method is the only reasonable one.) Notably infrequent are attempts to assess the child's representation of pain experience—his or her appraisals, self-assessments, implicit theories, expectancies, causal scenarios, pain-related goals, and other cognitive contents, structures, or processes relevant to the assimilation and expression of pain information. Yet whatever gaps and insufficiencies there may be in Context II assessment, it is a vital and active domain largely occupied by behavioral scientists.

Finally, Context III reflects the dynamic nature of the person–environment dialectic. The perception of pain intensity cannot occur independent of factors in the internal environment of the body or the external social environment (Nuttin, 1984; Pennebaker, 1982). Nor do behavioral expressions of pain exist apart from the situations that evoke or respond to them. The focal question of Context III is: What difference does the experience of pain make?" It is asked in relation to the seven facets noted in Table 15.3. These relationships provide the "meaning" of pain, for both the child and the observer (assessor). The temporal dimension (IIIa) defines pain in terms of the unfolding of actions, reactions, beliefs, opinions, and social transactions over time. The motivational dimension (IIIb) considers pediatric pain in relation to the child's goals—both normative (going to school, playing with friends, building a model airplane) and rehabilitative (taking one's medication on schedule, doing special range-of-motion exercises, etc.). The relationship of pediatric pain to mental health indices is also considered (IIIc). Similarly, the meaning of pain is often related to the place of its expression (IIId). For youngsters, the impact of pain's intensity, its physical disfigurement potential, its demoralization potential, and the like are most dramatically demonstrated in the school setting (IIIe) and within the home (IIIf). Finally, we note that pain's meaning is also a personal interpretation subject to representation-driven processing (again see Fig. 15.1 and Tables 15.1 and 15.2). The task of sense making in chronic illness often falls to parents and teachers, but children themselves also carry this burden. Despite the view that children do not construct systematic life scripts until adolescence (McAdams, 1985), it may well be that young children with chronic pain are forced by bodily events and social forces (their doctors, their parents, their teachers) into at least rudimentary pain theory building, the contents of which feed forward in an action-steering capacity. For further discussion of Context III, see Karoly and Jensen (1987).

Although the emphasis thus far has been upon the specific contents or targets of pediatric pain assessment, it should be understood that a comprehensive measurement approach involves a coordinated explication not only of what, but also of *why* (assessment goals) and *how* (assessment methods). A consideration of the whys and hows will comprise the remainder of the chapter.

Assessment Purposes

The term *assessment* has many meanings. To some it is equivalent to diagnosis of underlying (causal) pathology. To others it implies the objective measurement of overt signs or symptoms. Still others consider assessment to include the cataloging of a person's skills and values as well as his or her particular skill deficiencies associated with current adaptive failure(s). In pediatric pain, all purposes are potentially (contextually) valid.

Typically, one or more pain facets are selected for assessment, varying in terms of their level of abstractness or, more correctly, in terms of the *unit of study* (neuronal, organ system, person, or person in interaction), the *unit of observation* (discrete vs.

continuous responding), or the *mode of analysis* (system description, functional analysis, or the prediction of outcome or covariation) (cf. Karoly, 1985). Pediatric pain has usually been assessed for purely descriptive or classificatory purposes, to assist in treatment planning and evaluation, or to assist in pinpointing pain antecedents, consequences, and/or mediators (which must also be measured). The descriptive, predictive, and functional or explanatory purposes cut across all three pain contexts. They yield a number of specific objectives, some of which are listed in Table 15.4. When assessing pain complaints not readily associated with disease, injury, or medical or dental treatment, the need for functional or explanatory analyses is heightened.

Assessment Procedures

Strategies of assessment in pediatric pain can currently be categorized as follows:

1. Child interview methods
2. Self-report procedures
    a. pain specific
    b. event specific
    c. multifaceted

TABLE 15.4. CLINICAL OBJECTIVES IN THE NONMEDICAL ASSESSMENT OF CHRONIC PAIN

1. Identifying and classifying preliminarily the pain problem (acute vs. chronic)
2. Clarifying medical history and its impact on current expectations, plans, and goals
3. Quantifying the disruptiveness versus the benefits of the pain problem in the social, academic, and recreational arenas
4. Estimating the patient's premorbid functioning (motoric, social, cognitive, etc.)
5. Prioritizing the foci of the initial intervention(s)
6. Establishing a performance baseline from which to evaluate change
7. Evaluating the patient's resources (coping skills, social support systems, etc.)
8. Clarifying the situational antecedents and cognitive mediators of pain reactivity
9. Differentiating the situational from the sensory antecedents of pain
10. Selecting intervention strategies matched to patient needs and resources
11. Forecasting possible negative "side effects" of successful treatment
12. Determining programmatic treatment alterations
13. Assessing posttreatment life-style modification
14. Regulating the patient's use of pain or nonpain medications
15. Evaluating the patient's satisfaction with pain treatment program(s)
16. Evaluating familial satisfaction with pain treatment program(s)
17. Assessing the patient's self-regulatory motives and skills, particularly in regard to pain control
18. Assessing the nature and adjustive impact of the patient's implicit pain theory (schema, script, model)

Table adapted from Karoly (1985).

3. Standardized observational techniques
4. Self-monitoring methods
5. Parent or clinician judgment or attribution
6. Physiological and neurochemical procedures
7. Projective and drawing methods
8. Cognitive process analyses

To reiterate a point made earlier in this chapter, it would seem advisable to employ several methods rather than one; but the choice of methods should be dictated by the assessment purpose and, of course, the facet of pain being targeted. There is no logical reason invariably to include a behavioral, self-report, and physiological index in every assessment—as if these methods will somehow (magically) converge upon the truth. If, for example, the goal is to understand a child's representation of his or her pain as it relates to goal directedness, to what use will a neurochemical assay be put?

Interview Methods. The clinical interview is perhaps the most flexible assessment procedure and the most likely to provide data relevant to Context III. Because they are open ended, some interview protocols are capable of eliciting from children their *causal scenarios* (Read, 1987), or their interpretations of sequences of behavior and thought over time and across contexts. However, typically, interviews are used to gather life history (factual) data, children's perceptions of their circumstances, their descriptions of pain, their preferences regarding treatment, and the like. When the goal is to determine how the child puts the facts together, I refer to such assessment as cognitive process analyses. Usually, however, the interviewer collates and interprets the separate bits of information in accordance with his or her guiding conceptualization(s). For research purposes, many interviewers combine open-ended with closed-ended questions (the latter being defined here as *self-report* methods), sharing primarily the scorable or structured responses in their published papers (cf. Beales, Keen, & Holt, 1983).

Ross and Ross (1984a, 1984b) conducted semistructured interviews with a large cohort of children 5 to 12 years old in California (N = 994), hoping to transcend the adult-centeredness of the pediatric pain literature through the use of a generate-response (open-ended) format. As they note (Ross & Ross, 1984a):

> It was clear that for most children a one-to-one relationship existed between the format of the question and the caliber, and often the content, of the answer. There was unequivocal evidence that given the appropriate interview framework, young children are a rich source of information pertinent to a diverse group of pain experiences. (p. 72)

Illustrative of how the content of a child's response can vary with question format is the finding (Ross & Ross, 1984a) that, while only 5 percent of the sample (8 children) spontaneously reported using self-initiated coping reactions of any kind in response to pain, fully 81.4 percent of the sample (130 children) indicated in reply to a "leading question" that they had tried "not to think about the pain." Indeed, in answering the open-ended question "When you had the pain was there anything you tried to do *yourself* so that it wouldn't hurt so much?" the most common response was that the child did nothing.

Also of interest is the finding that a mostly open-ended interview with youngsters of varying pain backgrounds (healthy to chronic blood dyscrasia cases), between 5 and 12 years of age, almost equally split between boys and girls, failed to yield age trends or gender differences (Ross & Ross, 1984b). In view of the fact that other studies (e.g., Bibace & Walsh, 1981; Perrin & Gerrity, 1981), using healthy children participating in open-ended interviews, have tended to find an age progression in subjects' understanding of *illness in general*, the experience of pain appears to be a leveling one, undercutting the expected age-graded cognitive differentiation found in so many other areas of knowledge.

Pain interviewing with children should not usually be expected to produce data that conform to those derivable from parent (or other adult) informants. The absence of convergence should be seen as reflecting not necessarily unreliability, but rather uniqueness of perspective (cf. also Achenbach, McConaughy, & Howell, 1987). The motivational aspects of Context III and the self-regulatory attitudes and skills of youngsters in pain are not as likely to be directly monitored as some of the other facets (see Table 15.3). Similarly, children's theories of pain and their "if–then" rules for pain schematization are certainly less accessible to observers than to youngsters themselves. Unfortunately, many of the most salient aspects of pain processing may be automatic, implicit, or beyond the child's normal self-monitoring capabilities. Thus whether a child doesn't know, doesn't notice, or knows differently (compared to other sources of information) is never easy to discern. Further, there are no ready criteria against which to validate child interview data. Perhaps the key requirements of interview-based assessment are that it be reliable (test–retest over short intervals) and that it yield information of use in the design and evaluation of pain treatment programs.

Self-Report Procedures. Self-report procedures can be directed at a patient's direct perceptions, evaluations, estimates (judgments), and monitoring of pain and discomfort (pain-specific reports) or they can attempt to assess similar appreciations of pain's antecedents, consequences, correlates, or conscious mediational operations (event-specific reports). Combinations of the two (multifaceted self-reports) are also possible (Karoly, 1985). Among the most popular pain-relevant *events* in the adult assessment literature are moods (particularly depression and anxiety), situational "triggers" of pain, activity level, and pain-contingent interpersonal reactions (presumably fostering invalidism via "secondary gains"). The literature on child pain assessment has focused almost exclusively on specific reports of sensory experience—particularly intensity and body location (cf. Varni et al., 1986).

The Visual Analogue Scale (VAS) is among the most reliable and simple self-report measures available, particularly useful with children because it minimizes reliance upon verbal facility. As described, for example, by Abu-Saad (1984), the VAS requires the child to mark the space along a 10-cm line that best describes the current experience of hurt. The scale is anchored by a 0, and the phrase "I have no pain" to the left of the line, and a 10, along with the words "I have very severe pain" on the right. Abu-Saad's instructions are: "If 0 means no pain at all, and 10 means you have very severe pain, can you place a mark on this scale that indicates how badly you hurt now?" (p. 165). Using a small, convenience sample of 10 surgical patients between the ages of 9 and 15, Abu-Saad obtained multiple measures over 2 postoperative days. She reported that VAS responses were related to behavioral indicators and word descriptors.

Children can often employ verbal descriptors to gauge the experience of their pain. Abu-Saad (1984) obtained 18 different words in an open-ended inquiry of children 9 to 15. Interestingly, 17 out of 18 were sensory in nature (e.g., *burning, pinching, stabbing,* etc.). Savedra, Gibbons, Tesler, Ward, and Wegner (1982) provided a list of 24 words to a group of 100 hospitalized and 114 nonhospitalized children between the ages of 9 and 12. The hospitalized children chose the words *sickening, uncomfortable, horrible,* and *tiring* and the phrases *like a pinch* and *like a sting* to describe their pain significantly more often than did the nonhospitalized children (who tended to use the word *biting* significantly more often than did the hospitalized youngsters). It is not known how reliable children tend to be in their choice of words, or the extent to which children merely mimic the descriptors that are most used by parents, doctors, or other children. Hence verbal labels may be of less use than visual analogue scales or simple numerical rating scales ("Rate your pain from 0 to 100"). Nonetheless, consistency of word use tends to increase with age (Tesler, Ward, Savedra, Wegner, & Gibbons, 1983), so older children may be trustworthy reporters of pain via verbal descriptors.

Often, self-reports (via numerical rating scales or visual analogue scales) are recommended for children 9 years old and up, under the presupposition that younger children are unreliable self-monitors or careless (thoughtless) in their data giving. However, the question of a child's reliability should be an empirical one. If, during a 20-minute interview with a 5-year old, the question "How much do you hurt right now?" (using a VAS or a 3-, 4-, or 5-point rating scale) is asked several times, the interviewer can readily ascertain the stability of the response. If, further, an analgesic is orally administered during the interview period, the clinician can take note of the extent of reduction in pain report (obviously, if an injection is used, the child will report an *increase* in pain due to the needle stick). Contextual effects should also be explored. For example, do children's self-reports vary with place, time of day, and the presence or absence of parents, doctors, nurses, and/or peers? Clinicians should also consider the possibility of training their young patients to be reliable self-reporters of pain sensation, rather than simply bemoaning their patients' inconsistency, and forgoing a potentially useful source of data.

Among the critical "events" related to pain that have been examined, if only on a limited basis, is the child's coping response. Tesler and colleagues (1983), in their Pediatric Pain Questionnaire, ask school-age children (9 to 12) "What helps you feel better when you are in pain?" In one study, two-thirds of the children (182 out of 263) were able to identify at least one coping activity (Tesler, Wegner, Savedra, Gibbons, & Ward, 1981). Hospitalized youngsters identified fewer coping responses than nonhospitalized children, and the most common strategies selected were the taking of medications and the use of rest, sleep, or relaxation.

The most studied attributional aspect of pain experience is the child's perception of pain causality. As already noted, numerous investigators have taken a Piagetian perspective on illness understanding, discovering an age-related pattern of cognitive maturation (from egocentric to abstract). Focusing specifically upon pain and utilizing a wide age spectrum (5 to 14), Gaffney and Dunne (1987) have reported on 680

Irish schoolchildren's response to the item "A person gets a pain because. . . . " A 12-category coding scheme was devised which yielded a 91 percent interrater agreement. Almost half of the sample (44 percent) cited causes that related to personal transgression or "self-causality." As the authors note: "The importance of 'transgression' interpretations of pain and illness presumably derives from the assumption that these ideas evoke guilt and notions of punishment which, as negative psychological variables, would tend to augment the experience of pain" (p. 98).

Indeed, the study of any event-specific aspect of pain is justified to the extent that pain-related perceptions are implicated in the process of children's long-term adjustment. Unfortunately, few pain events have been clearly identified as causally linked to pain adaptation. On a research level, longitudinal studies are required. From a clinical assessment perspective, it is suggested that multiple pain indicators be assessed over repeated testings in order that functional relationships (or conditional probabilities) can be established beyond the assumptive level.

Finally, with respect to multiple measures, it can be stated that, increasingly, the pediatric assessment community has opted for more than single indicators. In addition to the Pediatric Pain Questionnaire noted earlier, the Varni-Thompson Pediatric Pain Questionnaire (which I shall call the VT-PPQ to distinguish it from the measure of Tesler et al.) has recently been introduced (cf. Thompson & Varni, 1986; Varni, Thompson, & Hanson, 1987). The VT-PPQ, modeled after the McGill Pain Questionnaire, has a child form, an adolescent form, and a parent form containing a combination of open-ended questions, verbal descriptors, rating scales, color codings, visual analogue–type indices, and pictorial items. The VT-PPQ seeks to assess the sensory, evaluative, and affective focal qualities of pain, along with pain location, activities, and (for parents) family health history.

At this time, many gaps exist in the self-report assessment of pediatric pain, involving not only unattended facets of the pain experience but unexplored empirical relationships as well. For example, stress as a precipitant of pain, social support as a stress buffer, and self-regulatory skills as a mediator (or protective factor) remain to be systematically investigated.

Observational Techniques. Patterns of overt motor behavior indicative of wellness and of pain have been the traditional targets of behavioral assessment specialists (cf. Keefe, 1982). Of the various methods available for indexing overt response patterning—including global ratings made by judges and indirect measures, such as medication requests and days of school missed—the use of trained observers recording and coding ongoing activities in specified situations has been the most reliable and the most popular (Katz, Varni, & Jay, 1984).

Pain occurring in youngsters undergoing bone marrow aspirations (BMAs) was the target of several investigations, each utilizing a structured observational protocol. The Procedure Behavior Rating Scale (PBRS) was first developed by Katz and colleagues (1980) to permit the quantification of 25 categories of pain response in pediatric oncology patients. Acts such as crying or screaming were given clear operational definitions, and they proved to be capable of reliable recording. Differentiating between anxiety and sensory pain indicators (two central but distinct aspects of Context II) was not easily accomplished, however. "The distinction between the constructs is important from both a theoretical and clinical point of view. For example, methods used to reduce distress related to pain are often different from those used to reduce anxiety" (Schacham & Daut, 1981, pp. 468–469).

The Observation Scale of Behavioral Distress (OSBD), a revision of the PBRS, has been employed by Jay and her colleagues (e.g., Jay, Ozolins, Elliott, & Caldwell, 1983) to assess anxiety and pain reactions of children. The term *behavioral distress* is used to encompass both the sensory pain and anxiety components of children's responding in acute clinical contexts (such as BMAs or dental procedures). To refine the PBRS further, the developers of the OSBD employed: (1) 15-second recording intervals; and (2) a weighting system (e.g., screaming = 4.0, muscular rigidity = 2.5, and information seeking = 1.5). Jay and associates found the 11-category OSBD to be correlated significantly with trait anxiety scores and ratings of anticipated and experienced pain in a group of pediatric cancer patients (Jay et al., 1983).

The Pain Behavior Checklist (PBCL) is an 8 category observation system employed by LeBaron and Zeltzer (1984). Occurrence of such actions as screaming, crying, physical resistance, verbalized anxiety, verbalized pain, need for physical restraint, verbal stalling, and muscle tension or body stiffness is recorded, along with observer ratings of the intensity of each (from 1 = very mild to 5 = extremely intense). Like the previously noted procedures, the PBCL can be used reliably. The PBCL correlates highly with children's self-ratings and with global observer ratings of pain.

Observational techniques for pediatric pain assessment are not "fast and dirty." They require observer training and reliability and accuracy monitoring. However, they can provide a valuable source of information about the way children "display" pain and distress, and they may be particularly helpful with preverbal or nonverbal youngsters. Nevertheless, it is important to bear in mind that social enactments are not equivalent to internal state processing. LeBaron and Zeltzer (1984) suggest corroborative data collection from parents or other knowledgeable informants as well as assessing the child patient across time and across distinct health-relevant settings.

Self-Monitoring of Pain. Because the experience of pain is subjective and because pain can be felt at times and places not easily subjected to external surveillance, there is a need to make use of ongoing, in vivo (rather than one-shot, retrospective) patient-centered reports. Self-observation diaries are the most common form of portable, context-sensitive self-reporting. Real-life pain self-monitoring often involves little more than the use of familiar self-report procedures (verbal ratings, visual analogues, numerical ratings, etc.) at selective times of the day and outside the direct supervision of an adult. Not surprisingly, diaries are most useful with co-operative youngsters capable of remembering when and how to make diary entries. Few examples of diary methods are available for children under 8 years of age; the most common format appears to be the Headache Diary (e.g., Joffe, Bakal, & Kaganov, 1983).

For our present purposes, a few main points need to be underscored. First, headache symptoms are not the only potential sensory targets of a pain diary. Further, focal pain experience need not be the sole focus of a diary-based assessment.

Meaning-level dimensions and action-level aspects (see Fig. 15.1) are viable targets, along with recordings of nonpain, health-engendering responses, such as coping, medication taking, goal pursuits (social or recreational), and social support.

The ability of pain diaries to capture the phenomenology of pain (the descriptive function), to help match children's needs to modes of therapeutic intervention (the prescriptive function), to assist in untangling causal networks (the explanatory function), and to forecast clinical outcomes (the predictive function) should be established empirically and not by fiat. Clinicians must be prepared also to train their child self-monitors to be accurate and to provide meaningful reward contingencies for children's continued collaboration.

Informant Ratings or Judgments. Quite apart from examples of trained observers using structured time-sampling procedures to record specific, overt pain responses, the clinical literature is replete with instances of global judgments made by adults about the *quality* of pediatric pain reactions. If one has misgivings about the utility of children's subjective reports, he or she must certainly doubt the wisdom of subjective reports *one body removed* from the source of the internal experience.

Currently, however, global informant ratings are principally used not as a source of verification of children's perceptions, but rather as a unique source of data about children's adaptive functioning (Achenbach et al., 1987). Because parents and teachers so often set the standards (or criteria) for acceptable performance across a variety of goal categories, their qualitative judgments should carry a good deal of potential weight in any descriptive, prescriptive, or predictive pain assessment.

The Varni-Thompson Pediatric Pain Questionnaire (VT-PPQ), for example, has a parent form that requests, among other things, a family health history, a listing of "major life stresses in the family situation," and an accounting of how the child's pain affects family adjustment (e.g., "if your child's pain were suddenly to disappear, how would it change his/her life? How would it change your life?"). While the parent is also asked (with questionable justification) to indicate for cross-validation purposes how the child feels pain, much of the parent form is more aptly directed at contextualizing the pediatric pain problem in the family setting. Unfortunately, the authors of the VT-PPQ have as yet published little on the relationship of the open-ended (qualitative) responses on the inventory to clinical process or outcome indices. Thus the utility of parent and physician reports remains to be demonstrated.

Physiological and Neurochemical Procedures. Molecular, body-centered indices of pain in pediatric assessment have not seen widespread application outside the medical literature. Some procedures, like percutaneous neurography (wherein nerve fiber transmission is measured via insertion into the skin of an epoxy-coated wire), are painful and dangerous as well as being more relevant to the assessment of acute or laboratory-induced pain as compared to chronic pain conditions. On the other hand, the measurement of *physiological arousal* via *noninvasive* techniques (such as electromyography or evoked potential measurement) is certainly feasible. Additionally, autonomically activated organ systems can be the assessment target. Heart rate, GSR, blood pressure, skin temperature, pupil dilation, and the like are systemic indicants of bodily arousal that have served psychologists very well over the years. When several autonomic indicators are assessed together, patterns of reactivity are sometimes discovered with the potential for discriminating among various painful medical conditions (at least in adults) (cf. Karoly & Jensen, 1987).

Feuerstein, Barr, Francoeur, Houle, and Rafman (1982) sought to identify possible autonomic factors associated with recurrent abdominal pain (RAP) by investigating children's reactions to cold pressor stress (immersion of the hand in ice-water). Ten youngsters between 9 and 14 diagnosed with RAP, 10 healthy matched controls, and 9 hospital controls (nonpain patients) were compared in terms of heart rate, digital blood volume pulse, forearm EMG, subjective intensity (visual analogue scale), and facial expression (reliably coded from videotapes by a blind rater) across a baseline, cold pressor, and recovery period. Contrary to expectations, there were no differences across the three groups of children (thus failing to support the hypothesis that RAP children are differentially predisposed to or are unable to recover from stress). The study nonetheless illustrates the use to which autonomic analyses can be put in testing hypotheses about pediatric pain.

Finally, neurochemical aspects of pediatric pain have been the subject of recent research investigations, following upon the animal and human research on endogenous opiates begun in the 1970s. Although preliminary, immunoassay findings on children under stress are beginning to reveal biochemical substrates of pediatric pain reactivity (cf. Varni et al., 1982).

Projective and Drawing Methods. When Joann Eland conducted her master's thesis research on children's communication of pain (Eland, 1974), she elected to use a projective technique because "it permitted an almost unlimited variety of possible responses" (p. 16). Because so little was known about the ways children think about pain, a cartoon dog character in five different situations was a reasonable vehicle for eliciting youngster's reactions. An alternative approach to the use of structured TAT-like stimuli is to ask children to draw pictures representing their pain (e.g., "Draw a picture of your pain" or "Draw a picture of you when you are in pain"). Unlike the projective analyses of adults, techniques such as those just described do not rely exclusively upon psychodynamic assumptions concerning unconscious, psychosexual meanings ascribed to (or "projected onto") the stimuli. Rather, it is assumed that young children may be unable to express their emotional reactions either in words or in numbers, but (1) can represent their experiences "intuitively" via colors or shapes and/or (2) can be prompted to talk about their feelings more openly than usual if childlike media (cartoons or stick figures) are employed.

Intensity and affective response have been major targets of projective pain assessment. In her pioneering study, Eland (1974) showed children 5 to 8 years old a series of pictures of a dog cartoon figure. In one, the dog was resting atop a doghouse. In others, the dog was shown falling off the doghouse, getting hit in the nose by a swing, and getting a paw caught in a car door. The child was asked (among other things) to rank-order the pictures from least to most hurt, and to then select the picture best representing his or her current pain level (intensity). Parent corroboration was also elicited. While children could recognize that the dog was hurting, they did not agree about how to rank-order the pictures. Within children, there was some consistency–19 of the 25 children studied by Eland provided the same rankings over successive days. "It would seem," Eland (1974) concluded, "as though using cartoon pictures of a dog has face validity as a method to measure pain in children" (p. 31). Eland's indices of validity were mothers' rankings of pain (which agreed 95 percent of the time with children's pain-level choices) and decreases in children's pain ratings from the time of surgery to a postoperative interview.

Later, Eland used a chimpanzee cartoon character (presumably a stimulus with which children more readily identified) and found similar trends. However, she ultimately abandoned cartoons because children tend to see a variety of catastrophic events occurring to cartoon characters on television with no apparent long- or short-term harm. Thus Tom and Jerry put the cartoon pain projective device out of business.

Eland and others (Scott, 1978; Stewart, 1977) then used a *color spectrum approach*, requiring youngsters to scale pain intensity on a color scale (with red representing the most severe pain and green representing no pain). A method called the Poker Chip Tool (Hester, 1979), which requires children to use one to four poker chips to represent pain, was found to correlate more highly with behavioral responses than did the more abstract methods like cartoon choices. Based on the work of Petrovitch (1957), Lollar, Smits, and Patterson (1982) devised perhaps the most elaborate projective procedure, called the Pediatric Pain Inventory (PPI), which uses 24 pictures representing medical, recreational, daily living, and psychosocial settings of pain or upset, and which requires children to make (1) intensity ratings via a three-color spectrum scale (red, yellow, green = much, some, or little pain), and (2) duration ratings ("How long would the hurt last?) in seconds, days, weeks, and the like.

The empirical and clinical yields of projective devices such as described here are relatively small, particularly in terms of the time required to conduct the assessment. The methods are only moderately reliable (test–retest and internal consistency). The methods have also focused rather narrowly upon the Context II facets of intensity and affect, and have not proven themselves more useful or cost-effective in gauging these dimensions than other procedures (e.g., numerical ratings or behavioral observations). While projective methods are often aimed at preverbal youngsters, the procedures nonetheless require the child to comprehend verbal instructions. Finally, studies of the predictive validity of projective methods are almost nonexistent.

It would be incorrect, I feel, to conclude that projective devices are of no use in pediatric pain assessment. If (as the present information processing model asserts) pain experience is partially schema driven, then some way is needed to assess children's inference-building operations. Projectives may be the "right" method (or be part of a family of right methods) heretofore applied to the "wrong" set of questions. A consideration of alternate questions is presented next.

Cognitive Process Analyses. Cognitive processes such as attentional focus, bodily state labeling, expectancy, perceived self-efficacy, and the like can affect sensory processing—including the perception of pain or distress symptoms. Similarly, sensory arousal (such as in anxiety and pain) can affect the content and efficiency of cognitive operations such as problem solving, concentration, memory, and the like (cf. Pennebaker, 1982; Revelle, 1986). Because of the traditional algesimetric interest in molecular spheres of analysis (pain intensity perceptions, pain tolerance times, etc.) and because of the avoidance of higher-order (complex) tasks in the study of child pain, the two-way link between cognition and sensory encoding has not been widely explored.

The framework presented earlier in this chapter (and the gate-control model from which it derives) provides a reasonable heuristic justification for developing a technology for the analysis of Context IIf (Table 15.3)—the internal symbolic code, model, or abstraction of pain experience that helps organize attention, memory, decision making, and action. Such a technology should be developmentally grounded (age appropriate) and sensitive to the effects of individual differences, the influence of settings, and the role of motivation. To date, the assessment of children's pain experience at the sensory level and at the action level has developed far in advance of any serious attempt to measure children's pain schemata or representations. Any such representational assessment, should it be accomplished, could inform us not only about *what* children think and perceive, but also about *how* they organize their pain knowledge and use said knowledge to make plans and achieve goals (adaptive and maladaptive) linking sensation to action.

A potential benefit of a dynamic representational assessment might well be the integration of our knowledge about the pain experience across the now dissociated sensory, cognitive, and behavioral planes. Of course, any attempt at mental model building is likely to offend some powerful factions in pain research, including purists within the operant camp and psychodynamicists within the psychosomatic medicine camp. I would urge, on the other hand, that my upcoming proposal be evaluated on logical grounds (in the absence of data), and that its ultimate offensiveness be derived solely from its empirical shortcomings.

It should also be apparent by now that the philosophical "bottom line" of a cognitive process analysis is nothing like the traditional biomedical and physicalistic search for a number that would inform us what the child (or adult) is actually feeling or sensing. Human beings are simply not equipped to read their internal states cleanly, in the way a light meter detects the presence and intensity of physically definable phenomena in nature. Rather, we often make *inferences* about what is occurring internally, based on past experiences and current setting conditions. Further, "the encoding of sensory data may be the result of selective search. Alternatively, subjects may simply [make] educated guesses concerning their sensations rather than perceiving them at all" (Pennebaker, 1982, p. 49). Particularly in the case of chronic pain states (such as RAP or migraine headache), the goal is to understand how the child constructs the experience and not how the pain is directly given. The child's pain representation thus need bear no direct correspondence to any physical reality detectable, say, by an EMG. It is the language of thought, not the "mirror of nature," which is being sought (cf. also Gardner, 1985; Pylyshyn, 1984).

Having briefly stated the goals, assumptions, and philosophical tenets that undergird the analysis of children's complex cognizing about pain, a consideration of assessment methods is in order. To do this, I will make use of an organizing framework discussed by Landau and Goldfried (1981), Neisser (1976), and Schank and Abelson (1977).

Assuming that cognitive processing mechanisms exist at varying levels of complexity and may be hierarchically organized, these authors suggest that at the highest level of generality are so-called *cognitive maps*, and, at the lowest are *semantic schemata*. Between the cognitive map, defined as a representation of the physical environment, and the semantic schema, defined as a representation employed to help categorize objects or events, are intermediary structures called *plans* and *scripts*. Plans are general models for goal satisfaction, while scripts are representations of specific, stereotyped action sequences designed to move the person toward a particular goal. Two other types of postulated knowledge structure are: *goals*, or the reinforcers in the person's life; and *themes*, or bundles of related goals (called *life themes*, *interpersonal themes*, and *role themes*). Landau and Goldfried (1981) also subdivide scripts into *situational scripts*, *instrumental scripts*, and *personal scripts*.

The representational or knowledge structures hypothesized and investigated to date have been employed in the analysis of social inference, as vehicles to explain how people (mostly adults) make sense of their own or other people's actions in the world. It is here being argued that such analytic tools can also be used to help clarify *causal reasoning about bodily events*—particularly pain—and the *relationship between somatic occurrences and their perceived antecedents and consequences*. Further, it is being asserted that children's representations can be studied in addition to those of adults.

Thus might not children with persistent pain make use of *cognitive pain maps*, depicting their environment in terms of safe or unsafe locations (people or events) or attainable and unattainable goals? More specifically, might children with chronic pain utilize general *pain coping* or *pain display plans*, consisting of mental representations of sequences of thoughts and actions capable of bringing about pain reduction (coping plan) or solicitude (display plan)? Similarly, *pain scripts* would focus even more sharply on the achievement of pain goals in regular, predictable places—the "pain in school" script, the "pain at grandmother's house" script, the "pain tolerance if the doctor threatens to send you to the hospital for tests" script, and the like. Semantic *pain schemata* for categorizing felt pain or other sensations represent another core explanatory construct that has heretofore been operationalized only in terms of intensity, frequency, or duration but that may be found to include meaningful associations to sensory experience (e.g., along the semantic differential dimensions of potency, activity, and evaluation).

Strategies for the assessment of these different types of knowledge structure would include procedures in which many children, even as young as 5, would be capable of participation. Maps have been assessed via interviews, and, when the psychological structure of the perceived environment is the target, multidimensional scaling procedures have been used. The latter may be cumbersome for the assessor to employ (in the absence of computer facilities), but importantly, the child's task is merely to rate the similarity or dissimilarity among pairs of stimuli (cf. Kruskal & Wish, 1978). More interesting perhaps are the possible methodologies for the elicitation of children's plans, scripts, goals, and themes. Here, some variation on structured "projective" methods might serve quite well. Drawings, pictures, or even videotapes of children in pain-relevant contexts, displaying pain or pain control behaviorally or verbally, could be presented to youngsters with pain symptoms. The respondents might be required to describe what they see, to tell why a particular stimulus yielded a particular response (e.g., sight of needle producing tears), to infer general, "if–then" rules, to identify the actor's goals, and so on. Less projectively, the child in pain could be required to do these same things in response to a videotape of himself or herself in a pain situation. The assessor's task, of course, would be to develop codes for categorizing children's responses.

Models for such scoring schemes are illustrated in Galambos, Abelson, and Black (1986), Graesser and Clark (1985), and Read (1987).

SUMMARY

This chapter has offered an information control–action system model of pain, a three-dimensional assessment framework, and a review of both existing and needed measurement procedures for child pain analysis. Although much of what has been presented is speculative, the constructs are grounded in contemporary cognitive science and are consistent with research findings in the domains of information processing and cognitive social learning. Throughout the chapter it has been asserted that many levels of analysis are potentially useful in our efforts to describe, predict, or explain the course of pain and to determine the most suitable match between a child's needs and the available therapeutic operations. Parochialism in the choice of assessment tools or assessment targets is contraindicated by the restricted clinical and empirical orbit of the extant literature on pediatric pain and by the vastness of the as-yet-uncharted territory that our model, among others, opens up for exploration.

References

Abu-Saad, H. (1984). Assessing children's responses to pain. *Pain, 19,* 163–171.

Achenbach, T. M., McConaughy, S. H., & Howell, C. T. (1987). Child/adolescent behavioral and emotional problems: Implications of cross informant correlations for situational specificity. *Psychological Bulletin, 101,* 213–232.

Angell, M. (1982). The quality of mercy. *New England Journal of Medicine, 306,* 98–99.

Beales, J. G. (1982). The assessment and management of pain in children. In P. Karoly, J. J. Steffen, & D. J. O'Grady (Eds.), *Child health psychology: Concepts and issues*. New York: Pergamon.

Beales, J. G., Keen, J. H., & Holt, P. J. L. (1983). The child's perception of the disease and the experience of pain in juvenile chronic arthritis. *Journal of Rheumatology, 10,* 61–65.

Bibace, R., Walsh, M. E. (1981). Children's conceptions of illness. In R. Bibace & M. E. Walsh (Eds.), *Children's conceptions of health, illness, and bodily functions*. San Francisco: Jossey-Bass.

Breakwell, G. (1986). *Coping with threatened identities.* London: Methuen.

Carey, W. B. (1982). Clinical use of temperament data in pediatrics. In R. Porter & G. M. Collins (Eds.), *Temperament differences in infants and young children: Ciba Foundation Symposium 89*. London: Pitman.

Carey, W. B. (1986). Temperament and pediatric practice. In S. Chess & A. Thomas (Eds.), *Temperament in clinical practice*. New York: Guilford.

Chess, S., & Thomas, A. (1984). *The origins and evolution of temperament*. New York: Brunner/Mazel.

Coleman, W. L. (1984). Recurrent chest pain in childhood. In M. D. Levine (Ed.), Symposium on recurrent pain in children. *The Pediatric Clinics of North America* (Vol. 31). Philadelphia: Saunders.

Craik, F. I. M., & Lockhart, R. S. (1972). Levels of processing: A framework for memory research. *Journal of Verbal Learning & Verbal Behavior, 11,* 671–684.

Craik, F. I. M., & Tulving, E. (1975). Depth of processing and the retention of words in episodic memory. *Journal of Experimental Psychology: General, 104,* 268–294.

Eland, J. M. (1974). *Children's communication of pain.* Unpublished master's thesis. College of Nursing, University of Iowa.

Eland, J. M., & Anderson, J. E. (1977). The experience of pain in children. In A. Jacox (Ed.), *Pain: A sourcebook for nurses and other professionals.* Boston: Little, Brown.

Feuerstein, M., Barr, R. G., Francoeur, T. E., Houle, M., & Rafman, S. (1982). Potential biobehavioral mechanisms of recurrent abdominal pain in children. *Pain, 13,* 287–298.

Flor, H., & Turk, D. C. (1985). Chronic illness in an adult family member: Pain as a prototype. In D. C. Turk & R. D. Kerns (Eds.), *Health, illness, and families: A life-span perspective.* New York: Wiley.

Gaffney, A., & Dunne, E. A. (1987). Children's understanding of the causality of pain. *Pain, 29,* 91–104.

Galambos, J. A., Abelson, R. P., & Black, J. B. (Eds.) (1986). *Knowledge structures.* Hillsdale, NJ: Erlbaum.

Gallistel, C. R. (1980). *The organization of action: A new synthesis.* Hillsdale, NJ: Erlbaum.

Gardner, H. (1985). *The mind's new science.* New York: Basic.

Graesser, A. C., & Clark, L. F. (1985). *Structures and procedures of implicit knowledge.* Norwood, NJ: Ablex.

Guyton, A. C. (1982). *Human physiology and mechanisms of disease* (3rd ed.). Philadelphia: Saunders.

Harter, S. (1987). The determinants and mediational role of global self-worth in children. In N. Eisenberg (Ed.), *Contemporary topics in developmental psychology.* New York: Wiley.

Hawley, D. D. (1984). Postoperative pain in children: Misconceptions, descriptions and interventions. *Pediatric Nursing, 10,* 20–23.

Hester, N. K. (1979). The preoperational child's reaction to immunization. *Nursing Research, 28,* 250–255.

Jacox, A. (1981). The assessment of pain. In W. L. Smith, H. Merskey, & S. C. Gross (Eds.), *Pain: Meaning and measurement.* New York: S P. Medical.

Jay, S. M., Ozolins, M., Elliott, C. H., & Caldwell, S. (1983). Assessment of children's distress during painful medical procedures. *Health Psychology, 2,* 133–147.

Joffe, R., Bakal, D. A., & Kaganov, J. (1983). A self-observation study of headache symptoms in children. *Headache, 23,* 20–25.

John, E. R. (1976). A model of consciousness. In G. E. Schwartz & D. Shapiro (Eds.), *Consciousness and self-regulation* (Vol. 1). New York: Plenum.

Karoly, P. (1985). The assessment of pain: Concepts and procedures. In P. Karoly (Ed.), *Measurement strategies in health psychology.* New York: Wiley.

Karoly, P., & Jensen, M. P. (1987). *Multimethod assessment of chronic pain.* New York: Pergamon.

Katz, E. R., Kellerman, J., & Siegel, S. E. (1980). Behavioral distress in children with cancer undergoing medical procedures: Developmental considerations. *Journal of Consulting & Clinical Psychology, 48,* 356–365.

Katz, E. R., Varni, J. W., & Jay, S. M. (1984). Behavioral assessment and management of pediatric pain. In M. Hersen, R. M. Eisler, & P. M. Miller (Eds.), *Progress in behavior modification* (Vol. 18). New York: Academic.

Keefe, F. J. (1982). Behavioral assessment and treatment of chronic pain: Current status and future directions. *Journal of Consulting & Clinical Psychology, 50,* 896–911.

Konorski, J. (1967). *Integrative activity of the brain.* Chicago: University of Chicago Press.

Kruskal, J. B., & Wish, M. (1978). *Multidimensional scaling.* Beverly Hills: Sage.

Landau, R. J., & Goldfried, M. R. (1981). The assessment of schemata: A unifying framework for cognitive, behavioral, and traditional assessment. In P. C. Kendall & S. D. Hollon (Eds.), *Assessment strategies for cognitive-behavioral interventions.* New York: Academic.

Lavigne, J. V., Schulein, M. J., & Hahn, Y. S. (1986). Psychological aspects of painful medical conditions in children. I. Developmental aspects and assessment. *Pain, 27,* 133–146.

LeBaron, S., & Zeltzer, L. (1984). Assessment of acute pain and anxiety in children and adolescents by self-reports, observer reports, and a behavior checklist. *Journal of Consulting & Clinical Psychology, 52,* 729–738.

Leventhal, H., & Everhart, D. (1979). Emotion, pain, and physical illness. In C. E. Izard (Ed.), *Emotions in personality and psychopathology.* New York: Plenum.

Lollar, D. J., Smits, S. J., & Patterson, D. L. (1982). Assessment of pediatric pain: An empirical perspective. *Journal of Pediatric Psychology, 7,* 267–277.

Martindale, C. (1981). *Cognition and consciousness.* Homewood, IL: Dorsey.

McAdams, D. P. (1985). *Power, intimacy, and the life story: Personalized inquiries into identity.* Homewood, IL: Dorsey.

Melamed, B. G., & Siegel, L. J. (1975). Reduction of anxiety in children facing hospitalization and surgery by use of filmed modeling. *Journal of Consulting & Clinical Psychology, 43*, 511–521.

Melzack, R., & Wall, P. D. (1965). Pain mechanisms: A new theory. *Science, 150*, 971–979.

Melzack, R., & Wall, P. D. (1983). *The challenge of pain*. New York: Basic.

Mennie, A. T. (1974). The child in pain. In L. Burton (Ed.), *Care of the child facing death*. London: Routledge & Kegan Paul.

Miller, S. M., & Green, M. L. (1985). Coping with stress and frustration. Origins, nature, and development. In M. Lewis & C. Saarni (Eds.), *The socialization of emotions*. New York: Plenum.

Neisser, U. (1976). *Cognition and reality*. San Francisco: W. H. Freeman.

Nuttin, J. (1984). *Motivation, planning, and action*. Hillsdale, NJ: Erlbaum.

Pennebaker, J. W. (1982).*The psychology of physical symptoms*. New York: Springer-Verlag.

Perrin, E. C., & Gerrity, P. S. (1981). There's a demon in your belly: Children's understanding of illness. *Pediatrics, 67*, 841–849.

Petrovitch, D. V. (1957). The pain apperception test: A preliminary report. *Journal of Psychology, 44*, 339–346.

Powers, W. T. (1973). *Behavior: The control of perception*. Chicago: Aldine.

Poznanski, E. O. (1976). Children's reactions to pain: A psychiatrist's perspective. *Clinical Pediatrics, 15*, 1114–1119.

Pylyshyn, Z. W. (1984). *Computation and cognition*. Cambridge, MA: MIT Press.

Rasmussen, J. (1986). *Information processing and human-machine interaction: An approach to cognitive engineering*. New York: Elsevier-North Holland.

Read, S. (1987). Constructing causal scenarios: A knowledge structure approach to causal reasoning. *Journal of Personality & Social Psychology, 52*, 288–302.

Revelle, W. (1986). Motivation and the efficiency of cognitive performance. In D. R. Brown & J. Veroff (Eds.), *Frontiers of motivational psychology: Essays in honor of John W. Atkinson*. New York: Springer-Verlag.

Rodin, J. (1982). Biopsychosocial aspects of self-management. In P. Karoly & F. H. Kanfer (Eds.), *Self-management and behavior change: From theory to practice*. New York: Pergamon.

Ross, D. M., & Ross, S. A. (1984a). The importance of type of question, psychological climate and subject set in interviewing children about pain. *Pain, 19*, 71–79.

Ross, D. M., & Ross, S. A. (1984b). Childhood pain: The school-aged child's viewpoint. *Pain, 20*, 179–191.

Ruble, D. (1987). The acquisition of self-knowledge: A self-socialization perspective. In N. Eisenberg (Ed.), *Contemporary topics in developmental psychology*. New York: Wiley.

Savedra, M., Gibbons, P., Tesler, M., Ward, J., & Wegner, C. (1982). How do children describe pain? A tentative assessment. *Pain, 14*, 95–104.

Schank, R., & Abelson, R. (1977). *Scripts, plans, goals, and understanding*. Hillsdale, NJ: Erlbaum.

Schechter, N. L. (1984). Recurrent pains in children: An overview and an approach. *Pediatric Clinics of North America, 31*, 949–968.

Schechter, N. L. (1985). Pain and pain control in children. *Current Problems in Pediatrics, 15*, 1–67.

Schechter, N. L., Allen, D. A., & Hanson, K. (1986). Status of pediatric pain control: A comparison of hospital analgesic usage in children and adults. *Pediatrics, 77*, 11–15.

Schwartz, G. E. (1984). Psychobiology of health: A new synthesis. In B. L. Hammonds & C. J. Scheirer (Eds.), *Psychology and health: The master lecture series* (Vol. 3). Washington, DC: American Psychological Association.

Scott, R. (1978). "It hurts red": A preliminary study of children's perception of pain. *Perceptual & Motor Skills, 47*, 787–791.

Semmer, N., & Frese, M. (1985). Action theory in clinical psychology. In M. Frese & J. Sabini (Eds.), *Goal-directed behavior: The concept of action in psychology*. Hillsdale, NJ: Erlbaum.

Shacham, S., & Daut, R. (1981). Anxiety or pain: What does the scale measure? *Journal of Consulting & Clinical Psychology, 49*, 468–469.

Stewart, M. L. (1977). Measurement of clinical pain. In A. Jacox (Ed.), *Pain: A sourcebook for nurses and other health professionals*. Boston: Little, Brown.

Swafford, L. I., & Allen, D. A. (1968). Pain relief in the pediatric patient. *Medical Clinics of North America, 52,* 133–139.

Tesler, M., Ward, J., Savedra, M., Wegner, C., & Gibbons, P. (1983). Developing an instrument for eliciting children's description of pain. *Perceptual & Motor Skills, 56,* 315–321.

Tesler, M., Wegner, C., Savedra, M., Gibbons, P., & Ward, J. (1981). Coping strategies of children in pain. *Issues in Comprehensive Pediatric Nursing, 5,* 351–359.

Thompson, K. L., & Varni, J. W. (1986). A developmental cognitive–biobehavioral approach to pediatric pain assessment. *Pain, 25,* 283–296.

Varni, J. W. (1983). *Clinical behavioral pediatrics: An interdisciplinary biobehavioral approach.* New York: Pergamon.

Varni, J. W. (1984). Pediatric pain: A biobehavioral perspective. *The Behavior Therapist, 7,* 23–25.

Varni, J. W., Jay, S. M., Masek, B. J., & Thompson, K. L. (1986). Cognitive–behavioral assessment and management of pediatric pain. In A. D. Holzman & D. C. Turk (Eds.), *Pain management: A handbook of psychological treatment approaches.* New York: Pergamon.

Varni, J. W., Katz, E. R., & Dash, J. (1982). Behavioral and neurochemical aspects of pediatric pain. In D. C. Russo & J. W. Varni (Eds.), *Behavioral pediatrics: Research and practice.* New York: Plenum.

Varni, J. W., & Thompson, K. L. (1986). Biobehavioral assessment and management of pediatric pain. In N. A. Krasnegor, J. D. Arasteh, & M. F. Cataldo (Eds.), *Child health behavior: A behavioral pediatrics perspective.* New York: Wiley.

Varni, J. W., Thompson, K. L., & Hanson, V. (1987). The Varni-Thompson Pediatric Pain Questionnaire: I. Chronic musculoskeletal pain in juvenile rheumatoid arthritis. *Pain, 28,* 27–38.

Von Cranach, M., Mächler, E., & Steiner, V. (1985). The organisation of goal-directed action: A research report. In G. P. Ginsburg, M. Brenner,, & M. Von Cranach (Eds.), *Discovery strategies in the psychology of action.* London: Academic.

Winfrey, L. L., & Goldfried, M. R. (1986). Information processing and human change process. In R. E. Ingram (Ed.), *Information processing approaches to clinical psychology.* Orlando, FL: Academic.

16

Pain Assessment in Children II: Understanding Recurrent Abdominal Pain

MORGAN T. SAMMONS

In the previous chapter the argument was made that pediatric chronic pain can be most adequately conceptualized in terms of information processing and action control. Using a levels-of-processing model, Karoly made the point that acute pain is processed at a shallow level as it is stimulus activated, requires minimal subjective interpretation, and evokes a restricted range of behavioral response. On the other hand, chronic pain is processed deeply. It is ambiguous, multifaceted, and subjective, and is not tied to a limited number of behavioral responses. The chronic pain experience is organized around the individual's representational schemata of pain. These schemata control both the interpretation and the response to pain. Erroneous information contained in individual schemata may result in misinterpretation and dysfunctional responses to pain. Thus chronic pain may involve dysfunctional information systems that help to shape pain schemata.

It was also argued that it is necessary to analyze pain in the context in which it occurs, and that three primary contexts for pain exist. Context I involves biological and medical facets. Context II focuses on the sensory, affective, and cognitive experience of pain. Context III examines the interpretation of pain in relation to developmental, familial, and situational dimensions. By expanding and operationally defining the contextual model of pain behavior first advanced in operant theories of pain, the author has provided a more fully articulated framework in which to analyze chronic pediatric pain.

The purpose of this chapter is to illustrate the utility of this expanded contextual model in the analysis of recurrent abdominal pain, a common, chronic condition of childhood. Whereas the tenor of the previous chapter was theoretical and speculative, this chapter will be largely descriptive. Previous attempts to explain recurrent abdominal pain using single-factor models will be briefly reviewed and critiqued from the perspective of Karoly's (Chapter 15 in this volume) tripartite contextual model of pain. More recent efforts to explain RAP in a biopsychosocial context will be examined. Suggestions for further elaboration of such models will be advanced.

Recurrent abdominal pain was chosen as the topic of this chapter because it presents particular challenges to investigators and clinicians in pediatric health psychology. Most studies comprising the RAP literature are based on psychogenic pain constructs that posit single-factor etiologies. Assessment devices used to measure physiological and psychological variables in these works are often unstandardized, and sample selection is often arbitrary. As a result, the reader is confronted with what is primarily a body of clinical observations. Because of the diversity of issues addressed and lack of standardization, these observations contribute little to theoretical understanding or treatment efficacy. The principal thesis of this chapter is that utilization of an appropriately developed biopsychosocial investigative rubric can produce a more coherent body of data and ultimately influence clinical outcome.

RAP is particularly suited to study from a biopsychosocial perspective. It is a very common pediatric illness and one of the most frequent presenting complaints in pediatric practice. It rarely has an identifiable organic cause. Its development is influenced by a combination of individual, environmental, and cultural factors, all of which interact in poorly understood ways to produce the illness in children who are, for reasons largely unknown, at risk. In other words, the three questions that Green (1986) identifies as research foci in behavioral medicine (why some persons become ill when others do not, why the symptoms of a particular disorder predominate in certain individuals, and why certain stressors produce such a broad array of symptoms) are immediately encountered in an investigation of RAP.

Psychological factors almost certainly play a role in the etiology of RAP. However, research attempting to pinpoint a unitary psychological or physiological variable has been singularly unsuccessful. In part, this lack of success is due to uncertain methodologies. A larger consideration is that most studies examining either organic or psychological elements of RAP have focused on single explanatory factors, such as negative life events or lactose intolerance. Not surprisingly, results of these investigations suggest that the variable under examination can account for the symptoms of a generally small percentage of the children under study. A few more recent analyses have abandoned the search for single explanations and have focused instead on multidimensional models, as in the confluence model of RAP proposed by Levine and Rappaport (1984). Such models have more heuristic and practical utility than those that posit a causal relationship between single organic or psychologic factors and RAP symptoms. However, while they are able to account for more of the variance than single-factor models, they have the distinct disadvantage of leaving the exact contribution of each variable unknown. It is thus questionable whether such models are analytically superior to the earlier approaches. This issue becomes particularly germane in light of the near impossibility of designing an investigation that can statistically account for the myriad of factors hypothesized to be involved in the etiology of disorders such as RAP. Nevertheless, failure of single-factor models indicates that a trial of the new multidimensional perspectives, however imperfect, is warranted. It is, in fact, illogical to expect perfection from such models at this stage in their development. Furthermore, the shift from single-factor explanations to a multidimensional investigative perspective is not a phenomenon isolated to health psychology or the study of psychophysiologic disorders. It is part of a trend occurring throughout psychology and the behavioral sciences wherein the positivistic expectations engendered by single-factor empirical investigation are being rejected in favor of a more complex (but less deterministic) systems view of the problem under study.

THE RECURRENT ABDOMINAL PAIN SYNDROME

Recurrent abdominal pain is one of the most common illnesses of childhood. Estimates of the incidence of the disorder vary, in part because no standard definition exists (Lavigne, Schulein, & Hahn, 1986b). The most frequently cited statistic estimates its incidence at approximately 10 percent in a school-age population (Apley, 1975). Others have corroborated this figure or have reported slightly higher percentages in populations surveyed. In a long-term longitudinal analysis of 11,000 British 7-year-olds, 14 percent of boys and 15.7 percent of girls reported symptoms concordant with a diagnosis of RAP (Pringle, Butler, & Davie, 1959). Most estimates are that between 10 and 15 percent of all schoolchildren will experience RAP symptoms at some point (Levine & Rappaport, 1984). Incidence of symptoms appears to peak at 9 to 10 years old (Green, 1967). Apley (1975) found that more than 25 percent of 9-year-old girls experienced clinical symptoms. The disorder is rare before age 5, although there are reports in the literature of symptoms occurring as early as 1 or 2 (Bain, 1974).

Most investigators have employed Apley's (1975) operational definition of RAP (Barr & Feuerstein, 1983). Apley's criteria limit the syndrome to children who have experienced at least three episodes of abdominal pain over a period of longer than 3 months. Pain must be severe enough to affect activities (Apley, 1975). This definition has established a precedent in terms of minimum criteria for inclusion in studies of RAP, but has been criticized as incomplete. Quality of pain, duration of painful episodes, alleviating factors, and physical conditions between episodes are not addressed (Lebenthal, 1980). Also, this definition does not address the distinction between RAP of organic etiology and that which is not.

Differentiation between organic and nonorganic abdominal pain is often problematic (Galler, Neustein, & Walker, 1980; Lebenthal, 1980). This is in part due to the large number of causes of abdominal pain, more than 80 of which were identified by Bain (1974). Lack of agreement on a uniform set of procedures also complicates the diagnostic picture (Galler et al., 1980). Further, the terms used to separate organic and nonorganic pain are not uniformly applied. As Barr and Feuerstein (1983) note, "the phrase *organic cause* is ambivalent. It may refer either to organic disease as producing the pain symptom or to normal physiological functioning resulting in pain symptoms" (p. 17). To resolve confusion surrounding terminology, Barr (1983) has proposed a tripartite classification system of organic, psychogenic, and dysfunctional pain. In this scheme, the term *dysfunctional pain* refers to pain generated in the abdomen as a result of normal physiological functioning. This is the case in lactose intolerance, in which ingestion of normal quantities of milk in the absence of sufficient quantities of the intestinal enzyme lactase causes abdominal pain. Insufficiency of lactase is not a disease-related phenomenon, since lactase naturally disappears from the intestinal tract as children age. Barr, therefore, classifies pain resulting from the ingestion of milk in the absence of lactase as dysfunctional pain, since neither organic pathology nor psychological factors can account for it.

Nonorganic RAP is usually a chronic condition, but the pain associated with the syndrome is benign and intermittent. This complexity has made it difficult to classify RAP accurately. RAP is not listed in the most complete taxonomy of pain syndromes available (International Association for the Study of Pain, Subcommittee on Taxonomy, 1986). However, two related conditions are. Irritable bowel syndrome, which is thought to be the adult equivalent of RAP (Latimer, 1983; Stone & Barbero, 1970), is listed as a dysfunctional or psychophysiological pain disorder. It is important to distinguish this classification from pain regarded to be of psychological origin (conversion hysteria or depressive hallucinations). Abdominal migraine (also known as the periodic syndrome), a rare disorder of uncertain diagnosis (*Painful Young Bellies*, 1978), is also listed. The legitimacy of abdominal migraine as a diagnosis has been questioned (Cooperman, 1976), but some regard it as a possible organic cause of RAP.

RAP remits spontaneously in some children, but persists in others (Lavigne, Schulein, & Hahn, 1986b). Long-term studies also indicate that a sizable portion of samples treated with psychotherapy are not responsive. Christensen and Mortensen (1975) found that significantly greater numbers of subjects who had experienced RAP during childhood continued to have abdominal symptoms as adults when compared to a non-RAP control group. Follow-up at 28 to 30 years after initial examination of the patients indicated that one-half the children with RAP, even after psychotherapeutic intervention, continued to suffer from pain symptoms as adults. (One-fourth of children without RAP symptoms developed abdominal problems as adults.) Apley and Hale (1973) reported on 30 RAP children at long-term follow-up (8 to 20 years) who had been treated with reassurance and explanation. Twelve continued to have abdominal pain, and another 9 had developed other symptoms. Equivalent numbers of a control group (who had received no reassurance or explanation) also continued to experience symptoms. Elsewhere, Apley (1975) reported more long-term follow-up data on 18 RAP children and 18 healthy controls. In the RAP group, 8 of 18 cases continued to experience abdominal symptoms. Similar pain symptoms developed in another 6. No members of the control group developed abdominal pain. One group that reported a high incidence of RAP (approximately 25 percent) among 6-year-old children in a British planned community (Faull & Nicol, 1986) found that 25 of 26 subjects were symptom free at the time of a second survey 6 to 8 months later (Davison, Faull, & Nicol, 1986). However, follow-up in 6 to 9 months is probably not sufficient to gauge chronicity of RAP. Why this group was able to document such a high number of cases with such rapid symptom resolution remains unclear. Some investigators (Friedman, 1972; Heinild, Malver, Roelsgaard, & Worning, 1959) have reported high percentages of symptom resolution at follow-up of 1 to 3 years, but not at the level reported by Davison and colleagues.

Stickler and Murphy (1979) provided follow-up data (minimum of 5 years) on 161 children with RAP. Organic pathology (inflammatory bowel disease) accounting for painful symptoms developed in only 3 children over a 5-year period. Symptoms resolved in 123 of the 161 children followed. Thirty-eight failed to resolve abdominal pain. Additional symptoms, classified as psychosomatic, developed in 18 percent.

Analysis of long-term follow-up studies of RAP children suggests that nonorganic abdominal pain persists in at least one-third of all patients (Barr, 1983). There also appears to be a positive correlation between the percentage of individuals who continue to experience abdominal problems and length of time at follow-up, as the study by Christensen and Mortensen (1975) indicates.

Children with RAP have an elevated risk of undergoing unnecessary medical or surgical procedures. Bain (1974) reported that normal appendixes were removed from 52 of 82 children who underwent appendectomies after other organic causes of pain had been ruled out. (Although some abnormality was observed in the remaining 30 appendixes, no cases of acute appendicitis were discovered.) Of the 38 children in the Stickler and Murphy (1979) study who failed to resolve abdominal pain, 14 underwent surgical procedures of doubtful necessity. Overall, the authors found that 20 percent of their total sample underwent possibly unnecessary surgical or medical procedures.

As mentioned, RAP is a possible precursor of adult irritable bowel syndrome, and children with RAP may be prone to the development of somatization disorder (Briquet's syndrome) later in life as well (Ernst, Routh, & Harper, 1984; Routh & Ernst, 1984). In any event, if symptoms persist into adulthood, patients with abdominal pain remain at elevated risk for unnecessary surgery, in part due to the chronic nature of the disorder (Latimer, 1983b). DeVaul and Faillace (1978) found that 72 percent of patients surveyed in a polysurgery group (more than five surgeries) had undergone abdominal or pelvic procedures. Joyce and Walsh (1980) presented a case study of a family with abdominal pain. The mother had undergone seven surgeries over the course of 35 hospital admissions for abdominal pain. Her five children had 25 hospitalizations for similar complaints. Healthy appendixes had been removed from three.

Ill-advised surgery does nothing to ameliorate symptoms of abdominal pain (Sarfeh, 1976), and frequently worsens them (Lennard-Jones, 1983). Once surgery is contemplated or has been performed, the patient often becomes convinced that an organic basis to symptoms does in fact exist. Such patients may continue to demand surgical intervention or traipse perpetually from doctor to doctor in the vain hope of encountering an organic cure.

RAP IN CONTEXT I: BIOMEDICAL ASPECTS

Of the many possible organic models of RAP, one of the most thoroughly investigated has been the lactose intolerance hypothesis. As noted above, this hypothesis holds that an insufficiency of the intestinal enzyme lactase, which is responsible for the metabolization of milk sugar (lactose), exists in the GI tracts of many RAP children. Ingestion of lactose in the presence of a lactase deficiency causes abdominal pain, gas, cramping, and diarrhea. As has been said, it is difficult to classify lactase deficiency as a true organic cause of RAP, since lactase naturally disappears from the intestinal tract as children age.

While many individuals with a lactase deficiency do suffer abdominal pain after ingesting lactose, this is not universally true. Barr, Levine, and Watkins (1979) found that a history of pain, diarrhea, or avoidance of (or preference for) milk was not helpful in distinguishing between lactose-tolerant and lactose-intolerant groups. A breath hydrogen test, considered to be indicative of lactase insufficiency if positive after ingestion of lactose, was used to separate the two groups. Of 80 children with RAP assessed by these authors, only 40 percent indicated lactose intolerance as measured by breath hydrogen analysis. A greater percentage of lactose intolerance was found among the small Black (N = 16) and Hispanic (N = 5) subsamples studied (75 and 80 percent, respectively). Other investigators have reported similar figures (70 percent) for lactose intolerance in Black populations (Bayless & Huang, 1971).

Lebenthal, Rossi, Nord, and Branski (1981) investigated the association of lactase deficiency to RAP in a controlled double-blind study. Like Bayless and Huang (1971), Barr and colleagues (1979), and McGrath, Goodman, Firestone, Shipman, and Peters (1983), they found similar rates of lactase deficiency in both RAP and non-RAP groups. They administered lactose to RAP children with and without lactose intolerance, and 46 percent of lactose malabsorbers and 23.5 percent of lactose absorbers reported increases in pain over regular diet. However, in diet trials with substances not containing lactose, 33.3 percent of malabsorbers and 23.5 percent of absorbers reported increased pain. After 12 months of a lactose-free diet, 40 percent of lactose-intolerant subjects and 38.4 percent of lactose-tolerant subjects reported symptom resolution. Thus neither ingestion of lactose nor the presence of a lactase deficiency seemed related to onset or relief of abdominal pain. The authors concluded that the role of lactose intolerance in RAP was marginal. This conclusion seems justified. Yet the study of Lebenthal and colleagues (1981) can be criticized on the grounds that, while it was well designed in general, the authors erred in using a control group composed of patients with nonpainful GI symptoms (chronic diarrhea, failure to thrive, suspected malabsorption, and recurrent vomiting). These symptoms often mimic those of the RAP syndrome. It is possible that these children also experienced some pain but failed to report it because of stoic natures or lesser perceived severity. As the authors noted, the RAP syndrome is as yet poorly defined, and the control group's symptoms may in fact be pathognomonic of a larger syndrome of which pain symptoms are but a part.

Other studies investigating organic causes of RAP have focused on the role autonomic nervous system dysfunction plays in the production of symptoms. Few such studies exist, and their results are difficult to interpret. Apley (1975) proposed a constitutional sensitivity to stress as a possible contributor to RAP. In general, such sensitivity has been investigated in the context of autonomic hyperreactivity resulting in changes in blood flow to the colon or changes in gastric motility. For example, Dimson (1971) argued that organic causes of RAP may be more responsible for symptoms than is currently believed. He found constipation and delayed transit time to be common in a group of 306 RAP children. Dimson also found that migraine headache existed coincidentally with RAP in 96 of his 306 subjects. He therefore hypothesized a common autonomic imbalance as causal of many RAP symptoms.

In another report of ANS imbalance, Heinild and colleagues (1959) radiologically examined 81 Danish RAP children at initial hospitalization and at 3-year follow-up. Demonstrable changes in gastric mucosa and peristalsis existed for significantly more RAP children than controls. These changes persisted in 75 percent of subjects at follow-up. However, two-thirds of RAP children reported subjective improvement at follow-up. Several observations can be made about these data. First, the existence of changes in gastric mucosa or peristalsis does not necessarily point to an organic cause of RAP. Second, it seems evident that subjective symptoms of RAP may be reported independent of the existence of demonstrable physiological changes.

The best designed and most complete study of ANS dysfunction in RAP children is the report of Feuerstein, Barr, Francouer, Houle, and Rafman (1982). These investigators attempted to ascertain whether RAP children demonstrated ANS deficits or behavioral or physiological hyperreactivity to pain. Groups of pain-free controls and controls suffering from nonpainful organic conditions were included. The authors found that neither physiological, subjective, nor behavioral responses to acute laboratory-induced pain were different among any of the three groups. While the study did not support differences in ANS reactivity among RAP children, the authors noted that this finding did not rule out allied hypotheses, that is, that there is a specific target organ system response to stress in RAP children that is perhaps mediated by social learning factors. The authors also acknowledged that behavioral differences in response to pain are usually expressed in context, and may not occur in response to acute pain induced in a laboratory setting.

Epilepsy has been thought by some to be implicated in RAP. The only well-designed study investigating the role of epilepsy in the disorder is that of Papatheophilou, Jeavons, and Disney (1972). While 11 of 50 RAP children in their study showed electrical abnormalities suggestive of epilepsy, these authors concluded that findings of EEG abnormalities in association with RAP should not be taken as evidence of epilepsy.

RAP IN CONTEXT IID: INTERPERSONAL DIMENSION

Social modeling is often presumed to be important in the genesis of childhood abdominal pain (Apley, 1975; Craig, 1978; Whitehead; 1986). In general, it is assumed that a dysfunctional somatic response to stress in a parent (mother is almost always identified) is observed and reproduced by a child. Cases of multiple siblings with RAP are apparently rare. Why any particular child in a family is susceptible to modeled pain behaviors is unclear, although birth order, being the only boy or girl in a large family, or constitutional sensitivity have all been implicated in placing a child at risk. While a social modeling theory makes a certain amount of a priori sense, research indicating higher incidences of RAP in families with histories of abdominal pain is inconsistent.

Studies supporting a social modeling theory were cited by Galler and colleagues (1980), who provided an excellent review of available observations on RAP. These authors noted that a family history of abdominal or other pain is often present. They also cited data indicating higher rates of other psychogenic disorders, such as migraine headache or allergy, in families of RAP children. Likewise, Berger, Honig, and Liebman (1977) found RAP-like abdominal symptoms in the parents of children with RAP. The children in Christensen and Mortensen's (1975) study with parents who had suffered from RAP in childhood were no more likely than normals to display abdominal symptoms. However, their data did indicate a higher incidence of abdominal pain in children of parents who were complaining of abdominal discomfort at the time of the investigation. This temporal relationship between symptom display in parents and children has been interpreted as providing empirical support for a social modeling theory of RAP (Barr, 1983; Feuerstein et al., 1982). Oster (1972) found that the parents of children with pain were less likely to be pain free (of head, limb, or stomach pain) both in childhood and at the time of the investigation than parents of pain-free children. Stone and Barbero (1970) found that as many as 50 percent of mothers of children with RAP complained of functional gastrointestinal symptoms. (These authors also reported that 46 percent of fathers of RAP children had some type of gastrointestinal illness. The finding of high rates of GI illness in fathers of RAP children is unique to this study.)

Green (1967) speculated that RAP is indicative of a familial pattern of hypochondriasis. Further evidence supporting the intergenerational transmission of functional GI disorders can be found in case studies and surgical histories of families with such disorders, as in the Joyce and Walsh (1980) family case history presented earlier, or in the case of a female with recurrent vomiting, reported by Brady (1986). Jackson and Yalom (1966) studied patterns of illness in the families of eight children with ulcerative colitis. While ulcerative colitis and RAP appear to be independent disorders afflicting the same organ system, the anecdotal evidence presented is striking in its similarity to reports of illness in families of RAP children. For instance, five of eight mothers in this group had one or more abdominal surgeries accompanied by numerous other physical or emotional complaints. Two others had unspecified bowel trouble.

Evidence contrary to the social modeling hypothesis is presented by McGrath and colleagues (1983). In this study no significant differences between RAP children and their families and control groups were noted on psychological variables thought to be implicated in RAP (marital adjustment and family pain history). These findings are at variance with those of most published works on RAP. However, this study is also exceptional in that it is one of very few that has utilized standardized assessment devices to gather data rather than relying primarily on clinical observation. In a more recent report, McGrath and Feldman (1986) again found little support for a family modeling theory of RAP.

Aside from methodological criticisms regarding instrumentation and data collection procedures in studies showing a high family incidence of abdominal pain, a more substantive argument counter to this assumption exists. This is that, even in those studies of RAP that focus on familial patterns of illness, usually only in a quarter to a third and at most half of all cases are corresponding symptoms between parent and child found (Liebman, 1978; Oster, 1972; Stone & Barbero, 1970). Thus a social modeling hypothesis leaves unexplained a large percentage of all RAP cases.

While it has yet to be conclusively demonstrated that RAP occurs in pain-prone families (Lavigne et al., 1986b), social modeling obviously plays a major role in the intergenerational transmission of pain syndromes (Payne & Norfleet, 1986). However, it is not the only family dynamic affecting the transmission of pain. Parental abuse and lack of affection may be contributory factors (Violon, 1985), in addition to socioeconomic status, family size, and other factors. If chronic pain is to be understood in a multidimensional perspective, it is necessary that some reliable way of measuring family variables exist (cf. Turk, Rudy, & Flor, 1985). The recurrent abdominal pain questionnaire devised by Levine and Rappaport (1984) does attempt to measure parental and child pain behavior, and the Varni-Thompson Pediatric Pain Questionnaire (Varni & Thompson, 1985) also attempts to incorporate these factors. Both of these instruments have the potential to provide indirect empirical support for a social modeling hypothesis. As of yet, neither tool has been used sufficiently to provide relevant data. Their existence represents a considerable advance toward understanding pediatric pain syndromes, but techniques to assess other family dynamics are sorely needed.

RAP IN CONTEXT IIF: COGNITIVE–REPRESENTATIONAL DIMENSIONS

Compliance, Perceived Vulnerability, and Recurrent Abdominal Pain

A good part of the pediatric health psychology literature is devoted to the subject of enhancing compliance to a medical regimen. This objective has largely been approached from the perspective of increasing levels of perceived vulnerability in target populations (Gochman & Saucier, 1982). On the other hand, the task faced by investigators examining RAP and similar disorders with a strong psychological component is to delineate variables resulting in the misinterpretation of benign physical symptoms and the overreliance on health care services. As Gochman and Saucier (1982) remarked:

> Perceptions of being vulnerable to health problems are not associated with preventive beliefs, attitudes, or behaviors in a consistently happy way. A more compelling objective would be the determination of what the *optimum* levels of perceived vulnerability are as bases for preventive attitudes and behaviors. (p. 152)

The point is that intervention models that focus only on increasing perceived vulnerability are not liable to help most individuals become efficient seekers of health care. It is suggested that a more appropriate way to help individuals utilize health care services effectively is not to seek to increase vulnerability but instead to increase the individual's overall competence in seeking medical attention. In pediatric health behavior, competence has been defined to include characteristics that allow the child to resist negative influences such as poor family functioning or higher stress levels. Karoly (1982) has also emphasized that problem-solving skills and self-regulatory abilities are necessary to the development of competence in seeking health care.

The issue of competence in health care seeking is important in the analysis of RAP, in that painful but nonthreatening symptoms are commonly misinterpreted as harbingers of grave physical illness. Issues of competence and compliance are also important in light of evidence suggesting that misinterpretation of symptoms and overreliance are easily transmitted from parents to their children. Therefore, models of compliance will be briefly discussed.

The health belief model has been widely used in the investigation of health beliefs and compliance in pediatric illness (Varni, 1983a). Most studies using the health belief model have investigated pediatric health beliefs almost exclusively from the perspective of increasing compliance. This is logical in that the model was developed with the purpose in mind of understanding failure to take preventive measures against disease (Janz & Becker, 1984). Basic components of the model are derived from theory hypothesizing that individual behavior depends on the value placed on a particular goal and the estimate of the likelihood that a given action will achieve a valued goal. Regarding health behavior, this hypothesis is stated in terms of the individual's desire to avoid illness (or if ill, to get well), and the belief that specific health actions will prevent or ameliorate illness (Janz & Becker, 1984). The health belief model holds that individuals vary in their conceptions of illness along four basic dimensions: perceived susceptibility, perceived severity, perceived benefits, and perceived barriers.

Janz and Becker reviewed 30 health belief model studies published between 1974 and 1984. Most of these studies examined clinic underusage or other phenomena related to the underestimation of symptoms. Based on the number of positive and significant findings from the combined studies, their review concluded that the most important of the four dimensions in determining health-related action was the perceived barriers dimension. This was followed by the benefits, susceptibility, and severity dimensions, in descending order. Therefore, the susceptibility dimension ranked third out of the four in order of importance in determining health behavior. However, a study examining relationships between mothers' health beliefs and utilization of pediatric services found that mothers who viewed their children as more vulnerable took them to clinics more often for acute illness and less often for preventive checks than mothers who viewed their children as less vulnerable (Becker, Nathanson, & Drachman, & Kirscht, 1977, cited in Janz & Becker, 1984).

Cummings, Becker, and Maile (1980) examined 14 theoretical models that have been used to explain individual health behavior. They statistically condensed more than 100 variables thought to be of importance in accounting for health behavior into a three-dimensional array with six clusters of variables. Groups into which variables were clustered were: (1) accessibility of health services (ability to pay, awareness of availability of services); (2) attitudes toward treatment (benefits of treatment and perceptions of quality of care); (3) threat of illness (perception of symptoms and beliefs regarding vulnerability to, and consequences of, illness); (4) knowledge about disease; (5) social interaction, norms, and social structure; and (6) demographic characteristics. A close proximity existed between items concerning knowledge of disease and those dealing with perceptions and evaluation of symptoms with items on social interaction. The authors therefore speculated that knowledge of illness might be emphasized through social interactions, and that this information might be used to judge severity of symptoms and the threat of disease.

Studies with the health belief model and those using other models to examine health beliefs such as cited in Cummings and colleagues (1980) generally examine the health beliefs of adults as they pertain to children. Those studying children do so mainly on the basis of mothers' perceptions and reports. However, children undoubtedly play a more active role in determining levels of compliance than previously recognized (see Bush & Davidson, 1982).

One of the few investigations of the health belief model with children is that of Dielman, Leech, Becker, Rosenstock, and Horvath (1980). They found that younger children reported a greater degree of concern regarding health in general, and that children's health beliefs may be fairly consolidated by the third or fourth grade. Older children were seen to be more sensitive to or perceptive of parental concerns regarding the child's illness. On the issue of perceived vulnerability, they found evidence suggesting that this may not be a unitary concept for children. Three relatively independent factors were isolated from this category. These factors included general susceptibility, individual estimation of the likelihood of experiencing symptoms, and a third cluster that was a mix of the first two. The authors found significant age effects on all but one factor, suggesting that levels of concern decrease with increasing age (sample age ranged from 6 to 17 years). In another investigation of children's health beliefs by the same group, Dielman, and colleagues (1982) differentiated health beliefs from health behaviors. Results of this study indicated that parental health behaviors were the primary predictors of children's health behaviors. Parental health beliefs also influenced children's health beliefs, but to a lesser extent than parental behaviors influenced child behaviors. As was the case with health beliefs, children's health behaviors were seen to have strong developmental correlates.

Analysis of health beliefs and health behaviors using the health belief model has some inherent limitations. In particular, predication of causal relationships between health beliefs and compliance is not possible on the basis of the model alone. Fear and anxiety, among other psychological factors, may either increase or decrease compliance to treatment. This phenomenon is not specifically addressed in the health belief model (Olson, Zimmerman, & Reyes de la Rocha, 1985).

RAP IN CONTEXT IIIA: DEVELOPMENTAL–TEMPORAL DIMENSIONS

Analysis of children's conceptions of pain and illness has received considerable recent attention. Most studies to date indicate that children's concepts do develop systematically and predictably (Thompson & Varni, 1986). Burbach and Peterson (1986) summarize the major findings of the cognitive–developmental literature regarding children's concepts of illness. Older children are generally seen to conceptualize illness in terms of specific symptoms and disease. Younger children have more global and nonspecific conceptions. Older children tend to be cognizant of psychological aspects of illness, whereas younger children are not. Younger children are largely unable to differentiate causes of illness. Cognitively mature children rely on internal cues to determine health and illness, while less mature children are more external. The notion of contagion is grasped by mature children and poorly differentiated by immature children.

Within the past few years attempts have been made to classify children's conceptions of illness according to the stages of causal reasoning in Piagetian developmental theory (Bibace & Walsh, 1980, 1981). Bibace and Walsh found that conceptualizations of illness causation and cure were compatible with predicted stages of cognitive maturation. For example, 4-year-old children (presumed to be in the prelogical stage of development) most commonly gave responses containing the concept of contagion, regardless of the nature of transmission of the disease in question. Illness was thought by these children to be transmitted by some unknown and possibly magical mechanism from persons or inanimate objects proximal to the child. Older children gave increasingly sophisticated responses, the most mature of which indicated awareness of both psychological and physical elements of the disease process. Children at the stage of formal logical operations indicated awareness of psychological and physiological aspects of illness causation (Bibace & Walsh, 1980). Bibace and Walsh used normal, healthy children in their studies and presented them with examples of acute childhood illness, as well as pain, headache, heart attack, or personal illness in the child. The question remains whether such conclusions are generalizable to chronic, benign disorders like RAP.

A small number of studies have examined cognitive development and illness conceptualizations in chronically ill children (for descriptions of these studies, see Varni, 1983b; Thompson & Varni, 1986). These authors found that, in general, such studies support that notion that chronically ill children's cognitive and psychosocial development approximated that of normal healthy children. To my knowledge, no developmental studies have been performed using subjects with chronic nonorganic illness, such as RAP. While there may be an implicit assumption that such children are in some way psychologically or developmentally abnormal, the failure to find specific psychopathology in many RAP children does not support this point of view.

It remains to be investigated whether children with RAP interpret pain and illness causation in a similar fashion to children with chronic, organic illness. In doing so, theories of cognitive development and locus of control may be able to explain some features of the course of RAP in individual children. For instance, the most common period for onset of RAP symptoms is 5 to 6 years (Apley, 1975), when the child is presumably in the later phases of the preoperational stage. If Bibace and Walsh's scheme applies to these children, it may be that abdominal pain is perceived to be transmitted via unknown mechanisms from persons proximal to the child. That is, a child whose parent(s) or schoolmates suffer from frequent abdominal pain may interpret such symptoms as contagious (due to proximity) and thus be predisposed to display similar symptoms. A related phenomenon is the decline in the frequency and severity of RAP symptoms as children age. Investigations of RAP from a cognitive–developmental perspective may yield data indicating that, as the child's conception of illness grows more sophisticated, internal self-regulatory mechanisms exert a more powerful influence on symptom control. The analysis by Dielman and colleagues (1982) indicates that this may be the case, in that younger children were found to view themselves as more susceptible to illness than older children. A 13-year-old who has achieved a formal operational level may, as Bibace and Walsh suggest, discern a psychological component to the illness process and take some form of positive self-regulatory action to correct it.

Locus of control is also thought to be developmentally linked to the cognitive maturation process, and may be implicated in children's conceptions of illness. Neuhauser, Amsterdam, Hines, and Steward (1978) concluded that children at higher levels of cognitive development display a more internal locus of control and have greater perceived control over the healing process. If this is indeed so, development of an internal locus may be related to perceived control over the illness process. A preoperational 5-year-old therefore would perceive less control over symptoms than a formal operational 12-year-old. This may also be a factor in explaining patterns of symptom onset and severity in RAP children, as well as the longitudinal course of the disorder.

Another hypothesis that has an apparent connection to cognitive–developmental processes involves individual tendencies toward introspection (Mechanic, 1983, 1986). Mechanic argued that adolescents (and presumably children) impress clinicians as psychosomatic simply because they are uncertain about how to interpret symptoms. According to Mechanic's hypothesis, adolescents who develop introspective tendencies are more emotionally reactive and are prone to define common bodily sensations as symptoms.

RAP IN CONTEXT IIID, IIIE, AND IIIF: SITUATIONAL, VOCATIONAL–ACADEMIC, AND FAMILIAL DIMENSIONS

Unusual pressure to succeed in athletics was reasoned to be a cause of RAP symptoms in two case studies of 10- and 11-year-old boys reported by Adler, Bongar, and Katz (1982). Symptoms resolved when parents (in both cases the father) were persuaded to modify what were seen as inappropriate goals for the children.

Other situational precipitants of RAP have been presented by Schmitt (1971) and Berger (1974), who believed RAP to be a symptom masking the serious underlying problem of school phobia. But given this etiological hypothesis, the questions remain as to why stress is expressed via physical illness in some children and not in others, and why the GI tract is the target organ system in some, but not all, children experiencing similar stressors. Also, chronic abdominal pain that persists for months or years needs to be differentiated from pain expressions used as a mechanism for short-term school avoidance. This is not to deny that a certain percentage of RAP cases are reflections of school phobia or other situational factors. In the majority of cases of RAP, however, it appears that the expression of abdominal pain usually bears no common relationship to any particular factor (Bain, 1974) or stressful situation (Green, 1967).

Onset of the symptoms of RAP has been linked to separation from or illness in a family member. Chronic parental depression, alcoholism, and the onset of financial stress may also play an etiological role (Berger et al., 1977). Marital discord or divorce may be more common in RAP families than in others (Lambert, 1941; Liebman, 1978). In seven of the eight families in Jackson and Yalom's (1966) study of ulcerative colitis patients, onset of symptoms followed parental conflict or desertion, other family disruption, or maternal illness. Jackson and Yalom also found that fathers in the families studied were generally passive and uninvolved in family affairs, and were seen as vocational failures. Berger (1974) noticed the presence of devalued or isolated fathers in families with a RAP child as well. Also common in case histories of four such families were overprotective attitudes toward the patient and a major change in the family (departure of an older sibling from the home in three of four cases).

Green (1967) believed that RAP symptoms resulted from identification with a family member who had experienced similar pain. He found common factors predisposing onset of RAP to be anticipation of death or actual death of an important person in the child's life, parental separation or divorce, desertion by a parent, prolonged absence of another family member, or the child's own fear of death.

Chronic depression and alcoholism in parents were also observed. Green provided a concise picture of some of the major assumptions about RAP, but his conclusions were observationally based and did not result from systematic investigation.

Life events are situational factors that have been the focus of several recent investigations of RAP. However, when life events are subject to systematic assessment, their role in the etiology of RAP becomes uncertain. Greene, Walker, Hickson, and Thompson (1985) reported significantly higher levels of mean negative life events in children with nonorganic pain when these were compared to others in an outpatient sample. Higher levels of stress and negative life events in RAP children were also reported by Hodges, Kline, Barbero, and Flanery (1984). Children were assessed using a modified version of the Coddington Life Events Inventory, which measures events in the previous year. Parents of RAP children, who were given a modified form of the Schedule of Recent Experience and the Life Experiences Survey, showed a greater tendency to report issues involving changes in health or personal injury and illness, but this did not reach levels of significance. Raymer, Weininger, and Hamilton (1984) found no significant difference in life event scores between children with organic pain, children with nonorganic pain, and pain-free controls.

In a report of interest because of its cross-cultural implications, Singh, Gupta, and Agrawal (1972) reported many characteristics of Indian RAP children that are similar to those seen in western RAP groups. Children in their study were able to identify a precipitating psychosocial cause for abdominal pain in half the cases studied. However, the authors did not provide details as to the exact nature of precipitating causes. Overall, there are many methodological problems in reports correlating higher stress levels with the incidence of RAP. None of these reports utilized the same schedule for assessing life events. Also, Barr and Feuerstein (1983) have commented that the temporal proximity or sequential relationship of stressors to symptom onset is often ignored in such studies. Barr and Feuerstein point out an additional confounding factor that confuses the relationship of stressful life events and RAP symptom onset. This is that stressful events apparently increase the likelihood that a child will be seen by a physician, whether or not the stress is related to the presenting symptoms (Meyers & Haggerty, 1973; cited in Barr & Feuerstein, 1983). Because of this and other potential confounds, a convincing argument that stress is a definitive etiological factor in RAP cannot as yet be made, although some form of relationship is undoubtedly present.

Parental psychopathology has been noticed in a fairly high percentage of families studied for this variable. A recent investigation in which behaviorally disordered and RAP children were compared found no significant difference in depression scores between RAP children and healthy controls on the Children's Depression Inventory and the Child Assessment Schedule. Depression scores for both groups were significantly lower than for the behaviorally disordered group. However, mothers of both RAP and behaviorally disordered children had significantly higher depression scores than the mothers of healthy children. This suggests that depressive family characteristics may be important in the development of the RAP syndrome, even though depression is not liable to be a major part of the presentation of RAP in affected children (Hodges et al., 1985).

Routh and Ernst (1984) interviewed mothers of children with either organic or functional abdominal pain. They detected a higher proportion of psychiatric illness among families of RAP children (attention deficit disorder, alcoholism, antisocial or conduct disturbance, or somatization disorder). However, differences were significant only in the case of somatization disorder. "Unhealthy attitudes" toward children were found in 79 percent of parents by Singh and colleagues (1971). Again, such attitudes were left unspecified.

The evidence for involvement of parental psychopathology in the etiology of RAP is somewhat more compelling than that supporting a case for a social modeling theory. Numerically, larger percentages of parents with psychopathology are reported than parents with abdominal pain. Also, slightly more studies investigating this factor have been empirical in nature. Again, however, most published reports are strictly anecdotal. Also, an explanatory theory involving parental or familial psychopathology may make the dangerous assumption of the existence of psychopathology in the RAP child. Until recently, there have been no controlled studies examining psychological disorders in children with stomach pain (McGrath, 1983). This situation appears to be changing. In the controlled study by Raymer, Hamilton, and Weininger (1984), significantly higher levels of depression and low self-esteem were present in children with nonorganic abdominal pain when compared to pain-free controls, but depression and low self-esteem were also higher for a group with organic abdominal pain (Crohn's disease and ulcerative colitis). These findings are at variance with other published reports (usually nonempirical) examining such factors. Barr and Feuerstein (1983) and Apley (1975) have pointed out that substantial portions of the RAP population do not exhibit signs of psychopathology, and others (McGrath, 1983) have not found RAP children to be different from normals. Most investigators are careful to deny an etiology based on psychological factors alone in light of failure to identify characteristic personality types or common forms of psychopathology among RAP children.

Birth order, number of siblings, gender, intelligence levels, and behavioral disorders have been implicated in the development of RAP in a particular child. Other family-related features, such as family size and social class, have also been identified in the development of pain syndromes (Violon, 1985). A number of authors have reported that birth order seemed significant in the etiology of RAP, with many children being either the first or last in the family (Berger et al., 1977; Liebman, 1978; Singh et al., 1972; Stone & Barbero, 1970). Other investigators (Friedman, 1972) have found no relationship between birth order and incidence of RAP complaints, and in general it has not been carefully examined. Berger and colleagues (1977) found that often RAP children were the only boy or girl of a large family. They also found RAP patients to be more emotionally immature than other children, an observation also reported by Hughes and Zimin (1978). Unspecified behavioral disorders in RAP children were reported by Lambert (1941) and Heinild and colleagues (1959).

The study by Friedman (1972) is one of only three that systematically examine IQ in RAP children. Friedman found the mean IQ for boys in his sample to be 99 as measured on the WISC (SD = 18; range = 60 to 137). Mean IQ for girls was 97 (SD = 15; range = 66 to 118). Lambert (1941) used the Binet scales to measure IQ in his sample of RAP patients, and found IQ scores to be markedly elevated. Median score on the Binet was 110, with a range of 80 to 143. In contrast, less than 1 percent of his control group scored over 110 on the Binet scale. On the other hand, Singh and colleagues (1971) found mean IQ scores for their RAP sample to be somewhat below average for Indian children at large.

RAP IN A MULTIDIMENSIONAL CONTEXT

The preceding analysis should make it clear that an understanding of the complexities of RAP cannot be achieved if the separate components that contribute to the disorder are analyzed in isolation. Neither organic causes, psychosocial variables, nor individual characteristics can account for the manifestations of RAP if these elements are considered alone. To account for the majority of cases, which occur in the absence of physiologic or psychologic disturbance, it is useful to return to the dysfunctional category of abdominal pain proposed by Barr and Feuerstein (1983) in which no assumption of psychological abnormality is made, and in which the presence of symptoms is not presumed to imply the presence of organic disease.

The dysfunctional category proposed by Barr and Feuerstein has merit, and it clearly can be used to bring together a number of factors involved in RAP. The concept is also useful clinically, as in reassuring anxious parents or children that a bout of stomach pain does not signal onset of a severe organic problem. The dysfunctional definition is perhaps less powerful in a theoretical conceptualization of RAP, largely because it does not account for the influence of environmental or cognitive factors in the process of the disorder.

Levine and Rappaport (1984) have developed a compelling biopsychosocial model for RAP that incorporates the dysfunctional category suggested by Barr and Feuerstein (1983). In place of single-factor etiologies examined by earlier investigators, these authors proposed that multiple predisposing factors converged to produce symptoms of the RAP syndrome. Their model suggests that life-style patterns, somatic predispositions, learned response patterns, and environmental factors act together in such a way that:

> a somatic propensity toward pain localized to the abdomen occurs in a living milieu that itself is affected in part by critical life events. The milieu may or may not trigger or intensify the pain. The child's own habits and style of life are also influential forces either promoting or counteracting symptom development. Finally, there is a repertoire of temperamental traits and patterns of response that promote pain appreciation. The four forces influence each other and become specific targets for evaluation and patient management. (p. 971)

This model is both compelling and workable; it has the capability to incorporate individual targets of earlier research into an equation that may have explanatory power in analyzing the etiology of RAP. With adequate assessment procedures, it may have real predictive ability in determining children at risk for developing RAP. However, the model's explanatory power can be increased by the addition of another element that has been scantily investigated to date. Given the discussion presented in the previous section of this chapter, Levine and Rappaport's model seems incomplete without the addition of a category encompassing cognitive and developmental processes that are important in determining susceptibility to illness, symptom interpretation, and the ability to cope with pain. The current author has examined this variable in terms of irritable bowel syndrome in adults (Sammons & Karoly, 1987). Table 16.1 shows how these elements can be incorporated into a theoretical explanatory conception of RAP. In the following section, strategies for the assessment of each of these categories will be outlined.

TABLE 16.1.

RAP symptom expression =	(*f*) somatic predisposition
	+ life-style
	+ learned response patterns, social modeling influences, individual psychological characteristics, and family dynamics
	+ environmental factors
	+ cognitive–developmental processes

ASSESSING RAP IN CHILDREN: GENERAL CONSIDERATIONS AND FUTURE DIRECTIONS

All aspects of the pain experience need to be considered in order to facilitate a complete understanding of the RAP syndrome and to aid in treatment. Although physical pathology is an infrequent cause of RAP, such factors must be ruled out before effective psychological management (if indicated) can begin. A rapid accounting of physical problems alleviates fears shared by parents, patient, and clinician. The timing, performance, and reporting of results of physical elevations represent critical moments in determining the ease with which psychological interventions may be initiated. Parents who believe that their child has been incompletely evaluated or is being dismissed because the presenting complaint is psychogenic are likely to be dissatisfied and seek medical attention elsewhere. When this occurs, the child goes without consistent treatment, distress is magnified, and the risk of unnecessary surgery increases.

The medical literature contains numerous suggestions pertaining to the prevention of this unhappy chain of events. First, parents and patient must be reassured that the pain is real, and that pain due to stress hurts no less than pain due to physical pathology (Bain, 1974). Lennard-Jones (1983) and Stark and Blum (1986) suggest that a psychosocial history be taken as part of the initial consultation when a strong psychosomatic component is suspected, as a later interest in psychological factors, when organic causes have been ruled out, can arouse hostility. Establishment of a supportive relationship is essential so that the problem can be constructively redefined in nonorganic terms (Berger et al., 1977). In the case of "psychosomatic" families, where reliance on medication or surgery to alleviate distress may be a way of life, a carefully orchestrated approach is necessary to ensure that the child receives proper treatment (Hughes & Zimin, 1978). Diminution of parental anxiety and alleviation of stress upon the child should be emphasized as treatment goals in their own right (Farrell, 1984). Hospitalization for evaluation and a multidisciplinary team approach to diagnosis have been advocated in such difficult cases (Dunger et al., 1986). Dunger and his colleagues found that detection of factors such as marital problems, parental alcoholism, and distress surrounding bereavement was more valuable than organic workup in providing clues as to the nature of RAP symptoms presented. Hospital admission for diagnostic workup provided valuable information as to the interactions between the child's behavior and frequency of symptoms in the presence or absence of family members. Dunger and colleagues reported that, although physicians had suggested that psychological factors were significant in 10 of 12 cases referred for evaluation, parents in all cases had refused to accept this explanation and sought further organic workup. This group commented that in most cases organic evaluation in excess of the basic procedures already undertaken serves only to confuse, rather than clarify, diagnosis.

Three phases in organic workup of RAP patients have been identified (Galler et al., 1980). The first, which is confined to laboratory work and is highly effective in ruling out most organic causes, consists of blood and urine analyses and stool testing for ova and parasites. If the physician is still concerned, blood tests are repeated, and lactose intolerance tests, barium enema, EEG, and/or other more specific tests are ordered. Endoscopy has been recommended at this phase, but caution in the use of invasive procedures is recommended because of the possibility of psychological or physical trauma to the child (McGrath & Feldman, 1986). The third phase involves exploratory surgery, and is used only in very rare cases. Trials of diet therapy, maintenance of a close physician–patient relationship, and the passage of time between the first and second phase of evaluation are highly recommended (McGrath & Feldman, 1986; also see Levine & Rappaport, 1984).

The sensory experience of pain in RAP has not been widely investigated (Masek, Russo, & Varni, 1984). As these authors commented, the available evidence does not indicate that RAP children respond differently than others to laboratory-induced pain (see the study by Feuerstein et al., 1982, discussed earlier). Levine and Rappaport (1984) have developed an instrument for standardized measurement of characteristics of RAP children, which includes pain assessment, but data with this new instrument have yet to be produced. No other instruments specific for RAP are known to exist. Varni and Thompson's (1985) Pediatric Pain Questionnaire includes sensory, affective, and evaluative qualities of pain as well as family history and environmental events mediating pain (Thompson & Varni, 1986). While the Pediatric Pain Questionnaire seems to focus primarily on the sensory aspects of pain, its existence signifies a considerable advance in how pediatric pain is conceptualized and measured.

How pediatric patients cope with their pain can also be objectively assessed, as Jay (1985) has demonstrated. Jay investigated ability to cope with pain in the context of acute pain in children afflicted with chronic fatal disease (cited in Jay, 1985). The painful episodes she examined were connected with medical procedures (bone marrow aspiration). It may be argued that pain behavior in such circumstances is different from ongoing chronic pain because the event is predictable and takes place with the expectation that pain is necessary to ameliorate the condition. The situation with RAP is distinct, in that the pain is endogenous and unpredictable, and of unknown origin to the child.

However, there is at least one report in the literature concerning children's coping styles in response to chronic benign pain. Dunn-Geier, McGrath, Rourke, Latter, and D'Astous (1986) have analyzed the behavior of children with chronic benign pain (50 percent of whom had stomach pain) and their mothers. Subjects were videotaped while participating in laboratory tasks designed to simulate activities in which the child experienced pain. Noncopers were found to engage in significantly more negative behaviors than coping children. Also, noncopers tended to emit more verbal expressions of pain. They found mothers of noncoping children to be overinvolved with the children's behavior. They also found that mothers of noncopers tended to discourage coping behavior. (However, no differences in family or personality variables for copers and noncopers emerged when these were measured using standardized self-report devices).

Just as instruments like the Pediatric Pain Questionnaire provide replicable and reliable sources of data on pediatric pain, the assessment of individual and familial psychological characteristics has increasingly benefited from the use of standardized assessment devices since Apley's early investigations in the late 1950s. The recent investigation of Hodges and colleagues (1985, cited earlier) exemplifies the use of such well-constructed devices as Achenbach's Child Behavior Checklist and structured DSM-III interviews for children.

Because of the apparent importance of social modeling and learned illness behaviors, the assessment of familial variables is arguably of greatest importance in understanding the *development* of RAP. Yet it is in this area that the largest advances need to be made. Primary obstacles here are a set of poorly operationalized theoretical constructs and the failure to address how dysfunctional family interactions are translated into specific physical symptoms (Turk et al., 1985). While family intervention has been used to treat RAP (Liebman, 1978), some (McGrath & Feldman, 1986) object to the use of such approaches. In the absence of research supporting the efficacy of family therapy to treat chronic benign pain (Roy, 1985), such objections should be given some consideration.

While some work on cognitive variables in pediatric illness has been accomplished (largely through versions of the health belief model and stage theory conceptions of development), more is clearly needed. Two points are particularly salient here. First, most work in children's health beliefs has focused on the health beliefs of parents rather than children themselves (Bush & Davidson, 1982). More work is clearly needed to provide insights into how children interpret illness, illness vulnerability, and the various facets of the doctor–patient relationship that determine self-regulatory ability and compliance to treatment. Second, research exists to indicate that many children with chronic physical illness achieve normal developmental progress, despite the special conditions imposed by chronic illness (Varni, 1983b; also see Russo, 1986). However, developmental processes in children with chronic benign pain are largely unexplored. Are such children able to achieve developmentally normal interpretations of illness? If so, why does such a large percentage of this population continue to display self-regulatory problems (accurate interpretation of physical symptoms) in adulthood?

In conclusion, the assessment of pediatric pain has come a considerable distance in recent years. Standardized devices are becoming available to measure pain in its different representational and environmental contexts, and the importance of assessing pain in the circumstances in which it occurs is increasingly acknowledged. However, the applicability of our emerging knowledge to painful disorders that are chronic and benign remains uncertain. As this chapter has attempted to demonstrate, this uncertainty cannot be resolved without utilization of well-developed biopsychosocial models.

References

Adler, R., Bongar, B., & Katz, E. R. (1982). Psychogenic abdominal pain and parental pressure in childhood athletics. *Psychosomatics, 23,* 1186–1189.

Apley, J. (1975). *The child with abdominal pains* (2nd ed.). London: Blackwell.

Apley, J., & Hale, B. (1973). Children with recurrent abdominal pain: How do they grow up? *British Medical Journal, 3,* 7–9.

Bain, H. W. (1974). Chronic abdominal pain in childhood. *Pediatric Clinics of North America, 2,* 991–1000.

Barr, R. (1983). Recurrent abdominal pain. In M. D. Levine, W. B. Corey, A. C. Crocker, & R. T. Gross (Eds.), *Developmental behavioral pediatrics*. Philadelphia: Saunders.

Barr, R. G., & Feuerstein, M. (1983). Recurrent abdominal pain syndrome. In P. McGrath & P. Firestone (Eds.), *Pediatric and adolescent behavioral medicine*. New York: Springer.

Barr, R. G., Levine, M. D., & Watkins, J. B. (1979). Recurrent abdominal pain due to lactose intolerance. *New England Journal of Medicine, 300*, 1449–1452.

Bayless, T. M., & Huang, S. S. (1971). Recurrent abdominal pain due to milk and lactose intolerance in school-age children. *Pediatrics, 47*, 1029–1032.

Becker, M. H., Nathanson, C. A., Drachman, R. H., and Kirscht, J. P. (1977). Mothers' health beliefs and children's clinic visits: A prospective study. *Journal of Community Health, 3*, 125–135.

Berger, H. G. (1974). Somatic pain and school avoidance. *Clinical Pediatrics, 13*, 819–826.

Berger, H. G., Honig, P. J., & Liebman, R. (1977). Recurrent abdominal pain. *American Journal of Diseases in Children, 131*, 1340–1344.

Bibace, R., & Walsh, M. E. (1980). Development of children's concepts of illness. *Pediatrics, 66*, 912–917.

Bibace, R., & Walsh, M. K. (Eds.) (1981). *Children's conceptions of health, illness, and bodily functions*. San Francisco: Jossey-Bass.

Brady, J. P. (1986). Behavioral analysis of a case of psychogenic nausea and vomiting. *Journal of Behavior Therapy & Experimental Psychiatry, 17*, 221–224.

Burbach, D. J., & Peterson, L. (1986). Children's concepts of physical illness: A review and critique of the cognitive developmental literature. *Health Psychology, 5*, 307–325.

Bush, P. J., & Davidson, F. R. (1982). Medicine and drugs: What do children think? *Health Education Quarterly, 9*, 209–224.

Christensen, M. F., & Mortensen, O. (1975). Long term prognosis in children with recurrent abdominal pain. *Archives of Diseases in Children, 50*, 110–114.

Cooperman, E. M. (1976). The child with recurrent abdominal pain. *Canadian Medical Association Journal, 115*, 973–974.

Craig, K. D. (1978). Social modeling influences on pain. In R. Sternbach, (Ed.), *The psychology of pain*. New York: Raven.

Cummings, K. M., Becker, M. H., & Maile, M. C. (1980). Bringing the models together: An empirical approach to combining variables used to explain health actions. *Journal of Behavioral Medicine, 3*, 123–145.

Davison, I. S., Faull, C., & Nicol, A. R. (1986). Temperament and behavior in six year olds with recurrent abdominal pain: A followup. *Journal of Child Psychology and Psychiatry, 27*, 539–544.

DeVaul, R. A., & Faillace, L. A. (1978). Persistent pain and illness insistence. *American Journal of Surgery, 135*, 828–833.

Dielman, T. E., Leech, S. L., Becker, M. H., Rosenstock, I. M., & Horvath, W. J. (1980). Dimensions of children's health beliefs. Health Education Quarterly, *7*, 219–238.

Dielman, T. E., Leech, S., Becker, M. H., Rosenstock, I. M., Horvath, W. J., & Radius, S. M. (1982). Parental and child health beliefs and behavior. *Health Education Quarterly, 9*, 156–173.

Dimson, S. B. (1971). Transit time related to clinical findings in children with recurrent abdominal pain. *Pediatrics, 47*, 666–674.

Dunger, D. B., Pritchard, J., Hensman, S., Leonard, J. V., Lask, B., & Wolff, O. H. (1986). The investigation of atypical psychosomatic illness. *Clinical Pediatrics, 25*, 341–344.

Dunn-Geier, B. J., McGrath, P. J., Rourke, B. P., Latter, J., & D'Astous, J. (1986). Adolescent chronic pain—The ability to cope. *Pain, 26*, 23–32.

Ernst, A. R., Routh, D. K., & Harper, D. C. (1984). Abdominal pain in children and symptoms of somatization disorder. *Journal of Pediatric Psychology, 9*, 77–86.

Farrell, M. K. (1984). Abdominal pain. *Pediatrics, 74* (Suppl.), 955–957.

Faull, C., & Nicol, A. R. (1986). Abdominal pain in six-year-olds: An epidemiological study on a new town. *Journal of Child Psychology & Psychiatry, 27*, 251–260.

Feuerstein, M., Barr, R. G., Francouer, T. E., Houle, M., & Rafman, S. (1982). Potential biobehavioral mechanisms of recurrent abdominal pain in children. *Pain, 13*, 287–298.

Friedman, R. (1972). Some characteristics of children with "psychogenic" pain. *Clinical Pediatrics, 11,* 331–333.

Galler, J. R., Neustein, S., & Walker, W. A. (1980). Clinical aspects of recurrent abdominal pain in children. *Advances in Pediatrics, 27,* 31–53.

Gochman, D. S., & Saucier, J. F. (1982). Perceived vulnerability in children and adolescents. *Health Education Quarterly, 9,* 142–155.

Green, M. (1967). Psychogenic recurrent abdominal pain. *Pediatrics, 40,* 84–89.

Green, M. (1986). Developmental psychobiologic implications for pediatrics. In N. Krasnegor, J. Arasteh, & M. Cataldo (Eds.), *Child health behavior: A behavioral pediatrics perspective.* New York: Wiley.

Greene, J. W., Walker, L. S., Hickson, G., & Thompson, J. (1985). Stressful life events and somatic complaints in adolescents. *Pediatrics, 75,* 19–22.

Heinild, S. V., Malver, E., Roelsgaard, G., & Worning, B. (1959). A psychosomatic approach to recurrent abdominal pain in childhood. *Acta Paediatrica, 48,* 361–370.

Hodges, K., Kline, J., Barbero, G., & Flanery, R. (1984). Life events in families of children with recurrent abdominal pain. *Journal of Psychosomatic Research, 28,* 185–188.

Hodges, K., Kline, J. J., Barbero, G., & Flanery, R. (1985). Depressive symptoms in children with recurrent abdominal pain and in their families. *Journal of Pediatrics, 107,* 622–626.

Hughes, M., & Zimin, R. (1978). Children with psychogenic abdominal pain and their families. *Clinical Pediatrics, 17,* 569–573.

International Association for the Study of Pain Committee on Taxonomy (1986). Classification of chronic pain. *Pain, 24* (Suppl. #3).

Jackson, D. D., & Yalom, I. (1966). Family research on the problem of ulcerative colitis. *Archives of General Psychiatry, 15,* 410–418.

Janz, N. K., & Becker, M. H. (1984). The Health Belief Model: A decade later. *Health Education Quarterly, 11,* 1–48.

Jay, S. (1985). Pain in children: An overview of psychological assessment and intervention. In A. Zeiner, D. Bendell, & C. Walker (Eds.), *Health psychology: Treatment and research issues.* New York: Plenum.

Joyce, P. R., & Walsh, J. W. B. (1980). A family with abdominal pain. *New Zealand Medical Journal, 92,* 278–279.

Karoly, P. (1982). Developmental pediatrics: A process oriented approach to the analysis of health competence. In P. Karoly, J. Steffen, & D. O'Grady (Eds.), *Child health psychology: Concepts and issues.* New York: Pergamon.

Lambert, J. P. (1941). Psychiatric observations on children with abdominal pain. *American Journal of Psychiatry, 69,* 451–454.

Latimer, P. (1983a). Irritable bowel syndrome. *Psychosomatics, 24,* 205–217.

Latimer, P. (1983b). *Functional gastrointestinal disorders: A behavioral medicine approach.* New York: Springer.

Lavigne, J. V., Schulein, M. J., & Hahn, Y. S. (1986a). Psychological aspects of painful medical conditions in children I: Developmental aspects and assessment. *Pain, 27,* 147–169.

Lavigne, J. V., Schulein, M. J., & Hahn, Y. S. (1986b). Psychological aspects of painful medical conditions in children: II. Personality factors, family characteristics, and treatment. *Pain, 27,* 147–169.

Lebenthal, E. (1980). Recurrent abdominal pain in childhood. *American Journal of Diseases in Childhood, 134,* 347–348.

Lebenthal, E., Rossi, T. M., Nord, K. S., & Branski, D. (1981). Recurrent abdominal pain and lactose absorption in children. *Pediatrics, 67,* 828–832.

Lennard-Jones, J. E. (1983). Functional gastrointestinal disorders. *New England Journal of Medicine, 308,* 431.

Levine, M. D., & Rappaport, L. A. (1984). Recurrent abdominal pain in school children: The loneliness of the long distance physician. *Pediatric Clinics of North America, 31,* 969–990.

Liebman, W. M. (1978). Recurrent abdominal pain in children. *Clinical Pediatrics, 17,* 149–153.

Masek, B. J., Russo, D., & Varni, J. W. (1984). Behavioral approaches to the management of chronic pain in children. *Pediatric Clinics of North America, 31,* 1112–1130.

McGrath, P. J. (1983). Psychological aspects of recurrent abdominal pain. *Canadian Family Physician, 29,* 1655–1659.

McGrath, P. J., & Feldman, W. (1986). Clinical approach to recurrent abdominal pain in children. *Developmental & Behavioral Pediatrics, 7*, 56–61.

McGrath, P. J., Goodman, J. T., Firestone, P., Shipman, R., & Peters, S. (1983). Recurrent abdominal pain: A psychogenic disorder? *Archives of Disease in Childhood, 58*, 888–890.

Mechanic, D. (1983). Adolescent health and illness behavior: Review of the literature and a new hypothesis for the study of stress. *Journal of Human Stress, 9*, 4–13.

Mechanic, D. (1986). The concept of illness behavior: Culture, situation, and personal predisposition. *Psychological Medicine, 16*, 1–7.

Meyer, R. J., & Haggerty, R. J. (1962). Streptococcal infections in families. *Pediatrics, 29*, 539–547.

Neuhauser, C., Amsterdam, B., Hines, P., & Steward, M. (1978). Children's concepts of healing: Cognitive development and locus of control factors. *American Journal of Orthopsychiatry, 48*, 335–341.

Olson, R., Zimmerman, J., & Reyes de la Rocha, S. (1985). Medical adherence in pediatric populations. In A. Zeiner, D. Bendell, & C. Walker (Eds.), *Health psychology: Treatment and research issues*. New York: Plenum.

Oster, J. (1972). Recurrent abdominal pain, headache, and limb pains in children and adolescents. *Pediatrics, 50*, 429–436.

Painful young bellies. (1978). *British Medical Journal, 1*, 1090–1091.

Papatheophilou, R., Jeavons, M. P., & Disney, M. E. (1972). Recurrent abdominal pain: A clinical and electroencephalographic study. *Developmental Medicine & Child Neurology, 14*, 31–44.

Payne, B., & Norfleet, M. A. (1986). Chronic pain and the family: A review. *Pain, 26*, 1–22.

Pringle, M. L. K., Butler, M. R., & Davie, R. (1966). *11,000 7 year olds: First report of the National Child Development Study*. London: Longmans.

Raymer, D., Weininger, O., & Hamilton, J. R. (1984). Psychological problems in children with abdominal pain. *Lancet*, February 25, pp. 439–440.

Routh, D. K., & Ernst, A. (1984). Somatization disorder in relatives of children and adolescents with functional abdominal pain. *Journal of Pediatric Psychology, 9*, 427–437.

Rowat, K. M. (1985). Assessing the "chronic pain family." *International Journal of Family Therapy, 7*, 284–296.

Roy, R. (1985). Family treatment for chronic pain: State of the art. *International Journal of Family Therapy, 7*, 297–309.

Russo, D. C. (1986). Chronicity and normalcy as the psychological basis for research and treatment in chronic disease in children. In N. Krasnegor, J. Arasteh, & M. Cataldo (Eds.), *Child health behavior: A behavioral pediatrics perspective*. New York: Wiley.

Sammons, M. T., & Karoly, P. (1987). Psychosocial variables in irritable bowel syndrome: A review and proposal. *Clinical Psychology Review, 7*, 187–204.

Sarfeh, J. (1976). Abdominal pain of unknown etiology. *American Journal of Surgery, 132*, 22–25.

Schmitt, B. D. (1971). School phobia: The great imitator. *Pediatrics, 48*, 433–441.

Sholevar, G. P. (1982). The role of the family in psychosomatic disorders. In R. Gallon (Ed.), *The psychosomatic approach to illness*. New York: Elsevier.

Singh, M. V., Gupta, S., & Argrawal, H. C. (1972). Sociopsychological basis of abdominal pain in children. *Indian Journal of Pediatrics, 39*, 33–36.

Stark, T., & Blum, R. (1986). Psychosomatic illness in childhood and adolescence: Clinical considerations. *Clinical Pediatrics, 25*, 549–554.

Stickler, G. B., & Murphy, D. B. (1979). Recurrent abdominal pain. *American Journal of Diseases of the Child, 133*, 486–489.

Stone, R. T., & Barbero, G. (1970). Recurrent abdominal pain in childhood. *Pediatrics, 45*, 732–738.

Thompson, K. L., & Varni, J. W. (1986). A developmental cognitive–biobehavioral approach to pediatric pain assessment. *Pain, 25*, 283–296.

Turk, D. C., Rudy, T. E., & Flor, H. (1985). Why a family perspective for pain? *International Journal of Family Therapy, 7*, 223–234.

Varni, J. W. (1983a). Children's cognitive development, conceptualizations of illness and health beliefs.

In J. W. Varni (Ed.), *Clinical behavioral pediatrics: A multidisciplinary biobehavioral perspective*. New York: Pergamon.

Varni, J. W. (1983b). Pediatric chronic disorders: Introductory overview. In J. W. Varni (Ed.), *Clinical behavioral pediatrics: A multidisciplinary biobehavioral perspective*. New York: Pergamon.

Varni, J. W., & Thompson, K. L. (1985). The *Varni-Thompson Pediatric Pain Questionnaire*. Unpublished manuscript.

Varni, J. W., & Thompson, K. L. (1986). Biobehavioral assessment and management of pediatric pain. In N. Krasnegor, J. Arasteh, & M. Cataldo (Eds.), *Child health behavior: A behavioral pediatrics perspective*. New York: Wiley.

Violon, A. (1985). Family etiology of chronic pain. *International Journal of Family Therapy, 7*, 235–246.

Whitehead, W. (1986). Pediatric gastrointestinal disorders. In N. Krasnegor, J. Arasteh, & M. Cataldo (Eds.), *Child health behavior: A behavioral pediatrics perspective*. New York: Wiley.

17

The Psychological and Psychiatric Evaluation of Asthmatic Children

DAVID A. MRAZEK
MARY D. KLINNERT

This chapter reviews the current literature that addresses the interaction of psychological stressors and asthmatic illness as a framework for understanding the psychological assessment of the asthmatic child. The medical assessment procedures that should accompany the psychological evaluation will also be reviewed, with an emphasis on the value in integrating these two efforts. This will be followed by a section on more formal psychological assessment procedures as well as a discussion of the psychotropic actions of antiasthmatic medications and a consideration of the use of psychopharmacological agents with asthmatic children. Finally, cases will be presented that illustrate the advantage of a multidisciplinary team approach for the evaluation of emotionally disturbed children with severe asthma.

LITERATURE REVIEW

Despite a long tradition of theoretical and empirical work, the incidence of psychological disturbance in asthmatic children has been difficult to determine.

Epidemiological studies have shown that, when considering an entire sample of children with a range of severity of illness, the incidence of behavioral and emotional problems is similar to or only slightly higher than that for other children (Graham, Rutter, Yule, & Pless, 1967; McNichol, Williams, Allan, & McAndrew, 1973). McNichol and colleagues found that those asthmatics who showed behavioral disturbances suffered from severe asthma and suggested that failure to consider severity might account for mixed reports on the incidence of problems in this population. Norrish, Tooley, and Godfrey (1977) addressed this question directly and found no relationship between asthma severity as defined by medication requirement and the presence of psychological problems, but they did find an association with medical utilization that in other studies has been used as a measure of severity of the disease. Mrazek, Anderson, and Strunk (1985) found a high incidence of emotional and behavioral problems within a group of severely asthmatic preschoolers when compared to a control group of nonasthmatic children. This high incidence was in part felt to be related to the uniformly severe nature of the asthma, which required both high levels of medication and multiple hospitalizations.

Variations in the estimation of the incidence of psychopathology in asthmatics and the role of severity in its genesis are in part a reflection of the evolution of new paradigms or models for the conceptualization of the relationship between asthma and emotional factors. Stereotypes of perfectionistic, internalizing children, overdependent on their overprotective mothers, have not held up under scrutiny (Gauthier et al., 1977). Similarly, the concept of maternal rejection, which at one point was put forward as universal (Miller & Baruch, 1948), has been considerably modified and found in only a minority of families (Cernelc, Skuber, & Kos, 1968). The early view that psychological issues led to asthma has been replaced largely by the perspective that asthma is a medical problem, the occurrence of which causes psychological problems for sufferers (Siegel & Rachelefsky, 1985). Yet both clinical experience and a small but consistent scientific literature have continued to support the contributory role of emotional reactions in asthmatic episodes (Cohen & Lask, 1983). Thus there exists a continued recognition of a complex relationship between childhood asthma and psychological problems. The question of directionality of effects, whether emotional problems exacerbate asthma or whether the presence of asthma leads to emotional problems, is difficult to demonstrate, in part because the mechanism is probably reciprocal.

The relationship between emotional problems and asthma has been looked at in a variety of ways. Steinhausen, Schindler, and Stephan (1983) examined correlates of psychopathology in two groups of chronically ill children, asthmatics and cystic fibrosis patients, and in a group of psychiatrically disturbed children. The children with cystic fibrosis showed a high relationship between the severity of psychological problems and the frequency of disease-related events. In contrast, the asthmatics were similar to the psychiatric population in that the severity of psychopathology was related to factors such as social problems, parents' marital problems, disturbed parenting, and fathers' individual psychopathology. These data can be interpreted to mean that, for the CF children, psychological problems seem to result from having the disease. The asthmatics, in contrast, are similar to other children with psychiatric disturbance in that high child psychopathology is related to increased parent problems. In a different approach, Block, Harvey, Jennings, and Simpson (1966) divided asthmatic children according to the role of allergies in their asthma and found that the group with low allergic potential was more likely to have emotional difficulties and to come from families characterized by anxiety and conflict.

It is important to distinguish severity of disease, as measured by medication requirements, from poorly controlled disease, often measured by increased medical utilization. Although these concepts have frequently been confounded, the mechanism by which asthma severity likely affects psychological adjustment is different from the composite of ways in which psychological problems and poor symptom control might interact. Norrish and colleagues (1977) found asthma severity unrelated to psychological disturbance, as noted earlier, but did find that emotional or conduct disorders were significantly more frequent among children whose asthma was poorly controlled by medication. Similarly, the occurrence of death due to asthma in children and adolescents has been found to be related to emotional and social factors, as well as to medical compliance and other aspects of illness management (Strunk, Mrazek, Fuhrmann, & LaBrecque, 1985).

It seems feasible to conclude that, while there may be only a slightly increased incidence of psychopathology in the entire asthmatic population, for asthmatic children whose illness is difficult to control, there is a higher incidence of psychological problems. These emotional problems do not result solely from the disease process, although it may be contributory. The combination of asthma and psychological problems is related to a greater likelihood that the asthma will be poorly controlled. These children may have had more severe asthma to begin with, or it may be that poorer control, which is associated with psychological problems, results in their being assessed as more severely asthmatic. In addition, the experience of having severe asthma, involving not only the impedance of normal activities but also the threat to physical integrity, provides an independent stimulus for feelings of depression or anxiety.

Given this current understanding of psychological factors and asthma, assessment of those factors in asthmatic children is both more complex and simpler than previous knowledge dictated. No longer is the task as simple as identifying internalizing children or those with rejecting mothers. The range of psychological problems in asthmatic children appears to be as broad as the range in other children with psychological difficulties. At the same time, knowledge of child development, childhood psychopathology, and family functioning can be employed, in concert with an understanding of the specific mechanisms through which a child's emotional problems can be intertwined with his or her asthma.

Understanding the role of psychological factors in a child's asthma follows the same procedure as assessment in any population of children. A child's functioning at any particular age must be understood within the context of the developmental tasks facing a child at that stage of growth. Once there is an understanding of the child's functioning, including any difficulties he or she might be having, it is possible to relate it to the specific problems involved in managing that individual's asthma. However, each child must be looked at individually to assess how emotional stressors affect airway function and how asthmatic symptoms affect emotional equilibrium.

PEDIATRIC ASSESSMENT

An understanding of the basic pathophysiologic processes associated with bronchoconstriction (i.e., narrowing of the bronchial airways) provides a framework with which to understand emotional and behavioral reactions. The simultaneous assessment of both physical and psychological parameters of the illness creates the possibility that the teams will guide each other's assessment. A simple set of illustrations can clarify this principle. If the pediatric team learns, as a result of the initial portion of the psychological workup, that the child is intentionally missing steroid doses in order to maintain a more slender appearance, such information is likely to alter the course of the medical workup dramatically. Similarly, if the pediatrician communicates to the psychosocial team evaluating the family that the child has had two nearly lethal episodes, this will affect how the level of anxiety and care-seeking behaviors of the family are interpreted. More extensive discussions of the medical features of the assessment of asthma are available (Talavera & Alexander, 1986). Only the basic components of the pediatric evaluation that have more direct psychological implications will be discussed here.

Differential Diagnosis

The first step in the evaluation process is firmly to establish the correct diagnosis. This is particularly true in cases in which a condition that is treatable is incorrectly labeled as a chronic problem. In young children, aspiration of a small foreign object would fall into this category, while in older patients, dysfunction of the vocal cords is critical to exclude as a cause of wheezing that can mimic asthma (Christopher et al., 1983). While this is primarily the domain of the pediatrician, psychological parameters are important to consider. One of these is the degree of anxiety associated with the process of establishing a diagnosis. A second is dealing with the initial effects of a misdiagnosis. It is particularly difficult to help families respond adaptively to the consequence of a misdiagnosis that has resulted in unneeded medical treatment. Clearly, this is a sensitive problem that must be dealt with openly and with the child's best interests kept squarely in focus.

Historical Data

In order to understand the potential psychological implications of asthma, it is critical to have an appreciation of what the illness experience of the patient has been. The medical history includes much data that are of importance. Basic characteristics of the course of the asthma including onset, frequency of attacks, and duration of hospitalizations give a perspective on how much the illness has interfered with normal development. A review of the precipitants that trigger an attack provides an early indication of the degree to which emotional factors contribute to the illness as well as how much of the exposure to known triggers is within the control of the child and family. Additionally, patterns of avoidance of perceived triggers may have had unfortunate emotional sequelae, if the child has been consequently unable to establish normal peer relationships. The degree to which exercise has played a role in aggravating episodes of asthma may also explain delays in the child's motor development and sense of self-confidence.

Genetic considerations are important and often missed. If the parents have asthma, their level of concern and personal interpretation of the symptoms of the illness may well affect their behavior in regard to their child's disease. Furthermore, on having one asthmatic child, they may feel the need to consider methods for decreasing the potential risk for subsequent children, and they may have a wide variety of emotional reactions regarding their own behavior that they believe may have put their asthmatic child at increased risk. A classic example of this phenomenon is the asthmatic mother who, for pragmatic reasons, has made the entirely appropriate decision not to breast-feed the child despite her allergist's suggesting to her that breast-feeding might have a protective effect for the baby. Independent of the strength of the evidence that breast-feeding is an effective method for preventing the onset of symptoms, this woman may be at some increased risk for feelings of guilt and self-blame. Potentially stressful circumstances are apparent from a review of the medical history, but would not be a standard component of the preliminary psychological history.

Pulmonary Function Testing

Measurement of the parameters of breathing is an important component of both the diagnosis and the treatment of asthmatic children. While a large number of different types of measurements are possible, in practice a relatively small number are employed.

The easiest measurements to grasp conceptually are those of the volume of the respiratory system. For example, *tidal volume* is simply the amount of air contained in the normal breath of an individual. In contrast, *vital capacity* is the volume of air that can be exhaled using maximal effort and is more reflective of lung pathology. However, volume measures alone are of only limited value in the assessment of asthma, as it is a functional disorder resulting primarily from the narrowing of the airways. Based on this knowledge, measurement of the volume of air that can be forced through the narrowed airways in a fixed period of time becomes more relevant. An example of this type of measurement is the *forced expiratory volume* expelled in one second (FEV 1 second) which would be decreased during bronchoconstriction. The ratio of the FEV 1 second to the forced vital capacity (FVC) yields a composite measure that has been used as one index of airflow obstruction and referred to as FEV_1 percent.

The flow of air has been measured using a number of creative formulas to highlight specific aspects of breathing. In each case, the basic measure is volume per time. The *peak expiratory flow rate* (PEFR) occurs at the beginning of the expiration and is highly dependent on the cooperation of the subject to make a maximal effort. In contrast, the flow rate achieved in the mid-stage of exhalation is less likely to be affected by problems in optimum compliance. This measurement begins after 25 percent of the volume has been exhaled and ends after 75 percent of the volume has been exhaled. The primary advantage of peak flow rates is that they can be determined frequently using inexpensive hand-held meters, thus providing an easily obtained objective measure of flow in cooperative patients.

By studying the inhalation of the patients in addition to the exhalation, more subtle airway obstruction can be documented. Dynamic changes in the caliber of the airways vary so that at maximal expiration, the airways are contracting slightly, while at maximal inspiration they are expanding. If both phases of respiration are plotted together, a *flow volume loop* is created that can be used to determine whether obstruction is more predominantly of the upper or lower airways.

In addition to establishing the presence of airway obstruction, pulmonary function testing is a useful tool for demonstrating the specific characteristics of the reactivity of the airways. The most straightforward method is to do a baseline measurement and then repeat the assessment after giving the patient a bronchodilator. Reversibility of airway obstruction is the hallmark of asthma and easily demonstrated using this technique. Using a similar strategy, potential bronchoconstrictive agents can be given that induce bronchoconstriction. The inhalation of increasingly large doses of methacholine to establish the concentration that induces a decrease in pulmonary function has been put forward as an objective method for identifying hyperreactivity of the airways. This is particularly useful during periods of time when the patient may be asymptomatic. Similar exposures to exercise, cold air, or specific inhaled antigens are diagnostic procedures that can be used to identify substances or conditions that may lead to asthmatic attacks. An alternative strategy for identifying possible triggers of attacks is to use skin testing with standardized antigenic substances to identify potential precipitants of asthma. The primary therapeutic response to successful identification is avoidance of the substance, but where this is not possible, desensitization through immunotherapy is an alternative strategy.

Antiasthmatic Medications

While the rationale for the use of antiasthmatic medications is straightforward, a complete mastery of the pharmacology of these substances is not necessary to complete the psychological evaluation. However, it is helpful to have an appreciation of the correlation between the use of specific medications and both the severity and the prognosis of the disease process. Children whose symptoms can be controlled with a single agent, such as theophylline or any of the beta-2 adrenergic agonists, have relatively mild asthma and are probably at less risk for emotional disturbance. In contrast, those children who require multiple medications, including cromolyn and corticosteroids, are more likely to have problems. Finally, those children who have become steroid dependent have usually suffered from the most distressing respiratory symptoms and are most at risk for the development of a number of specific medical side effects. These include shortness of stature and weight gain, which can be particularly difficult for adolescents who are normally more sensitive to issues of body image. Other specific psychotropic effects of antiasthmatic medications are discussed later in this chapter.

PSYCHOLOGICAL ASSESSMENT

Emotional Contributions to Asthma

To understand the interplay between psychological functioning and asthma, it is necessary to have a grasp of the ways in which asthma is affected by emotional factors. Like other psychological processes, these functions can rarely be directly observed, but rather must be inferred from associations between specific events and behavior within the context of what is known of a child's and his or her family's functioning. Nevertheless, certain emotional interactions occur with some regularity in asthmatic children.

Emotional Triggers. Strong emotions can trigger bronchial constriction, which is the hallmark of asthma (Cohen & Lask, 1983). The exact mechanism by which this occurs is as yet unclear, and empirical evidence is limited. However, individual case reports and clinical experience support the observations that the experiences of anger, excitement, fear, sadness, and anxiety can serve as triggers. Additionally, experimental studies have demonstrated the possibility of provoking an attack in response to emotional stimuli in selected subjects (Dekker & Groen, 1956; Masuda, Notske, & Holmes, 1966). For some children, the irregular breathing pattern associated with emotional expressions such as laughing or crying may be the actual trigger.

The relationship between the emotional expression and the emotion-eliciting events can be quite apparent. Children, their parents, or observers are often quite aware of the emotional triggers. Their reports of how the onset of the wheezing is temporally linked to the occurrence of emotional stressors can be crucial in understanding the mechanism of attacks, leading to the development of management strategies. Sometimes wheezing occurs in anticipation of an emotional event. Wheezing attacks the evening before an exciting event are well enough recognized by some parents that they arrange the announcement of news to accommodate the attack. Anxiety or excitement often appears to be related to wheezing that occurs prior to the first day of school, or in preparation for discharge after a lengthy hospital stay. Wheezing may also be set off in conjunction with an emotional expression. For example, parents of young children may be able to report the onset of wheezing at the time of a temper tantrum. Finally, emotional responses may follow the onset of wheezing related to some other trigger. For example, a child may begin to wheeze after exercising and subsequently become frightened. The panic reaction may in turn exacerbate the bronchospasm.

Ongoing Exposure to Persistent Emotional Stressors. The chronic stressful experience is conceptually different from exposure to acute emotional triggers. Emotional triggers are specific events that elicit a response, and the wheezing associated with them is often tied directly to the experience of the emotion. In contrast, persistent stressors seem to affect wheezing in a less specific manner. This type of stressor is the product of an ongoing situation that is unpleasant and potentially overwhelming. Parental conflict would present such a stressor for most children, while an adult might experience job insecurity in this way. The identification of stressors that lead to wheezing is often only accomplished restrospectively, after the onset of an attack. The role of persistent stressors was emphasized by Purcell and colleagues (1969) in his studies of children whose asthmatic symptoms rapidly remitted when they lived away from home at some distance from hypothesized family stressors.

Children differ greatly in the extent to which they perceive events as stressful to them and in how well they cope with stressors. The occurrence of stressful events, particularly if linked to family relationships, should signal the examiner to look closely at the coping strategies of the child.

Secondary Gain. The concept of secondary gain refers to the positive reinforcement that children may receive for having asthmatic symptoms. This is not a unitary process. Positive reinforcement can take different forms and is dependent on the meaning of a reinforcer for the child. Reinforcement would include receiving time and attention from parents, friends, and peers as well as avoiding unwanted experiences, such as school, difficult physical activities, or challenging social situations. The sense of being a vulnerable child can become internalized as a part of the sense of self. Consequently, interactions consistent with this view can be experienced as positive while healthier connotations can be experienced as at odds with this self-view and therefore negative.

A variety of illness behaviors can be increased by reinforcement. It is possible for a child to avoid taking medications in order to remain ill, which results in more parental caretaking. A child may ignore early signs of tightness or fail to attend to wheezing, resulting in full-blown attacks that elicit even more concern and attention. It is possible to exaggerate or simulate asthmatic symptoms in order to elicit caring responses. Subsequently, the physiological response of wheezing can become cued to environmental stimuli through the mechanism of conditioning.

The presence of secondary gain can be detected through a behavioral analysis of wheezing episodes that documents the circumstances under which wheezing is typically triggered. Key factors include the role the child takes in responding to symptoms and the nature of responses elicited from parents, siblings, peers, and teachers. The child's perception of the extent to which his or her needs are being met and the range of relationships that are supportive to him or her can be revealed through behavioral observation, interviews with the child or parents, and projective testing.

Medical Compliance. The manner in which a child participates in the management of his or her illness provides an illuminating perspective on the relationship between psychological functioning and asthma. An asthmatic child grows up with asthma. It is part of his or her self-image, in terms of both body image and self-attributes. It takes on meaning within interpersonal relationships, either as helpful or as obstructive. The experience of having asthma becomes incorporated into the development of a child's internal awareness. In the same way that other children learn to recognize that a stomachache may be due to hunger, nausea, or nervousness, asthmatic children learn the meaning of sensations associated with tightness and wheezing. Asthma subsequently becomes integrated into a child's self-help repertoire. Just as all children learn to bathe themselves, comb their hair, and dress themselves, asthmatic children learn to take their pills, sit through their respiratory treatments, and remember their exercise pretreatments. The various aspects of the asthma self-care regimen, from recognition of wheezing to follow-through with medications, can be seen as integral parts of a child's functioning. Because asthma self-care represents a range of knowledge and behaviors that are integral to general development, an appraisal of a child's ability to respond to symptoms yields important data about his or her psychological status.

Age-appropriate expectations for asthma self-care can be generated based on personal care capacities in other areas. Managing the illness typically involves: (1) taking regular medications; (2) avoiding triggers; and (3) responding appropriately to tightness or wheezing either behaviorally by slowing down or by taking medications prescribed for symptom relief. Infants and young children are dependent on their parents or other adult caretaker for administration of medications. Older children can be expected to learn to ask for their regular medications just as they initiate routine tasks such as washing hands before dinner. Parents will typically remind young children a great deal at first, and less as a routine becomes established. As children reach 9 or 10 years of age and are spending more time away from home, they can be completely responsible for one medication time each day. Adolescents should be able to manage their own regular medications with supervision and support.

A similar developmental progression occurs in the area of avoiding triggers. Young children need to be removed from cats or dogs if this leads to wheezing. In contrast, older children can be expected to cope with these circumstances (e.g., "I can't pet your cat, but I can watch from here"). By middle school age, many children are able to carry a nebulizer with them for preexercise treatments.

Coping with wheezing symptoms follows the same developmental steps. Some preschoolers may recognize when they are wheezing, but most will require vigilant adults to identify the tightness and to intervene. At this age, children can be helped to play quietly and relax by redirecting their attention or engaging them in joint activities. Medications or respiratory treatments occur at the discretion of the caretaker. By the school years, children are able to recognize their own tightness and make preliminary decisions regarding courses of action prior to being checked by a supervising adult. Adolescents can be expected not only to know when they are having tightness or wheezing, but to decide independently on appropriate action, which may include asking for help from adults or contacting their physicians.

Knowledge of age-appropriate expectations for asthma self-care allows the identification of deviations from a normal developmental progression. Resistance to learning or carrying out the tasks is frequently a diagnostic indicator of problems for the child or family in adjusting to the illness. Various diagnostic techniques may be necessary to gain a complete understanding of the nature and extent of the difficulty. A child's difficulty learning about asthma self-care may reflect a developmental delay, a learning disability, or a memory or attention problem. Other children may have difficulty focusing on their internal states as a direct result of having developed styles of coping based on denial of affect or self-states.

Poor medical self-care can also indicate a problem in the relationship between the child and parent. An oppositional child may choose the emotionally charged area of asthma medication to refuse to comply with caretakers' expectations. Alternatively, a parent may be unwilling to allow a child to take age-appropriate responsibility for his or her own care. Finally, inability to learn information, to remember medication, or to demonstrate self-care follow-through can be indicative of difficulty in accepting the disease itself. Thus denial of the reality of the severity and chronicity of the disease can be manifested in inconsistent compliance.

Emotional Interactions with Asthma

Anxiety. High levels of anxiety are common in asthmatic children. Fears and worries can be focused on the asthma or generalized to other life circumstances. At the simplest level, the experience of having difficulty breathing is frightening and may result in panic reactions. These reactions often lead to maladaptive coping, such as overuse of a medihaler rather than attempting to slow down and relax. A particularly vivid maladaptive response is hyperventilation, which directly results in increased bronchoconstriction.

Although even mild asthmatics may fear death, the fear of dying is especially prevalent in children who have had near-death experiences related to their asthma. Respiratory arrests, hypoxic seizures, and losses of consciousness represent concrete evidence to children that their asthma can overcome their bodily functions. Often children are reluctant to talk about their fears, revealing them primarily through maladaptive behaviors or by projective responses. However, some children speak openly about these worries, as exemplified in the report of a child who described keeping himself awake night after night in an effort to prevent dying by maintaining conscious control of his breathing.

In contrast to specific fears, anxiety disorders also occur in asthmatic children, and complicate their asthmatic condition. Separation anxiety develops in some asthmatic children as part of an overdependent adaptation to the illness. These children may express morbid ideation and fears of death, together with the classic inability to be separated from their parents. They can be distinguished from other overdependent, fearful asthmatic children by their worry about the well-being of the attachment figure in addition to their anxiety about their own well-being. Separation anxiety must be distinguished from school phobia based on the focus of the anxiety. For a child who is school phobic, asthma difficulties can be a convenient vehicle to avoid facing dreaded activities. On the other hand, a child who has missed a great deal of school due to illness may find it difficult to return because of having fallen behind academically or having to face questions or teasing from peers.

Generalized anxiety reactions can raise complicating issues for asthmatic children. The high arousal level of a child who is preoccupied with worries may increase the likelihood that other triggers or allergens will precipitate wheezing. At the same time, a child who is generally anxious is likely to have difficulty managing symptoms and medications in an effective manner.

Depression. The fact that a child has asthma can in itself lead to a depressive reaction. This is especially likely for a child who has severe physical problems that restrict experience. An example would be a steroid-dependent asthmatic teenage boy with osteoporosis who experiences an acute depressive reaction in response to his doctor's recommendation that he not play contact sports. Similar reactions can occur when adolescents who had clung to the hope that they would outgrow their disease find their breathing problems persist. This often occurs in response to a specific event that creates a new level of awareness of limitations and is experienced as an acute sense of loss.

In contrast are those children who develop depressive reactions as a consequence of life circumstances. Family stressors may include marital conflict, alcoholism, physical or sexual abuse, or parent depression. Such conditions may be directly harmful to children through inflicting physical or emotional injury, or indirectly harmful in that the parents' own concerns limit their availability to their children. Whatever the contributing factors, children who manifest significant depression and who also have asthma appear to be at increased risk for complications with their asthma. Emotional distress itself may be associated with increase in the severity of the disease and precipitation of wheezing. Alternatively, ongoing stresses may lower the child's threshold for bronchoconstriction in response to allergies or other triggers. The self-care required by asthmatics often deteriorates in individuals experiencing the lethargy, low motivation, and hopelessness characteristic of depression. Suicide through failure to secure treatment is an option for children who see no reason to go on living. This is particularly dangerous if there is no vigilant caretaker who is aware of the child's emotional state and can take over the administration of the medical treatment. In studying the course of children who died from asthma, depression was found to be central among a constellation of psychological and social factors that characterized this group (Strunk et al., 1985).

Conduct Problems. Asthmatic children with conduct problems can be extremely difficult to manage medically. Their poor impulse control, difficulty tolerating frustration, and tendency to break rules contribute to poor medication compliance and inconsistent responsiveness to symptoms of tightness or wheezing. Maintaining a regular intake for drugs such as theophylline is a serious problem for a conduct-disordered child. Sitting through the 15 minutes required for a nebulized breathing treatment is a great challenge for a child with low frustration tolerance. In contrast, there would be a high likelihood of overusing prn inhalers because they provide immediate relief and require no anticipation or planning ability. The poor self-esteem that is often associated with behavioral disturbance is antithetical to the positive regard for self that provides ongoing motivation for following a treatment regimen. These are the children most likely to say "Who cares, anyway?" and who subsequently jeopardize their own well-being through angry acting out against caretakers. It is probable that these children's inability to modulate their affective states contributes to disregulation in their physiological states as well, as manifested by emotional reactions triggering their wheezing.

While the individual characteristics of these children impede the effective management of their asthma, the picture is greatly compounded by the family situations from which these children often come. Inconsistency in the parents' physical or emotional presence results in poor medical supervision. Similarly, inconsistent parents are typically unable to foster in their children planning skills, capacity to delay gratification, or self-esteem. Not only are they unable to provide protection and foster healthy development and coping, but these parents' own problems, such as conflict and instability in relationships, substance abuse, and difficulties with impulse control, add to the stresses experienced by their children and contribute to the stress-induced component of wheezing. It is noteworthy that characteristics of this group of children, including family dysfunction and interpersonal conflict for both the children and the parents, were also prominent among the factors found to be related to asthma death in Strunk and colleagues' (1985) study.

Assessment Methods

An understanding of the ways in which emotional factors can affect asthmatic symptoms should guide the general assessment of the child's psychological functioning. The goal of the assessment is to be able to answer questions about: (1) the specific concerns of the parent or physician who requested the evaluation; (2) the child's general developmental progression and level of functioning within the family, at school, and with peers; and (3) the child's overall adjustment to the asthma. In regard to the last goal, the evaluator should have a clear view of several asthma-specific issues. First, emotional stressors that are contributors to wheezing exacerbations should be identified. Next, individual or family factors contributing to maladaptive asthma self-care that may result in either under- or overmedication should be determined. Specifically, the identification of dysphoric feelings or maladaptive behavior resulting from overidentification with the disease should be noted. Finally, the use of asthmatic symptoms in negotiating developmental tasks or interpersonal relationships should be explored.

Physician Referral Information. As previously discussed, the referring physician often provides data that are pertinent to the psychosocial evaluation. The physician has typically worked with the child and the child's family in an ongoing fashion and has had a chance to observe the child's behavior across time. Often the medical treatment team has observed specific symptoms, such as a short attention span or unexplained crying. Given the importance of these data as well as the physician's need to understand problems that the child and family may have with the treatment plan, mutual ongoing collaboration should be standard practice.

Parent Interview. It is sensible to interview both parents and absolutely imperative to meet with at least one of them. Such an interview provides a historical perspective, medical data, and an opportunity to assess the parents' attitudes toward the child. Additionally, information about the parents' emotional involvement in caring for the child, as well as their intellectual level, psychological insight, and overt psychopathology, is a necessary part of the evaluation.

It is helpful to begin the parental interview with a simple explanation regarding the relationship between asthma and emotions, such as: "Asthma affects how children feel about themselves, and how children feel can affect their asthma." Providing more information may not be desirable until there has been an opportunity to understand the parents' own views on the role emotions play in the course of their child's asthma. An initial exploration of concerns about the effect of the child's asthma should follow, establishing whether emotional expressions trigger asthma attacks. Defining the sequential relationship between emotional triggers and wheezing will help to clarify this issue. Many parents have an opinion regarding whether their children respond to stressors with increased asthma symptoms. However, defining a broader picture of how recent life events and difficult stressors have affected the child and family often leads to a new understanding of how specific wheezing episodes and emotional stressors are related.

Exploration of the adequacy of asthma self-care can occur with the parents alone or with the parents and child together. In either case, one can establish who has specific responsibility for ensuring accurate compliance with the medication plan. Probing questions focused on where the medication is kept, who gets the specific dosage out and at what time, and who is responsible for maintaining the supply can provide helpful information about the developmental appropriateness of the balance of responsibility between the parent and child, the organization in the home, and the availability of necessary resources.

After beginning with asthma-specific concerns, it is useful to explain that a complete picture of how the child has developed and is functioning currently will provide more information about how emotions and asthma may be interacting. Developmental histories that focus not only on normative milestones but also on the history of illnesses and the development of the asthma often reveal the genesis of current interactions around the asthma.

Within the family unit, adequacy of functioning is integrally related to the child's developmental level. For example, establishing autonomy is a central issue throughout development. Thus clarifying how negotiation of control within the family is established can give a good indication of whether the child is functioning on a developmentally appropriate level. Overvaluing a child's dependency and failing to encourage striving for personal competence are indications of difficulties within the family. A high level of conflict is another major risk factor. This may focus on simple household tasks or more dangerous disagreements about taking medications properly or avoiding allergens. Emotional availability of parents to children and general supportiveness need to be assessed, as does tension between parents.

In addition to obtaining information about within-family adjustment, it is helpful to obtain an overview of significant family milestones and events. It is not unusual for the worsening of a child's asthma to occur following a significant loss or other stressful event. While dramatic losses such as the death of a family member are obvious, less clear-cut changes such as a family move from an established neighborhood or decrease in visitation with the noncustodial parent may result in a deterioration of the child's physical status. Divorces and remarriages are almost always significant stressors for children, and often result in changes in the severity or controllability of asthma.

Parents are usually able to provide information about a child's school adjustment and how it has been affected by asthma. Little knowledge of school adjustment and discrepant views from the child's or the school's report are indicators of potential problems. Significant absence from school is a clear risk for developmental problems and should be explored. Issues regarding absenteeism should be discussed that include the family's view of what is sufficient reason to stay home from school, how that decision is made, and whether there is any reason why the child may wish to avoid going to school. For those children regularly attending school, it is helpful to inquire about how the parents and child have worked with the school to provide routine medications, exercise pretreatments that may be necessary for participation in physical education, and decide upon contingency treatment for sudden exacerbations. A parent who goes to the school every day to administer medication is doing little to encourage the child's sense of independence and competence. In contrast, the child who is sent to school with an inhaler and no help in how to deal with teachers or peers about wheezing episodes is at increased risk for developing a pattern of denial of wheezing or inhaler abuse. The parents should also be able to report on the child's academic progress. This should include their view of the child's performance level relative to his or her ability and their knowledge of the current teacher's assessment of the child's performance. If there are problems, it is important to learn how the parents understand them, whether evaluations have been recommended or completed, whether the child receives any special help, and to what extent the parents are involved in remediation strategies.

The parental interview can also be used to gain a general idea of the child's peer relationships. While the amount and quality of interactions change with normal development, an assessment of social skills should be a component of the evaluation. The parents should be able to provide information about best friends and favorite activities. In addition, the parents should be able to provide information about how the child informs his or her peers about the asthma and the nature of the responses the child receives.

Child Interview. An interview with the child is the most important component of the evaluation and must be understood within a developmental context. As pointed out by Edelbrock, Costello, Dulcan, Kalas, and Conover (1985), children between 6 and 9 are less reliable in reporting behavioral symptoms than their parents. As the children grow older, their reports increase in reliability while those of the parents decrease. Even though younger children are not the most reliable reporters of behavioral symptoms, their perception of events, affective state, defensive strategies, and coping skills can still best be assessed through direct observation.

Depending on the age of the child, the evaluator's specific techniques for eliciting information will vary. Older children and adolescents can be interviewed more directly. They are able to provide reliable reports about their own behavioral symptoms (Edelbrock et al., 1985), and their abstract reasoning skills and self-awareness allow them to talk about their feelings and attitudes. In contrast, younger children are more concrete and egocentric. Their reasoning skills are less well developed, and their reports are more related to transient events and feelings (Bierman, 1984).

As with the parent interview, the child interview should begin by establishing the reason for meeting. This may include clarifying who the evaluator is with a statement such as "I am a psychologist. That is someone who talks with children about their troubles and helps them with them." Some children will deny that they have any troubles. A helpful response can be "Your doctor told me that you have asthma, and having asthma causes trouble for a lot of children. Let's talk about whether it causes any trouble for you."

Regardless of developmental level, the child's own description of asthma is invaluable in assessing how he or she is coping with the disease. By obtaining this verbal, pictorial, or demonstrated description of what asthma means to the child, the evaluator can establish a common understanding with the patient. Frequently, serious misconceptions are identified. It is helpful to establish with children just how serious they believe their asthma to be. One child might report, "It's no big deal; I just have to take some medicine," while another whispers with wide eyes, "Sometimes I just about died!" To determine the meaning of such statements, they must be considered within the context of an objective account of the seriousness of the child's disease. When asked, children can typically report a worst incident, such as "when they put that tube down in me to help me breathe." In contrast, other children with equally serious histories may provide innocuous answers. Something is learned regardless of whether the child presents an accurate account, a minimization, or an overdramatization. Questions about what are the good parts about having asthma and what are the bad parts can be especially effective with young children who are as yet unaware of the stigma attached to secondary gain and can be quite candid about the benefits of wheezing (e.g., "I like my asthma because when I wheeze I get to stay at home with my mom").

Understanding the child's interpersonal world in a more general sense is also part of a complete evaluation. Defining the child's perspective of his or her family is basic. The child can relate who is in the family, with whom he or she spends time, what they do together, and who is available to listen to troubles. Similarly, the child should be asked about friends, favorite activities, dreams, and wishes. It is important to ask children about school, since this is the second most important domain in their lives. Children are typically candid in reporting their grades and how their performance compares to their parents' expectations.

Throughout the course of the interview, the evaluator must establish and build rapport with the child. A preliminary assessment of cognitive functioning, affective state, organization of thought processes, motor behavior, and verbal skills can be accomplished, but further testing or assessment after an initial interview is usually required.

Psychological Testing. Psychological testing can be a helpful tool for the clarification of specific questions. Projective drawings are a useful technique for establishing rapport and providing assistance to younger or less verbal children. Drawings of the self and the family are time-honored tools for exposing unspeakable feelings about one's self and one's role in the family system. Some clinicians find it useful to ask children to draw an asthmatic child and a healthy child to highlight attitudes about the disease. Such pictures can graphically illustrate a child's fears of bodily disintegration (e.g., torn, bloody lungs superimposed on an otherwise intact latency-age boy), of medical involvement and dependency (e.g., IVs in every limb), or of denial (e.g., there is no difference between children with asthma and those without it).

Sentence completion tasks are also useful as a semistructured means of directing an interview toward relevant issues. When administered in an interactive mode, the evaluator is able to observe long latencies or conflicted responses to certain stem phases. Standard sentence completion formats allow asthmatic children to respond in terms of their own issues and views of the world even though such formats do not specifically address the asthmatic condition. An example would be "When I am sick I . . . get scared." Additionally, some stems are helpful in eliciting responses about general life stresses, such as "When I see my mother and father together, I . . . I can't answer that one. I never see them together. I've never seen my dad." Other projective techniques, such as the Rorschach or thematic story tasks, may be helpful for further elucidation of personality structure, defensive patterns, or interpersonal connectedness and for gaining a better understanding of the child's underlying affect and perception of his or her role in the world.

Intellectual testing is necessary when there are questions related to cognitive functioning. A typical problem might be a child who is having difficulty learning age-appropriate asthma self-care. It is important to establish, by means of a standard intelligence test such as the Revised Wechsler Intelligence Scale for Children, the level at which the child is functioning intellectually and whether there are any specific learning difficulties or areas of deficit. Identified deficits can then be dealt with therapeutically. Since asthmatic children may have school difficulties if they have missed significant periods, an assessment of school problems should include an evaluation of intellectual abilities.

A more asthma-specific problem is the possibility of learning or performance deficits being due to medication side effects or resulting from trauma due to hypoxic episodes or seizures. It is not unusual for parents to point to increased motor activity or attention problems as resulting from theophylline medications. An assessment of attention or behavioral side effects requires that testing or behavioral observation take place both while the child is on medication and during medication-free periods, preferably in a double-blind ABAB design. If this is not possible, the child can be tested and his or her behavior and cognitive functioning described, but a correlation between medication side effects and child functioning cannot be drawn. Possible central nervous system damage secondary to hypoxic episodes should be ruled out using neuropsychological testing. Memory deficits can be assessed through a combination of current testing of memory functions, records regarding functioning prior to the hypoxic episodes, and careful historical documentation of the episode itself. Serious damage following the hypoxic episode is often associated with behavioral changes or less subtle cognitive regressions.

For adolescents some of the interviewing can be shortened or supplemented by a test battery that was originally developed for adults to assess patterns of attitudes toward asthma. The Battery of Asthma Illness Behavior (BAIB) consists of three psychometric instruments: the Minnesota Multiphasic Personality Inventory (MMPI), the Respiratory Illness Opinion Survey (RIOS), and the Asthma Symptom Checklist (ASC) (Kinsman, Dirks, & Jones, 1980). The standard MMPI scales, together with several derived scales, are used to assess the asthmatic's general functioning, with specific attention to the tendency to panic. At a more illness-specific level, the RIOS assesses attitudes toward illness and its treatment, resulting in scores on five scales reflecting, for example, optimism or attitudes toward medical staff. The ASC is used to assess subjective experiences and symptoms during an asthma attack. Patterns of scale scores on these instruments were found to relate to psychomaintenance behaviors in adult asthmatics seen at National Jewish Hospital (Kinsman et al., 1980). *Psychomaintenance* refers to maladaptive patterns of self-care in response to asthma symptoms. Such patterns can be at the denying, minimizing end of the spectrum, or at the overresponding, overinvested end where a variety of needs are met through the illness. In either case, Kinsman and colleagues have shown that patients identified as showing psychomaintenance patterns are highly likely to require hospitalization or medical care beyond what would be expected based on objective measures of their asthma severity. While the entire BAIB package has not been validated specifically for all adolescents, the standardization sample for the RIOS and ASC included adolescents age 15 and older, and separate MMPI norms are available for adolescents. Thus this instrument package provides a means of assessing for this age group the same types of issues that must by necessity be assessed in less formal ways for younger children.

PSYCHIATRIC CONSIDERATIONS

Differential diagnosis of psychiatric illness is a central part of the evaluation process. The use of a multiaxial system such as the one defined in the *Diagnostic and Statistical Manual of Mental Disorders* (APA, 1982) is particularly helpful, as it clarifies the simultaneous occurrence of specific psychiatric syndromes with the child's asthma. While a complete review of the process of establishing a differential diagnosis is beyond the scope of this discussion, it should be emphasized that this is an important aspect of the evaluation. Similarly, a complete mental status examination should be conducted if psychiatric disturbance is suspected. Rather than focus on these more basic aspects of psychiatric assessment, this review will look specifically at how medication can affect mental status.

Psychotropic Effects of Antiasthmatic Medication

Three commonly used classes of antiasthmatic medications affect children's behavior and affect. Major reactions will be reviewed. However, less common side effects may occur as well, necessitating a high degree of alertness for possible psychotropic effects of antiasthmatic medications that are introduced into a child's treatment protocol.

Theophylline. Theophylline has been reported to be associated with problems in attention span and hyperactive behavior in a small number of children with serum levels of the medication well within usually accepted therapeutic limits (Furukawa, 1984). These symptoms are quite frequently observed in children who inadvertently receive excessive doses of this drug. However, a larger number of children have nonspecific problems with this medication, which include irritability and restlessness. A quite frequent problem is disturbance of sleep patterns, which can be particularly difficult in children with affective disturbances.

In those children whose parents provide a history of persistent behavioral reactions to theophylline, the use of double-blind clinical trials with good monitoring of behavior is the preferred method of investigation. However, the substitution of an alternative antiasthmatic medication in children with relatively mild disease is an acceptable alternative.

Sympathomimetics. The use of a beta-agonist in either oral or inhaled forms can result in disturbances of mental status. Ephedrine is no longer used in children, but even the newer beta-sympathomimetics such as metaproteranol, albuterol, and terbutaline can produce symptoms in sensitive children. Key among these problems are hyperactivity, restlessness, and sleep disturbances. Tremor is a fairly frequent side effect when these medications are given at higher doses. This can be a frustrating problem for children, particularly if the tremor is misinterpreted by caretakers as a symptom of anxiety. Tricyclic antidepressants and phenothiazines that have prominent anticholinergic actions should be used with care as they interact additively with these agents to shift the balance between the sympathetic and the parasympathetic systems. The use of monoamine oxidase inhibitors is contraindicated in these patients because of the possible risk of hypertensive crisis.

Corticosteroids. A large clinical literature exists suggesting that affective symptoms may be associated with the use of corticosteroid medications. Lerner, Mrazek, and Strunk (1986), in a study of severely asthmatic children, noted that an increase in behavioral problem scores on a maternal report checklist was associated with steroid use in the previous 6 months. Affective symptoms have long been reported in the literature and include both depressive and manic episodes. Some children may become dependent on the sense of well-being sometimes associated with steroid treatment and can experience depressive features on withdrawal. Other children may become distressed as a consequence of visible side effects, such as weight gain, and impulsively discontinue their treatment. In extreme cases, psychotic ideation can be precipitated by steroid administration. While this occurs most frequently in children with previous psychiatric disturbance, it can occur in patients with no former history of disturbed thinking or affect. Fortunately, these more serious symptoms frequently resolve with the withdrawal of the drug. Given the potentially serious and pervasive psychotropic properties of steroids, mental status changes in children using these preparations should be considered in light of a possible iatrogenic etiology.

Indications for Psychotropic Medications

Independent of the pharmacologic effects of antiasthmatic medications, it is important to consider the appropriate use of psychotropic medication for underlying psychiatric disturbance. Indications for prescribing psychotropic medications become apparent with some regularity in the course of the assessment of more seriously asthmatic children. Three common conditions for which the use of psychotropic medication is indicated will be considered.

Depression. The most frequent symptom that presents in seriously asthmatic children is depressed affect. The primary criterion for referral for antidepressant treatment is severity of the depressive symptoms rather than any specific diagnostic category of affective disturbance. While the use of antidepressive medication should be considered for any pervasively depressed child, a number of specific criteria are important to consider. Primary among these is estimation of the suicidal risk for the child given the reality that severely asthmatic children have access to two lethal suicide methods. The first is an overdose of their antiasthmatic medication, while the second is deliberate noncompliance coupled with self-exposure to precipitants of severe asthma. Vegetative symptoms that include disturbances in appetite and sleep should be seen as additional phenomenological evidence indicating the appropriateness of antidepressants. A family history of depressive illness, particularly if affected family members have had a good response to pharmacological treatment, is also helpful information in considering treatment. A number of special considerations in the use of antidepressants should be weighed before instituting these medications (Mrazek, 1987). It is also important to be aware of the possibility that tricyclic antidepressants may have a direct antiasthmatic effect (Sugihara, Ishihara, & Noguchi, 1965).

Attention Deficit Disorder. In those children with persistent problems of attention, with or without symptoms of hyperactivity, stimulant therapy must be considered. A family history can identify similar pathology within first-degree relatives who may have been successfully treated. In the case of a seriously asthmatic child, the careful correlation of behavioral symptoms with the administration of antiasthmatic medications is particularly important. This can be facilitated through the use of standardized checklists that have been designed to be completed by parents and teachers that can be used to monitor behavior during either a trial to confirm the effects of an antiasthmatic medication thought to be producing behavioral side effects or a clinical trial of a stimulant medication to look for a therapeutic response.

Thought Disorder. The presence of a psychotic disturbance in thinking, whether or not it is associated with behavioral disturbance, is sufficient indication for referral for consideration of neuroleptic treatment. Family history of psychotic illness and drug response is an important consideration in this assessment, as is the nature of the psychotic ideation. In patients with bipolar illness, lithium may have a specific effect on respiratory function that can result in modification of the antiasthmatic treatment.

Borderline Personality Disorder. While children with relatively pure conduct disorders are unlikely to benefit from medication, those with transient or persistent thought disturbance should be considered for neuroleptic therapy. In this regard, adolescents with features of borderline personality disorder are a particular clinical group that is at high risk for self-destructive behavior and in whom medication may be effective. Given the impulsive and often self-destructive symptomatology of such children, a clinical trial of neuroleptics should be conducted either on an inpatient service or with very supportive and extensive outpatient support for the family.

CASE ILLUSTRATIONS

RICHARD

Richard was an 8-year-old asthmatic referred for an evaluation of depressive symptomatology and possible family dysfunction. He was the younger of two children from an intact family. His respiratory problems began at birth, but his asthma was first diagnosed at age 6. His physical condition had worsened over the past year, beginning with three hospitalizations in the month of March a year ago and leading to the use of steroids over the intervening year. Richard had been considered to have mild asthma with no history of cyanosis, losses of consciousness, or respiratory arrests.

For the past year, Richard was described as exhibiting depressive symptoms that included frequent but not daily crying, recurrent thoughts of death, sleep disturbances, low energy, and poor self-esteem. The symptoms were precipitated by the death from cancer of a middle-aged maternal aunt. Since his aunt's death, Richard had experienced a dramatic increase in fears around bedtime. Frequent nightmares often resulted in his sleeping in his parents' bed. Despite numerous school absences over the year, Richard had generally done well in school.

Additional stressors related to Richard's increased depressive symptoms involved his mother's short-term hospitalization for gynecological problems during the month after his aunt's death and his subsequent multiple hospitalizations for asthma. Following his own hospitalizations, Richard became preoccupied with the fear that he might die from his asthma. His parents disclosed that when Richard was 4, he witnessed the death of his cousin who was hit by a car. The mother reported that the entire family was upset by this death, and she could not remember how Richard coped with it because she herself was too overcome with grief.

The parental interview revealed the family to be close-knit. They had strong fundamentalist religious convictions, believed in strong discipline, and had very definitive ideas about children's behavior. The family was very focused on Richard's asthma and spent much time and energy caring for him medically. His mother appeared overprotective. She completely managed his medication and restricted him from outdoor physical activities. She had quit her job a year ago to care for Richard and had arranged for him to attend a special air-conditioned school. Richard's older brother also showed particular concern for Richard's health and stayed in to be with him.

In the child interview, Richard appeared depressed as indicated by teariness, low energy, and sad affect. His overall response to the assessment was one of great compliance and a desire to please. He made a quick attachment to the examiner and expressed the desire to see her during evening hours and on the weekend. However, he also showed evidence of anxiety during the testing, as indicated by his making frequent requests to go to the bathroom, asking for feedback about his performance, and fidgeting.

Richard expressed a number of fears related to going to sleep both at home and at the hospital. He reported being worried by nightmares about being kidnapped or physically hurt and was frightened that he might die from his asthma. Richard also expressed sadness about the fact that his mother could not stay with him overnight at the hospital. He said that this made him feel even more frightened because he could not turn to her for comfort and help. Finally, Richard communicated a great deal of sadness and ongoing worries about his aunt's and cousin's deaths. While he denied any overt suicidal ideation, he asked numerous questions such as "What really happens when someone dies?" and expressed confusion about the difference between sleep and death and between the diseases of asthma and cancer.

The interview was supplemented with an incomplete sentence task, thematic stories, and the Rorschach. Results of projective testing showed that Richard experienced a significant amount of long-standing depression and emotional distress. He showed evidence of having limited available coping resources and of tending to rely on the external world to provide structure and to meet his basic needs. Richard also tended to overestimate his capacities and to try to accomplish more than he was able. When presented with emotionally charged and ambiguous stimuli, Richard responded in a very concrete and oversimplified manner, which resulted in extremely poor reality testing at times. His affect was highly constricted, and he made consistent attempts to avoid feelings of anger and sadness in particular. Richard's primary conflict was seen as centering around his difficulty dealing with issues of closeness and separation.

Diagnostically, Richard was seen as suffering from a primary affective disorder and, secondarily, separation anxiety. The long-standing depression appeared to have been an outgrowth of the cousin's death when he was 4. His own capacity to deal with this death was negatively affected by the entire family's difficulty in managing feelings around the loss. The aunt's death, his mother's hospitalization, and his own hospitalizations then served as precipitants for a more reactive component of the depression.

The medical history suggests that Richard was predisposed to respiratory problems, and that wheezing symptoms developed within 2 years of a serious trauma and in the context of ongoing stress. The mild symptoms became more serious following the stresses of the additional loss and repeated separations. This all occurred in an overprotective family context that provided minimal encouragement for independent coping and where the mother's attempts to deal with her own grief and loss were manifested in her vigilance and protection of her vulnerable child. Thus as a latency-aged boy Richard was emotionally immature, with coping skills consisting of relying on his mother for comfort. The emotional traumas he experienced resulted in depression and anxiety as well as in unrealistic fears for his safety and a confused understanding of his asthma. He was not learning to manage his own affect, nor was he learning to manage his asthma medications and symptoms. Recommendations included: (1) individual psychotherapy to help Richard deal with his losses and improve his coping skills; (2) family therapy to promote grieving that might allow the family to let Richard be more independent while maintaining closeness; and (3) education for Richard and his family regarding the realities of asthma and age-appropriate self-care.

VERA

Vera was a 15-year-old girl whose asthma began when she was 3 months old. She missed much of the previous year of school because of persistent asthmatic attacks and had been hospitalized five times in the previous 3 months. She had been treated aggressively with theophylline, cromolyn, respiratory treatments with alupent, a ventalin inhaler, and daily steroids. Despite this aggressive protocol, she presented at the emergency room nearly every week because of frightening attacks. From this history alone, it was clear that Vera was a very severely asthmatic girl whose illness was almost completely out of control.

Vera reported a history of exacerbations of asthmatic symptoms with seasonal increased exposure to pollen. However, her skin testing to these substances was negative. Her total serum immunoglobulin E level was within normal limits, and she showed no serum eosinophilia, which suggested that she was less likely to have an atopic form of asthma. However, she did show positive skin tests to a variety of foods. From these findings, it is difficult to categorize her illness as extrinsic despite some positive findings.

While both Vera and her mother denied there was any problem with her compliance to the medication plan, an initial serum theophylline level was well below the therapeutic range when assessed on admission. Once the previously prescribed dosage of theophylline was instituted on the unit, her serum theophylline levels were found to exceed the therapeutic range, and her dosage level was subsequently decreased. Strong suspicion of inconsistent compliance to the medication protocol was subsequently corroborated by Vera, who also admitted to excessive use and emotional dependence on her ventalin inhaler.

Parental screening questionnaire scores completed by her mother were not helpful, and behavioral difficulties were minimized by both parents. ASC and RIOS results suggested that Vera used excessive denial and was specifically low in the panic–fear dimension. This finding corroborated her admittedly poor medical compliance, and suggested that this would be a critical area for therapeutic effort.

An initial family session was not particularly revealing. Father was dominant and continued strongly to deny any distress within the family. He idealized Vera and refused to acknowledge any problems related to her considerable school absence. Mother was largely silent while Vera smiled throughout the session and was perceived as quite mature. An early observation was that she was allowed by both parents to have complete control of her own treatment. Furthermore, neither parent provided even minimal supervision of her self-care despite her medical instability.

During the first week of her admission, Vera became markedly depressed and increasingly agitated. She was admitted to a pediatric intensive care unit when her serum sodium level mysteriously dropped. During her first night on this service, she became acutely delusional and suicidal, threatening to jump out of the window into a nonexistent bonfire. In reviewing the medical record, there was little documentation of risk factors that could have predicted this acute decompensation.

Subsequent to her sudden onset of suicidal ideation, a psychiatric interview revealed pervasive depressive symptoms that had been present for over a year since the death of her grandmother. Additionally, obsessive preoccupation with demonic possession and supernatural forces was elicited. The diagnosis of primary affective disorder was made, and the possibility of her having a borderline personality disorder was raised. Substance abuse was strongly considered in the differential diagnosis, but was later thought to be unlikely in light of a negative drug screen and the absence of corroborative evidence of illegal drug use. Suicidal precautions and a series of diagnostic interview sessions were initiated.

Psychological testing included cognitive assessment, which was initiated due to concerns about problems at school. Vera was found to be of normal intelligence but a few months behind her expected level on standardized tests of school performance. Projective testing confirmed clinical impressions of a persistent morbid and depressive ideation.

While only minimal concern was evoked by the results of the screening questionnaire and family session, the individual evaluation of Vera revealed more profound disturbance. In retrospectively reviewing the diagnostic process, it became evident that the referring physician had noted some disturbance within the family, but this had not been well communicated to the assessment team. Once the clinical assessment reached the point of individual evaluations, the degree of psychopathology that had been suppressed as a result of the family's pervasive denial became apparent. Subsequent family sessions were helpful in defining multiple previous areas of denied family dysfunction.

Manipulation of antiasthmatic medications did not result in improvement in Vera's mental status. A trial of amitriptyline was complicated by physical side effects and little improvement. In contrast to this essentially unsuccessful first psychotropic trial, low doses of a phenothiazine resulted in considerable improvement in her thought disorder and were accompanied by an improvement in her depressive affect as well. Of considerable interest was the finding that her asthmatic symptoms became very much more easily controlled as her mental state improved. This was most probably the result of a number of factors, but improved compliance and more modulated emotional responsivity were major contributors. During the course of an extended hospitalization, her steroid dosage was reduced by more than 50 percent, and she was able to decrease her risk for medical side effects by shifting from a daily to an every-other-day protocol. Major advances in family therapy resulted in her parents taking a more active role in her treatment. This was a particularly positive outcome as it allowed for a more optimistic prognosis for her course after discharge.

Fortunately, children with a disturbance as severe as Vera's problem are rare. However, the "atypical" nature of her presentation highlights the need for thorough assessment and the dangers of timesaving shortcuts that can miss serious psychopathology.

SUMMARY

This chapter has focused on practical considerations in the assessment of seriously asthmatic children. It should be clear that much of the evaluation is based on primary principles of more generic psychological and psychiatric assessment. However, our objective has been to demonstrate concretely how to proceed in the assessment of an asthmatic child in a manner that provides the maximum information regarding the effect of the illness on the child's and the family's ability to cope with the disease. Throughout this review it has been emphasized that this evaluation is best conducted in close interactive collaboration with the pediatric medical team that is evaluating or treating the asthmatic child.

References

American Psychiatric Association (1982). *Diagnostic and statistical manual of mental disorders* (3rd ed.). Washington, DC: Author.

Bierman, K. L. (1984). Cognitive development and clinical interviews with children. In B. Lahey & A. E. Kazdin (Eds.), *Advances in psychology*. New York: Plenum.

Block, J., Harvey, E., Jennings, P. H., & Simpson, E. (1966). Clinicians' conceptions of the asthmatogenic mother. *Archives of General Psychiatry, 15,* 610–618.

Cernelc, D., Skuber, P., & Kos, S. (1968). The medical and psychological study of children with asthma—Controlled study of allergic and psychological background of asthmatic children. *Allergie und Asthma, 14,* 33–43.

Chirstopher, K. L., Wood, R. P., Eckert, R. C., Blager, F. B., Raney, R. A., & Souhrada, J. F. (1983). Vocal-cord dysfunction presenting as asthma. *New England Journal of Medicine, 308,* 1566–1570.

Cohen, S. I., & Lask, B. (1983). Psychological factors. In J. H. Clark & S. Godfrey (Eds.), *Asthma* (2nd ed.). London: Chapman & Hall.

Dekker, E., & Groen, J. (1956). Reproducible psychogenic attacks of asthma. *Journal of Psychosomatic Research, 1,* 58–67.

Edelbrock, C., Costello, A. J., Dulcan, M. K., Kalas, R., & Conover, N. C. (1985). Age differences in the reliability of the psychiatric interview of the child. *Child Development, 56,* 265–275.

Furukawa, C. T., Shapiro, G. G., Bierman, C. W., Kraemer, M. J., Ward, D. J., & Pierson, W. E. (1984). A double-blind study comparing the effectiveness of cromolyn sodium and sustained-release theophylline in childhood asthma. *Pediatrics, 4,* 453–459.

Gauthier, Y., Fortin, C., Drapeau, P., Breton, J., Gosselin, J., Quintal, L., Weisnagel, J., Tetreault, L., & Pinard, G. (1977). The mother–child relationship and the development of autonomy and self-assertion in young (14–30 months) asthmatic children. *Journal of the American Academy of Child Psychiatry, 16,* 109–131.

Graham, P. J., Rutter, M. L., Yule, W., & Pless, I. B. (1967). Childhood asthma: A psychosomatic disorder? Some epidemiological considerations. *British Journal of Preventive and Social Medicine, 21,* 78–85.

Kinsman, R. A., Dirks, J. F., & Jones, N. F. (1980). Psychomaintenance of chronic physical illness: Clinical assessment of personal styles affecting medical management. In T. Millon, C. Green, & R. Meagher (Eds.), *Handbook of clinical health psychology*. New York: Plenum.

Lerner, J. A., Mrazek, D. A., & Strunk, R. C. (1986). Prednisone use is associated with psychiatric disturbance in asthmatic children. In *Proceedings for Papers and New Research Posters*. Thirty-third annual meeting of the American Academy of Child Psychiatry, Los Angeles.

Masuda, M., Notske, R. N., & Holmes, T. H. (1966). Catecholamine excretion and asthmatic behavior. *Journal of Psychosomatic Research, 10,* 255–262.

McNichol, K., Williams, H., Allan, J., & McAndrew, I. (1973). Spectrum of asthma in children. III. Psychological and social components. *British Medical Journal, 4,* 16–20.

Miller, H., & Baruch, D. W. (1948). Psychosomatic studies of children with allergic manifestations. I. Maternal rejection: A study of sixty-three cases. *Psychosomatic Medicine, 10,* 275–278.

Mrazek, D., Anderson, I., & Strunk, R. (1985). Disturbed emotional development of severely asthmatic preschool children. In J. Stevenson (Ed.), *Recent research in developmental psychopathology. Journal of Child Psychology and Psychiatry Book Supplement No. 4*. Oxford: Pergamon.

Mrazek, D. A. (1988). Asthma: Psychiatric considerations, evaluation, and management. In E. Middleton, C. E. Reed, & E. F. Ellis (Eds.), *Allergy: Principles and practice* (3rd ed.). St. Louis: Mosby.

Norrish, M., Tooley, M., & Godfrey, S. (1977). Clinical, physiological, and psychological study of asthmatic children attending a hospital clinic. *Archives of Disease in Childhood, 52,* 912–917.

Purcell, K., Brady, K., Chai, H., Muser, J., Molk, L., Gordon, N., & Means, J. (1969). The effect on asthma in children of experimental separation from the family. *Psychosomatic Medicine, 31,* 144–164.

Resh, M. G. (1970). Asthma of unknown origin as a psychological group. *Journal of Consulting and Clinical Psychology, 35,* 429.

Siegel, S. C., & Rachelefsky, G. S. (1985). Asthma in infants and children: Part I. *Journal of Allergy and Clinical Immunology, 76,* 1–14.

Steinhausen, H., Schindler, H., & Stephan, H. (1983). Correlates of psychopathology in sick children. An empirical model. *Journal of the American Academy of Child Psychiatry, 22,* 559–564.

Strunk, R., Mrazek, D. A., Fuhrmann, G. S. W., & LaBrecque, J. F. (1985). Physiologic and psychological characteristics associated with deaths due to asthma. *Journal of the American Medical Association, 254,* 1193–1198.

Sugihara, H., Ishihara, K., & Noguchi, H. (1965). Clinical experience with amitriptyline (tryptanol) in the treatment of bronchial asthma. *Annals of Allergy, 23,* 422–429.

Talavera, W., & Alexander, S. (1986). Asthma. In S. H. Young, J. M. Rubin, & H. R. Daman (Eds.), *Psychological aspects of allergic disorders*. New York: Praeger.

18

Assessment of Eating and Elimination Disorders

C. EUGENE WALKER
WILLIAM SHAW

ASSESSMENT OF ELIMINATION DISORDERS

Enuresis

Definition and Prevalence. According to DSM-III (American Psychiatric Association, 1980), functional enuresis is defined as: (1) repeated involuntary voiding of urine by day or at night; (2) at least two such events per month for children between the ages of 5 and 6, or at least one event per month for older children and (3) not due to a physical disorder (p. 80). Involuntary voiding of urine during the day is referred to as diurnal enuresis, while wetting the bed at night is referred to as nocturnal enuresis. DSM-III suggests 5 or 6 as the earliest age for diagnosing enuresis. This represents a reasonable compromise. Some clinicians have diagnosed enuresis in children as young as age 3, while others prefer to wait until the child is 6 or 7. The third diagnostic criterion listed in DSM-III refers to the fact that the disorder is not caused by organic factors, thus justifying the term *functional* enuresis. Many clinicians use *urinary incontinence* as the general term and reserve the term *enuresis* exclusively for cases of functional incontinence. A distinction is sometimes made between *primary* and *secondary* enuresis. The term *primary enuresis* refers to a situation in which the child has never been dry for a significant period of time, while *secondary enuresis* refers to a child who was toilet trained for a period of time but began to wet subsequent to that. Generally, a dry period of from 6 months to a year is used to distinguish between primary and secondary enuresis. However, these two types of enuretics do not appear to respond differently to treatment, so the distinction is largely an academic one (Walker, 1978).

Between 15 and 20 percent of 5- and 6-year-olds are enuretic, 5 percent of 10-year-olds, and about 2 percent of 12-, 13-, and 14-year-olds (Lovibond & Coote, 1970; Oppel, Harper, & Rider, 1968). A little more than 1 percent of adults suffer from nocturnal enuresis (Doleys, 1977). Boys are approximately twice as likely as girls to be enuretic (Pierce, 1980). Nocturnal enuresis is much more common than diurnal enuresis. Nocturnal enuresis commonly occurs alone. However, most cases of diurnal enuresis will coincide with nocturnal enuresis in the same child. Primary enuresis is much more common than secondary enuresis, especially at younger ages. The spontaneous remission rate for untreated enuresis is approximately 14 to 16 percent of the remaining cases each year from ages 5 to 19 (Forsythe & Redmond, 1974).

Etiology. There are three major sources of urinary incontinence. These are organic disorder, emotional disturbance, and learning problems. Organic disorders that may cause urinary incontinence include structural problems of the bladder or urinary tract, infections of the bladder or urinary system, central nervous system impairment such as spinal cord lesions or epilepsy, and various chronic diseases such as diabetes mellitus and diabetes insipidus. Some authors have even mentioned food allergies as a possible cause of urinary incontinence (Henderson, 1976). It is generally agreed that 90 percent or more of the cases of urinary incontinence in children are caused by other than organic factors (Pierce, 1972). These would correctly be called enuresis, which is, by definition, a functional disorder.

The idea that enuresis is linked to emotional disorder originally developed in psychoanalytic and psychodynamic theory. According to this approach, enuresis was a form of psychosomatic symptom that resulted from sexual conflicts or other neurotic problems that expressed themselves by affecting the genitourinary system. Unfortunately, while there are a few case studies, there are virtually no research data that substantiate this theory. In contrast, several studies have indicated that the vast majority of enuretic children are not neurotic or emotionally disturbed (e.g., Cullen, 1966; Tapia, Jekel, & Domke, 1960). In addition, the majority of emotionally disturbed children are not enuretic. Thus the presence of the symptom of enuresis is not synonymous with neurosis or emotional disturbance. On the other hand, there is evidence that a general increase in stress in a child's life may result in enuresis (Walker, 1978). Thus a child experiencing school problems or living in a household where divorce occurs may begin to wet the bed, having been continent prior to the stressor. This bed-wetting, however, appears to be due to the fact that stress increases the frequency of urination in all individuals. Psychological stressors also distract the child from the viligance necessary to control urination. In sum, increased stress in children may precipitate enuresis, but the presence of enuresis is not synonymous with neurosis or emotional disturbance.

The third view regarding the cause of enuresis, and the one that has the most support from research and treatment experience, is the learning or behavioral explanation (Walker, 1978). According to this approach, children wet because they have not learned sufficient control of the urination process. In infants, urination is reflexive and occurs automatically when sufficient urine has accumulated. As the child matures, he or she is called upon to control the reflexive activity of the bladder and retain urine until appropriate times to void. This process of learning is difficult for some children and the performance, once learned, may deteriorate under stress.

Assessment Prior to Treatment. Assessment of the enuretic child should be careful and thorough, including both medical and psychological factors.

Since some behavioral treatments for enuresis can be harmful if physical pathology is present, it is important that each child treated for enuresis be first seen by a physician for examination. The medical screening will evaluate the patient for obvious neurologic and urologic abnormalities as well as for infection or kidney disease. If the following signs are observed at any time during the assessment or treatment of enuresis, they *suggest organic pathology* and should be investigated by a competent physician: presence of blood in the urine; discoloration of urine; unusual odors of the urine; signs that the size and velocity of the urine stream are being interfered with; daytime dribbling; painful urination; excessively frequent urination; and burning or itching after urination.

Following the medical examination, the mental health professional will undertake a clinical interview with the child and the family. The first task of the clinical interview is to determine whether there are serious emotional or behavioral problems present. Some clinicians, noting serious psychopathology, may use enuresis as an excuse for a referral, assuming that the psychologist will note these other symptoms and deal with them. This is not a good practice, but it often occurs because it allows the person making the referral to avoid direct confrontation with the family concerning the difficulties noted. If serious pathology is present or suspected, a thorough personality evaluation may be required. Any of the standard assessment instruments for child evaluation may be used in this process (see Chapters 9 and 10, this volume).

Assuming that serious psychopathology is not present, the clinician will require information in several other areas before beginning the treatment program for enuresis (Ciminero & Doleys, 1976). For example, a complete description of the nature of the symptom must be obtained. The following questions should be asked: Is the wetting during the day, at night, or both? How many wettings per day and night? Does the child wet during every 24-hour period or only intermittently? How many times during the day and the night does the child use the bathroom for urination? Is there a great deal of urgency when the child must urinate? Is the enuresis primary or secondary? If secondary, when was the child toilet trained and when did the wetting resume? If the child stays overnight with a friend or relatives, such as grandparents, is he or she able to remain dry on those occasions? What is the child's reaction to the problem—is he or she embarrassed, concerned, and interested in overcoming the problem, oblivious to the problem, or actively resistant to attempts to do anything about it? Certain symptoms such as encopresis, somnambulism, nightmares, and persistent requests to sleep in the parents' room may occur with enuresis and should be inquired about.

Brief inquiry should be made into the developmental history of the child. Has the child been slow in acquiring other skills? Are there evidences of learning disability, poor coordination, or similar problems? Many times these are correlated with delayed toilet training and problems of enuresis.

The depth of sleep of the child should also be investigated. While research data are conflicting, bed-wetting children are often described by their parents as heavy sleepers or children who are difficult to arouse at night.

If the enuresis is of the secondary type, one should inquire into the possible stressors that are present and may be contributing to the difficulty. These may involve school problems, family problems, sexual abuse, or a host of others. This is also a good time to explore the child's relationship with parents and peers as well as his or her self-concept and the degree of anxiety or depression present.

It is wise to evaluate the degree of anger and hostility that has been generated in the parents as a result of the child's failure to achieve control. Parents often feel that the child is not trying or that the wetting is deliberately calculated to make more work for them. Parents also are often at odds, with one parent holding one view of why the wetting is occurring while the other holds a different view. Such attitudes and misperceptions must be dealt with to pave the way for successful treatment. It is often useful to ask why the parents are seeking treatment at this particular time. It may be because the relationship with the child is deteriorating as a result of failure to resolve this problem, or because they are seriously at odds and the family is being disrupted, or simply because the child wants to be able to go to summer camp. Depending on the desperateness of the situation, the treatment program may vary. This point in the interview is also a good time to ask the parents whether or not they had problems with enuresis. Enuresis is known to run in families, and the motivation of the parents to pursue treatment is influenced by what seemed to be helpful to them and the approximate age at which they became dry.

Finally, the clinician will want to explore the previous attempts of the parents to deal with the problem. Both the initial attempts at toilet training and the attempts to deal with the enuresis once it was specifically defined as a problem are of importance. In selecting a treatment, it will be necessary either to avoid methods that the parents tried without success or to explain clearly why the treatment to be employed can be expected to work this time, since it did not in the past. It is also important to discuss the preferences of the child and parent for various approaches to treatment. Sometimes parents and/or their children have read or heard about a treatment that they are convinced is the best one. This should be seriously considered, and either it should be employed as part of the program, or a clear reason should be given as to why it will not be employed. Taking time to do this will greatly improve compliance with the program employed. Morgan and Young (1975) have developed a questionnaire having to do with compliance in enuresis treatment that has been found to be useful in predicting whether the family will continue with the treatment program or not.

Planning for Treatment. The assessment generally can be completed by the mental health professional in an hour or less (unless more serious psychopathology is found), and the total process including treatment instructions should take no more than an hour to an hour and a half for the average case. It is not possible within the confines of this chapter to go into details regarding successful treatment protocols; however, these are available from several other sources (Walker, 1978; Walker, Milling, & Bonner, in press). Unfortunately, there is no research on how to choose the most successful protocol based on patient variables.

At present, it is only possible to use the information obtained in the assessment in a general manner to plan a treatment intervention (Sorotzkin, 1984). For example, if a child is severely psychotic and in a chaotic home, it would generally be regarded as much more important that these problems be dealt with and that the enuresis treatment be delayed until later. Often during treatment of the more serious problems, the enuresis will spontaneously remit. If not, specific treatment may begin when the more serious problems are under better control. A young child, without other psychopathology, who exhibits excessive frequency and urgency of urination and who has not been tried on urine retention and sphincter control exercises may be started on a program of this sort providing the parents and child are willing to comply (Kimmel & Kimmel, 1970; Walker et al., in press). The urine alarm is generally not used with children under 4 years of age. However, urine retention and sphincter control or dry bed training can be used with even very young children. Elaborate programs such as the dry bed procedure (Azrin, Thienes-Hontos, & Besalel-Azrin, 1979) may not be suitable to parents who are lacking intellectual ability, who are disorganized, disturbed, or have limited time. An older child who either has tried retention exercises or does not show signs of small functional bladder capacity may be started on a pad and bell program immediately. Procedures that require that the parent exert a great deal of control or supervision over the child are generally not accepted by adolescents, who prefer methods that they can do largely on their own.

If children or parents have a strong preference for it, hypnosis may be tried, since such methods work better when there is a strong belief in the efficacy of the procedures.

Since most of the behavioral treatments require several weeks or months for success, medication may be an appropriate treatment if immediate results are required. In general, the clinician will have to use his or her own judgment in assessing the suitability of various treatments and the practicality of employing them with a given case based on the information collected.

Assessment During and Following Treatment. Assessment is also needed to evaluate treatment progress and outcome. This may include frequency counts of both correct toileting and wetting episodes, measurement of the size of wet spots on the clothing or bed, and bladder capacity. Ideally, these assessments should be collected for 4 to 6 weeks before treatment begins. However, in most clinical settings, this is a luxury. Requiring the patient to wait that period of time before treatment results in a great deal of attrition. Thus a more practical method is to send the parents a letter asking them to keep baseline data for the days or weeks prior to their first appointment and to bring that information with them. Information for a period of weeks can retrospectively be reconstructed while the family is in the office on their first visit. This method tends to be crude and subject to error, but it is generally satisfactory for routine clinical practice. The baseline information, however collected, will be useful in assessing progress in treatment and evaluating outcome. For example, the first sign that a treatment program for nocturnal enuresis is proving successful is that the size of the spot begins to become smaller. Later there will be occasional dry nights, followed by complete continence. A delay in the wetting time at night and an increase in spontaneous awakenings are also early signs that the treatment is having an effect. While most studies have not assessed the relationship of bladder capacity to continence, it is generally believed that bladder capacity will increase during treatment. It is often helpful if the parents, with the assistance of the clinician, prepare graphs of the data that will help them see even small improvements during treatment. Doleys, Schwartz, and Ciminero (1981) have proposed a system of classifying the seriousness of enuresis (on a scale of 1 to 10 depending on the frequency and pattern of wetting) that is helpful in evaluating progress. Providing feedback to the parents and the child serves to keep them motivated to work on the program. However, if one approach does not result in success it may be necessary to conduct a brief additional assessment and try another method.

Since there is generally a high relapse rate in the treatment of enuresis, often as high as 40 percent (Doleys, 1977), it is important to inform the parents that relapse may occur and encourage them to contact the clinician for additional instructions should such be the case. Also, occasional phone calls to check on the child are worthwhile. If the parents and child are not informed about possible relapse, they may be very upset and discouraged if it does occur.

Encopresis

Definition and Prevalence. DSM-III (American Psychiatric Association, 1980) defined functional encopresis as: (1) repeated voluntary or involuntary passage of feces of normal or near-normal consistency into places not appropriate for that purpose in the individual's own sociocultural setting; (2) at least one such event a month after the age of four (3) not due to physical disorder (p. 82). In contrast to the first part of the DSM-III definition, the soiling involved in encopresis may range from a pasty stain in the underclothing to complete bowel movements. Encopresis is diagnosed and treated at age 4, in contrast to enuresis, which is not diagnosed or treated until 5 or 6, because bowel control is generally achieved earlier than bladder control. Also, untreated encopresis, if due to constipation, can result in damage to the intestine, whereas little damage or danger generally occurs with wetting. Encopresis may be diurnal or nocturnal, but is almost always diurnal. Instances of nocturnal soiling are rare but do occur. Encopresis may also be termed primary (continuous) or secondary (discontinuous). As is the case with enuresis, *primary* soiling occurs with a child who has never been continent, whereas *secondary* encopresis occurs with a child who was continent for at least 6 months and then became incontinent. An epidemiological study in Sweden (Bellman, 1966) found that 8.1 percent of 3-year-olds, 2.8 percent of 4-year-olds, and 2.2 percent of 5-year-olds soiled their clothing with fecal material. Soiling does occur in teenagers and adults, but is rare unless there is specific organic pathology present. Encopresis is four to five times more common in males than in females. Encopresis appears to be more underreported than enuresis. Psychologists who routinely inquire about soiling in their child patients are amazed at the number of cases that are reported only when information regarding this is specifically requested.

Etiology. Fecal incontinence can occur in a number of diseases; from structural abnormalities of the intestinal system and anal sphincters; and as a result of neurological dysfunction. If organic factors are present, the term *fecal incontinence* should be used rather than *encopresis*. The term *encopresis* should be reserved for cases in which there is no organic pathology sufficient to account for the symptom.

There are two major theories regarding the etiology of functional encopresis. One, as in the case of enuresis, is that the presence of encopresis indicates psychopathology, generally of a neurotic type, that results in conflicts being expressed in physical reactions in the gastrointestinal tract. The underlying conflict is sometimes thought to be related to a lack of parental love, separation anxiety, aggression toward a hostile world or the parents, fear of the loss of feces, and so forth. However, as is the case with enuresis, there are virtually no research data to support these contentions (Walker, 1978). Other psychological theories focus on excessively severe or early attempts at toilet training and the power struggle that can develop between parent and child at this time. Some clinicians and researchers have also commented on the general chaos and turmoil of some families in which children become encopretic (e.g., Anthony, 1957; Bemporad, Pfeifer, Gibbs, Cortner, & Bloom, 1971; Hoag, Norriss, Himeno, & Jacobs, 1971). However, the majority of encopretics are not emotionally disturbed and the majority of emotionally disturbed children are not encopretic. Mental health professionals often doubt this assertion, but that is because they tend to see cases that have been specifically referred for mental health treatment. If cases are selected from the general population or from the pediatrician's office, it readily becomes apparent that most encopretic children are not emotionally disturbed. Nevertheless, some forms of emotional reaction may predispose one to encopresis. Notable among these appear to be depression and family turmoil. It is possible for depression to compromise the functioning of the intestine, producing constipation that later results in soiling. In families where there is considerable turmoil the depression in the child is often further complicated by little consistent effort of the parents to toilet train the child. Either of these factors may then result in encopresis.

The behavioral explanation of the etiology of encopresis (Walker, 1978) emphasizes the failure to learn cognitive control over the bowel or a loss of this control following the development of chronic constipation. The majority (more than 90 percent) of cases of fecal soiling actually begin with the child becoming constipated (Levine, 1975). There can be a number of reasons for the development of constipation, some of which are emotional, others which are not. For example, as noted earlier, a child who is depressed may respond to that by developing constipation; however, an unfortunate choice of diet may also produce constipation. Some individuals appear to have a physical predisposition to develop constipation rather easily. Even outdoor play on hot summer days may result in mild dehydration that results in constipation. Unfortunately, constipation is often not noticed by parents because a reduction in bowel movements is not as readily observed as a wet bed. As a result, the constipation may become chronic, resulting in a severely impacted colon. Eventually the colon will become stretched and enlarged; this condition is referred to as *psychogenic megacolon*. When this condition is present, the contents of the intestine (which are liquid) proceed through the intestine to the point of the impaction, where they then form a pool and eventually trickle passively around the impacted material and leak out the anus. This results in staining of the underclothing. On occasion, large masses of the impacted material will be expelled, resulting in very large bowel movements. Presence of constipation sufficiently compromises the functioning and the control of the bowel that the child either is unable to establish cognitive control or loses cognitive control that was previously present. This theory of etiology has the largest body of support in terms of research findings and treatment success.

Walker (1978) has proposed a three-category system of classifying functional encopresis. The first and major category accounting for most of the cases is retentive encopresis based on constipation as just described. However, a smaller number of cases appear to be classifiable as a type of irritable bowel syndrome in which anxiety and stress produce mild diarrhea and incontinence. A third category proposed by Walker has to do with encopresis that is manipulative in nature. This appears to be the least frequent, though it is often commented on in the clinical literature. In this category, children delay bowel movements and initiate them at times that are calculated to manipulate their environment successfully. They may soil in order to force their parent to come to school and take them home, or at times when they are angry with their parents and wish to embarrass them, or to make a mess that must be cleaned by the mother, and so forth.

Assessment Prior to Treatment. Since there are many organic disorders that may cause encopresis, a thorough medical examination is required before behavioral treatment is attempted (Doleys, 1979). This examination will involve a careful abdominal and rectal examination by the physician. The possibility of structural abnormalities or blockages in the intestinal tract will be evaluated. Also, there will be a brief neurological evaluation performed as a part of this examination to determine the integrity of the nervous system with respect to the elimination process. The possibility that a seizure disorder is involved will be explored, and other diseases that may have adverse affects on the functioning of the gastrointestinal system will be ruled out as well. For example, the physician will attempt to rule out the presence of Hirschsprung's disease (aganglionic megacolon) which is a condition in which a band of the colon is lacking sufficient nerve innervation to propel the fecal material past it and out of the body (Nixon, 1964). As a result, the material backs up at the point where the innervation is lacking and serious impaction occurs. Very serious cases of this sort are detected shortly after birth and are corrected surgically. (The deficient section of the colon is removed and the remaining sections are reconnected.) However, minor cases may escape detection until later in the child's life.

If no organic problem is detected, behavioral intervention is the treatment of choice. When seen by a mental health professional, the encopretic child should be evaluated using a clinical interview and psychological testing as needed. Initially, there should be a general assessment of the child's emotional status. If serious emotional problems are noted, these should be evaluated using standard psychological assessment instruments. If the presence of severe problems is noted, it is generally best to treat these first. Often there is considerable pressure on the clinician to do something about the soiling problem. However, it is unwise to attempt treatment of this problem prematurely because it only increases the stress on the child and is generally not successful. However, if only minor problems are noted, it may be best to treat the encopresis immediately. Often emotional or behavioral problems are secondary to the encopretic problems and improve remarkably following successful treatment of the former.

The overall integrity of the family and the relations of the parents with each other and to the child must be assessed. In addition, the intellectual ability along with the emotional stability of the parents, their work schedule, the time available for treatment, and their willingness to follow instructions must be assessed since the success of most treatment programs will depend on strong parent cooperation. If the family is disorganized or tends to be overly aggressive with respect to the child, it may be necessary to delay the attempt at treating the encopresis until these factors can be reduced, making successful treatment possible. Even then the treatment should proceed with careful supervision so that the child is not subjected to abuse as a part of the treatment.

The attitudes of the parents toward the problem as well as previous attempts to treat the problem should be elicited and discussed. Inquiry should be made about constipation, encopresis, or other bowel problems in family members of the encopretic child. Abrahamian and Lloyd-Still (1984) found that 55 percent of the patients in their study had a positive family history for constipation. Since family members often consider the child's symptoms as more or less serious depending on their reaction to their own symptoms, information of this sort will have a strong bearing on the acceptability of a given treatment program and their likelihood to follow through on the program.

The clinical interview should include a careful exploration of the nature of the child's symptoms. For example, it is important to establish how frequently the soiling occurs; the times of day or night that the soiling occurs; and whether the soiling is primary or secondary in nature. The clinician will want to know something about the nature of the fecal material that is passed. Is there staining of the underclothing, or complete bowel movements, or both? Are the stools, when passed, unusually large in diameter for a child of the age involved? Stools larger than expected for a child of a given age suggest the presence of psychogenic megacolon. Are the stools unusually hard and difficult to pass? Is the odor particularly foul? Is the color dark? These may suggest constipation and stools that have been retained. The child should be asked whether the bowel movements are painful because hard stools are often abrasive.

Some inquiry should be made with respect to complaints about abdominal pain or gas in the child because these are frequently present with constipation. The possibility that the child is also enuretic should be explored. Abrahamian and Lloyd-Still (1984) found that 13 percent of their patients who were encopretic were also enuretic. A classic article on the characteristics of encopretic children and symptoms related to encopresis has been provided by Levine (1975). In this study he found that 31 percent of the encopretic children were also enuretic.

The possibility that the child has a bathroom or toilet phobia should be investigated (Ashkenazi, 1975; Doleys & Arnold, 1975; Gelber & Meyer, 1965; Walker & Werstlein, 1980). Various factors may produce a bona fide phobia about toileting. For example, excessively aggressive or abrasive attempts at toilet training, painful bowel movements, and small amounts of blood from passing hard stools have been known to produce toilet phobias in children.

The child's feelings about bowel functioning and privacy should be explored. Some children have been known to develop constipation followed by encopresis because they were embarrassed to ask the teacher to go to the bathroom, or because they were embarrassed to use toilets in their schools that did not have doors on the stalls, or because other children teased them about odors, and so forth.

The child's reaction to the soiling problem should be elicited. Most children are embarrassed and would like to get over the problem, but are frustrated and fearful that they will not be able to do so. The amount of discouragement and the degree of fear they have may influence compliance with the treatment program.

In young children, it is wise to inquire about whether they are able to unfasten their clothes skillfully enough to avoid soiling. In older children the clinician may want to ask the parents if the child has learned to hide underclothing that is soiled to cover up accidents. This will be important for accurate reports of progress.

Planning for Treatment. A number of very effective treatment programs have been developed for encopresis. Since these are discussed extensively elsewhere (e.g., Doleys, 1979, 1981; Walker, 1978) they will not be detailed in the present chapter. The first step in choosing a treatment plan is to determine, through the assessment process already outlined which of the three types of soiling (retentive, irritable bowel, or manipulative) is present.

If the soiling is of the manipulative type, some suitable intervention must be planned to eliminate the manipulative use of soiling and to promote better communication, cooperation, and understanding between the child and other family members. Various family therapy and behavioral therapy approaches are useful in dealing with this type of problem.

If the soiling is a result of stress that results in an irritable bowel–type syndrome, the program will generally involve symptomatic treatment by various medications that can be prescribed by a physician along with psychotherapy and stress management training by the psychologist. There is an increase in literature on stress inoculation, stress reduction, and stress management that can provide much useful information for a treatment program for this problem (Walker, 1975; Woolfolk & Lehrer, 1984).

If the problem is a result of retention and constipation, as are the large majority of the cases, there are a number of behaviorally oriented treatment programs that may be employed. Some of these are highly structured and involve administration of suppositories, enemas, and other substances by the parents. Others work primarily by reinforcing appropriate toileting and/or punishing soiling accidents. Both types of programs frequently use changes in diet to increase bulk or fiber. In general, the aggressive programs using cathartics and intensive parental involvement are necessary for more serious cases that have not yielded to other attempts at treatment. However, since the application of suppositories and enemas, as well as observing the stools, which is usually called for in these programs, may be very embarrassing and upsetting to older children (especially in their teens), these programs are sometimes not practical for older children. Thus for less severe cases of all ages and for older children who resent intrusive measures by parents, the programs selected will likely rely much more on responsibility by the patient and emphasize positive reinforcement for appropriate toileting. If a phobia has been identified as part of the problem, standard systematic desensitization techniques will be appropriate in reducing the phobia prior to training in toileting.

If, as is often the case, a great deal of hostility and power struggling has developed between the parents and child as a result of the symptom of encopresis, some parental and family counseling may be necessary to neutralize the effects of these negative interactions in order to obtain compliance with the program and for the overall better adjustment of the child.

Since most of the programs for encopresis involve fairly elaborate measures such as changes in diet, use of cathartics, establishment of habits or regularity in toileting, and so forth, a major problem in treatment has to do with compliance both by the parents and the child. The treatment approach must be geared to the expected level of motivation and compliance. Primarily, this will influence the degree and nature of supervision required by the therapist to ensure successful treatment.

Assessment During and Following Treatment. As was the case with enuresis, it is ideally wise to collect baseline data for 4 to 6 weeks before treatment begins. However, in a clinical setting this is often not practical. As a result, the parents can be informed in a letter to keep baseline data for the days or weeks prior to the time of the appointment, and the therapist can assist them in reconstructing additional baseline information from memory. This method has obvious shortcomings in terms of accuracy but is more practical and has generally been found to be adequate for clinical as opposed to research purposes.

Various types of data may be of interest to the clinician as treatment progresses. Such things as the number of soilings per day, the nature and amount of soiling each time, the size and consistency of the stools, and similar information will enable the clinician to determine whether the impaction is being removed and whether the colon is beginning to return to its normal size and function.

If dietary changes are employed, it is important to have the parents record the number of grams of fiber that have been consumed by the child each day. Textbooks on nutrition contain charts for various foods indicating the amount of fiber present. Likewise, an accurate recording of any cathartics used and the results from these is important. If the program is based on positive reinforcement for appropriate toileting, careful records should be kept of the number of occasions of toileting and the rewards earned.

The general reaction of the child to the program is important. Many children are enthusiastic at first but become discouraged and begin to sabotage the program after a period of time. These kinds of issues should be noted and can be dealt with by revisions of the program through use of more potent reinforcers, reduction of noxious aspects, and further explanation of the necessity for the components of the program.

Certainly, the ultimate criterion for success is the elimination of soiling. Careful records should be maintained of the number of soils per day. Successful treatment should result in complete elimination of all soiling and staining. It should be noted that some children are found to fail to clean themselves properly after a bowel movement and this may be mistaken for a soiling incident. If there is any suspicion that this may be occurring, use of commercial products such as Tucks may be recommended. The child can be instructed in the use of these to ensure complete cleanliness at the end of the bowel movement.

Most cases, with proper treatment, will be free of soiling at the end. However, relapses do occur. This should be discussed with the patient and his or her parents so that they will contact the clinician in such instances.

ASSESSMENT OF EATING DISORDERS

Definition and Prevalence

Children and adolescents are affected by numerous eating disorders. Because there is such a wide variety of eating disorders, several disciplines have been involved in their study and treatment. As a result, a standard classification system does not exist, and it is difficult to determine the incidence of these disorders with any degree of reliability (Palmer, Thompson, & Linscheid, 1975). The best estimate is that between 25 and 35 percent of children have recognized or reportable eating problems, and the actual incidence may be higher (Kessler, 1966; Palmer & Horn, 1978). These estimates pertain to a specific group of feeding problems most commonly found in infants, preschoolers, and occasionally in older children: mealtime tantrums; unusual food habits; refusal to eat solids or particular types of foods; multiple food dislikes; delay or difficulty in chewing, sucking, or swallowing; delay or refusal to self-feed; pica (the repeated eating of a nonnutritive substance for a period in excess of a month that is not due to a mental or physical disorder); overeating; excessively low intake of food; and rumination (repeated regurgitation without nausea or gastrointestinal illness that persists for a month, follows a period of normal functioning, and leads to weight loss or failure to achieve expected weight gain). Although occasionally found in older children, these disorders are essentially feeding problems of infancy and early childhood.

Childhood and adolescent obesity is a problem related to eating behavior that has serious health consequences. Childhood and adolescent obesity may be defined as the excessive deposition and storage of body fat. However, weight alone may underestimate obesity in the younger child or overestimate it in the teenager because of the changing fat composition of the body. Thus the literature lacks a consistently accepted operational definition for childhood and adolescent obesity, as well as agreement on the appropriate cutoffs for excess weight, especially in terms of important factors such as age, height, sex, and body structure. The incidence of childhood and adolescent obesity is, again, difficult to estimate. Two respected researchers in the field, Brownell and Stunkard, estimated the incidence to be as high as 25 percent (1978).

Anorexia nervosa and bulimia, as well as disorders featuring elements of both, also represent a range of eating disorders commonly brought to the attention of psychologists. Although it may have its onset at any age during adolescence or young adulthood, anorexia nervosa is most commonly diagnosed in the early teens. There is some evidence that younger children are now being affected as well. Bulimia, on the other hand, has its onset generally in later adolescence and may persist well into adulthood. Since these disorders may occur in patients who fall outside the usual age groups, age should not be a criterion for the diagnosis of either anorexia nervosa or bulimia.

The *Diagnostic and Statistical Manual of Mental Disorders* (APA, 1980) treats anorexia nervosa and bulimia as separate diagnostic entities. The criteria for anorexia nervosa are: "(1) an intense fear of becoming obese which does not diminish even as the patient loses weight; (2) a disturbance of body image, that is, claiming to feel fat even when emaciated; (3) weight loss of at least 25% of original body weight, or, if under 18 years of age, weight loss from original body weight plus projected weight gain expected from growth charts may be combined to make the 25%; (4) refusal to maintain body weight over a minimal normal weight for age and height; (5) no known physical illness which would account for the weight loss" (p. 69).

Bulimia, which means "ox hunger," is sometimes referred to as the sister disorder of anorexia nervosa. The DSM-III criteria for bulimia are: "(1) recurring episodes of binge eating (rapid consumption of a large amount of food in a discrete period of time, usually less than 2 hours); (2) at least three of the following: (a) consumption of high-caloric, easily ingested food during a binge; (b) inconspicuous eating during a binge; (c) termination of such eating episodes by abdominal pain, sleep, social interruption, or self-induced vomiting; (d) repeated attempts to lose weight by severely restricted diet, self-induced vomiting, or the use of cathartics or diuretics; (e) frequent weight fluctuations greater than 10 pounds due to alternating binges and fasting; (3) awareness that the eating pattern is abnormal, and the fear of not being able to stop eating voluntarily; (4) depressed mood and self-deprecating thoughts following eating binges; and (5) bulimic episodes that are not due to anorexia nervosa or any known physical disorder" (p. 70–71). Although anorexia and bulimia are considered separate diagnostic entities, it should be noted that a large subgroup of anorexic patients alternate their periods of severe dietary restriction with periods of bulimia (gorging). This may lead the patient to restrict her intake severely for several days following the binge episode or to purge through the use of self-induced vomiting or laxatives. This group of patients is thought to represent a distinct subtype of the anorexia nervosa syndrome (Garfinkel, Moldofsky, & Garner, 1977).

Good epidemiological data regarding anorexia nervosa and bulimia are lacking. In part, this results from inconsistent definitions of anorexia nervosa and bulimia in the professional literature. Furthermore, the majority of studies that have been conducted have been drawn not from the general population but, rather, from selected populations such as clinics, hospitals, and universities. These studies reflect a bias due to factors that may apply specifically to those populations such as age, educational level, and socioeconomic background. For example, Crisp, Palmer, and Lacey (1976) surveyed several schoolgirl populations at various times, and found that approximately 1 in 200 girls (1 in 100 girls above the age of 16) in independent private schools reported symptoms of anorexia nervosa. Hawkins and Clement (1980) found that 79 percent of a sample of college women and 49 percent of a sample of college men binged. However, these binges, as reported, may not constitute the full bulimic syndrome, but may represent the occurrence of a specific behavior that is part of the syndrome. The absence of other diagnostic criteria in such reports might lead to inaccurate estimates of the incidence of the full syndrome. Applying DSM-III criteria to 500 students at a university mental health clinic, Strangler and Printz (1980) found 3.8 percent of the patient sample to be bulimic. Halmi, Falk, and Schwartz (1981) surveyed 355 college students. Of this sample, 13 percent reported the major symptoms of bulimia according to DSM-III. Of those reporting such behavior, 87 percent were female. These researchers, as well as Hawkins and Clement (1980), found that as many as 10 percent of college students sampled vomit following binges. Therefore, bingeing and vomiting may be fairly common among college students, but good data regarding the incidence of bulimia are still lacking.

Many studies of the incidence of anorexia nervosa have involved the use of case registers (Jones, Fox, Babigan, & Hutton, 1980; Kendel, Hall, Hailey, & Babigan, 1973; Theander, 1970). These studies were conducted in Sweden, New York State, and Scotland, respectively. The reported incidence ranged from 0.24 per 100,000 to 1.6 per 100,000. Nylander (1971) studied dieting behavior among Swedish teenagers and the extent to which they reported feeling fat. The results suggested that 1 in 155 Swedish teenagers in 1971 were seriously anorexic and about 10 percent were found to be moderately so.

In summary, the epidemiological data for all feeding problems and eating disorders are of limited reliability due to inconsistent definitions, vague or inconsistent descriptions of the behavioral manifestations of the disorders, or studies of selected populations. Obviously, this is an area in which a great deal of work is yet to be done.

ETIOLOGY

The etiology of feeding problems in infancy and childhood is multidetermined. While virtually all childhood feeding problems may be due to behavioral mismanagement, most of them may also be the result of other factors, notably neuromotor dysfunction, mechanical obstruction, or medical and genetic abnormalities. With respect to the behavioral mismanagement, Linscheid (1983) noted that the problems related directly to the food may be only a small part of the entire spectrum of the child's problem. In other words, mealtime may provide the time and place in which such things emerge as inconsistent parental discipline, lack of parental awareness regarding nutrition and good food practices, inappropriate use of food as a punishment or reward, or a number of other factors. It would be inappropriate to lay blame completely on parents since it may be quite likely that the parents are generally quite competent in this and other areas. The particular child affected may be an unusually difficult child for other reasons. The parental responses may be inappropriate for that particular child but not necessarily indicative of deficiencies on the part of the parents (see Chapter 7 for a discussion of temperament).

The theories regarding the etiology of obesity can be divided into two groups, biological and psychosocial. They are not mutually exclusive. The biological theory has enjoyed a great deal of popularity historically and many considered obesity to be a disorder of metabolism. However, Kaplan and Kaplan (1957) conducted a review of the literature and found no relationship between various metabolic factors and obesity. Fewer than 5 percent of the cases they reviewed could be attributed to glandular abnormalities. Mayer (1968) argued convincingly for the role of heredity as a causal factor in obesity. Mayer noted that hereditary factors are readily accepted as an explanation for the amounts of adipose tissue in animals, but that heredity is not accepted as an explanation for obesity in humans. Mayer further pointed out that certain hereditary diseases such as Tay-Sachs disease are characterized by excessively large accumulations of adipose tissue in certain parts of the body. He further notes that amounts and distribution of fat tend to be fairly consistent within certain third world tribes. It is Mayer's contention that no environmental explanations would suffice to explain these phenomena.

A relatively recent theory concerning obesity proposed the existence of a biologically determined set point (Nisbett, 1972). According to this theory, hereditary factors combine with early nutritional factors to determine the total number of fat cells. This number of fat cells is determined very early in life and, according to the original theory, cannot be subsequently altered. Weight gain or weight loss is achieved by increasing or decreasing the size of the cells. Therefore, according to this theory, since the number of cells remains the same, the body will attempt to maintain a consistent weight necessary to provide appropriate nutrition for all the cells.

As one may note, all the biological theories emphasize the onset of factors leading to obesity very early in life, perhaps at birth. Therefore, attempts at weight loss that manipulate only environmental factors and that cannot alter these early biological influences have virtually no chance of success according to the biological theories.

The psychosocial theories are quite varied. Kaplan and Kaplan (1957) noted that, in the psychoanalytic literature, at least 28 unconscious "meanings" of overeating were suggested. They concluded that the numerous causes reported in the literature to influence overeating probably mean that any emotional conflict may eventually lead to overeating, and that the dynamic explanations for obesity are, at best, nonspecific. Central to the dynamic theories is the belief that eating serves an anxiety-reducing function. Holland, Masling, and Copley (1970) concluded, from interview data, that obese individuals eat in response to emotional turmoil, particularly anxiety and depression, rather than in response to hunger. In another study, also conducted through interviews, Leon and Chamberlain (1973) compared eating habits of normal-weight individuals with those of obese individuals. The normal-weight respondents cited hunger as the primary stimulus for eating as opposed to the obese individuals who cited arousal states such as anger, boredom, or excitement. Although the effects of emotions on eating are uncertain, especially in view of the unreliability of interview data, there is evidence that obese individuals are more emotionally reactive than normal-weight individuals (Abramson & Wunderlich, 1972; Rodin, 1973).

Schachter (1967, 1971) proposed the external-cue hypothesis. This theory holds that food consumption of normal-weight people relates to internal, visceral factors such as gastric motility and hypoglycemia. In contrast, obese individuals are thought to be controlled by external, cognitive, and social cues such as the taste and smell of food, the time of day, the modeling influence of others eating, and so forth. A number of studies have provided support for this view (Pliner, Meyer, & Blankstein, 1974; Rodin, 1973; Ross, 1969; Schacter, Goldman, & Gordon, 1968; Schacter & Gross, 1968; Stunkard & Koch, 1964).

The precise etiology of anorexia nervosa is unclear. It is commonly thought that a variety of factors interact resulting in anorexia nervosa, but the means by which these various factors interact is unclear. The primary manifestation is the drive for thinness, which dominates the patient's life. The drive for thinness and fear of losing control over eating are two important patterns of obsessional thinking in the anorexic. The drive to be thin pushes the patient to extreme starvation and illustrates what Garner and Bemis (1982) referred to as dichotomous thinking, that is, the difficulty the anorexic encounters dealing with degrees of difference and the tendency to think only in extremes: "If I am not perfect, I am bad"; "If I am not the best in class, I am a failure"; "If I am not as skinny as possible, I am fat." The patient's fear of losing control of her (or his) eating illustrates what Bruch (1973) described as an overwhelming sense of ineffectiveness in these patients. Crisp (1970) and Selvini-Palazzoli (1974) state that the anorexic patient is aware of this basic conflict, that is, the demand to be perfect in the face of a pervasive sense of incompetence. Furthermore, they believe that the anorexic is aware that this conflict will become more severe as she grows older. This conflict is thought to be central to the psychopathology of anorexia nervosa. Crisp believes that the patient equates the complex problems of emerging psychosexual maturity with increasing physical maturation. She then becomes convinced that she can control the crises inherent in growing up by controlling her weight, and, in effect, slowing or arresting her physical maturation. Selvini-Palazzoli believes that the patient's excessive control and rigid, compulsive behavior patterns, including eating pattern, represent a rejection of those specific aspects of her femininity that are thought to be the source of potentially serious problems.

Bruch (1973) emphasizes the patient's deficits in recognizing and responding effectively to internal cues and visceral processes and believes it to be another major component in the onset of anorexia nervosa. This particular deficit is not, however, clearly noted premorbidly and may be a function of the disorder rather than a cause of it.

The current cultural emphasis on thinness is often thought to be a contributing factor in the development of anorexia nervosa in what appear to be larger numbers of patients. Yet the condition existed long before such emphasis occurred, and was also reported during times when the ideal body image was more full figured. So while some people who rely on physical, external signs of personal worth may be strongly influenced by these standards, and we know that anorexics are strongly bound to external standards to measure self-worth, the present cultural ideals do not satisfactorily explain the development of the disorder in all cases (Boskind-Lodahl, 1976; Bruch, 1973, 1978; Ryle, 1939).

The family role in the etiology of anorexia nervosa has been the object of much study over the years. In the nineteenth century, Lasegue (1873) cautioned against "an erroneous idea of the disease by confining ourselves to an examination of the patient" (p. 265). Garfinkel and Garner (1982) provide a fine summary of the family literature. They stress that the data are still very unclear in spite of all the definitive statements made recently regarding the role of the family in the etiology of anorexia nervosa and bulimia. The family may be involved in two ways. First of all, the family may represent and magnify the values and influences of the culture at large. Second, anorexia nervosa may develop or its symptoms become more elaborate due to specific patterns of behavior within the family.

Biological factors have also been investigated regarding the etiology of anorexia nervosa. Weiner (1983a, 1983b) noted that there is evidence in the literature that the hypothalamic–pituitary–adrenal axis is activated in anorexic patients, and that they are highly responsive to stimulation of adrenal glands by adrenocorticotrophic hormone. Weiner also noted evidence of the involvement of the hypothalamic–pituitary–ovarian axis, but the factors in these phenomena are unclear. However, the interaction of neurological, endocrinological, and psychological factors remains an interesting and potentially productive area of research.

The etiology of bulimia also is, according to present data, multidetermined. Psychoanalytically oriented investigators (Boskind-Lodahl, 1976; Bruch, 1973; Szyrynski, 1973) emphasized early childhood experience as leading to confusion of sex roles, inability to establish a female identity, and confusion regarding the psychosocial role of women in modern society. Either anorexia or bulimia may result, but bulimia is thought to be more likely in those patients who are less perfectionistic and more impulsive or who have been required to behave in excessively traditional feminine ways. The patient is thought to have difficulty resolving the traditional feminine role with those more traditionally masculine qualities of assertiveness and independence thought to be necessary for success in today's society.

The psychoanalytic explanations are inadequate. Generally speaking, they fail to explain bulimia in males and they do not identify the goals of therapy or assist in the application of the theoretical constructs to the process of therapy. The conflicts noted may well be present, but the psychoanalytic explanations fail to elucidate how these conflicts lead to the symptoms seen in bulimia.

Cognitive–behavioral theories have also been proposed. Cognitive–behavioral orientation examines the antecedent variables that serve as cues to elicit the conditioned physical and emotional responses. These responses, in turn, serve as cues to perpetuate the cycle. Prolonged dieting, feelings of deprivation, limited coping skills, anxiety, stress, depression, and guilt have all been identified as cues for binges. Theoretically, the binge distracts the patient from these unpleasant antecedents and is, therefore, negatively reinforced. However, the overeating perpetuates thoughts of self-reproach, feelings of guilt, and panic regarding eating and weight gain. Vomiting relieves these negative emotions and is also negatively reinforced. However, the vomiting itself leads to guilt, depression, self-criticism, and disgust with one's behavior and lack of discipline. Excessive steps may then be taken to control oneself such as strict dieting, excessively rigid resolutions, or self-denial, which serve as cues to binge, thus perpetuating the cycle.

The cognitive–behavioral explanations seem to be supported by clinical experiences and can be more easily adapted to a treatment program. These theories must, however, be expanded to include the developmental aspects of bulimia. In addition, the process by which the panic and conflict experienced by these patients grow to such overwhelming proportions must be more fully defined.

There have been attempts to link bulimia to neurological deficits, but these attempts lack any substantial research support at this time. An avenue of research that does seem to warrant continued study is that dealing with the effect of stress on eating behavior. Several studies have noted that stress seems to have pronounced effects on the physiologic mechanisms that regulate eating behavior, leading to increases in the amount of food eaten and the speed of the response in experimental animals (Leibowitz, 1980; Lytle, 1977; Risch, Cohen, Janowsky, Kallin, & Murphy, 1980). Such explanations may also be helpful in understanding the role of stress or anxiety in the development of obesity. Therefore, there is some evidence that physiological factors warrant further investigation in the understanding of the etiology of bulimia.

In summary, the major feeding problems and eating disorders all appear to have significant psychological and physiological factors involved in their onset. Assessment must be comprehensive, employing several appropriate instruments and techniques to examine all relevant factors.

Assessment Prior to Treatment

Assessment of the young child's feeding problems must begin with an understanding of the development of normal eating patterns. For coverage of this important topic, the reader is referred to Ilg and Ames (1953) and Knobloch and Pasamanick (1974). Medical and nutritional evaluations should be part of the assessment. They should have as their purpose the identification and treatment of those medical and dietary factors that may contribute to the feeding problem or that may result from it.

The essential component of the psychological assessment of feeding problems is a behavioral analysis. Three aspects of the child's eating pattern must be analyzed: food preferences; current intake; eating-related behaviors. The food preferences and current intake may be directly observed or measured by self-report (if the child is old enough and reliable enough) or by parental report. As would be expected, the direct measures are preferable.

Several methods have been proposed and used to identify preferences. The child or parent may simply keep a record of foods eaten over a period of time. However, this method does not control for the possibility that availability of foods is limited to those selected by someone else, eliminating the chance that other foods might be preferred by the child if they were available. Another method is to have children select from foods put in front of them, progressively narrowing the selection by pairing previously chosen foods until the clear preferences are identified and the others eliminated.

Food intake can be measured most accurately by weighing the food to be eaten and then by weighing the amount left uneaten. Another method is to count the number of bites or sips that the child takes. However, as would be expected, the amount consumed in each bite or sip cannot be controlled. A third method is to measure changes in the child's weight over time. This method is also less direct than might be desirable for the most accurate measure of food intake.

Linscheid (1983) noted that the actual food consumption process may be only a small part of the child's eating problem. The behaviors that are related to eating problems fall into two categories: those behaviors that interfere with food consumption (such as tantrums, rumination, crying, etc.) and those that must be learned to allow self-feeding (use of utensils, etc.).

When assessing behaviors that interfere with food consumption, it is important clearly to define the problem behavior and to measure the frequency, intensity, and duration of the defined behavior. Often the measure must be made in relation to some other standard since, as Linscheid pointed out, a purpose of assessment is to ascertain whether a behavior is, in fact, a problem in need of modification. Therefore, a tantrum may be measured by its duration relative to the total amount of time at feeding or regurgitation of food may be measured by the amount spit up compared to the total amount eaten (Riordan, Iwata, Wohl, & Finney, 1980; Thompson, 1977; Thompson & Palmer, 1974).

When delay or refusal to self-feed is the problem, it is important to do two things in the assessment: first, define what the child should be doing, and second, determine whether the child is in a setting where the appropriate behavior could occur. The child's behavior can then be monitored and recorded, paying special attention to the presence or absence of reinforcement for the appropriate or inappropriate behaviors. Linscheid (1983) cited the need for an evaluation of the interaction between the child and feeder to determine what the effect of certain interactive patterns may be on the child's eating behavior. Unfortunately, no procedure has emerged as uniquely applicable to this measurement.

More traditional assessments may be carried out using standardized tests, projectives, questionnaires, and evaluation of play to diagnose psychopathology that may play a part in the onset and maintenance of the feeding problem. These do not, however, address the core features of the feeding problem, but such information may be very helpful in planning a comprehensive treatment program.

The assessment of childhood obesity also requires a comprehensive evaluation including a medical examination. Then the early feeding history must be assessed, including the point at which the parents began to tell the difference between cries of hunger and those of loneliness, fatigue, or discomfort. This will help identify the point at which the parents were able to respond more appropriately to the child's needs using things other than food. Second, the attitude of the parents about food, including their own attempts to control eating and weight, must be assessed. It is also important to note the extent to which the parents have typically used food as a reward or punishment for the child's behavior. Third, a child's food habits must be examined. This would include those foods that the child prefers, the extent to which food serves as the focus of social activities, and the extent to which eating serves as the response to hunger as opposed to the degree to which it serves as a response to boredom, anger, excitement, and other states of arousal. Fourth, the food purchasing and supply practices of the family should be examined to determine whether high-calorie foods are selected primarily due to a limited range of choices. Fifth, the nature and extent of the child's routine physical activity should be examined. Sixth, the child's current psychological status may provide useful information, especially any recent or continuing life events that may have an effect on the child's eating and weight. Seventh, the nature of the child's social relationships should be examined to determine the degree of support or interference by family and friends on attempts at weight control. Eighth, the family history with respect to obesity and psychopathology may provide useful information from both an environmental and a hereditary perspective. As noted previously, important psychological factors have been identified as contributing to obesity. These include anxiety, depression, personality disturbance, excessive responsiveness to external cues, and poor role models (Bruch, 1979; Schachter, 1971) and should be assessed using the appropriate techniques and instruments.

The assessment of anorexia nervosa and bulimia can be extensive due to the complexity of these disorders. Adequate assessment should always involve a complete medical and nutritional evaluation as well as a psychological evaluation. For a summary of the nutritional factors to be considered, including the physical, laboratory, and metabolic conditions often associated with anorexia nervosa, the reader is referred to Mellendick (1983). Excellent reviews of the physical and nutritional evaluations appropriate to anorexia nervosa and bulimia may be found in Shenker and Shaw (1986) and Kilbourne (1986).

From a psychological perspective, the diagnostic interview, consisting of a psychosocial history and mental status examination, is necessary as the first step in the assessment process. Throughout the evaluation, the psychologist should be aware of the patient's tendency to deceive or minimize problems. During the interview, the psychologist must attempt to link the behavioral pattern to important etiological and developmental factors that have been identified as playing a major role in the development of anorexia nervosa. These would include the following: the development of self-concept largely dependent upon weight; the patient's sense of ineffectiveness, often in spite of evidence to the contrary; the obsession with self-control through rigid dieting and exercise, and the fear of losing control if one deviates from the rigid routine; the depression frequently associated with anorexia nervosa and due in part to poor nutrition in cases of moderate to extreme starvation; the compulsive drive to be perfect, well liked, and beyond reproach in the face of nagging doubt and self-criticism.

In the assessment of bulimia, the psychologist should attempt to identify the functions served by the binge–purge cycle. The binge–purge cycle may serve one of three purposes: a means of controlling the habit of overeating; a means of reducing interpersonal stress; and a means of reducing anxiety.

In the eating habit control model, the patient thinks of herself (or himself) as a compulsive overeater, one who is unable to control her periodic binges. However, she believes that she can at least control the effect of her eating by purging, thus negating the effects of the food. Thus, the binge–purge cycle allows her to maintain a level of control over the effects of her eating, if not the eating itself.

In the interpersonal stress reduction model, the binges are triggered by stressful events that stimulate a variety of negative emotions: fear, depression, anger, and so on. The binge distracts the patient and reduces the stress, filling the void in the patient's coping strategies and assuming a general stress reduction power that is applied broadly and indiscriminately. The purge eliminates the negative effects of the binge, including guilt, self-criticism, and uncomfortable physical sensations. The driving force for these patients is the ability of the binge to reduce stress. The purge is used merely to offset the effect of the binge.

In the anxiety reduction model, the purge, usually vomiting, reduces the anxiety associated with eating even if the amount eaten is moderate. Thus the vomiting permits even binge eating since the patient often gives herself permission to eat only after she has given herself permission to vomit and has arranged her setting and schedule accordingly.

Johnson (1985) presents a comprehensive and systematic outline for conducting the initial session with anorexia nervosa and bulimia patients. Stressing the importance of the first meeting, especially the first few minutes, Johnson urges that the process be presented to the patient as a "collaborative inquiry" into her eating problem and its associated effects on her life. The inquisition-style interview, lacking in understanding and empathy from the therapist, is to be avoided. The specific areas to be investigated are well defined, comprehensive, and structured.

First, Johnson explores with the patient her weight history and body image. Then her dieting behavior is reviewed, including the reasons for dieting, the kinds of diets followed, the short- and long-term effects of the diets, and the nature and extent of reinforcement received. The degree to which successful dieting has been equated with self-esteem is very important to evaluate.

Next, Johnson examines the patient's attitude toward exercise and body measurement, including weighings, measuring of hips, stomach, thighs, and so on. The patient's general eating pattern is discussed with special attention paid to binge–purge episodes. With respect to the binge–purge cycle, the therapist seeks to understand the antecedent events, both internal and external, the time of onset, frequency, duration, methods, and effects.

As noted earlier, the high correlations between eating disorders and affective disorders require that the therapist assess the possible presence of primary affective disorder as opposed to psychological depression (Strober, Salkin, Burroughs, & Morrell, 1982). In addition to affective disorders, other types of impulse disorders must be assessed, including chemical abuse, sexual promiscuity, explosive episodes, and shoplifting.

Sexual and menstrual histories are important from a psychological as well as an endocrinological perspective. A patient may be hesitant to discuss these issues with individuals who are not physicians or nurses. Such reluctance is usually due to a failure to understand the effect of disrupted eating patterns and poor nutrition on the menstrual cycle. A brief explanation usually is sufficient to elicit the patient's cooperation.

The patient's family history is important since familial patterns of interaction, including how affect is expressed, the demands and expectations for performance and success, and the rigidity of family rules, can be a major force in the etiology of eating disorders. A family history for other psychopathology such as affective disorders and chemical abuse should be reviewed along with the family's overall medical history.

The development of anorexia nervosa or bulimia is often indicative of disruption in other areas of life. Thus Johnson (1985) advises the psychologist to explore overall life adjustment, including social, marital, educational, occupational, and leisure adjustment.

The patient's medical history may be reviewed. This may seem unnecessary if the patient has been seen by a physician or other health professional, but unless the patient will be followed at regular intervals throughout the treatment by a health professional the psychologist must be prepared to monitor such things as gastrointestinal problems, sleep disturbances, fatigue, dizziness, nausea and vomiting, symptoms of hypertension or of electrolyte imbalances, and so forth. When indicated, the psychologist much be prepared to arrange for medical consultation.

Psychological testing can be an important aid in the assessment of the patient. Certain instruments can be useful in evaluating the specifics of the eating disorder, while other instruments can be useful in assessing the associated personality factors and psychopathology. The widely divergent ways in which anorexia nervosa and bulimia have been studied and conceptualized have limited the ability of psychological testing to contribute greatly to the understanding of these disorders. Small (1984) contended that projective tests have been underutilized in furthering our understanding of anorexia nervosa, especially in light of the amount of literature identifying ego deficits as a major factor in the etiology and maintenance of anorexia. Small contended that projective tests could be extremely valuable due to their theoretical foundations and their suitability for evaluating ego function and object relations. But Small properly noted that the specific application of projective tests to anorexia nervosa and its associated symptomatology, such as disturbed body image, has not been studied from a consistent clinical or theoretical framework to yield what might be referred to as an anorexic profile. As a result, clinicians who wish to use projectives should do so with the understanding that specific pathogonomic signs or patterns indicative of anorexia nervosa are yet to be found.

Several studies do provide a basis for understanding important aspects of the anorexic personality that may be quite useful in the overall treatment planning. Strober and Goldenberg (1981) found a sample of 20 anorexic females to have deficits in ego boundaries as evidenced by excessive or highly personal elaborations of responses. They also found indications that members of their sample attempted rigidly to define ego boundaries, possibly as a defense against the frequently noted tendency of anorexics to fail at developing a clear sense of autonomy and independence. Sugarman, Quinlan, and Devenis (1982) also noted a failure by 12 anorexic subjects to maintain boundaries between the self and others as well as constriction of cognitive processes. Projectives may be useful in revealing depression, psychosis, isolation, impaired reality testing, thought disturbances, and associated indicators of borderline personality disorder (Selvini-Palazzoli, 1971; Rowland, 1970; Small,

Teagno, Madero, Gross, & Ebert, 1982). However, the validity of projectives in understanding, describing, and predicting outcome in anorexia nervosa is yet to be determined.

Standardized, empirical tests have been used in several studies with anorexic patients. These studies have found similar patterns to those found in studies employing projective techniques or clinical interviews. Wingate and Christie (1978) found anorexic subjects to have less ego strength as indicated by lower scores on the E scale of the MMPI when compared to normal controls. They also found anorexics will overestimate body size, a finding similar to that of Pierloot and Houben (1978). The latter found no relation between this overestimation of body size and patterns on the MMPI or Rorschach. It should be noted that the control groups in these two studies were different. The subjects in the Wingate and Christie study were compared to normal controls but the experimental group in the Pierloot and Houben study was compared to a sample of persons who had been diagnosed as psychoneurotic.

Pierloot, Wellens, and Houben (1975) found that a lower overall profile on the MMPI was suggestive of a better treatment outcome. This finding is not surprising in view of the fact that a lower overall profile is generally indicative of less psychopathology and better overall adjustment. In addition, these investigators found that elevation on the Schizophrenic scale seemed to be predictive of a worse prognosis. Small and colleagues (1982) found no difference in the MMPI profiles of 20 inpatient anorexics when compared to a sample of schizophrenic patients. The collective profile of the anorexic patients suggested chronic thought disorder and depression. Norman and Herzog (1983) differentiated between restricting anorexics, anorexics who binged and purged, and normal-weight bulimics using the MMPI. The anorexic who periodically binged and purged appeared to be more depressed and suffer more severe personality disorder as indicated by a higher elevation of the Pd scale. These patients also appeared to be more psychologically disturbed overall than were the other two groups. This study suggested that the differentiation between anorexic restricters and bingers has important clinical significance.

The Eysenck Personality Inventory has been used to assess the neuroticism of anorexic patients. Smart, Beaumont, and George (1976) and Garner, Garfinkel, Stancer, and Moldofsky (1976) used the EPI along with the 16 PF and Layton Obsessional Inventory in comparing anorexics to a control group. Both studies found the anorexic patients to be more introverted than the controls. But Garner and colleagues failed to find their sample to be as neurotic and obsessional as that of Smart and colleagues. Hood, Moore, and Garner (1982) used the EPI as well as a modification of Rotter's I-E Scale, the 16 PF, the Restraint Scale, the Eating Attitudes Test, the Beck Depression Inventory, and a body image measure. Seeking to assess the degree of ineffectiveness felt by anorexics, they found that the high external scores, indicative of a sense of ineffectiveness, increased with age and were not characteristic of all anorexics. An additional important finding was that the sense of ineffectiveness did not exist independently, but was correlated with high levels of suspiciousness, insecurity, tension, emotional instability, and lack of self-discipline.

Although objective measures help identify associated pathology, as noted in these and other studies, they have generally been of little use in understanding the primary diagnostic features of anorexia nervosa. For example, Rybicki and

Lepowsky (1984) compared the profiles of 21 bulimic women to those of 27 normal females on the MMPI, the FIRO-B, the Beck Depression Inventory, the Moos Family Environment Scale, BEM Sex Role Inventory, and the Conte Borderline Syndrome Index. No differences were found on the Family Environment Scale, the BEM, or the FIRO-B. On the MMPI, the bulimics had significantly higher 2-4-7 elevations indicating depression, rigid personality dysfunction, obsessive–compulsive features, and anxiety. The Beck Depression Inventory indicated a moderate to severe level of depression in bulimics compared to normals.

Thus the most commonly used projective and objective measures of personality are useful in understanding the more global personality features of patients suspected of having eating disorders as well as in diagnosing the associated psychopathology. However, these tests have failed to be of much value thus far with respect to the specific diagnostic criteria of anorexia nervosa and bulimia.

The two most common procedures for assessing the specific features of anorexia nervosa and bulimia are questionnaires and the diagnostic interview. Through the questionnaires or through the interview, a third type of measurement can be conducted, that is, behavioral analysis. In addition to conducting a behavioral analysis on the basis of the patient's recall and self-report, the therapist may choose to do a behavioral analysis *in vivo*. *In vivo* behavioral analysis is especially helpful with bulimic patients who may be able more accurately to identify and report those cognitions and feelings that serve as cues to binges and vomiting in situations closely approximating real life. However, it should be noted that comprehensive behavioral analysis of the problematic eating patterns has received virtually no attention in the professional literature. Therefore, the clinician would be hard-pressed to find readily available models to conduct such behavioral analysis, although it would appear to have a great utility with respect to the most discrete aspects of the eating disorders.

Gandour (1984) listed several questionnaires that have been used to assess bulimia and its diagnostic criteria. References for the instrument, format, the basis for item selection, scoring, validity, and reliability data as well as factor analysis results are also presented. These questionnaires have been designed to assess specific aspects of bulimia: the binge behavior, the tendency toward compulsive eating, the cognitive factors associated with dieting. Reindl and Gerstein (1984) developed a questionnaire to assess the bulimic's pattern of interpersonal relationships over time and across categories of familial and social relationships. Hsu and Lieberman (1982) designed an instrument to measure the level of social and sexual functioning of anorexic and bulimic patients. The Eating Attitudes Test (Garner & Garfinkel, 1979) measures the broad range of anorexic symptoms, not merely symptoms resulting from refusal to eat. As such, it has been reported to be an accurate means of predicting the degree to which the patient's symptom complex is consistent with the symptom complex of anorexics in general. The Eating Disorders Inventory (Garner & Olmsted, 1984) is a 64-item self-report questionnaire designed to measure eight behavioral and psychological traits commonly found in anorexic or bulimic patients: the drive for thinness; bulimia; body dissatisfaction; ineffectiveness; perfectionism; interpersonal distress; interoceptive awareness; and maturation fears.

With respect to the Eating Disorders Inventory, the authors see it as a multipurpose instrument that can be an aid when used with other information in establishing the specific diagnosis of anorexia nervosa or bulimia. Both the Eating Attitudes Test and the Eating Disorders Inventory have been designed to assess eating disorders broadly. Therefore, they are useful screening tools in assessing individual patients with a wide range of eating disorders. However, the responsible clinician must remain cognizant of the fact that the results of these tests are not, by themselves, diagnostic. They must be used only as aids and be supplemented by other diagnostic measures to establish a valid diagnosis.

A comprehensive interview is a critical part of the assessment of the eating disorders. Because the eating disorders are, as noted frequently, multidetermined, it is necessary that an interview be broad in scope and yet focus on specific aspects of the disorder when necessary. Johnson (1985) provided a standardized interview format called the Diagnostic Survey for Eating Disorders. While a structured, standardized interview would be necessary in the conduct of research on eating disorders, the clinical literature would be well served, as would the individual clinical case, by the use of standardized interviews. Such an interview would provide us with data that could be more easily compared across cases and across studies since the data would be gathered in a more consistent fashion. The use of an interview format such as that described by Johnson has considerable merit in both research and clinical work.

Bruch (1961, 1962, 1973, 1978) noted three main psychological characteristics of anorexic patients. These characteristics have provided a good general framework for understanding the overall personality structure of the anorexic patient over several years and in a variety of clinical settings. Bruch noted that the anorexic patients tend to have, first, significant distortions of their body image, a finding that is to many authorities in the field one of the critical markers in the diagnosis of anorexia nervosa. Second, Bruch noted that anorexic patients tend to have significant interoceptive disturbances, that is, a marked inability accurately to identify internal sensations such as hunger. Researchers and clinicians have been somewhat puzzled by anorexic patients' denials that they experience hunger. It has been unclear whether anorexics are unable accurately to identify the sensations of hunger, whether they are able to identify them but also able to marshal a remarkable degree of discipline to keep themselves from satisfying these sensations, or whether, in fact, they fail to experience sensations of hunger. It does appear that anorexics in more advanced stages of starvation do not experience hunger, but it remains unclear at what physiological or psychological level this failure to experience hunger occurs. The third characteristic noted by Bruch is an overwhelming and pervasive sense of ineffectiveness. These patients frequently have a very poor self-concept and little self-confidence. This particular aspect of their personality is particularly notable since many people consider them to be quite capable and competent individuals, persons whose accomplishments are often easily and objectively identified. However, many of these patients report that their standards are so high that reaching their goals is seen as minimal success since they have been expected to do so all along. Failure to reach the highest goals, even though they may enjoy a significant degree of success and accomplishment, is seen as failure. So the sense of ineffectiveness and incompetence may be due not to objective failure but rather to repeated inability to measure up to their own excessively high standards. Psychologists have developed and applied a variety of techniques to assess these characteristics, thus gathering data that allow for the measurement and quantification of very important personality dimensions found in anorexia nervosa and in certain bulimics.

A number of studies have used a technique called the moveable caliper (Reitman & Cleveland, 1964) to measure the amount of distortion of body image by anorexics. Although the differentiation of the anorexic groups from the controls was inconsistent, within the groups of anorexic subjects it was consistently noted that increased distortion was related to poor prognosis and more psychopathology (Ben-Tovim, Whitehead, & Crisp, 1979; Button, Fransella, & Slade, 1977; Casper, Halmi, Goldberg, Eckert, & Davis, 1979; Crisp & Kalucy, 1974; Goldberg, Halmi, Casper, Eckert, & Davis, 1977; Russell, Campbell, & Slade, 1975; Slade & Russell, 1973). In 1975, Askevold described a technique in which the subject imagines she is facing a mirror and marks her estimate of the width of various parts of her body, such as hips, on a long sheet of paper mounted on the wall. Results of studies using this technique show similar results to those using the moveable caliper (Pierloot & Houben, 1978; Strober, Goldenberg, Green, & Saxon, 1979; Wingate & Christie, 1978). In addition, Garner and colleagues (1976) and Garfinkel, Maldofsky, Garner, Stancer, and Coscina (1978) showed that there is a broad distribution of self-estimates of body size across patients and that the significance of distortion of body size must be determined in each individual case.

In summary, the formal psychological tests that a psychologist may choose to use in addition to the diagnostic interview will depend largely on his or her own theoretical orientation. The self-report instruments such as the Eating Attitudes Test or the Eating Disorders Inventory can be valuable measures to identify specific core features of anorexia nervosa and bulimia. Objective measures such as the MMPI or the EPI can help identify the nature and extent of associated psychopathology and, as such, can be sources of important information and treatment planning. Projective techniques have a similar utility, but, as noted by Small (1984), consistency of assessment procedures and therapeutic orientation requires that the projectives be used to assess the disturbances in which impairment of ego functioning is prominent. Since many theorists have noted ego deficiencies in both major eating disorders, the projective techniques, when used with proper attention to validity and reliability, may be important tools in assessing the associated pathology of anorexia nervosa and bulimia. Without attention to reliability and validity, however, the use of such techniques runs the risk of further clouding the diagnostic picture.

The use of measures of perceptual distortion may also be helpful in establishing the degree of distortion of body image and the prognosis for each individual case. This will permit appropriate design of therapeutic intervention.

Finally, some additional techniques have been devised to study or measure areas that have been noted to be important clinically. One of the most prominent is the study of family structure and patterns of interaction. Based on the work of Selvini-Palazzoli (1974) and Minuchin, Rosman, and Baker (1978), a variety of observational and other techniques to assess family patterns of interaction and pathology have been developed. None has shown specific application to families of anorexic or bulimic patients in terms of the core features of these disorders. However, in a recent study, Humphrey, Apple, and Kirschenbaum (1986) employed a technique called the Structural Analysis of Social Behavior (Benjamin, Foster, Giat-Roberto, & Estroff, 1983). It is an interpersonal observational system that the authors found discriminates anorexic–bulimic families from normal control families on measures of interpersonal dynamics and emotional interactions. Impairment in these areas, as identified and measured by the SASB, is suggestive of family pathology and allows for the specification of this pathology in such a way that therapy may be more precisely planned. While the dimensions are not specific to eating disorders, the ability of the technique to discriminate shows some potential as a research and clinical assessment tool.

Planning and Treatment

Most contributions to the literature concerning the treatment of childhood feeding disorders have focused on retarded children rather than on normal children. The work on childhood obesity has been primarily concerned with the behavioral approaches to weight reduction. However, effective treatment can be designed based on the assessments conducted as described earlier. Linscheid (1983) divided feeding problems into those unrelated to the quantity of food eaten and those related to intake and quantity. Those problems that are not related to quantity include conduct problems at mealtime, unwillingness to eat solid foods, unusual food habits, delays in self-feeding, and multiple food dislikes.

When the assessment of the associated pathology identifies important developmental or psychopathological processes such as childhood depression, hyperactivity, developmental delays, and so on, the appropriate therapies can be initiated to deal with these difficulties. However, a behavioral program can be designed based on the behavioral analysis of the feeding problem. Using the behavioral analysis, the therapist can, first, specify those goals to be achieved in behavioral and nutritional terms. Second, a means of measuring progress can be devised, possibly using the techniques employed during the assessment phase including direct observation, self-report, or parental report, to measure progress. Third, the assessment can help specify those particular procedures that will be designed to increase the child's appropriate behavior, decrease the child's inappropriate behavior, and establish fair and consistent reinforcement and punishment criteria.

In treating childhood obesity, the assessment is vital. Those nutritional, physical, and psychological factors contributing to and maintaining the obesity can be identified and treated. Of course, any physical disease that has been identified will be treated by appropriate professionals. Psychopathological disorders of childhood, such as oppositional disorder, are not directly associated with obesity but may identify important patterns of behavior, thinking, and emotional reactivity that are an important part of the child's total adjustment and that must be addressed insofar as they may contribute to the obesity by, for example, having mealtime become a battleground where the child attempts to assert his or her will over that of the parents. The dynamically oriented approaches are more suited to the associated pathologies than to the obesity itself. The treatment of the obesity will usually involve more direct or indirect behavioral interventions. The target behaviors, the stimuli, and the contingencies that are identified as part of the treatment program should be those identified during the behavioral analysis.

One of the most important contributions of the assessment can be to identify the setting in which the treatment can best be carried out and the type of therapy best suited to the particular case in question. Serious disruption in the home might indicate the use of inpatient hospitalization. The identification of strong family influences may lead the therapist to consider family therapy as the treatment of choice.

The multidetermined nature of anorexia nervosa and bulimia demands a flexible set of treatment options: individual therapy, family and group therapy, medications, nutritional therapy. Inpatient therapy is an option until the overall situation is stabilized.

Inpatient hospitalization is needed when the assessment reveals one or more of the following: serious medical complications due to low weight; refusal to eat or excessive use of purgatives; seriously disturbed family or other inadequate social supports outside the hospital; serious affective disorders with suicidal risks; complex unresolved diagnostic issues; a binge–purge cycle that is extreme in frequency, intensity, and/or duration and that can be effectively interrupted only by hospitalization.

The effects of starvation or extremely poor nutrition in the anorexic are of primary importance. Starvation can be related to depression and, therefore, the patient's nutritional status must be stabilized and improved before psychotherapy can be beneficial. The therapist's analysis of the antecedent events, stimuli, mediating variables, response patterns, and consequences can allow for the structuring of a behavioral program to aid in refeeding and renourishing the anorexic patient. The specifics of treatment planning would, of course, be dependent on the skill, orientation, and resources of the psychologist as well as the needs of the patient as they are determined in the assessment. One may consult the work of Garfinkel and Garner (1982) on anorexia nervosa and Garner and Garfinkel (1985) for a comprehensive view of psychotherapy with both anorexics and bulimics.

As treatment progresses, the therapist must assess progress and must base this assessment on the data gathered in the pretreatment assessment. As weight is restored to the anorexic or as the binge–purge cycle is reduced in the bulimic, the motivation and reinforcers for the pathological eating behaviors should be addressed, especially those other than control or reduction of weight. Specific recommendations regarding caloric and nutritional needs should be provided, even to the point of setting up specific diets and exercise regimens. The therapist must remain aware of the obsessive–compulsive features of the patient's fears and anxieties over what may be perceived as a reduction in her sense of control.

The assessment should help the therapist anticipate the core features of the disorder that are unique to each patient. The Eating Disorders Inventory can be helpful in specifying which of these may be the most prominent in a given patient.

Associated pathologies must also be treated. Therapists must be prepared to treat the depression, even though the major signs of affective disorder may remit with improved nourishment. In such a case, the interpersonal, behavioral, and cognitive patterns associated with the depression may persist. The therapist must continue to assess the extent of other forms of psychopathology and behavior disorder as they emerge in the course of treatment such as features of the borderline personality disorder, anxiety, patterns of chemical abuse, and so on.

The type of therapy most suited to a specific patient may be identified through the assessment. For example, one type of therapy is group therapy. Yalom (1975) reviewed several studies and noted characteristics associated with high dropout rates in group therapy: extreme denial; preoccupation with somatic complaints; poor motivation; lack of social skills and discomfort with social situations; lack of psychological sophistication and insight. These characteristics are frequently found in anorexic patients and, when revealed in the assessment, may indicate a poor prognosis for group therapy. Yalom addressed the anorexic patients specifically and indicated those who are most likely to profit from group therapy. The criteria cited are quite broad and may also be applicable to bulimics. They are: (1) patients who are not severely ill and whose weight is stable; (2) patients who are highly motivated; (3) patients who have experienced progress and success in other treatments; (4) patients who are not withdrawn or isolated; (5) patients who are open and sensitive to others and who display some level of psychological sophistication; (6) patients whose physical or psychological needs now require another therapeutic setting; (7) patients who have the potential to be liked by peers. Gandour (1984) stated that group therapy has little evidence to support its use as the sole treatment for bulimia since it has little demonstrated effect on the core features of bulimia, that is, the binge–purge cycle.

When the assessment identifies the family system as a major force in the onset or maintenance of an eating disorder, family therapy may be the most appropriate type of therapy. Minuchin and colleagues (1975, 1978) identified the five predominant characteristics of families with anorexic members. Using their guidelines, family therapy would be the treatment of choice when the analysis reveals the enmeshment, overprotectiveness, rigidity, lack of conflict resolution, and involvement of the patient in unresolved parental conflict, all of which are the characteristics cited by Minuchin and his group. Since these characteristics have been applied to psychosomatic families in general, Schwartz, Barrett, and Saba (1985) suggested that they may be applied to the family of bulimic patient as well.

Assessment During Therapy

Since there are no proven psychometric tests that address the core features of the feeding or eating disorders, assessment of progress during therapy must focus on the measurement, either directly or indirectly, of the target behaviors and improvement in the associated pathology. The direct or indirect assessment of improvement in the target behaviors can be made through self-report, if the child is reliable enough, or through the report of the parents. Direct measurement may be made of the child's eating and feeding behaviors if the child is in a setting where it is feasible to do so. The techniques employed to measure the improvement in the behavior should parallel those used in the assessment of the problem. For example, if the problem focuses on mealtime temper tantrums, the same measurements used to identify and specify the problem, such as duration of the tantrum, should be used to measure progress and improvement. The most reliable evaluation is that done by several people.

Changes in the associated pathology, such as anxiety or depression, may be measured using those instruments sensitive to changes over brief periods of time such as the State-Trait Anxiety Inventory or the Children's Depression Inventory, the children's version of the Beck Depression Inventory.

When assessing improvement in childhood obesity, the therapist must be sensitive to the speed with which certain changes can be expected to appear. Weight changes may appear more slowly than changes in the amount or quality of food eaten. But the best measurements of improvement in childhood obesity would, of course, be direct measurements in the caloric value of food, the increase in physical activity, and weight change. The therapist and the child, as well as family, must be aware that weight change can be a function of a number of different influences and that short-term improvement is less important than modification of more permanent factors such as eating habits, selection of food, exercise routine, and so forth. When the problem is childhood obesity, the assessment of progress through measurement of associated pathology must take into consideration those problems that are the result of obesity and those that may be contributing to it. For instance, the assumption that improvement in weight will lead to improvement in self-esteem may be erroneous if poor self-esteem existed prior to the obesity and may have contributed to its onset by virtue of the child's restricting his or her activities, staying away from peers, remaining at home, and spending large amounts of time eating. In assessing progress in the treatment of childhood obesity, it is very important for the therapist to address the problem, that is, the obesity, but also to treat and measure improvement in other areas closely associated, such as self-esteem, social involvement, and so on.

In summary, since the literature lacks substantial information on the treatment of eating disorders and obesity in children, it also lacks substantial information regarding the assessment of change during therapy. The psychologist, therefore, must use his or her expertise to design a means of assessing improvement that addresses changes in the core pathology as well as the associated pathologies. The measurements used during therapy should be based on those used during the assessment of the patient prior to therapy, that is, in the problem identification stage. The therapist must also give proper consideration to issues of validity and reliability regarding the measurement of progress.

The assessment of progress in the treatment of anorexia nervosa or bulimia poses similar problems. During therapy, the assessment can be conducted in a variety of ways. Most simply, patients may be asked how well they are doing. Any clinician experienced in treating eating disorders is aware of the tendency of these patients to deny and conceal, generally out of fears of losing control and the belief that others don't understand their need to lose weight and wish to control their lives. Self-report measures must be used cautiously and the data confirmed through other means.

Psychological tests described earlier, including questionnaires designed to assess factors central to the eating disorder and instruments designed to assess associated pathologies, may be used at varying intervals to assess progress. The therapist may also note, as will family members, that the patient may become more emotionally expressive as she progressively controls her eating disorder. Problems may be acknowledged and emotions previously denied may be expressed, a development for which family members must be prepared so they may view this change to a more assertive behavior pattern as a necessary and appropriate step in recovery. It is essential that the psychologist using objective, empirical tests or projective tests to assess progress differentiate those aspects that are characterologic, such as obsessive–compulsive patterns, and that are therefore less likely to show significant short-term change, from those such as affective symptoms that may change more rapidly. Furthermore, effective therapy requires that the therapist acknowledge the eating patterns to be the most obvious symptoms and those that must be changed first. However, the associated pathology will be a primary focus of therapy once the eating patterns and nutrition have stabilized. Therefore, measures to assess the eating pattern will be important at the onset of therapy and should also be used at regular intervals as the therapy progresses to prevent relapse. At the same time, measures to assess depression, such as the Beck Depression Inventory, can be used early since progress in nutrition usually contributes to some improvement in affect. Other measures such as the MMPI, EPI, Rorschach, and so on are useful when the eating patterns have been brought under control. As noted earlier, there are insufficient research data showing correlation of these test profiles with improvement of the core symptoms of anorexia nervosa or bulimia.

A number of authors have reported the use of outcome data other than psychological tests. A frequently used method is that recommended by Hsu (1980). Hsu advised in-depth face-to-face follow-up interviews, examining basic skills and living arrangements as a means of assessing overall adaptation. The criteria will depend largely on the emphasis in therapy such as the orientation, type of therapy, and setting. For instance, Schwartz and colleagues (1985) use a family therapy approach and assess outcome by rating the patient in four areas: (1) symptom control; (2) change in family relationships; (3) change in life goals or careers; and (4) changes in behavior in extrafamilial relationships. Anderson, Hedblom, and Hubbard (1983) emphasized the need for a multidisciplinary treatment approach. In their follow-up, they assess the patient's percentage of ideal body weight, regularity of menstrual cycle, binge–purge cycle, food rigidity, occupational status, and social adjustment.

The degree of progress in various areas makes sense only in the context of what might be expected based on studies of progress reported in the literature. The patient's weight may stabilize rather quickly. Dally (1969) found that 97 out of 140 patients stabilized their weight and more than 80 percent regained a stable weight within 3 years of the onset of the disorder. Dally reports that patients may have a weight loss shortly after discharge from an inpatient treatment program. Theander (1970) reported that infrequently patients may relapse after a year or more. Many studies have reported that patients will achieve a more normal weight following effective treatment (Dally & Gomez, 1979; Garfinkel et al., 1977; Hsu, Crisp, & Harding, 1979; Morgan & Russell, 1975; Pertschuk, 1977; Theander, 1970). These studies also reported that obesity is relatively uncommon.

In assessing progress, the therapist should be aware that some patients tend to maintain a degree of concern about their weight and fears of losing control and becoming fat. Morgan and Russell (1975) noted that 65 percent of their patients continued to express concern about the appearance of their bodies. Thirty percent of the patients felt fat, and 40 percent reported still being afraid of obesity. Hsu and colleagues (1979) found that 46 percent of their patients continued to display some form of dietary restriction, and that only approximately 35 percent had what might be referred to as normal eating patterns. Thus it is important that the therapist place these fears in proper perspective.

Finally, adequate assessment should provide some insight regarding the prognosis. Factors that have been related to prognosis, both favorable and unfavorable, should be understood. Crisp, Kalucy, Lacey, and Harding (1977) and Bemis (1978) examined the specific factors related to outcome in anorexia nervosa. Patients who have a more favorable prognosis tend to be those who are younger at the time of onset, unmarried, have no prior history of treatment failures, and are presenting with an illness of shorter duration. Vomiting has been associated with a poorer prognosis, although the data have been inconsistent. Data are also inconsistent with respect to laxative abuse, with some studies showing that the prognosis is not significantly impaired as a result of laxative abuse, but with other studies showing that patients who have abused laxatives tend to have poorer outcomes. Patients who do not have a prior history of obesity tend to have a more favorable prognosis, as do those in whom an external precipitant or cause for the disorder can be identified. Success in school prior to the onset of the disorder also appears to be predictive of a favorable outcome. Those patients who have a stronger tendency toward somatization tend to have a poorer prognosis.

Hsu and colleagues (1979) reported that outcome at 1-year follow-up is predictive of long-term prognosis. However, the therapist must consider the type of therapy being employed since some therapies are, by definition, more long-term. In these therapies, the patient may still be at a mid-point or intermediate stage of therapy after a year.

References

Abrahamian, F. P., & Lloyd-Still, J. D. (1984). Chronic constipation in childhood: A longitudinal study of 186 patients. *Journal of Pediatric Gastroenterology & Nutrition, 3*, 460–467.

Abramson, E. E., & Wunderlich, R. A. (1972). Anxiety, fear and eating: A test of the psychosomatic concept of obesity. *Journal of Abnormal Psychology, 79*, 317–321.

American Psychiatric Association. (1980). *Diagnostic and statistical manual of mental disorders* (3rd ed.). Washington, DC: Author.

Anderson, A. E., Hedblom, J. E., & Hubbard, F. A. (1983). A multi-disciplinary team treatment for patients with anorexia nervosa and their families. *International Journal of Eating Disorders, 2*, 181–192.

Anthony, E. J. (1957). An experimental approach to the psychopathology of childhood encopresis. *British Journal of Medical Psychology, 30*, 146–175.

Ashkenazi, Z. (1975). The treatment of encopresis using a discriminative stimulus and positive reinforcement. *Journal of Behavior Therapy & Experimental Psychiatry, 6*, 151–157.

Askervold, E. (1975). Measuring body image. *Psychotherapy & Psychosomatics, 26*, 71–77.

Azrin, N. Y., Thienes-Hontos, P., & Besalel-Azrin, V. (1979). Elimination of enuresis without a conditioning apparatus: An extension by office instruction of the child and parents. *Behavior Therapy, 10*, 14–19.

Bellman, M. (1966). Studies on encopresis. *Acta Pediatrica Scandinavica (Suppl.), 170*, 1–137.

Bemis, K. M. (1978). Current approaches to the etiology and treatment of anorexia nervosa. *Psychological Bulletin, 85*, 593–617.

Bemporad, J. R., Pfeifer, C. M., Gibbs, L., Cortner, R. H., & Bloom, W. (1971). Characteristics of encopretic patients and their families. *Journal of American Academy of Child Psychiatry, 10*, 272–292.

Benjamin, L. S., Foster, S. W., Giat-Roberto, L., & Estroff, S. E. (1983). Breaking the family code: Analyzing video tapes of family interactions by structural analysis of social behavior. In L. S. Greenburg & W. M. Pinsof (Eds.), *Psychotherapeutic process: Research handbook*. New York: Guilford.

Ben-Tovim, D. I., Whitehead, J., & Crisp, A. H. (1979). A controlled study of the perception of body width in anorexia nervosa. *Journal of Psychosomatic Research, 23*, 267–272.

Boskind-Lodahl, M. (1976). Cinderella's step-sisters: A feminist perspective on anorexia nervosa and bulimia. *Signs: The Journal of Women in Culture & Society, 2*, 342–356.

Brownell, K. D., & Stunkard, A. J. (1978). Behavioral treatment of obesity in children. *American Journal of Diseases in Children, 132*, 403–412.

Bruch, H. (1961). Conceptual confusion in eating disorders. *Journal of Nervous & Mental Disorders, 133*, 46–54.

Bruch, H. (1962). Perceptual and conceptual disturbances in anorexia nervosa. *Psychological Medicine, 24,* 187–194.

Bruch, H. (1973). *Eating disorders: Obesity, anorexia nervosa and the person within.* New York: Basic.

Bruch, H. (1978). *The golden cage: The enigma of anorexia nervosa.* Cambridge, MA: Harvard University Press.

Bruch, H. (1979). Anorexia nervosa. *Key, 60,* 7–8.

Button, E. J., Fransella, F., & Slade, P. D. (1977). A reappraisal of body perception disturbance in anorexia nervosa. *Psychological Medicine, 7,* 235–243.

Casper, R. C., Halmi, K. A., Goldberg, S. C., Eckert, E. D., & Davis, J. M. (1979). Disturbances in body image estimation as related to other characteristics of outcome in anorexia nervosa. *British Journal of Psychiatry, 134,* 60–66.

Ciminero, A. R., & Doleys, D. M. (1976). Childhood enuresis: Considerations in assessment. *Journal of Pediatric Psychology, 4,* 17–20.

Crisp, A. H. (1970). Premorbid factors in adult disorders of weight, with particular reference to primary anorexia nervosa (weight phobia): A literature review. *Journal of Psychosomatic Research, 14,* 1–22.

Crisp, A. H., & Kalucy, R. S. (1974). Aspects of perceptual disorder in anorexia nervosa. *British Journal of Medical Psychology, 47,* 349–361.

Crisp, A. H., Kalucy, R. S., Lacey, J. H., & Harding, B. (1977). Long-term prognosis in anorexia nervosa: Some factors predictive of outcome. In R. Vigersky (Ed.), *Anorexia nervosa.* New York: Raven.

Crisp, A. H., Palmer, R. L., & Lacey, R. S. (1976). How common is anorexia nervosa? *British Journal of Psychiatry, 128,* 549–554.

Cullen, K. J. (1966). Clinical observations concerning behavior disorders in children. *Medical Journal of Australia, 1,* 712–715.

Dally, P. (1969). *Anorexia nervosa.* New York: Grune & Stratton.

Dally, P., & Gomez, J. (1979). *Anorexia nervosa.* London: Heinemann.

Doleys, D. M. (1977). Behavioral treatments for nocturnal enuresis in children: A review of the recent literature. *Psychological Bulletin, 84,* 30–54.

Doleys, D. M. (1979). Assessment and treatment of childhood enuresis. In A. J. Finch & P. C. Kendall (Eds.), *Treatment and research in child psychopathology.* New York: Spectrum.

Doleys, D. M. (1981). Encopresis. In J. Ferguson, & C. Taylor (Eds.), *The comprehensive handbook of behavior medicine: Vol. 2. Syndromes and special areas.* New York: Spectrum.

Doleys, D. M., & Arnold, S. (1975). Treatment of childhood encopresis: Full cleanliness training. *Mental Retardation, 13,* 14–16.

Doleys, D. M., Schwartz, M. S., & Ciminero, A. R. (1981). Elimination problems: Enuresis and encopresis. In E. J. Mash & L. G. Terdal (Eds.), *Behavioral assessment of childhood disorders.* New York: Guilford.

Forsythe, W. I., & Redmond, A. (1974). Enuresis and spontaneous cure rate: Study of 1129 enuretics. *Archives of Diseases in Childhood, 49,* 259–263.

Gandour, M. J. (1984). Bulimia: Clinical description, assessment, etiology and treatment. *International Journal of Eating Disorders, 3,* 3–38.

Garfinkel, P. E., & Garner, D. M. (1982). *Anorexia nervosa: A multidimensional perspective.* New York: Brunner/Mazel.

Garfinkel, P. E., Moldofsky, H., & Garner, D. M. (1977). The outcome of anorexia nervosa: Significance of clinical features, body image, and behavior modification. In R. Vigersky (Ed.), *Anorexia nervosa.* New York: Raven.

Garfinkel, P. E., Moldofsky, H., Garner, D. M., Stancer, H. C., & Coscina, D. V. (1978). Body awareness in anorexia nervosa: Disturbances in body image and satiety. *Psychosomatic Medicine, 40,* 487–498.

Garner, D. M., & Bemis, K. M. (1982). A cognitive–behavioral approach to anorexia nervosa. *Cognitive Therapy in Research, 6,* 123–150.

Garner, D. M., & Garfinkel, P. E. (1979). The Eating Attitudes Test: An index of the symptoms of anorexia nervosa. *Psychological Medicine, 9,* 273–279.

Garner, D. M., & Garfinkel, P. E. (1985). *Handbook of psychotherapy for anorexia nervosa and bulimia.* New York: Guilford.

Garner, D. M., Garfinkel, P., Stancer, H., & Moldofsky, H. (1976). Body image disturbances in anorexia nervosa and obesity. *Psychosomatic Medicine, 38*, 327–336.

Garner, D. M., & Olmsted, M. P. (1984). *Manual for Eating Disorders Inventory (EDI)*. Odessa, FL: Psychological Assessment Resources.

Gelber, H., & Meyer, V. (1965). Behavior therapy and encopresis: The complexities involved in treatment. *Behaviour Research & Therapy, 2*, 227–231.

Goldberg, S. C., Halmi, K. A., Casper, R., Eckert, E., & Davis, J. M. (1977). *Pretreatment predictors of weight change in anorexia nervosa*. In R. Vigersky (Ed.), *Anorexia nervosa*. New York: Raven.

Halmi, K. A., Falk, J. R., & Schwartz, E. (1981). Binge-eating and vomiting: A survey of a college population. *Psychological Medicine, 11*, 697–706.

Hawkins, R. C., & Clement, P. F. (1980). Development and construct validation of a self-report measure of binge eating tendencies. *Addictive Behaviors, 5*, 219–226.

Henderson, W. (1976). A review of the current medical aspects of enuresis. *Journal of Pediatric Psychology, 4*, 15–16.

Hoag, J. M., Norriss, N. G., Himeno, E. T., & Jacobs, J. (1971). The encopretic child and his family. *Journal of American Academy of Child Psychiatry, 10*, 242–256.

Holland, J., Masling, J., & Copley, D. (1970). Mental illness in lower class normal, obese, and hyperobese women. *Psychosomatic Medicine, 32*, 351–357.

Hood, J., Moore, T., & Garner, D. (1982). Locus of control as a measure of ineffectiveness in anorexia nervosa. *Journal of Consulting & Clinical Psychology, 50*, 3–13.

Hsu, L. K. G. (1980). Outcome of anorexia nervosa: A review of the literature (1964–1978). *Archives of General Psychiatry, 37*, 1041–1046.

Hsu, L. K. G., Crisp, A. H., & Harding, B. (1979). Outcome of anorexia nervosa. *Lancet, 1*, 61–65.

Hsu, L., & Lieberman, S. (1982). Paradoxical intention and the treatment of chronic anorexia nervosa. *American Journal of Psychiatry, 139*, 650–653.

Humphrey, L. L., Apple, R. F., & Kirschenbaum, D. S. (1986). Differentiating bulimic-anorexic from normal families using interpersonal and behavioral observational systems. *Journal of Consulting & Clinical Psychology, 54*, 190–195.

Ilg, F. L., & Ames, L. B. (1955). *Child behavior*. New York: Harper & Row.

Johnson, C. (1985). Initial consultation for patients with bulimia and anorexia nervosa. In D. M. Garner & P. E. Garfinkel (Eds.), *Handbook of psychotherapy for anorexia nervosa and bulimia*. New York: Guilford.

Jones, D. J., Fox, M. M., Babigan, H. M., & Hutton, H. E. (1980). Epidemiology of anorexia nervosa in Monroe County, New York (1960–1976). *Psychosomatic Medicine, 42*, 551–558.

Kaplan, H. I., & Kaplan, H. S. (1957). The psychosomatic concept of obesity. *Journal of Nervous & Mental Disorders, 125*, 181–201.

Kendel, R. E., Hall, D. J., Hailey, A., & Babigan, H. M. (1973). Epidemiology of anorexia nervosa. *Psychological Medicine, 3*, 200–203.

Kessler, J. W. (1966). *Psychopathology of childhood*. Englewood Cliffs, NJ: Prentice-Hall.

Kilbourne, K. A. (1986). Nutritional evaluation and management of anorexic and bulimic patients. In G. D. Comerci (Ed.), *Seminars in adolescent medicine: Eating disorders: Anorexia nervosa and bulimia* (Vol. 2). New York: Thieme.

Kimmel, H. D., & Kimmel, E. C. (1970). An instrumental conditioning method for the treatment of enuresis. *Journal of Behavior Therapy & Experimental Psychiatry, 1*, 121–123.

Knobloch, H., & Pasamanick, B. (1974). *Developmental diagnosis: The evaluation and management of normal and abnormal neuropsychologic development in infancy and early childhood*. Hagerstown, MD.: Harper & Row.

Laseque, C. (1873). De l'anorexie hysterique. *Medical Times Gazette, 2*, 265–266.

Leibowitz, S. F. (1980). Neurochemical systems of the hypothalamus: Control of feeding and drinking behavior and water-electrolyte excretion. In P. J. Morgane & J. Panksepp (Eds.), *Handbook of the hypothalamus* (Vol. 3A). New York: Marcel Dekker.

Leon, G. R., & Chamberlain, K. (1973). Emotional arousal, eating patterns, and body image as differential factors associated with varying success in maintaining a weight loss. *Journal of Consulting & Clinical Psychology, 40*, 474–480.

Levine, M. D. (1975). Children with encopresis: A descriptive analysis. *Pediatrics, 56,* 412–416.

Linscheid, T. R. (1983). Eating problems in children. In C. E. Walker & M. C. Roberts (Eds.), *Handbook of clinical child psychology.* New York: Wiley.

Lovibond, S. H., & Coote, M. A. (1970). Enuresis. In C. G. Costello (Ed.), *Symptoms of psychopathology.* New York: Wiley.

Lytle, L. D. (1977). Control of eating behavior. In R. J. Wortman & J. J. Wortman (Eds.), *Nutrition and the brain.* New York: Raven.

Mayer, J. (1968). *Obesity: Causes, cost, and control.* Englewood Cliffs, NJ: Prentice-Hall.

Mellendick, G. J. (1983). Nutritional issues in adolescence. In A. Hofmann (Ed.), *Adolescent medicine.* Menlo Park, CA.: Addison-Wesley.

Minuchin, S., Baker, L., Rosman, B. L., Liebman, R., Milman, L., & Todd, T. (1975). A conceptual model of psychosomatic illness in children. *Archives of General Psychiatry, 32,* 1031–1038.

Minuchin, S., Rosman, B. L., & Baker, L. (1978). *Psychosomatic families: Anorexia nervosa in context.* Cambridge, MA: Harvard University Press.

Morgan, H. G., & Russell, G. F. M. (1975). Value of family background in clinical features as predictors of long-term outcome in anorexia nervosa: Four year follow up study of 41 patients. *Psychological Medicine, 5,* 355–371.

Morgan, R. T. T., & Young, G. C. (1975). Parental attitudes and the conditioning treatment of childhood enuresis. *Behaviour Research & Therapy, 13,* 197–199.

Nisbett, R. E. (1972). Hunger, obesity, and ventromedial hypothalamus. *Psychological Review, 79,* 433–453.

Nixon, H. H. (1964). Hirschprung's disease. *Archives of Diseases of Childhood, 39,* 109–115.

Norman, D. K., & Herzog, D. B. (1983). Bulimia, anorexia nervosa and anorexia nervosa with bulimia. A comparative analysis of MMPI profiles. *International Journal of Eating Disorders, 2,* 43–52.

Nylander, I. (1971). The feeling of being fat and dieting in a school population: Epidemiologic interview investigation. *Acta Sociomedica Scandinavica, 3,* 17–26.

Oppel, W. C., Harper, P. A., & Rider, R. V. (1968). The age of attaining bladder control. *Pediatrics, 42* (4), 614–626.

Palmer, S., & Horn, S. (1978). Feeding problems in children. In S. Palmer & S. Ekvall (Eds.), *Pediatric nutrition in developmental disorders.* Springfield, IL: Thomas.

Palmer, S., Thompson, R. J., & Linscheid, T. R. (1975). Applied behavior analysis in the treatment of childhood feeding problems. *Developmental Medicine & Child Neurology, 17,* 333–339.

Pertschuk, M. J. (1977). Behavior therapy: Extensive follow-up. In R. Vigersky (Ed.), *Anorexia nervosa.* New York: Raven.

Pierce, C. M. (1972). Enuresis. In A. M. Freedman & H. I. Kaplan (Eds.), *The child* (Vol. 1). New York: Atheneum.

Pierce, C. M. (1980). Enuresis. In H. I. Kaplan, A. M. Freedman, & B. J. Sadock (Eds.), *Comprehensive textbook of psychiatry* (Vol. 3, 3rd ed.). Baltimore: Williams & Wilkins.

Pierloot, R. A., & Houben, M. E. (1978). Estimation of body dimension in anorexia nervosa. *Psychological Medicine, 8,* 317–324.

Pierloot, R., Wellens, W., & Houben, M. (1975). Elements of resistance to a combined medical and psychotherapeutic program in anorexia nervosa. *Psychotherapy & Psychosomatics, 2,* 101–117.

Pliner, P., Meyer, P., & Blankstein, K. (1974). Responsiveness to affective stimuli by obese and normal individuals. *Journal of Abnormal Psychology, 83,* 74–80.

Reindl, M., & Gerstein, L. (1984, April). *Bulimics and their relationships: The Bulimic Interaction Inventory (BII).* Paper presented at the First International Conference on Eating Disorders, New York.

Reitman, E. E., & Cleveland, S. E. (1964). Changes in body image following sensory deprivation in schizophrenia and control groups. *Journal of Abnormal Social Psychology, 68,* 168–176.

Riordan, M. M., Iwata, B. A., Wohl, M. K., & Finney, J. W. (1980). Behavioral treatment of food refusal and selectivity in developmentally disabled children. *Applied Research in Mental Retardation, 1,* 95–112.

Risch, S. C., Cohen, R. M., Janowsky, D. S., Kallin, N. H., & Murphy, D. L. (1980). Mood and behavioral effects of physostigmine on humans are accompanied by elevations in plasma beta-endorphine and cortisol. *Science, 209,* 1545–1546.

Rodin, J. (1973). Effects of distraction on performance of obese and normal subjects. *Journal of Comparative & Physiological Psychology, 83,* 68–75.

Ross, L. D. (1969). *Cue- and cognition-controlled eating among obese and normal subjects.* Unpublished doctoral dissertation, Columbia University.

Rowland, C. (1970). Anorexia nervosa: A survey of the literature and review of 30 cases. In C. Rowland, Jr. (Ed.), *Anorexia and obesity.* Boston: Little, Brown.

Russell, G. F. M., Campbell, P. G., & Slade, P., D. (1975). Experimental studies on the nature of the psychological disorder in anorexia nervosa. *Psychoneuroendocrinology, 1,* 45–56.

Rybicki, D. J., & Lepowsky, C. M. (1984, April). *An empirical assessment of bulimic patients using multiple measures.* Paper presented at the First International Conference on Eating Disorders, New York.

Ryle, J. A. (1939). Discussion on anorexia nervosa. *Proceedings of the Royal Society of Medicine, 32,* 735–737.

Schachter, S. (1967). Cognitive effects on bodily functioning: Studies of obesity and eating, In D. Glass (Ed.), *Neurophysiology and emotions.* New York: Rockefeller University and the Russell Sage Foundation.

Schachter, S. (1971). Some extraordinary facts about obese humans and rats. *American Psychologist, 26,* 129–144.

Schachter, S., Goldman, R., & Gordon, A. (1968). Effects of fear, food deprivation and obesity on eating. *Journal of Personality & Social Psychology, 10,* 91–97.

Schachter, S., & Gross, L. (1968). Eating and manipulation of time. *Journal of Personality & Social Psychology, 10,* 98–106.

Schwartz, R., Barrett, M. J., & Saba, G. (1985). *The treatment of bulimic individuals and their families.* New York: Guilford.

Selvini-Palazzoli, M. (1971). Anorexia nervosa. In S. Arieti (Ed.), *The world biennial of psychiatry and psychotherapy* (Vol. 1). New York: Basic.

Selvini-Palazzoli, M. (1974). *Self-starvation.* London: Chaucer.

Shenker, I. R., & Shaw, H. (1986). Diagnosis and early management of anorexia nervosa and bulimia. In G. D. Comerci (Ed.), *Seminars in adolescent medicine: Eating disorders, anorexia nervosa, and bulimia* (Vol. 2). New York: Thieme.

Slade, P. D., & Russell, G. F. M. (1973). Experimental investigations of bodily perception in anorexia nervosa and obesity. *Psychotherapy & Psychosomatics, 22,* 259–363.

Small, A. C. (1984). The contribution of psychodiagnostic test results toward understanding anorexia nervosa. *The International Journal of Eating Disorders, 3,* 47–59.

Small, A., Teagno, L., Madero, J., Gross, H., & Ebert, M. (1982). A comparison of anorexics and schizophrenics on psychodiagnostic measures. *International Journal of Eating Disorders, 1,* 49–56.

Smart, T., Beaumont, P., & George, G. (1976). Some personality characteristics of patients with anorexia nervosa. *British Journal of Psychiatry, 128,* 57–60.

Sorotzkin, B. (1984). Nocturnal enuresis: Current perspectives. *Clinical Psychology Review, 4*(3), 293–316.

Strangler, R. S., & Printz, A. M. (1980). DSM-III psychiatric diagnosis in a university population. *American Journal of Psychiatry, 137,* 937–940.

Strober, M., & Goldenberg, I. (1981). Ego boundary disturbance in juvenile anorexia nervosa. *Journal of Clinical Psychology, 37,* 433–438.

Strober, M., Goldenberg, I., Green, J., & Saxon, J. (1979). Body image disturbance in anorexia nervosa during the acute and recuperative phase. *Psychological Medicine, 9,* 695–701.

Strober, M., Salkin, B., Burroughs, J., & Morrell, W. (1982). Validity of the bulimia-restrictor distinction in anorexia nervosa: Parental personality characteristics and family psychiatric morbidity. *Journal of Nervous & Mental Disease, 170,* 345–351.

Stunkard, A. J., & Koch, C. (1964). The interpretation of gastric motility. *Archives of General Psychiatry, 2,* 74–82.

Sugarman, A., Quinlan, D., & Devenis, L. (1982). Ego boundary disturbance in anorexia nervosa: Preliminary findings. *Journal of Personality Assessment, 46,* 455–461.

Szyrynski, V. (1973). Anorexia nervosa and psychotherapy. *American Journal of Psychotherapy, 27,* 492–505.

Tapia, F., Jekel, K., & Domke, H. R. (1960). Enuresis: An emotional symptom. *Journal of Nervous & Mental Disease, 130,* 61–66.

Theander, S. (1970). Anorexia nervosa: A psychiatric investigation of 44 female cases. *Acta Psychiatrica Scandinavica, 214,* 1–194.

Thompson, R. J. (1977). Applied behavior analysis in the treatment of mealtime tantrums and delay in self-feeding in a multi-handicapped child. *Journal of Clinical Child Psychology, 6,* 52–54.

Thompson, R. J., & Palmer, S. (1974). Treatment of feeding problems—A behavioral approach. *Journal of Nutrition Education, 6,* 63–66.

Walker, C. E. (1975). *Learn to relax.* Englewood Cliffs, NJ: Prentice-Hall.

Walker, C. E. (1978). Toilet training, enuresis, encopresis. In P. R. Magrab (Ed.), *Psychological management of pediatric problems: Vol. 1. Early life conditions and chronic disease.* Baltimore: University Park Press.

Walker, C. E., Milling, L. S., & Bonner, B. L. (in press). Enuresis and encopresis. In D. Routh (Ed.), *Handbook of pediatric psychology.* New York: Guilford.

Walker, C. E., & Werstlein, R. (1980). Use of relaxation procedures in the treatment of toilet phobia in a 4-year-old child. *The Behavior Therapist,* 3(4), 17–18.

Weiner, H. (1983a). Psychobiological and psychosomatic aspects of anorexia nervosa and other eating disorders. In L. J. West & M. Stein (Eds.), *Critical issues in behavioral medicine.* Philadelphia: Lippincott.

Weiner, H. (1983b). Abiding problems in the psychoendocrinology of anorexia nervosa. In G. J. Bargman (Chairperson), *Understanding anorexia nervosa and bulimia: Report of the 4th Ross Conference on Medical Research.* Columbus: Ross Laboratories.

Wingate, B. A., & Christie, M. J. (1978). Ego strength and body image in anorexia nervosa. *Journal of Psychosomatic Research, 22,* 201–204.

Woolfolk, R. L., & Lehrer, P. M. (Eds.). (1984). *Principles and practice of stress management.* New York: Guilford.

Yalom, I. D. (1975). *The theory and practice of group psychotherapy.* New York: Basic.

19

Assessment in Childhood Arthritis and Related Disorders: The Human Side of Health-Illness Evaluation

J. GERALD BEALES

Any chronic childhood disease such as juvenile arthritis (JA) must inevitably exert its impact upon the patient as a whole, threatening not only physical but also social and psychological well-being during childhood itself and far beyond. In addition to the more immediate suffering caused by the illness and the associated treatment regime, disruption of normal upbringing and education can lead to major long-term problems, significantly affecting quality of life well into and perhaps throughout the adult years.

Although some children with JA recover within a relatively short period of time, the majority of patients with disease of early onset face a comparatively lengthy period of ill health and medical therapy, with consequent implications for intellectual and emotional development and the acquisition of interpersonal skills. Therefore, while proper clinical management can keep permanent joint damage within reasonable limits for a large number of youngsters, failure to attend to the wider needs of the child during important formative years can result in the patient's embarking upon adult life physically quite able, but socially and emotionally crippled (Beales, 1984).

A treatment plan that caters effectively to the whole child must relate not simply to the medical condition, but also to the manner in which the patient and parents perceive and adapt to the condition. And the successful implementation of such a plan itself requires comprehensive and ongoing assessment of the child and the immediate family along a wide range of dimensions. As the child becomes older, or the disease itself undergoes change, new problems and threats can arise, and if these are to be detected and dealt with quickly, the total assessment process has to be a continuous affair. This need for regular repetition of evaluation, the substantial number of factors to be assessed, and the importance of including parents and siblings as well as the patient himself or herself clearly mean that, in JA and related conditions, assessment is a massive and demanding undertaking. Because it is so massive and demanding, there is real danger that the assessment process itself will have a damaging effect upon the child and the family. The aim must be to create and operate an evaluation system that, in addition to being reliable, sensitive, and wide ranging, does the patient no appreciable harm.

During the period of active disease, the levels of physical discomfort and emotional distress experienced by children are very much influenced by their own perception of their condition. Where patients see their arthritis as effectively preventing attainment of key goals, or where they have exaggerated fears and fantasies about the nature of internal pathology, they are likely to focus attention upon joint pain and experience greater anxiety, unhappiness, and despair (Beales, Keen, & Holt, 1983). The means by which patients endeavor to minimize such immediate suffering can, in turn, greatly affect future physical and psychosocial prospects (Mattsson, 1972; Myers, Friedman, & Weiner, 1970).

Ideally, patients will compensate for the effects of arthritis by developing alternative goals that are compatible with their condition but are nonetheless "normal" for their age. They will maintain self-esteem by valuing personal characteristics and achievements that are not markedly affected by the disease, and, given their level of intellectual development, they will possess an understanding of the illness that avoids unnecessary fears and motivates them to cooperate with medical treatment. They will openly express inevitable worries, sadness, and frustration but will view their arthritis as more of a misfortune than a disaster. They will develop independence and satisfactory relationships with healthy peers. Their educational progress will be maintained.

In practice, of course, many patients may fall far short of this ideal, and it is by no means always the child with the most severe physical disease who responds in the least satisfactory way. When a child is ill, the family as a whole is affected, and the JA patient's response to arthritis is very much influenced by the manner in which parents attempt to cope with their own stress and anxiety. A common parental reaction is that of overprotection, encouraging the child to maintain an inappropriately high level of dependence upon the mother in particular, and substantially cutting the youngster off from the normal childhood world. And where overprotection and excessive comforting are offered, the young patient may well be inclined to collaborate as a means of achieving greater mental security from the threats posed by the disease and treatment. As a result, the patient can eventually find himself or herself having to face realities of adolescent and adult life for which the earlier years have left him or her totally unprepared.

Alternatively, the parents may endeavor to restrict their own fears by largely denying the fact, severity, or significance of their child's illness. At the same time, they may, deliberately or otherwise, promote a large measure of denial in the patient, thereby effectively discouraging compliance with the treatment regime—and good physical prognosis in JA is greatly dependent upon the child's total and active cooperation with what is often a quite complex combination of therapies.

In some cases, the strains upon the family will not be adequately contained, and some form of breakup will result. Intrafamily conflict can occur on many levels, up to and including formal separation of the parents, and aggravating the patient's problems still further. But if families are to be helped and kept together, it is essential to detect the danger signals early, before things get out of hand (Burton, 1975).

In fact, families can be very good at hiding their difficulties and conflicts from outsiders, and young patients themselves can be most effective at concealing their real thoughts and emotions from the professionals responsible for their medical care. Under a facade of indifference, children can be afflicted with a profound sense of hopelessness, causing them to withdraw from social relationships and give up on school work. They can entertain frightening beliefs and horrific fantasies about what is actually going on beneath the body surface (Beales, Holt, Keen, & Mellor, 1984) but give very little indication of these in their encounters with health care staff.

As well as obvious monitoring of the severity and extent of the physical disease, it is therefore necessary to undertake continuous evaluation of the child's emotional state, means of coping, intellectual maturation and school achievement, development of independence, self-esteem, understanding of the illness, and compliance with the treatment program. It is also essential regularly to assess the manner in which the parents are adapting to the child's condition, and the state of relationships between parents, patient, and siblings.

As children with juvenile arthritis and similar conditions have increasingly come under the care of multidisciplinary teams, including a psychologist member, greater opportunities for more formal and sophisticated assessment of the whole patient and the whole family, have become available. It is possible to make use of the improved tests and techniques that have been developed for the assessment of pediatric patients as a whole, which are described in other chapters of this volume. But the sheer scale of evaluation required means that such formal monitoring can never be adequate, and a major contribution to assessment has to be made by all members of the care team undertaking appraisal in the course of their own encounters with the child and family.

It has to be recognized that repeated formal psychological testing is not only time-consuming for the professional involved, but it can also have undesirable effects upon the individual who is the subject of the assessment. A clinical test to measure joint inflammation can be administered without appreciable risk that the test itself will produce change in the variable being measured. But this cannot be said of techniques designed to assess psychosocial factors. Continuous inquiry into the child's emotional response to arthritis can force him or her to give excessive thought to the more distressing implications of the condition; and persistent questioning into family relationships can result in the reopening of old wounds, or the highlighting of previously unrecognized areas of disagreement.

In the course of treating the child's disease, different care team members—doctors, nurses, physiotherapists, and others—have frequent opportunities to appraise many aspects of the patient and immediate family, with much less risk of producing unwanted side effects. It is, in fact, inevitable that, through their various encounters with child and parents, medical staff will make judgments about the type of response being made to the condition, and the impact the arthritis is having upon the child's life and development. They cannot help but come to conclusions on the basis of their own contacts and conversations. The problem is that such assessment can be undertaken in a less than deliberate manner, with little effort being made fully to exploit the enormous opportunities provided, and with conclusions being made on the basis of assumptions that have not been subjected to careful conscious thought. The aim must therefore be to ensure that appraisal that takes place through such encounters is undertaken in a skillful and organized manner, with the different assessments made being regularly and routinely combined with the results of more formal testing to provide a deep and wide understanding of the family and the child.

The intention here is to identify, consider, and suggest solutions to some of the main problems that, in practice, tend to limit the effectiveness of assessment that occurs as a virtual by-product of interactions between health professionals and patients, parents, and siblings.

THE INTRUSION OF PERSONAL VALUES

Overall assessment of patient and parents can be greatly distorted by the values placed upon particular behaviors and responses associated with illness. Different cultures have different standards and expectations, and the values of health professionals may sometimes vary from those dominating in the wider society. But there is little that the child may say or do that is not capable of generating approval or disapproval from members of the health care team.

Certainly, medical staff are not exempt from the tendency to applaud some reactions and deplore others, and emotions aroused by one incident or characteristic can go on to color general appraisal of the family and the child.

Concepts of the "good patient" and the "not-so-good patient" are widespread among health professionals, even if they are not always admitted. White Anglo-Saxon culture, of course, greatly esteems the chronically ill youngster who rarely complains about his or her ailment and displays an apparent determination to overcome difficulties and disabilities. Children who frequently indicate pain, and let their illness "get them down" are usually very much less admired. And it is hardly surprising if doctors and nurses share such values, for the child who openly announces discomfort and misery reminds them of their own shortcomings as healers. They are inevitably more comfortable with a young patient who succeeds in putting a brave face on things. In addition, they share society's expectations of proper behavior in patient–professional and child–adult encounters, and neither a show of gratitude nor an apparent lack of respect is likely to be received with absolute indifference.

Another feature health professionals have in common with the rest of humanity is a marked tendency to make general assumptions about the nature and character of an individual on the basis of minimal data. A pretty little girl who "looks bright" can be almost automatically assumed to be of higher than average intelligence and, therefore, to have a reasonable understanding of her illness, to be devoid of "silly" fears, and to have the sense to cooperate with prescribed treatment.

Attachment of a strong positive or negative value to one particular feature is especially likely to produce corresponding judgments about characteristics and behaviors on which little or no information is available. A child who is polite and manages to smile during consultations with the doctor or who tolerates venipuncture without tears is more likely to be assumed to be complying with medical treatment at home than a young patient whose behavior is the opposite of this.

Even where information relating, for example, to the child's compliance with treatment is available, there is real danger that it will not be recognized and interpreted with anything approaching objectivity, but that it will be perceived in the light of value judgments already made. Having concluded, even if not explicitly, that this youngster falls into the ranks of the "good" patients, there is a powerful tendency to force subsequent evidence to fit that categorization. The human brain seems to have a strong preference for consistency in its perception and appraisal of external phenomena, although human beings are rarely consistent in their own behavior. In considering a young patient, the doctor may unconsciously interpret his words and actions in the light of a previous assessment of him. Having been pleased by something about him, the doctor may manufacture a picture of him that is likable in many respects. Yet the reality is that children with a long-term condition such as JA, which affects all aspects of their lives and produces changing symptoms and disabilities, do not maintain a single, harmonious, integrated response.

Youngsters whose behavior in the consulting room evokes positive sentiments in medical staff do not necessarily follow instructions with enthusiastic obedience when they are safely back at home and in the company of their families. Different factors are at play, and children seen in the outpatient clinic can be very different from children on their own territory. Children may conform to their doctors' expectations when they are in direct contact with them, but elsewhere they may prefer to act in accordance with quite different expectations of parents or peers.

The various elements of children's responses to their arthritis are not determined by a single set of causal factors, nor is there any simple causal link between them. A girl who reports less pain than might be expected from her level of physical pathology might conceivably be doing so as a result of a personality trait that fosters a broad determination to adopt a positive outlook, to lead as normal a life as possible, and to cooperate with medical staff in combating the disease. And principal external influences upon her attitudes and behavior—the actions of parents and peers, for example—might also be such as to reinforce these responses. But, on the other hand, they might easily be working in the opposite direction; and, equally, the youngster's reluctance to admit pain might, in fact, be a consequence of a maladaptive response to the disease that involves overwhelming denial of the significance of the condition and the need for treatment (Beales, 1982).

It is important for all concerned with the medical care of the JA patient to recognize the ease with which judgment of a chronically ill youngster can become biased. Although the doctor and the nurse are obliged to try to repress emotional responses to their young patients, it is difficult to avoid liking some kids and disliking others. Some children seem so brave, and so downright nice, in the face of considerable misfortune during what adult society generally believes should be the happiest time of their lives, that it is hard to resist concluding that just about everything about them must be worthy of praise. If members of the health care team are to achieve adequate and useful assessment of their young patients, it is therefore essential that they be constantly aware of this danger of generalizing from personal value judgments, and that they endeavor always to guard against it. They have to scrutinize each and every evaluation they make, and consider whether it is validly based on reasonable interpretation of available data, or whether it is unduly influenced by emotional reaction to a show of courage, or respect, or even a pretty face.

If society and health professionals have their own views on what is desirable and undesirable in a chronically ill youngster, they also have firm values relating to the role of parents of such a child. The difference, perhaps, is that there is much less unanimity on what constitutes a "good" parent than on what constitutes a "good" young patient. Different doctors and different nurses will have their own standards on this, and assessments that they make of parents' response to and handling of their sick child can be determined as much by the nature of their own personal values as by the nature of the facts.

Although the subject of parental overprotection of severely ill and disabled children has received a good deal of analysis (Mattsson & Gross, 1966), and although it is unquestionably the case that the long-term well-being of JA patients can suffer if they are not allowed to develop a degree of independence in their early years, it is impossible to identify a single point at which parenting ceases to be generally beneficial to the child and becomes potentially harmful instead. In the absence of a clear, proven dividing line between responsible care and control of the child and actual overprotection, there is plenty of scope for health professionals to judge according to their own standards, and, where they have children of their own, to compare the behavior of the patient's parents with their own performance.

Single incidents in the consulting room can be taken as indicators of overall parental style, but phenomena that indicate overprotection to one member of the care team can be taken as signs of good parenting, or even neglect, by another. Such things as the amount of clothing a child is wearing on a wintry day, or the level of physical contact between parent and child, can be interpreted quite differently by different team members, and can lead to diametrically opposed assessments of the parent's response to the illness and general handling of the youngster.

Observation of frequent touching and cuddling of the child by the mother may generate an impression of a caring parent, sensitive to her child's anxieties in a threatening situation, keen to promote the welfare of her offspring, and likely to provide a secure home environment in which the youngster can adapt successfully to the illness. Alternatively, it may create a negative evaluation, causing the observer to assume that the mother is restricting her child's development of independence, and hindering the youngster's long-term adjustment to the arthritis. A mother who firmly directs her young child to a separate seat on entering the consulting room, and who insists that the youngster converse directly with the doctor without seeking constant parental reassurance or support, may be viewed by some as demonstrating a praiseworthy determination to prevent her sick offspring from becoming overdependent. But others may take this as evidence of withdrawal from, and rejection of, an ill and imperfect child, and their perception and evaluation of other items of information on this parent may be influenced accordingly.

Certainly, the ways in which the parent addresses and deals with the youngster in the presence of medical staff can provide important clues to his or her own reaction to the child's illness, and the extent to which he or she is helping the offspring to compensate for the effects of arthritis. Apparently trivial incidents can be important signs of developing problems, and it is essential that all members of the care team make deliberate effort systematically to observe the parent and patient whenever opportunity arises. But in interpreting observed phenomena, they must strive to be aware of their own value positions, and consciously endeavor to minimize the influence of these upon the assessment made.

THE ELEMENT OF SELF-DELUSION

Although much can be gained from observation and interpretation of behavior in the course of encounters with the JA patient and parents or siblings, it has to be appreciated that the behavior may be deliberately intended to deceive. The way the child and parents relate to each other when in the doctor's presence, for example, can be very different from their private interactions. Sometimes the family will put on a performance for the benefit of medical staff because they really do have something to hide: because the strain of the child's chronic illness is causing a serious breakdown in relationships, or because the parents are conspiring with the child to go against certain medical advice. Quite often, however, the motive is more innocent, reflecting social norms concerning "proper" behavior when in the presence of high-status professionals. But whatever the reason, the fact is that family members are frequently reluctant to allow themselves to be seen as they really are.

The same applies to what the patient or parents may say in conversation with health team members, and in response to direct questioning. Their verbal accounts of their own thoughts about, and reactions to, the illness may be a good deal less than honest. This may be because they fear criticism or disapproval if they admit the truth. But it may also be because they regard their own thoughts and feelings, or details of family life, as very much their private concern. Although such matters are of considerable importance for the successful management of the "whole patient" in a condition such as juvenile arthritis, the child and the parents may nonetheless consider them to be outside the legitimate sphere of concern of medical staff.

If patients and parents are to speak frankly, and confide in any members of the care team, they must first of all trust, respect, and just plain like them. They are certainly not going to confess their personal feelings, or describe family relationships, to people they find unpleasant.

Naturally, every doctor, nurse, physiotherapist, and everyone else concerned with the professional care of the JA patient believes that he or she is a friendly and likable person, even if certain other members of the care team do not fit into that category. Each individual prefers to feel that he or she has established a good relationship with child and parents, and where the relationship is manifestly poor, there is a powerful tendency to blame this upon the other party: the spoiled child, the overanxious mother, or the abusive father. Where the family is considered "nice," and is liked by members of the care team, each member is strongly motivated to believe that he or she is equally liked by the parents and child.

Since patients and parents will only confide in a team member for whom they have strong positive feeling, doctors who convince themselves that they actually are liked by the family are inevitably inclined to conclude that what family members say to them is generally frank and honest. To believe otherwise would be to acknowledge that they may not be trusted and admired quite as much as they would wish. And although health professionals may be reluctant to admit this, even to themselves, there can be a real sense of competition within treatment teams over the establishment of relationships with patient and parents, and the eliciting of intimate confessions. Being trusted confers prestige; and the team member who is specially selected to be told innermost feelings or family secrets undoubtedly gains in esteem. It is something of an honor to be singled out in such a way, but there is nothing to feel proud of in being deliberately deceived.

The more a family is highly valued by the treatment team, the more of an inbuilt tendency there is, therefore, for individual care team members to believe what they are told by the patient and parents, or are allowed to see of the family in action. And this element of self-delusion, creating a sense of complacency and weakening motivation to scrutinize the family more closely, can be catastrophic in its consequences.

It is by no means unknown for a family that appears to be coping admirably with the child's condition, displaying solidarity in the face of adversity, and providing a near perfect home environment for the young patient, suddenly to show signs of serious trouble. In fact, the suddenness is usually only apparent, problems having been building up over a long period of time. Mothers and fathers can sometimes maintain a convincing show of marital harmony despite considerable strains caused, in part at least, by their child's serious illness. And when their encounters with medical staff are characterized by displays of gratitude, friendliness, and an apparent willingness to answer questions without hesitation, it is easy for individual team members to conclude that they have been taken into the family's confidence, and would be told if any tensions and difficulties were to exist. When it is too late to do anything to help, they can find that the most pleasant and seemingly "open" people may have been concealing a disintegrating marriage, or a gradual shift of interest and affection from the sick child to a healthy sibling.

On reflection, of course, any member of the treatment team who assumes that he or she really enjoys the confidence of the patient or parents and is allowed to share their private fears and concerns is guilty of arrogance. However willing to talk they may seem to be, families never reveal all to the nurse or doctor. Assessment and evaluation have to be a progressive peeling away of layers, a gradual accumulation of insights, a painstaking building up of a partial picture, and there are no shortcuts. JA patients and their parents do not bare their souls to make it easy for the care team, although they may sometimes seem to be doing so. Members of the team must guard against ever taking it for granted that they can simply and straightforwardly believe what they see and hear. They must take care to avoid the conceit of imagining that they have been given privileged access to things people prefer to keep to themselves.

MINIMIZING FEAR OF DISAPPROVAL

Although it is important to appreciate that completely full and open access to the JA patient's innermost thoughts, and the family's private life, is rarely willingly given, it is certainly true that members of the care team can greatly influence the amount and quality of information children and parents provide about themselves in the course of their encounters with health professionals. It is all too easy to create a situation that discourages frank responses and disclosures, and deliberate effort has to be made to generate the kind of environment and relationship that facilitates adequate assessment of the patient and family. The manner in which the care team member interacts with child and parents over a series of encounters can greatly affect the extent to which important facts are withheld for fear of disapproval, for example.

One area in which there is often considerable reluctance to reveal the true state of affairs is that of compliance with prescribed treatment. The young JA patient may be faced with a quite complex therapy regime involving drugs that have to be taken in different dosages at different times, the wearing of splints day or night, and a program of physiotherapy exercises. Elements of the regime can be distressing and unpleasant for the youngster, or can simply demand time and effort the child would prefer to devote to more pleasant activities. And parents can find themselves in a considerable dilemma when confronted by resistance to some particular therapy. On the one hand, they may be anxious to ensure that the child complies in order that the disease be combated most effectively. But, on the other hand, they may wish to avoid causing their sick offspring additional distress. More often than not, they will attempt to deal with this clash of goals by resorting to compromise: rigidly enforcing those parts of the treatment regime where opposition from the child is weak or nonexistent, and being more indulgent where the child shows greater hostility or distress.

Recognizing that medical staff are unlikely to approve of such a solution, parents are naturally reluctant to reveal the compromise. But, as prognosis is very much dependent upon full and active compliance with the treatment program, it is essential that care team members ascertain the actual state of affairs in order to be able to provide appropriate counseling of parent and child. Resistance to particular regime components can be reduced, and parents can be shown how to ensure compliance at least cost to their sick child's happiness, if the specific points of difficulty are identified.

In the matter of treatment compliance or other issues, patients and parents are generally more inclined to hide the true state of affairs from health team members the more they feel themselves to be falling short of normal and expected standards of performance. If they imagine that their own behavior is substantially different from, and "worse" than, that of other JA families, they are understandably reluctant to reveal it to those responsible for the child's medical care. And in a comparatively rare condition such as juvenile arthritis, it is extremely easy for a family to convince itself that its own reactions are unique and inferior, and that every other family either has not had to face the same kinds of problems, or has come up with far better solutions to them.

Care team members can encourage patient and parents to be more open and honest by repeatedly expressing appreciation of the real difficulties JA families can face, and stressing desired responses as praiseworthy achievements, rather than hinting at disapproval of "substandard" performances. It may be tempting to threaten the child or the parents with some sort of sanction if it is discovered that, for example, drugs are not being taken as directed, or splints are not being worn at the proper times; but this kind of approach is unlikely to improve compliance, and it certainly does nothing to motivate frank disclosure. It is far better to provide constant assurance that, whatever the family's course of action, others will have gone down the same path for the same reason, and honest admissions, even of apparent failure or compromise, will be received with praise and appreciation rather than disapproval. Motivating the child and the parents to reveal more and more of their thoughts and actions means rewarding, not punishing, each disclosure. At the very least, this means thanking them every time they decide to say something about themselves, congratulating them for every positive achievement, not taking their willingness to talk for granted, and never responding with criticism. In fact, if families find that admission of some particular difficulty results in their being given positive encouragement and advice toward a more satisfactory solution, their motivation to produce further revelations will be additionally strengthened.

PROVIDING FOR SEPARATE CONTACT

A good deal can be learned from careful observation of patient, siblings, and parents in interaction in the course of consultations and other encounters with medical staff. Even accepting that what they do and say to each other will be greatly influenced by the fact that they are in the presence of a health professional, careful scrutiny can reveal important clues to family relationships and responses to the arthritis. But those clues can only be properly interpreted if, in addition to being seen together, each individual is also regularly seen alone. Furthermore, a good deal of information, either volunteered or in response to direct questioning, will only be made available if the child or parent is able to speak privately to a care team member without anyone else in the family being present. Unless they are given the opportunity of talking to someone alone, parents are often unwilling to voice their beliefs and worries about the child's condition, or to refer to marital conflict aggravated by the current stresses upon the family, for fear of distressing their offspring. And children may be equally reluctant to talk of relationship problems with siblings or parents, for example, for fear of provoking parental retribution.

In practice, the majority of outpatient contacts and consultations in JA seem to involve patient and parent remaining together, and in an endeavor to use every opportunity to glean information for assessment purposes, health professionals may, in fact, be tempted to question a child or mother on some potentially sensitive matter, regardless of the presence of the other person. In the case of questions directed at a parent, this may appear to be justifiable since the youngster seems to be paying no attention to, or to be incapable of comprehending, the grown-ups' conversation. But children with a serious illness like juvenile arthritis are usually eager to hear everything that is being said about their condition, and may even feign a lack of interest in a conversation between doctor and parent in order to encourage them to say things they might not want the youngster to hear. As one teenager confessed when describing her previous outpatient visits as a young child: "I used to sit quiet and listen very hard, and after a while they just seemed to forget that I was there." In such circumstances, however, it is easy for the youngster to mishear or misunderstand, and to experience unnecessary distress and anxiety as a result.

Questioning of a parent when the child is around, therefore, can at best produce an evasive or false response, but at worst it can aggravate the patient's suffering. Nor does posing the questions in a hushed voice eliminate the difficulties, although this is a device commonly resorted to. A whispered question may even be misheard by the person to whom it is directed, resulting in a misleading answer, and perhaps even causing the parent to believe that the doctor is hinting at some previously unthought-of complication or threat to the child's long-term well-being. One parent went away from such a whispered session convinced—quite incorrectly—that the doctor had asked if she had considered the possibility that the arthritis might damage her child's heart. Not unreasonably, she assumed that he had been trying to tell her something.

If reasonably truthful and accurate responses are to be elicited, and if the assessment process itself is not to cause unnecessary harm to the patient or anyone else in the family, effort has to be made, and time found, for each individual to be seen separately. Natural opportunities for one-to-one conversation have to be made full use of, and others have to be deliberately contrived. But even this has to be done with care and sensitivity, for children who are summarily ejected from the consulting room so that the doctor can talk to the mother alone are bound to fear that some bad news about the illness is being broken, and even the mother's subsequent assurances that this was not so many not be believed. Similarly, parents may resent an invitation to leave in order that the children and care team members can converse in private, unless the reasons for this are properly explained. Procedures for achieving individual questioning without producing annoyance or distress have to be worked out in advance, so that when it becomes evident in the course of a consultation, for example, that further useful information might be obtained by continuing with one family member alone, this can be quickly, smoothly, and plausibly achieved.

REMOVING THE FEAR OF RIDICULE

A reluctance to admit and describe some beliefs and fears often arises from a concern that the admission will be received not so much with disapproval by care team members as with ridicule. Children and parents frequently conceal worrying notions about the disease itself or its implications for future life simply because they imagine that someone outside the family, with a professional knowledge of juvenile arthritis, will consider these to be trivial or silly. In fact, some of the most significant causes of emotional distress and maladaptation in JA can be carefully witheld from medical staff for this reason.

Children generally come to realize quite early on in life that their own ideas and worries can be a source of great amusement to adults. They may see TV programs built on the fact that grown-ups find the child's eye view of the world inferior and funny, and most have experienced the personal humiliation of having their words and mistaken notions merrily recounted by parents for the pleasure of family friends or neighbors. And even in the consulting room, young JA patients can find that revelation of some quite serious concern of theirs can provoke condescending smiles or patronizing chuckles from the health professionals in attendance. Such a reaction, of course, will not be meant maliciously, and may well be seen by the smiling care team members involved as a means of promoting a more friendly and informal atmosphere. But the chances are that children will simply feel that they are being laughed at, they will find such an experience painful, and they will do what they can to avoid any repetition of it—keeping many of their thoughts to themselves in the future, and pleading with parents not to tell.

Children are aware that many of the things that matter to them are not taken seriously by adults, with play being a particular example. Almost by definition, play from the adult's point of view is a frivolous and inessential affair, but concern about a perceived inability to engage in certain pastimes can cause a young patient to avoid contact with peers, be miserable (and therefore unsuccessful) at school, and become increasingly dependent upon parents. It is quite essential that the JA patient's thoughts and responses regarding play be properly assessed, so that appropriate therapeutic counseling can, if necessary, be implemented; but this is one subject that youngsters may be especially reluctant to discuss.

Among teenagers, relationships with the opposite sex is another area that may be of desperate importance to the patient, but seen as being potentially a matter of amusement to members of the treatment team. Fear of rejection can cause JA patients in this age group to refrain from seeking possible relationships, and lead to a depression that may have wide implications for long-term well-being. An adolescent girl who believes that her arthritis will prevent her from ever having a boyfriend may consider this to be quite sufficient reason to give up altogether, and no longer cooperate with the medical treatment regime. Again, therefore, it is vital to be able to make an adequate assessment of the patient's thoughts and reactions relating to personal attractiveness, so that advice and counseling can be made available; but embarrassment and anticipation of a humiliating response from health professionals can make the patient exceedingly reluctant to speak the truth.

Children's fears and fantasies about their internal pathology are yet another area where it is important to identify the child's thinking, but where fear of ridicule can deter the patient from talking fully and frankly (Beales et al., 1984). Younger patients generally do not think of their arthritis as a matter of internal physical damage and disorder. Things like restriction of activities and subjective feeling states (such as pain or weakness) "are" the disease as far as they are concerned. But by the time they enter the teenage years, they are usually aware that these things are merely manifestations of unpleasant and abnormal events taking place out of sight beneath the skin surface. However, because their knowledge of disease processes and normal anatomy and physiology is usually very limited (Bibace & Walsh, 1980; Gellert, 1979; Perrin & Gerrity, 1981; Whitt, Dykstra, & Taylor, 1979), their images of the kind of joint damage involved in JA can be highly inaccurate. There is, perhaps, a tendency for teenage patients to assume that because the impact of the disease upon their lives is so great, the internal pathology must be correspondingly severe. It is difficult for them to appreciate that even microscopic changes in normal tissue can produce real pain and disability. Consequently, their fantasies about what is going on beneath the body surface can include such things as badly damaged bone, lacerated muscle, and the spilling of large quantities of blood into the joint. In addition to being highly distressing in themselves, such fantasies can result in internal sensations being given a new and disturbing meaning, and having attention focused upon them, so that the frequency, severity, and duration of pain episodes may be increased. They can also generate a diffuse anxiety, leading to a preoccupation with the arthritis and loss of motivation in other areas.

The need to elicit and (where necessary) correct patients' images of their internal condition is therefore clear, but teenagers are quite aware that their own knowledge of the disease is enormously inferior to that of medical staff, and that ideas that seem reasonable to them may sound ridiculous to the nurse or doctor. Consequently, they are likely to be very reluctant to describe their thoughts and fantasies, and, faced with direct questioning, may well deny that they have ever given any thought to the physical state of their joints.

Reluctance to describe beliefs about the physical disease is not confined to patients, however. Most parents also are aware that their own knowledge is very limited, and are often ashamed to admit thoughts and ideas about internal pathology that may, in fact, be greatly affecting their handling of the child. An undisclosed suspicion that the arthritis might involve brittle bones for example, can cause unnecessary restriction of the child's activities and independence for a considerable period of time.

If there is to be adequate assessment and evaluation of some vital aspects of the family's response to the arthritis, the child and parents have to be given regular reassurance that their beliefs about the illness, and concerns about its implications, will be taken seriously. They have to be persuaded that their lack of expertise on the medical aspects of the arthritis is entirely normal and understandable, and that their ideas about physical pathology will not be interpreted as signs of stupidity or low intelligence. And, however tempting it may be to smile at some of the things confessed by patients or their parents, strenuous efforts have to be made to maintain a straight face.

CONFLICTING CHILD–PARENT ACCOUNTS

There are many occasions when a young JA patient's account of symptoms or response to the arthritis is contradicted by the parent. Differing versions of events may be offered independently when child and parent are seen separately, but it also frequently happens that the parent will challenge the truth or accuracy of what the child has to say when the two are together in the consulting room. Sometimes differences between parent and child are clearly just a matter of differing points of view and experiences. But, as often as not, they relate to matters of fact. Is the patient really taking her medication properly? Does she have any friends among children of her own age? How much pain is she actually experiencing?

When disagreements over factual matters occur, care team members are faced with the question of whom to believe. And because it is common experience that youngsters in general are inclined to exaggerate or distort the truth (whereas grown-ups are supposed to be responsible and obliged to live in the "real world"), there is always a danger that health professionals will have a natural bias toward accepting the parental version in preference to that of the child. There are many factors, however, that can cause the parent of a JA patient to be unreliable as a reporter on the child, or to attempt deliberately to deceive the people responsible for the child's medical care, and contradict a reasonably truthful statement by the youngster.

The reporting of joint pain and discomfort serves as one particular example. Certainly it has to be acknowledged that children's reports of pain are not always accurate and truthful. There are occasions on which young patients will deliberately exaggerate the level of discomfort experienced, and others on which they will claim it to be less than it really is. It is necessary to be aware of the sort of factors that may motivate children to offer a less than honest report; but it is also essential that team members constantly question the validity of the criteria they use in deciding whether or not a patient should be believed.

The kind of value society places upon particular types of pain behavior must always have an influence upon patients' descriptions of their physical discomfort. In general, White Anglo-Saxon culture does not approve of frank admission of pain, particularly among males and, therefore, boys from such a cultural background may well feel that dignity and social approval depend upon verbal denial of discomfort. In fact, a belief that social approval depends upon denial of pain may well be reinforced by care team members themselves. The young patient may discover that the doctor or nurse is happy to praise the 'bravery' of a youngster who does not cry or complain as a result of some potentially painful procedure, such as venipuncture, but that tears and other manifestations of distress may be met with signs of apparent disapproval. The child may, therefore, be forgiven for assuming that if he has to hide his pain on some occasions in order to please those responsible for his medical care, the doctor may actually want an untruthful response when he or she asks how the youngster's joints have been feeling lately.

There is considerable evidence that different cultures have quite different attitudes toward the expression of pain (Zborowski, 1969), and such differences obviously have to be borne in mind when assessing a young patient's pain. But, on the other hand, it has to be recognized that considerable individual variations occur within ethnic and social groups, and health care team members must always guard against any tendency on their own part to make rigid assumptions about a youngster's "true" level of pain by reference to the child's cultural background or sex.

Among other things, JA patients' accounts of their pain may reflect their thoughts or fears about the likely consequences of their disclosures. Children are frequently reluctant to admit how they really feel because they are afraid that this may lead to more unpleasant treatment, investigations, or hospital admission. But, conversely, there are times when youngsters may associate a claim of pain with the prospect of reward, or the avoidance of punishment. JA patients are still kids, and when their behavior has not been the best, they can quickly learn to use their illness as a means of obtaining parental indulgence. Pain may be invented or exaggerated in order to avoid school, particularly when examinations are looming, or the child is suffering at the hands of classmates as a result of arthritis. However, it has to be appreciated that pain associated with school avoidance is not always fictional.

If a young girl is being subjected to taunts from fellow pupils, for example, her emotional distress can cause her to focus her attention upon her ailment, thereby augmenting sensations emanating from affected joints.

The ability of emotional distress and selective attention significantly to affect the frequency, duration, and sheer unpleasantness of pain means that severity of discomfort certainly cannot be inferred from the patient's clinical condition (Beales et al., 1983). It cannot be taken for granted that two youngsters with similar physical pathology must inevitably experience similar levels of pain, and that if one claims more discomfort than the other, somebody must be lying. Pain varies between individual patients, and even within the same child over time, depending upon mood and situation. If a boy is prompted by circumstances to dwell upon his ailment, he is more likely to notice sensations coming from his affected joints, and his state of mind is likely to cause him to perceive them as more nasty and unpleasant than he might otherwise have done. The same child on a happier day might not even be aware of such joint sensations, having better things to think about.

Because youngsters' levels of pain cannot be simply deduced from the state of their disease, and because children's reports of physical discomfort cannot always be relied upon, it might be felt that a more accurate assessment of a patient's pain is likely to be accomplished by asking the parents. Mothers might be assumed to be reasonably conscientious observers of their children, and to have a pretty fair idea of when their offspring are genuinely suffering and when they are attempting to deceive. But unfortunately, in reality, parents cannot be relied upon either to detect their children's level of pain, or to report their own assessments honestly (Beales, 1982). For instance much depends upon the manner in which parents are themselves responding to and attempting to cope with their youngsters' chronic illness. Some will develop quite considerable anxiety, and will be on the lookout for the slightest indication that the disease is becoming more widespread or severe. Others will become overprotective and offer immediate comfort and attempts at compensation whenever their children indicate distress. Such mothers and fathers will be inclined to believe any reports of pain their children care to provide, and will be eager to ensure that medical staff take each report seriously and act upon it. By attempting to wipe away their children's tears with gifts and cuddles, many parents actively reward pain reporting, and so increase the likelihood that patients will detect every unpleasant joint sensation, and from time to time, resort to invention when the genuine article is not to be found. In addition, they provide their youngsters with limitless opportunities to claim discomfort by constantly enquiring about how they feel.

But if some parents actively encourage their children to voice discomfort, there are others who act in opposite fashion. A proportion of parents endeavor to minimize their own distress and apprehension by denying the significance or severity of their youngsters' illness. They are, therefore, less inclined to accept, and pass on to health team members, the children's reports of discomfort. They are motivated to find reasons for doubting the genuineness of any announcement of joint pain, and may actively discourage the youngsters from volunteering how they are feeling by regularly accusing them of exaggeration and reprimanding them accordingly.

In addition, parents cannot always be relied upon to honestly relate their own assessments of their children's pain to care team members. There are times when parents are motivated to overstate their youngsters' levels of suffering in an attempt to ensure that the condition is taken completely seriously by medical staff, and that every effort is made to combat the effects of the disease. Where parents are especially anxious, and (however mistakenly) feel that care team members are not doing all they could, they can resort to exaggerated reports of pain in the hope of pressuring staff to devote more thought and effort to their children. On the other hand, in some circumstances, parents can themselves come under pressure from children to hide the actual level of physical discomfort from the health care team. Children who feel that an accurate report will result in a hospital admission or further unpleasant treatment can sometimes persuade their parents to be less than truthful in their dealings with the doctor. The mothers and fathers of children with long-term illnesses are commonly torn between a desire to cooperate with medical treatment in order to combat the disease and a wish to minimize their unfortunate children's total unhappiness. Some children, if they try hard enough, can occasionally succeed in drawing their parents into a temporary alliance against health care staff, to save them from some immediate misery.

Even when children and parents are in agreement, therefore, the truth of what they have to say cannot be taken for granted. And when parents' accounts differ from those of patients, it certainly cannot be assumed that, of the two, the adult is more likely to be speaking honestly and accurately. There are many occasions when a young JA patient may be motivated to deceive or mislead care team members on a wide range of matters, but the words and circumstances of both patient and parent must be scrutinized very carefully before coming to any conclusion that the youngster's account of his or her own actions, thoughts, feelings, and symptoms should not be believed.

COPING AND THE ASSESSMENT PROCESS

JA patients and their parents may endeavor to minimize the emotional impact of the disease by a variety of means, but whereas some coping styles are generally compatible with the child's immediate and long-term well-being, others may provide initial comfort at the expense of future welfare. Adequate and ongoing assessment of coping behavior is therefore necessary so that, where appropriate, counseling can be offered. Yet, in addition to being a subject of evaluation, the means by which family members attempt to cope exert a continuous influence upon the assessment process, by affecting the content of virtually all their communications with health care staff.

Some families maintain a beneficial or potentially disastrous solidarity—depending upon the particular strategy adopted—by uniting on one common coping technique. They may, for example, attempt to dispel their anxieties and distress by actively and enthusiastically engaging in alternative interests and pastimes that the affected child is capable of enjoying, and by working hard to try to ensure that the youngster has as normal a childhood and upbringing as possible. Or they may perhaps shut themselves off from the "healthy" world that reminds them of their misfortune, and become immersed in a process of mutual commiseration. But in many other families, the business of coping does not foster unity, but instead generates, or reinforces, conflict. While the mother may be endeavoring to deal with her fears and maybe a sense of guilt, by overprotecting her child and demanding the best attentions of care team members, the father may conceivably be relying on overwhelming denial, refusing to accept the diagnosis of JA or to acknowledge the implications of the disease for his child.

Where the parents are adopting different coping techniques, in addition to having potentially serious consequences for the well-being of the family and the patient, this can result in very divergent accounts of the youngster's symptoms and activities being presented to members of the care team. The overprotecting mother may present a picture of a miserable and pain-wracked child, cut off from friends and subjected to taunts and ridicule at school, whereas the denying father's portrayal of his child may largely ignore unpleasant features and events, and almost exclusively involve firm accounts of things the child can do well.

Faced with conflicting parental accounts, there is a risk that health professionals will be inclined to believe that one parent's version is nearer to the truth than that of the other. Some male doctors show signs of accepting what the father has to say more readily, since mothers are assumed to react in a more "emotional" fashion and therefore to exaggerate the young patient's problems. But a father who questions the diagnosis too aggressively may cause some care team members to develop a preference for the mother, who manifestly values their professional skills, and, therefore, to be biased in favor of her version of events.

Many factors can influence the credibility of a parent in the eyes of those responsible for the child's medical care, but it should be remembered that all parents attempt to cope by some means or another, and their words and actions are inevitably affected as a result. Care team members must always guard against becoming unwittingly inclined to believe one against the other, and rather than interpreting anything at face value, should always interpret what is said in the light of what has already been discovered on the individual's method of coping.

Although extreme denial is utilized by only a proportion of JA patients and parents, some use of this defense is common in the coping strategies of family members. There is frequently a failure to acknowledge the worst possible outcomes of the condition, trying to keep the more depressing features of the arthritis out of mind. In fact, successful adaptation to the JA may be dependent upon selective denial. When children and parents are questioned on potentially distressing matters for assessment purposes, their responses may reflect more their desire to shield themselves from additional misery than their desire accurately to report their thoughts and actions. A youngster who gives a simple "yes" in answer to a question such as "Do you have any friends to play with?", may be stating a straightforward fact; but alternatively he or she may be trying to keep discussion of an especially painful subject to the absolute minimum.

If real problems and concerns are to be identified, apparently reassuring responses cannot be accepted without further probing and exploration. But in endeavoring to move closer to the truth, shields erected by children and parents for their own emotional defense have to be broken down or bypassed. Adequate assessment and evaluation can involve causing additional distress and suffering in every family. For this reason, there must always be an immediate link between the assessment process and the provision of counseling and support. Assessment and evaluation are only justified where they are necessary for the maximization of the long-term well-being of the family. They have no value and justification in themselves. Therefore, when a young patient or parent is taken to the point at which he or she makes an upsetting disclosure, this is not the end of the road, and it is not yet time for self-congratulation. Help and advice must be made available immediately, to try to remove or ameliorate the cause of distress in a way most compatible with successful adaptation to the disease.

CONCLUSION

Because JA affects the child as a whole, assessment has to deal with physical, social, and psychological dimensions. But, whereas it is possible to be reasonably confident that tests of physical condition will yield reliable results without significant risk of causing harm, monitoring and evaluation of psychosocial factors yield results whose meaning is always open to interpretation, and can generate considerable suffering in patient, siblings, and parents. In addition, although the development of formal testing techniques may increasingly allow more precise analysis of psychosocial phenomena, the scale of the assessment task—monitoring many complex issues over a period of years, and involving the entire nuclear family—means that the greater part of evaluation has to be undertaken by the various care team members in the course of their normal encounters with parent and child.

In fact, it is inevitable that health care professionals will make judgments and evaluations of family members on the basis of their contacts with them, and it is therefore essential to ensure that any such assessment is undertaken in a deliberate manner, with the main difficulties and dangers being consciously recognized, and results regularly and formally combined to produce an increasingly comprehensive and detailed picture. Above all, care has to be taken to ensure that, when sensitive areas are revealed, and stress created, assessment leads directly to treatment, with appropriate counseling being speedily provided. In this way, the assessment process can contribute to the immediate and long-term welfare of the JA patient and do more good than harm.

References

Beales, J. G. (1982). The assessment and management of pain in children. In P. Karoly, J. J. Steffen, & D. J. O'Grady (Eds.), *Child health psychology: Concepts and issues*. New York: Pergamon.

Beales, J. G. (1984). Juvenile arthritis: The "whole child" approach. *Nursing* (2nd series), *2*, 908–909.

Beales, J. G., Holt, P. J. L., Keen, J. H., & Mellor, V. P. (1984). Children with juvenile chronic arthritis: Their beliefs about their illness and therapy. *Annals of the Rheumatic Diseases*, *42*, 481–486.

Beales, J. G., Keen, J. H., & Holt, P. J. L. (1983). The child's perception of the disease and the experience of pain in juvenile chronic arthritis. *Journal of Rheumatology*, *10*, 61–65.

Bibace, R., & Walsh, M. E. (1980). Development of children's concepts of illness. *Pediatrics*, *66*, 912–917.

Burton, L. (1975). *Family life of sick children*. London: Routledge & Kegan Paul.

Gellert, E. (1979). Children's conceptions of the content and functions of the human body. *Genetic Psychology Monographs*, *65*, 293–350.

Mattsson, A. (1972). Long-term physical illness and psycho-social adaptation. *Pediatrics*, *50*, 801–811.

Mattsson, A., & Gross, S. (1966). Adaptational and defensive behaviour in young hemophiliacs and their parents. *American Journal of Psychiatry*, *122*, 1349–1356.

Myers, B. A., Friedman, S. B., & Weiner, I. B. (1970). Coping with a chronic disability. *American Journal of Diseases of Children, 120,* 175–181.

Perrin, E. C., & Gerrity, P. S. (1981). There's a demon in your belly: Children's understanding of illness. *Pediatrics, 67,* 841–849.

Whitt, J. K., Dykstra, W., & Taylor, C. A. (1979). Children's conceptions of illness and cognitive development. *Clinical Pediatrics, 18,* 327–339.

Zborowski, M. (1969). *People in pain.* San Francisco: Jossey-Bass.

PART IV

SCREENING AND PREVENTION-CENTERED ASSESSMENT

20

Assessment for Accident Prevention

LOGAN WRIGHT
SALLY FLAGLER
ALICE G. FRIEDMAN

INTRODUCTION

The topic of psychological assessment for childhood injury encompasses two concepts. The first is assessment of the child who already has been injured, seeking to identify difficulties related to the accident. This typically involves standard psychological and medical assessment to aid in the development of a treatment strategy. The second is assessment prior to an accident, designed to identify psychological and related factors that are correlated with risk for accidental injury. Identification of these factors may provide the opportunity for preventive intervention and thus reduce the child's risk of injury. This chapter is primarily concerned with the second of these two concepts. It will examine accidents in childhood in order to describe the current state of knowledge and to serve as an impetus for further empirical work in the area of childhood accident prevention. It is hoped that this material will better equip the clinician with an approach to assessing for accident potential and serve a heuristic function by encouraging further research in the area.

We will begin by examining the scope of the problem of childhood injury including an examination of correlates to accidents. We will also examine the major areas of injury in an attempt to identify factors that may be predictive of injury. Next, we will examine models used to conceptualize these areas. These models will provide the framework for the development of an assessment strategy. Finally, we will provide a general approach for identifying children who are at risk for accidental injury, given the current level of knowledge in this area. We will describe the development of one instrument designed to gather information about accidental poisoning ingestion, in the hope of providing a prototype for the development of similar instruments in other accident areas.

SCOPE OF THE PROBLEM

Childhood injury has long been recognized as the leading cause of morbidity and mortality in childhood. However, only recently has the study of accidents and accident prevention been considered to fall within the province of psychology. Past efforts, led by physicians and epidemiologists, have focused on the physical cause, treatment, and rehabilitation of injury. Psychology's contribution was limited primarily to the evaluation of the psychological, neuropsychological, and educational *consequences of* injury. However, during the past decade, a multidisciplinary approach to the study of accidents has emerged that has increased awareness of psychology's potential contribution.

Within the behavioral sciences, the rapid growth of health psychology has stimulated the development of strategies designed to eliminate unhealthy habits and maintain healthy ones (Carter, Bendell, & Matarazzo, 1985). Many deaths from childhood injury are attributable to risky behavior, such as driving at excessive speeds, drinking while driving, and so forth. Certain of these risk-taking behaviors may be altered by minimal changes and thus are seen as highly amenable to intervention (Roberts, Elkins, & Royal, 1984). To date, most accident prevention efforts have targeted behaviors related to seat belt and child restraint usage (Christophersen, 1977; Christophersen & Gyulay, 1981; Roberts & Turner, 1984), pedestrian safety (Limbourg & Gerber, 1981), and fire safety (Hillman, Jones, & Farmer, 1986; Jones, Kazdin, & Haney, 1981; McLoughlin, Vince, Lee, & Crawford, 1982).

Contrary to expectation, studies examining the efficacy of prevention programs on decreasing risk behavior have been, for the most part, discouraging. Educational programs appear to increase knowledge about risk factors but show little evidence of changing behavior (Cliff, Catford, Dillow, & Swann, 1980). Interventions using reinforcement contingent upon desired behaviors appear to alter behavior initially, but the changes have proven difficult to maintain. These difficulties have prompted criticism of strategies that require individuals to alter their behavior (so-called active strategies; Williams, 1982) and encouraged a shift toward a passage of legislation to reduce environmental risk via methods that do not require behavioral changes (so-called passive strategies, e.g., air bags for automobiles, flame-resistant clothing, safety cap bottles; Carter et al., 1983). However, reliance solely upon passive preventive measures is probably insufficient, since there are numerous problems that are not amenable to passive interventions. The most effective approach to prevention may require a combination of active and passive strategies, with active interventions concentrated on populations at greatest risk. Obviously an ability to predict which children are at highest risk for accidental injury would have enormous implications for the health care system. Preventive interventions could be made more cost-effective by targeting the population at highest risk.

In summary, accidental injuries cause more deaths and suffering to children than the next six leading causes combined. From ages 1 through 4, injuries cause almost half of all deaths and result in three times as many deaths as the second leading cause (congenital anomalies; Baker, O'Neill, & Karpf, 1984). The most frequent childhood accidents are motor vehicle mishaps, drownings, burns, poisonings, and firearm-related occurrences. Accident rates in this area have not improved appreciably during the past 30 years, while death rates from tuberculosis, influenza and pneumonia, and gastric–intestinal disorders (the previous second, third, and fourth leading causes of mortality in children) have declined by more than 85 percent during the same period of time (Baker et al., 1984).

In the beginning, researchers viewed injuries as random, chance occurrences that couldn't be predicted or prevented (Rivara, 1982). As such, they were seen as essentially not amenable to either scientific study or change. Eventually researchers began to take an epidemiological view to conceptualizing this area. This approach typically relies heavily on an *agent–host–environment interaction* model. Studies employing this scheme attempt to identify the agent of injury as the form of energy that damages body tissue, the host as the injured individual, and the environment as the physical and psychosocial situation in which the injury occurs. According to this model, injuries occur when elements of host, agent, and environment come together in a critical manner at a precise time. Most of the agent–host–environment studies have concentrated on populations who have already sustained an injury (Haddon, 1968). Consequently, these studies rarely focused on accident prevention. Haddon (1980) has subsequently developed a set of problem-solving strategies that can analyze a particular injury and formulate ways in which human behavior can be modified to control injury rates. Such an approach allows for a systematic treatment of alternatives that might help researchers develop reliable assessment techniques. Robertson (1983) has demonstrated how these strategies can be utilized to study childhood injuries.

Most scholars in child injury behavior now feel that injuries can be prevented, and that children can be identified who are at risk for accidents. And a highly stressful environment has emerged as the strongest correlate for injuries in children (Brown & Davidson, 1978; Husband & Hinton, 1972; Plionis, 1977). Further, certain accidents appear to be prevalent among children possessing different demographic characteristics. Once psychosocial, developmental, and other demographic risk variables are identified, assessment and prevention programs can be designed that should impact on these at-risk individuals. The following section will identify the demographic and psychosocial variables associated with a high risk of specific types of childhood accidents. This information will provide a framework for developing an approach to the assessment of accidental risk. This in turn should lead to the design of strategies for prevention programs.

DEMOGRAPHICS

Developmental Correlates

Injury mortality in most categories tends to decrease sequentially from ages 1 to 10. For example, death rates in fires are three times higher for children 1 to 4 than for children 5 to 14 years old (Marcusson & Oehmisch, 1977). Aspiration, falls, and motor vehicle occupant deaths also decrease after the first year of life (Baker et al., 1984). Age-associated differences in accident incidence appear to be related to children's cognitive and motor development. Preschool children appear to have limited ability to make causal connections between accident agents (such as fire) and injuries (Coppens, 1986) but are likely to expose themselves to these agents while exploring their environment. In addition, young children often lack the motor control necessary to deal safely with the physical environment and the ability to govern their own behavior, even if they are aware of the dangers associated with their surroundings. For example, a child who understands that cars can be dangerous may lack the impulse control to resist running into the street while pursuing a ball (Maddux, Roberts, Sledden, & Wright, 1986).

Differences in cognitive development, physical stature, and motor skills may help explain differences in both type and prevalence of accidents among children of different ages. Assessment of these variables in similar-age children may shed additional light on why certain same-age children are more prone to accidents than others. Differences in rate of cognitive development, self-control, or understanding of cause and effect relationships may interact with overall development to increase the risk for some children.

Gender Differences

Boys appear to have higher overall injury rates than girls (Rivara, Bergman, LoGerfo, & Weiss, 1982), but sex differences vary for specific types of injuries. Males have a higher rate of vehicle injuries, homicides, and suicides. Overall, the death rate is more than twice as high for males as for females for unintentional injuries, and more than three times as high for intentional injuries (Baker et al., 1984). The higher rate of intentional injuries in boys may reflect a cultural expectation that males should exhibit more risk-taking behavior.

Behavioral differences between boys and girls have been studied in an attempt to explain sex differences in injury rates. Gould, Wunsch-Hitzig, and Dohrenwend (1981) summarized 25 American and 10 British studies that analyzed behavioral differences between males and females. They reported that in 22 of the 25 studies behavioral disorders for males exceeded the rate for females. More recent studies have supported this finding (Bosco & Robin, 1980; Jeanneret & Frutiger, 1980; McGee, Silva, & Williams, 1984). Manheimer and Mellinger (1967) found a significant relationship between injuries and behavioral indices such as anxiety, being an exploring, independent, or daring person, roughhousing, and athletic proficiency, all of which traditionally have been considered masculine characteristics. Other studies have shown that boys tend to be more hyperactive, impulsive, and aggressive than girls (Brown & Davidson, 1978; Brown & Wilson, 1972; Langley, McGee, Silva, & Williams, 1983; Sibert & Newcombe, 1977; Wright, Schaefer, & Solomons, 1979).

Higher accident rates among males have been demonstrated repeatedly; however, gender alone does not appear to constitute the major risk factor. Prospective studies are needed to examine which behavioral or other variables among boys significantly increase their risk of injury.

Family Concomitants

Many studies have reported positive correlations between family dysfunction on one hand and risk-taking behavior and injuries on the other (Bithoney, Snyder,

Michalek, & Newberger, 1985; Husband & Hinton, 1972; Padilla, Rohsenow, & Bergman, 1976; Plionis, 1977; Sibert, 1975). One study (Beautrais, Fergusson, & Shannon, 1982) identified the following factors as significantly related to injury rates: maternal educational level, stressful family life events, and sex of the child. A second study (Wadsworth, Burnell, Taylor, & Butler, 1983) found that the child's sex and frequency of changing residence were correlated with injuries requiring hospitalization.

Family instability appears to be a strong correlate to accidental injury. It is as yet unclear whether children from such households exhibit behaviors that increase their risk or whether family instability exposes them to situations (i.e., unsupervised play, faulty drug storage) related to higher risk. Assessment of both family functioning and the child's and caretaker's behavior may help explain how these variables interact to increase injury liability.

Psychosocial Factors

The relationship between psychosocial stress and accidental injury has been repeatedly demonstrated. In a prospective study of injury in seventh grade children, Padilla and colleagues (1976) reported that children with high scores on a measure of life stress had over twice as many accidents during a 5-month period as those with low scores. In a study examining correlates to burn injury, Martin (1970) found a significantly higher rate of marital discord and parental concerns among the families of burned children compared to those of healthy matched controls.

Behavioral Concomitants

The majority of research on accidental risk and behavioral variables has been retrospective. Nevertheless, a relationship between certain behavioral or emotional characteristics and a high propensity for accidental injury *has* been well demonstrated (Wright et al., 1979). Children with a history of accidental injury have been found to have a high activity level and are frequently described by parents as hyperactive or overactive (Husband & Hinton, 1972; Manheimer & Mellinger, 1967). In one of the few prospective studies in the area, Matheny, Brown, and Wilson (1971) reported a relationship between activity level at 1 year of age and propensity for accidental injury between ages 2 and 6. The study of 47 pairs of same-sexed twins showed that the twin with the highest frequency of accidents was also the more active, less attentive, and more temperamental of the pair.

Children who have high rates of accidents have also been rated as high in both actual and verbal aggression (Manheimer & Mellinger, 1967; Viney, 1971). Child accident victims have also been described as impulsive (Fuller, 1948; Husband & Hinton, 1972) and emotionally labile (Manheimer & Mellinger, 1967). Carey (1972) found that infants with "poor" temperaments (irregular rhythms, high intensity, negative mood, and low in approach and adaptability) had a higher frequency of lacerations requiring sutures in the first year of life than infants with more positive temperaments.

Children with a high frequency of accidents may be less likely to perceive a causal relationship between their own actions and an external event. In a study of college students, Williams and Nichels (1969) reported that those who were accident prone obtained high scores on Externality on Rotter's I-E Scale.

Socioeconomic Status (SES)

Several studies have examined the relationship between socioeconomic status (SES) and childhood injuries. Most have shown that lower SES children have more injuries than higher SES children (Husband & Hinton, 1972; McFarlane & Fox, 1978; Sobel & Margolis, 1965; Wise, 1983). Drownings and deaths by opiates are higher in high SES groups (Samkoff & Baker, 1982). However, accident rates on lower SES children may appear elevated because their injuries are more often treated in hospitals (and thus more often reported), while higher SES children are seen more often by private physicians (Berger, 1981).

Behavioral Factors

Behavioral and psychological characteristics appear to correlate with a high frequency of accidents. Children described as aggressive, impulsive, distractible, and inattentive appear to have a greater frequency of accidents than children without such characteristics. Children from families with a high level of stress, few resources, marital discord, and little supervision appear to be particularly vulnerable. While the discovery of these correlations has lead some researchers to suggest that certain children are "accident prone," it is also possible that these children live in environments that place them at greater risk for a variety of childhood injuries.

Having examined the relationship between both demographic and psychosocial variables and childhood accident rates, we can conclude that a relationship exists between many of these factors and risk for certain childhood injuries.

MAJOR AREAS OF INJURY IN CHILDREN

While identification of variables associated with accidental injury helps to identify individuals at risk, it typically provides little information about the specific type of injury they may encounter. The following section provides demographic information about the common accidents in childhood.

Motor Vehicle Occupant Injuries

Motor vehicle occupant injuries are the predominant cause of deaths in children. At the same time it is known that reduction of injury can be achieved by the use of seat belts and proper infant restraints. Ninety percent of all infant auto accident deaths and 75 percent of all injuries can be prevented by proper use of infant car seats (Christophersen & Sullivan, 1982). However, a minority of automobile occupants actually wear a belt; and in teenagers and low-income individuals, usage is almost nonexistent (O'Neill, Williams, & Karpf, 1983; Williams, Wells, & Lund, 1983). Even when seat belts are mandated, there is rarely police enforcement of the regulation. Consequently, usage rates do not rise substantially.

The vehicle occupant death rate for males is substantially higher than that for females and peaks between ages 16 and 19. Paradoxically, driver education classes may contribute to these mortality statistics because they may result in members of a high-risk group driving at a younger age. In some communities reduction in teenage crashes has been observed following a decrease in licensure after drivers education classes were discontinued (Robertson, 1980).

Occupant death rates are highest in the southern and western United States. Death rates from collisions with trains are highest in the Midwest; this may be due to the large number of open railroad crossings in these areas. In the Northeast a larger ratio of trains go over or under highways or have gates and signals. Collisions with trees and utility poles are highest in the East, which may reflect both the abundance of trees and the close proximity of poles to roadways. "Rollover" accidents occur more often in the mountain states, possibly because of the grade and curvature of roads and the absence of guardrails (Baker et al., 1984).

Passenger vehicle occupant fatalities are most common in the summer months and on weekend (Friday and Saturday) evenings. Alcohol-impaired driving is one of the leading causes of passenger vehicle crashes. One half of all fatal crashes involve drivers who are legally intoxicated. Studies of alcohol-related accidents are affected by the fact that fewer than 60 percent of all fatally injured drivers and only about 20 percent of all those seriously injured are tested for blood alcohol content (Haddon & Baker, 1981).

Asphyxiation

Asphyxiation by choking or suffocation on foreign materials is a major cause of fatal injury for children under 1 year (especially those under 6 months). It ranks fourth for all children 0 to 4 years of age (Baker & Fisher, 1980). Aspiration of foods (both solid and regurgitated) accounts for the majority of all asphyxiation deaths in the first year of life and half of all asphyxiation deaths in older children (Baker et al., 1984). Fatal choking in children usually involved round-shaped products such as hot dogs, candies, or improper pacifiers. Often suffocation occurs from plastic bags, entrapment in old refrigerators, crib strangulation, and wedging between crib rails or beneath a mattress. Suffocation by fallen earth causes a significant number of deaths (141 in 1980). Males ages 10 to 14 appear to have the greatest risk for this last cause (Baker et al., 1984).

Death rates for Blacks and Whites are similar for asphyxiation by food and suffocation. However, the rates for Blacks are twice those for Whites for airway obstruction. Death rates are highest for low-income subjects. Suffocation rates are four times higher in rural areas than in large cities (Baker et al., 1984).

Changing practices in coding sudden infant death syndrome (SIDS) deaths have contributed to a drop of about 85 percent of deaths coded aspiration or suffocation since 1968. Changes in refrigerator design seem also to have lowered these statistics.

The Consumer Product Safety Commission (CPSC) now sets minimum dimensions for pacifiers, rattles, and parts for toys. The agency has also established standards for crib safety and playpen safety. For example, crib slats must be less than 2¾ inches apart. The CPSC's "small parts" standard, which became effective in 1980, also precludes the manufacture of products whose components can be detached for children under 3 years of age. This is consistent with the finding of Baker and Fisher (1981) that the size and shape of objects seem to be important factors in childhood airway obstruction and subsequent injury.

The relationship of plastic bags and suffocation has been recognized for more than 25 years. Yet an average of 20 infants die each year of this cause (Blackbourne,

1974), and some researchers (e.g., Baker & Fisher, 1981) suggest that the incidence is much higher than reported.

Drowning

Submersion is the third most common cause of unintentional death, resulting annually in approximately 600 non–boat-related drownings and 1200 boat-related drownings in the United States. About 500 additional deaths per year are vehicle related, and another 1000 per year are probable suicide and intentional incidents (Baker et al., 1984). About 85 percent of these deaths are male (five times greater than females) with the highest incidence in the age range of 10 to 19 years. Among young children (in the age range of 1 to 4) rates for Whites are almost twice as high as for Blacks (Spyker, 1985). In older children the rates are highest among American Indians and Blacks. As might be expected, most drowning deaths of young children involve nonswimmers. With adolescents, however, mortality seems to be more a function of drug usage and/or daredevil behavior than lack of swimming ability. Many boating accident drownings are attributable to too few personal flotation devices being available and boats that do not stay afloat when tipped.

A majority of drownings (40 percent) occur on weekends when recreational activities are increased and alcohol consumption is higher. For non–boat-related drownings the rate is highest for children ages 1 to 2, and 85 percent result from falls into water (Baker et al., 1984). Drowning rates are highest among rural residents and boating deaths are highest in the South and Northwest. In a five-state study of 1201 drownings, fresh-water drownings outnumbered salt-water drownings (Press, Walker, & Crawford, 1968).

Infant drownings also occur in bathtubs and large pails. The bathtub ranks second to the swimming pool as a site of child drowning in the home (Spyker, 1985). It was shown in one study of bathtub submersions that fathers had responsibility for the infants in the majority of cases, but closer scrutiny of the data revealed that an older sibling actually had immediate care of the infant (Pearn, Brown, Wong, & Bart, 1979).

Children of older parents or children who are members of large families are at greater risk from submersion injury than are children in lower socioeconomic homes (Nixon & Pearn, 1978). Dietz and Baker (1974) found that 47 percent of the drowning victims in the state of Maryland had elevated ethanol blood levels. Of 600 drownings reported in Australia, over one-third were directly attributable to alcohol intake (Spyker, 1985).

Pedestrian Injuries

Each year 2000 children and youths in the United States are fatally injured when struck by motor vehicles. Another 110,000 receive nonfatal injuries (National Safety Council, 1984). Pedestrian injury rates are highest for children in the age group of 4 to 9 years and a second peak occurs in the range of 18 to 19 (Guyer, Talbot, & Pless, 1985). Most injuries occur on local roads in urban areas (often as a result of children running into streets in pursuit of objects). The rate of pedestrian accidents for boys is greater than for girls at each age. December is the peak month for pedestrian deaths, and Saturday is the peak day. Approximately 80 percent of all pedestrian injuries to children occur during daylight hours, most between noon and 6:00 P.M. For adolescents fewer than 50 percent occur during this period; more occur from 6:00 P.M. to midnight (Baker et al., 1984).

Alcohol intoxication plays a major role in pedestrian injuries and fatalities. Wolfe and O'Day (1982) found that 14 percent of all drivers involved in fatalities and 8 percent involved in all nonfatal pedestrian injuries had been drinking alcoholic beverages. Baker, Robertson, and O'Neill (1974) found that driver negligence was implicated in half of all collisions causing pedestrian deaths in Baltimore from 1968 to 1971, and 58 percent of the drivers had poor driving records prior to the accident.

Researchers disagree about whether educational approaches to pedestrian injury prevention are effective with young children. There is thus disagreement about whether preschoolers should be taught street-crossing skills or taught to avoid street crossings altogether. Limited empirical data are available on this topic.

Limbourg and Gerber (1981) have found that preschoolers did more poorly than very young school-age (5 to 6) children in pedestrian safety programs. This was attributed to greater impulsivity, difficulty in discriminating right from left, inability to access time and speed of autos, and a lack of cognitive skills to make valid and consistent judgments about crossing streets. Fortenberry and Brown (1982) taught children 6 to 7 years old basic rules for safe walking, crossing intersections, and understanding traffic signs and regulations. Pedestrian injuries for this group were reduced by 33 percent. However, studies of other programs have shown that traffic education programs did not change behavior or reduce pedestrian injuries (Guyer et al., 1985).

It may be that modifying driver behavior is a more efficacious method of lowering pedestrian injuries. Much publicity has been aimed at drunk drivers and most states, with the help of Mothers Against Drunk Driving (MADD), have developed stiffer penalties for drivers found under the influence. Driver education and training programs may have an effect on attitudes toward the rights and needs of pedestrians. Harano and Huber (1974) reported that drivers who were rewarded for accident-free driving with free extension of their licenses and reduction in insurance premiums had a 22 percent reduction in accidents.

Burns

Burns and fires cause more than 6000 deaths (1300 children) annually, and more than a million injuries requiring medical attention (National Safety Council, 1984). In addition, the financial cost for treatment is often staggering. Children from 1 to 4 constitute almost 20 percent of the fatalities (Baker et al., 1984). Mierley and Baker (1983) report that high blood alcohol concentrations are present in about one-half of the adults who die from burns.

House fires cause 3.1 percent of all childhood deaths, a majority occurring at night. Burns are most likely to occur on weekends and from December through March (Baker et al., 1984). Most victims die as a result of hypoxia (smoke inhalation). Children under 5 are more likely to die in a fire than their parents (Reisinger, 1980). Nearly one-half of all home fire deaths are a result of improper use of cigarettes and matches, but in recent years an increase in residential fires has been attributed to the use of wood-burning stoves and portable heaters (Berger, 1981). Among Blacks and American Indians, house fire death rates are more than twice the rates for Whites. Geographically, the highest death rates are seen in the East, especially the Southeast, and often in rural settings (Baker et al., 1984).

The second largest cause of burn deaths involves ignition of clothing. The problem is second only to scalds as a cause of hospitalization for burn injury. However, the problem has diminished greatly because of the Flammable Fabrics Act of 1953 and 1967 as well as the Children's Sleepwear Standards of 1971 and 1974.

Scalds are a major source of morbidity, especially for children ages 0 to 4, and hot water is the leading cause of scalds. Spilling food substances (coffee, grease) is second (Baker et al., 1984). Children 1 to 3 years old are particularly vulnerable to burn injuries (Baker et al., 1984). As children become older, burn injuries are more related to risk-taking behavior and curiosity. Several studies have shown a relationship among burn injury and low socioeconomic status, overcrowding, family mobility, and family size. Family stress and family instability (alcoholism, single parent, isolation, and emotional problems) are also related to childhood burn rates (Nixon & Pearn, 1978; Williams & Bowman, 1958; Jensen, 1959; Knudson-Cooper, 1984; Libber & Stayton, 1984; Noyes, Frye, Seyman, & Canter, 1979).

Falls

Falls are the most common cause of nonfatal injury in the United States. They are the fourth leading cause of death due to trauma to the spinal cord and brain (Barancik, Chatterjee, Greene, Michenzi, & Fife, 1983). Head trauma is present in the majority of falls causing death.

About 1800 fatal falls are known to occur each year in residential institutions for the elderly (Gryfe, Amies, & Ashley, 1977). While more than one-half of all fatal falls involve people over 75, there is also a high incidence of falls in early childhood. The *death* rate, however, is much lower (Gallagher, Finison, Guyer, & Goodenough, 1984) in the younger group.

Falls are more frequent among boys than among girls, and injuries tend to become more severe and to increase with age (Baker et al., 1984; Garrettson & Gallagher, 1985). Black children have a 67 percent higher death rate from falls than White children. This may be due to aging homes, concrete play areas, lack of window guards, living in high-rise buildings, and lack of adult supervision (Garrettson & Gallagher, 1985). Northern states generally have higher fall-related death rates. Falls occur more frequently in early evening. Young children fall more frequently in spring and early summer months.

Falls occur more often in homes than any other place and, for toddlers, falls usually are from structures (tables, beds, walkers, changing tables, windows, stairs, and steps). Older children and adolescents fall from trees, roofs, ladders, and often while involved in risk-taking or daredevil activities (Baker et al., 1984).

Poisoning

While a substantial number of injury deaths occur annually among children, childhood poisoning actually accounts for less than 3 percent of the total mortality statistics. Many more children, however, suffer mild to serious injuries as a result of toxic ingestion. In 1984 the American Association of Poison Control Centers reported that more than 450,000 children under the age of 5 had been exposed to toxic substances (Litovitz & Veltri, 1985). Poisonings are also one of the most common injuries reported to emergency rooms (Steele & Spyker, 1985). Many other cases are probably treated outside the hospital setting (Chafee-Bahamon & Lovejoy, 1983). Prescription and nonprescription drugs are responsible for the majority of poisonings, while household and personal care products and plants are the next two most commonly ingested categories of substances.

Ninety percent of all toxic ingestions involve children under the age of 5 and occur in the home. Males are predominant in ingestion rates. The majority of all cases occur during the second and third year of life (Wright, Schaefer, & Solomon, 1979). The high incidence at this age may correspond to developmental behaviors common to children during this period (i.e., high mobility, inquisitiveness, oral testing of new objects, and autonomy). A second elevation of the incidence rate appears during adolescence. Among this group, ingestion is generally an intentional suicidal attempt or related to drug and alcohol abuse. Adolescent males continue to account for a large proportion of deaths resulting from drug overdoses. Mortality is lower for adolescents under 15 and for persons over age 29, Males 20 to 29 years old had much higher death rates than any other age group (Samkoff & Baker, 1982).

The development of individual psychometric instruments designed to identify children who are at high risk for accidents has just begun. The lack of such measures constitutes a major barrier to the development of prevention programs.

MODELS OF ASSESSMENT

In general, assessment is the process of gathering data for the purpose of making decisions about or for individuals (Ysseldyke, 1979). Testing is only one part of this process. Since assessment facilitates different kinds of decisions, it is important to look at different models that produce different decisions and to find those models that have the most effective use with childhood injuries. Several models that have been utilized by health care personnel will be discussed.

Medical Model

This model defines problems in terms of biological symptoms of pathology. The model assumes biological causes, and views sociocultural factors as secondary and less essential to assessment and intervention. For example, a brain injury due to oxygen deprivation is diagnosed without attention to sociocultural factors. While there is often a need for medical assessment, prevention and intervention may require treatment of conditions other than medical or biological ones. Thus a medical model is usually not effective for preventive assessment, nor is it particularly effective in guiding the long-term psychological treatment of victims.

Process Deficit Model

This model defines problems in terms of information processing or ability deficits related to cognitive, motor, perception, discrimination, language, or attention weaknesses. Where accident consequences are concerned, stroke and head trauma victims might be assessed in terms of this model. Likewise, infants who have injuries that affect CNS functioning (falls, pedestrian accidents, motor vehicle occupant accidents) would fall within this category. Where accident risk is concerned, the focus is on the relationship between development in a given area and accident risk. Assessment within this model examines both strengths and weaknesses and also may measure hypothetical constructs when no clear-cut physiological parameters can be ascertained. Normed instruments are often used for this type of assessment, including the WISC-R, Stanford-Binet, and McCarthy Scales for older children; and the Bayley and Brazelton Scales for children up to 36 months of age. Neurological assessment often relies on such instruments as the Luria-Nebraska and Halstead-Reitan Tests for Children, both of which are comprehensive neuropsychological assessment tools.

Criticism of the process deficit model has focused on the question of whether or not accident-related behavior can be broken down into separate information processing areas and, if so, whether or not such processing components can be remediated. Further, few methodologically sound studies have documented the interaction between processing skills and behavior. The reliability of many measures within this model, particularly those that emphasize specific information processing skills (e.g., the Detroit Test of Learning Abilities, the Illinois Test of Psycholinguistic Abilities, and the Visual Motor Integration Test), is poor (Salvia & Ysseldyke, 1978).

The Task Analysis Model

A third model for accident assessment is the task analysis model. This scheme is employed primarily in educational and work settings. Following injury, the levels of skill related to the different aspects of the accident-related task are evaluated. This can be related to prevention by identifying those tasks to which children with insufficient developmental ability are exposed. Programs of remediation break new tasks into component parts (e.g., speech development, walking, feeding, math, and reading) and alter new task demands to fit the accident victim's level of current functioning.

A major problem with the application of this model to the prevention area is that it does not take into consideration the psychosocial dynamics of the situation and the victim. In many occasions it may also be difficult to ascertain the level of the victim's abilities prior to injury onset. Remediation models based on this rationale generally focus on developmental and cognitive skills, often ignoring the affective or other psychological components of the victim's injury.

Social Systems Model

The social systems model focuses primarily on the social expectations for a specific accident setting (Mercer, 1979). The patient presumably interacts with a variety of social systems (family, school, hospital, peer groups) and assumes a variety of social roles. His or her role in each of these social systems carries different expectations for behavior; and it is important to know which people in each setting are most influential. By knowing the diversity of roles and settings, one can presumably develop programs for: (1) encouraging interpersonal ties that could lower the risk of certain children; and (2) enhancing children's ability to function in particular roles without placing them in hazardous situations. Intervention within this model helps the victim to develop the knowledge needed more effectively to analyze situations in light of the relevant social variables.

The Ecological Assessment Model

This approach constitutes a somewhat more complex variation of the social systems approach. It is concerned primarily with the interaction of the structural, affective, and organizational components of accident-producing settings. One premise is that people adapt and act selectively toward their environment, either because of instinct or because they are reinforced for such activity. Thus specific environments are presumed to have predictable effects on specific individuals. Lack of adaptive flexibility will produce higher accident risk in new or changing environments.

Assessment within the ecological assessment model examines the individual's naturally occurring behavior, the environment immediately surrounding him or her, and the ways these two phenomena interact. This model has been employed in population-wide prevention (Caplan, 1964) such as legislated changes in infant crib construction, child-resistant caps, standards of toy construction, package warnings, and age-appropriate designations for toys. Mass media efforts related to this model include programs for swimming with a partner, for using seat belts, and for educating children to say "NO" to potential molesters. Gump (1978) suggests that assessment utilizing this model should encompass both the objects and people in a given environment and particularly any "built-in," accident-related reinforcement contingencies that might be inherent in a given situation.

The Epidemiologic Model

An epidemiologic approach to the study of accidents has been utilized for more than 30 years. Armstrong (1949), Cruikshank (1952), and Gordon (1949) were among the first to propose this perspective. Only in the past few years, however, have preventive measures based on this model been developed. In applying epidemiologic principles to the study and prevention of children's accidents, one must first identify a host, an agent, and the relevant developmental factors. Gibson (1961) was the first to identify the necessary aspects of injuries. He suggested that accident analysis include who was involved, when, where, and how it happened, as well as all the possible circumstances preceding and following the injury. Many early studies provided good epidemiologic data on age, sex, socioeconomic status (SES), and, in some instances, behavioral or family dynamics. However, these data were often drawn from samples that were not randomly representative and were so small that generalization was hampered. Too, much of the data were generated by second-person reporting and "tainted" judgmental decisions on the part of parents, teachers, and physicians.

Epidemiologic studies have tried to address the behavioral and developmental aspects of accident risk. Temperament factors (i.e., those measured by Thomas, Chess, & Birch's [1968] Behavioral Checklist) have also been used (within an epidemiologic framework) to assess the influence of variables such as bonding and parental interaction on accident behavior. Likewise, preventing accidents by preventing interaction between the child and the "agent" has been the purpose of several studies. In some instances this has been legislated (i.e., developing child-resistant closures for aspirin, making pajamas flame retardant, taking lead out of paint, etc.). Training children to recognize and avoid hazards is a second method of preventing child–agent contact. The American Academy of Pediatrics has established the American Standards Association and the Consumer Safety Prevention Program to monitor and change health hazards. The design and manufacture of furniture, carriages, and toys for children must now meet more rigid safety standards. Also, many manufacturers have incorporated human engineering data into the original design of equipment so that the features of these articles do not increase the likelihood of accidents as a result of incompatibility between equipment and children's level of development. Many toys today have recommended age of usage, particularly when hazards may be involved (as in swallowing of small toy components by infants and toddlers, etc.). Epidemiologic approaches often examine the location of injuries and the rate with which children frequent accident settings. For example, open stairs have long been identified as an environmental hazard that can easily be controlled by the use of a stair gate.

Behavioral Assessment Model

Only recently has a behavioral assessment model been used to address injuries. This model encompasses a variety of approaches that rely heavily on direct observation and measurement. It incorporates both the social systems and ecological assessment models and thus has a broader perspective than most of the models mentioned earlier. Assessment and observation focus on cognitive, affective, physiological, and behavioral variables within the child, the structural aspects of the environment, and the interaction between the patient and the various environmental settings. Typical assessment strategies include interviewing, rating scales, ethographic observations, analogue situations, self-evaluation, and mental status evaluation. Interventions are more often based on a social learning approach (Keller, 1981). A strength of this model is that, once a target is identified, a method for change can readily be developed. Roberts, Elkins, and Royal (1984) suggest such a model for use with children in high-risk situations. Many health psychologists have proposed intervention strategies based on this model that can be tailored to specific individuals (Matarazzo, 1982).

APPROACH TO ASSESSMENT

Our review of the research literature illustrates that, to date, a number of behavioral, psychological, and situational correlates to accidents have been identified. However, the strength of the correlations and the predictive value of the variables have yet to be determined. Differences in accident frequency among children appear to be accounted for by three global sources: parents, home environment, and the behavior of the child. The extent to which each variable contributes to injury liability may vary depending on the child's age and type of injury. In a longitudinal study of toddlers, Matheny (1986) identified characteristics related to the three sources of variance that were correlated with injury liability. Taken individually, however, these factors were only modestly related to injury. Combinations of characteristics of the mother and home *did* provide moderately strong correlations to accident liability.

A complete understanding of the "accident equation" (Matheny, 1986, p. 170) would permit prediction of which children run the highest risks for accidental injury. However, before such an equation is possible, more information is needed about which variables are most predictive of injury and how these variables interact. This information can be gathered via carefully controlled prospective studies and/or through assessment of children who have been involved in accidents. This information can then be compiled into a "risk registry" (Matheny, 1986, p. 175) that is developmentally specific and that can be used to screen children.

The following section will focus on assessment strategies that may be useful to the clinician as a method of assessing accident risk, and to the researcher who is interested in gathering normative data about variables correlated with injury.

Developmental Perspective

Children of different ages are vulnerable to different types of injury. Rapid changes in the child's cognitive, motor, and psychosocial functioning result in changes in exposure to health hazards and the child's ability to interact competently with the environment. Whereas an infant is most vulnerable to accidents caused by a caretaker's negligence or mistake, a toddler's mobility and exploratory behavior ensure exposure to hazards in the home and outdoors. On the other hand, the school-aged child is far less likely than the toddler to ingest toxins found in the home, but is more likely to be involved in accidents related to recreational activities and risk taking (Maddux et al., 1986).

Assessment for risk factors should be guided by a developmental perspective (Maddux et al., 1986). Since young children are most dependent on environmental and family variables, more emphasis should be placed on evaluating these potential sources of risk. Likewise, assessment for adolescents should place more emphasis on evaluation of risk-taking behaviors, drug and alcohol usage, and recreational interests.

Setting

Children and their parents come into contact with the health care system for a wide variety of reasons. Appointments for prenatal counseling, well child care, visits to the emergency room, and consultation for behavioral or psychiatric difficulties provide the opportunity for the health care worker to assess the child's risk for accidental injury. The extent of the evaluation and the instruments used will differ depending on the setting in which the evaluation is being undertaken. Prenatal counseling sessions and well child visits provide an opportunity for the clinician to intervene early in the life of the child. Brief screening questionnaires can be administered while the parent waits to see the physician. The physician or health care worker can utilize both general knowledge about child development and growth and specific information about the child to determine what hazards the child may encounter. This information can be used to alert the parent of these dangers and to provide anticipatory guidance. Follow-up assessment can be accomplished at the next scheduled appointment.

Assessment during emergency room visits can be the initial contact with a child who has already been injured. Screening can enable the clinician to determine whether the child is at risk before the child returns home. An appointment can then be scheduled for more complete evaluation and intervention at a later date. In such cases, siblings of the injured child should be included in the evaluation. In addition, many of the children who are at greatest risk for accidental injury are also at high risk for behavioral difficulties. Children who are overactive, aggressive, and/or impulsive often find their way into the health care system through referrals made by school personnel or parents. A main thesis of this chapter is that the probability of accidental injury should be considered when assessing these children for other difficulties.

ASSESSMENT INSTRUMENTS

The goal of assessment is to obtain information that can aid the development of strategies to minimize identified sources of risk. Assessment may be undertaken for research purposes or by the clinician who has concerns about a particular child. Screening questionnaires, whose items were derived from epidemiologic literature, can be helpful as a global measure to identify children who, statistically, have a greater likelihood of injury. Once these children are identified, further assessment can be tailored to the particular child. Once it has been determined that more extensive assessment is warranted, an adequate approach should include assessment of the range of variables shown to be related to increased injury liability, including: parental behaviors; psychosocial factors (particularly family stress); child behaviors; alcohol and/or drug usage by the family; and parental understanding of responsibility.

There are currently very few assessment instruments designed to identify children at risk. However, there are a number of instruments (such as the Parenting Stress Index and the Child Behavior Checklist) that have been developed and validated for other purposes (such as assessing family stress and child behavior) but *may* be helpful for the purposes of screening and assessing these children. Instruments designed to measure variables that have been shown to be correlated with accident frequency also provide a strategy, albeit indirect, for assessing risk. The conjoint use of such instrument and demographic information should provide an index of risk and suggest a strategy for decreasing the risk. Further research is needed to determine whether such instruments actually have predictive value.

Brief Screening Instruments—Risk Identification

Demographic Screening Checklist. This is an unpublished checklist (Wright, Flagler, & Friedman, 1986) of variables that epidemiologic studies have shown to be related to certain injuries. The checklist can be completed by a health care professional based on information derived from medical records or interviews. The form consists of a list of variables associated with increased risk, with letters representing each type of accident relevant to the variable at the right of each variable. The type of accident that the letter represents is listed on the top of the page. The respondent is asked to circle the letters next to each variable that are applicable to the child and family. The total number of each letter provides an indication of the type of injury for which the child is at greatest risk. Higher numbers represent greater risk. There are currently no standardized norms to facilitate decisions about a particular child. However, this list along with other information about the child, his or her environment, and the parents can be compared to the professional's internal norms to determine injury liability. The clinician may find that additional items particularly relevant to the local population need to be added to the checklist. Results of the checklist can then be compared against subsequent accident rates in an effort to compile correlates to accident injury for a given location. This checklist is shown in Figure 20.1.

The Framingham Safety Survey. This survey (FSS; Bass & Mehta, 1980) is one of the few instruments actually designed to identify parental behaviors and environmental hazards that could endanger the life of a child. The FSS comprises three surveys: one designed for use with parents of infants and two designed for use with the parents of toddlers and young children. Each questionnaire consists of approximately 20 developmentally appropriate questions concerning childhood safety.

The questionnaire was designed to be completed by parents while they wait for the physician during a well child visit. The questionnaire is brief and easy to read. Each survey actually consists of two copies. Endorsement of the appropriate (safe) response results in an "x" in a shaded square of the second copy. Thus potential difficulties are easily spotted. Once areas of difficulties are identified, the physician can educate the parent about steps that can be taken to minimize or eliminate the dangers. The parent should be contacted again soon after the appointment to assess whether the appropriate precautions were taken. The questionnaire should be administered initially while the child is an infant and yearly thereafter.

Assessment of Psychosocial Factors

Accidents are more prevalent among children who come from families with a high degree of stress or marital discord (Wright et al., 1979). Therefore, an adequate assessment of the parents' perceptions of family stress and difficulties is an essential part of the overall assessment. A number of instruments have been developed for the purpose of measuring family problems. What follows is a description of a few of the instruments that may facilitate the assessment. For a complete review of the psychometric properties of the following instruments, see Keyser and Sweetland (1979).

Family Stress Questionnaire. This 37-item questionnaire (Metz, Allen, Barr, & Shinefield, 1976) was designed to assess parental attitudes, experiences, and family events. While the questionnaire does not assess accidental risk per se, it appears to tap major events that presumably impact on family stress. The questionnaire is brief, has a true–false format, and should be comprehensible to individuals with an eighth grade reading level. While the questionnaire was designed to serve as a screening instrument to identify children at risk for emotional problems, the first section comprises questions pertinent to accidental injury. The questionnaire can be completed while the parent and child are waiting to see the health care worker. Responses to the questionnaire may suggest the need for further exploration

Assessment by Demographics Screening Checklist

This checklist consists of a number of demographic variables which are related to specific types of accidental injury. Read each demographic variable on the left. Circle all the letters to the right of demographic variable if that variable is appropriate to the child and/or the family. The letters represent the specific type of accident most closely associated with each demographic variable. After you have completed the checklist, count the number of times each letter is circled and put that total in the boxes at the bottom of the page. The higher numbers respond to the types of accidents for which the relative risk is highest. A large number of variables circled indicates higher overall risk for accidents in general. A checklist should be completed for each child within a family and repeated yearly if the family is seen again.

	All Accidents	Motor Vehicle	Pedestrian	Drownings	Falls	Poisoning	Asphixiation	Burns
(Category Code)	A	M	P	D	F	P	AS	B
Active	A							
Large Family				D				B
Older Parents				D				
0-4 years old				D	F	P	AS	B
4-9 years old		M						
15-19 years old		M		D		P		
Family problems/ Discord	A					P		B
Low SES/Education	A	M						B

FIGURE 20.1. Assessment by Demographic Screening Checklist.

	All Accidents	Motor Vehicle	Pedestrian	Drownings	Falls	Poisoning	Asphixiation	Burns
High SES				D				
Child Frequently home alone	A							B
No Seatbelt usage		M						
Teen Driver		M						
Drug/alcohol abuse/ Parents	A	M	P	D		P		B
Drug/alcohol abuse/ Child		M		D				
Rural Area							AS	B
Emigrant Family				D				
Urban			P					
Cigarette user/ In home								B
Mobile Family	A							B
Male	A							
TOTALS								

FIGURE 20.1. *(Continued)*

and/or assessment of problem areas. More complete information can be gathered via interview or one of the more extensive measures to be described.

Life Experiences Survey. This 57-item self-report inventory (Sarason, Johnson, & Siegel, 1977) was designed to assess an individual's perception of personal life stress during the preceding year. Respondents are asked to indicate which of 47 events were experienced during the preceding 12 months, and to rate the events according to how positive or negative they were and how strong an impact they had at the time of occurrence. It is presumed that the life events are stress inducing and require the individual to make life changes. Families with high scores on this questionnaire are presumed to be experiencing a high degree of stress.

This questionnaire provides little information about injury liability per se but may be used in conjunction with other measures to assess overall risk. Standard administration of this measure to families would facilitate development of a data base from which to assess which family stressors are correlated with specific accidents or occur among children of certain ages.

Parenting Stress Index. This 120-item questionnaire (Abidin, 1983) was designed to assess the magnitude of stress between a parent and child, and to identify the specific sources of the stress. The respondent is asked to rate items on a 5-point scale according to how accurately they describe his or her feelings. The questionnaire measures stress from three sources: child characteristics, parent characteristics, and life stress. The questionnaire is easily and quickly administered, scored, and interpreted. The questionnaire was designed for use with the parents of young children (below age 3) who may be at risk for developing problems. A high score on the instrument suggests the presence of significant stress and stressors in the family.

The Parenting Stress Index is currently used in medical settings as a screening tool for pediatricians. It is sufficiently comprehensive to cover many of the areas thought to be related to increased risk for both accidental and intentional injury. It is longer, more time-consuming, and more intrusive than some of the measures described earlier. Consequently, it is best administered to parents who, based on previous assessment, are having some difficulties. Reliability and validity data for the PSI are presented in the test manual. See McKinney and Peterson (1984) for a thorough review of the instrument.

Assessment of Drug and Alcohol Usage

A number of the leading causes of accidental injury are closely related to parental drug and alcohol use. At least half of all vehicle crashes involve alcohol. Alcohol, drugs, and risk-taking behaviors make the parent less available and less diligent as a caretaker.

Interviewing parents may provide some information about their own alcohol and drug practices. There are few instruments that reliably discriminate individuals who drink excessive amounts and those who do not. The McAndew Schedule of the MMPI does appear to have some utility for such purposes (McAndrew, 1965). While the scale was normed on a population of alcoholics, there is some evidence that it may be sensitive to drug usage as well (Graham, 1982). For parents with known alcohol or drug problems, the possibility that their children may be in danger should be seriously considered. These parents should be questioned about their driving and recreational habits and care practices for their children.

Child Behaviors

Numerous rating scales and checklists are available to assess child behaviors. Since a wide range of behavioral difficulties appear to be correlated with accident risk, a broad range of childhood behaviors should be assessed. Following are descriptions of child rating scales that appear to have adequate psychometric properties.

The Child Behavior Checklist. This checklist (Achenbach, 1979; Achenbach & Edelbrock, 1979) consists of 118 items designed to assess behaviors and an additional 20 items designed to assess social competency. Parents rate, on a 3-point scale, the degree to which each item describes their child. The checklist is easily administered, scored, and interpreted and can be used to assess children 4 to 16.

Elevations of scales measuring aggression, hyperactivity, and delinquency may be predictive of potential risk and should alert the clinician to the possibility that the child is at risk for accidental injury.

Revised Problem Checklist. This 89-item questionnaire (Quay & Peterson, 1967; Quay, 1977) is designed to evaluate children 5 to 15. The checklist yields scores on six dimensions for each child: Conduct Disorders, Socialized Aggression, Attention Problems—Immaturity, Anxiety—Withdrawal, Psychotic Behavior, and Motor Tension—Excess. Children who obtain elevations of Conduct Disorders, Socialized Aggression, Attention—Immaturity, and Motor Tension should be considered to be at risk for accidental injury.

Assessment of Cognitive Factors

The accident literature suggests a relationship between cognitive factors and injury liability. A child's understanding about the relationship between accident agents (i.e., fire) and injury may be an important predictor of injury liability. Children who perceive causal relationships and have knowledge about safety-related behaviors may be better equipped to avoid situations that place them at risk (see Coppens, 1986). However, impulsive children may be at great risk for accidents even if they perceive causal relationships. Likewise, adolescents who perceive little control over their environment and attribute life events to luck may be unlikely to take necessary precautions to avoid injury while engaged in recreational activities (Williams & Nichels, 1969). Finally, parents who perceive little control over events in their lives or do not view their child as susceptible to injury may have a poor understanding of the relationship between actions they take and their child's health. See Becker and Maiman (1975) for discussion of the health belief model.

Cognitive style, understanding of causal relationships, and perceptions of control represent difficult variables to assess and a challenge to researchers. Typically, researchers rely on experimental (rather than widely available) instruments to assess such characteristics. For example, in a recent study, Coppens (1986) used latency to first response and total errors on the Matching Familiar Figures Test (Kagan, Rosman, Day, Albert, & Phillips, 1964) as a measure of a child's tendency to be reflective or impulsive. Similarly, Coppens (1986) used sets of picture sequence cards and a gear movement task to assess children's ability to perceive causal relationships. Other strategies based on Piagetian principles may be equally useful. Questionnaires such as the Health Locus of Control Scale based on the health belief model (Becker & Maiman, 1975) may have some utility in assessing parental perceptions of the child's susceptibility to accidental injury. Rotter's Internal–External Scale, one of the few instruments designed to assess cognitive variables that is widely available, may be useful in assessing adolescent and parental perceptions of control of their environment.

The Internal–External Scale. This scale (I–E; Rotter, 1961) was designed to assess the extent to which an individual perceives a causal relationship between his or her own behavior and an outcome. The questionnaire may be helpful for identifying parents and adolescents who perceive little control over their own lives. The scale consists of 29 pairs of statements. Respondents are asked which of the two statements they more strongly believe. Responses are tallied and yield a score for Externality. The higher the score, the more the individual perceives that events are beyond his or her control. See Green (1985) for a review of this measure.

Individuals who are involved in repeat accidents have been shown to have elevated scores on the I–E Scale (Williams & Nichels, 1969). However, further research is needed on the relationship between this measure and propensity for accidents among adolescents and parents of young children.

Interpretation of Assessment Results

Once data about the child, parents, and environment are compiled, the clinician will be better equipped to make decisions about whether a particular child is at risk for injury, and if so, which variables constitute the greatest risk. Unfortunately, there are currently no standardized norms with which to evaluate the child. Rather, the clinician will have to rely on his or her internal norms and clinical acuity to assess level of risk. However, each assessment should add to the clinician's data base and thus should serve to increase the accuracy of the clinician's decisions. Once areas of difficulty are identified, strategies can be designed to alter the variables that constitute the greatest risk.

ASSESSMENT FOLLOWING INJURY

Once a child has been involved in an accident, the goal of assessment should include: (1) identification of the circumstances surrounding the accident; (2) investigation of previous accidents and injuries; and (3) determination of the potential for repeat accidents. Identification of the circumstances surrounding the injury can be accomplished by interviewing the child, parents, and others who may have witnessed the accident. These interviews may reveal environmental hazards or behavioral difficulties that increase the child's vulnerability to injury and ability to cope with the environment. Discussions with parents may reveal information about previously undiagnosed disabilities such as a sensory impairment or hyperactivity. Alternatively, the interview may reveal that the accident was symptomatic of more pervasive difficulties such as family problems or inadequate supervision. Further, the information obtained can be used to establish a more complete data base about accidental injury.

The investigation of previous accidents and injury has at least two purposes. First, repeat accidents increase the risk for future accidents (Wright et al., 1979). Secondly, the possibility that the child's injury may have been intentional rather than accidental must always be considered.

The assessment of potential for future accidents should be considered via interviews, questionnaires, or, if possible, home visits, or lab simulations.

DEVELOPMENT OF ASSESSMENT INSTRUMENTS

There are few assessment instruments designed to determine whether a child is at risk for specific accidental injuries. As should be apparent from the preceding discussion, such measures would have to be sufficiently comprehensive to assess each variable correlated with accidental injury. The Children's Repeat Poisoning Checklist (Wright, Flagler, & Litovitz, 1985) is a comprehensive checklist designed to be administered to families who have had poisoning incidents. The questionnaire is currently in the process of being validated, and it is described here in the hopes that it may serve as a prototype for development of similar questionnaires for assessment in different risk areas.

The Children's Repeat Poisoning Checklist is a 116-item questionnaire consisting of closed-ended questions. It was designed to be administered via an interview. Questions are worded simply, often requiring a "yes" or "no" response. The interviewer is instructed to rephrase the wording of the questions when the respondent is having difficulty understanding them. The questions were designed to be answered in response to a particular poisoning incident. However, provisions are made for multiple ingestions. Items inquire about circumstances surrounding the incident, parental reactions to the event, behaviors of the child, socioeconomic factors, and parental behavior.

Initial item selection was based on a review of the accident literature. Lists of variables that, based on research findings, appeared to predispose children to multiple poisoning accidents were compiled. The questionnaire was then sent to experts in the poison control field (pediatricians and directors of poison control centers in the United States) for review and suggestions. The questionnaire was modified in light of the recommendations of these experts. The questionnaire is currently being piloted in poison centers throughout the country. Once a sufficient number of responses are obtained, analysis will suggest which questions are actually related to accident liability. Questions that are unrelated to accidental injury will be eliminated. The shortened questionnaire will then be subjected to studies to determine the predictive and discriminative validity of the questionnaire. Further study of the interrater reliability of the questionnaire is currently under way.

The approach to the development of the questionnaire on repeat poisoning could be used to develop instruments designed to predict risk for a variety of different accidental injuries. Once the psychometric properties of the instruments are demonstrated, they could be used to target children who are at risk for specific accidents for intervention.

CONCLUSIONS

Assessment for accidental injury in children is in the formative stage. Accurate discimination of children who are at high risk for injury from those who are not would enable preventive efforts to be focused on the appropriate population; however, at present the tools for such an assessment are not available. This chapter, as well as a number of recent works (i.e., Roberts, Elkins, & Royal, 1984; Roberts, Maddux, & Wright, 1984) is an encouraging sign that the groundwork is being laid for the development of such assessment tools.

References

Abidin, R. (1983). *Parenting Stress Index manual.* Charlottesville, VA: Pediatric Psychology Press.

Achenbach, T. (1979). The Child Behavior Profile: An empirically based system for assessing children's behavioral problems and competencies. *International Journal of Mental Health, 7,* 24–42.

Achenbach, T., & Edelbrock, C. (1979). The Child Behavior Profile: II. Boys aged 12–16 and girls aged 6–11 and 12–16. *Journal of Consulting & Clinical Psychology, 47,* 223–233.

Armstrong, D. (1949). Accident prevention: Introduction. *Public Health Reports, 64,* 355–357.

Baker, S., & Fisher, R. (1980). Childhood asphyxiation by aspiration or suffocation. *Journal of the American Medical Association, 244,* 1343–1346.

Baker, S., O'Neill, B., & Karpf, R. (1984). *The injury fact book.* Lexington, MA: Lexington Books.

Baker, S., Robertson, L., O'Neill, B. (1974). Fatal pedestrian collisions: Driver negligence. *American Journal of Public Health, 64,* 318–325.

Barancik, J., Chatterjee, B., Greene, Y., Michenzi, E., & Fife, D. (1983). Northeastern Ohio trauma study: I. Magnitude of the problem. *American Journal of Public Health, 73,* 746–751.

Bass, J., & Mehta, K. (1980). Developmentally oriented safety surveys. *Clinical Pediatrics, 19,* 350–356.

Beautrais, A., Fergusson, D., & Shannon, F. (1981). Accidental poisoning in the first three years of life. *Australian Pediatric Journal, 17,* 104–109.

Becker, M., & Maiman, N. (1975). The health belief model and personal health behavior. *Health Education Monographs, 2,* (4).

Berger, L. (1981). Childhood injuries: Recognition and prevention. *Current Problems in Pediatrics, 61,* 1–59.

Bithoney, W., Snyder, J., Michalek, J., & Newberger, E. (1985). Childhood ingestions as symptoms of family distress. *American Journal of Disease in Childhood, 139,* 456–459.

Blackbourne, B. (1974). Accidental injuries in children. *Clinical Procedures of Children's Hospital National Medical Center, 30,* 83–91.

Bosco, J., & Robin, S. (1980). Hyperkinesis: Prevalence and treatment. In L. Whalen & G. Tinker (Eds.), *Hyperactive children: The social ecology of identification and treatment.* New York: Academic.

Brown, G., & Davidson, S. (1978). Social class, psychiatric disorder of mother and accidents to children. *Lancet, i,* 378–380.

Caplan, G. (1964). *Principles of preventive psychiatry.* New York: Basic.

Carey, W. (1972). Clinical applications of infant temperament measurement. *Journal of Pediatrics, 81,* 823–828.

Carter, B., Bendell, D., & Matarazzo, J. (1983). Behavioral health: Focus on preventive child health behavior. In A. Zeiner, D. Bendell, & C. Walker (Eds.), *Health psychology.* New York: Plenum.

Chafee-Bahamon, C., & Lovejoy, F., Jr. (1983). Effectiveness of a regional poison center in reducing excess emergency room visits for children's poisonings. *Pediatrics, 72,* 164–169.

Christophersen, E. (1977). Children's behavior during automobile rides: Do car seats make a difference? *Pediatrics, 60,* 69–74.

Christophersen, E., & Gyulay, J. (1981). Parental compliance with car seat uage: A positive approach with long-term follow-up. *Journal of Pediatric Psychology, 6,* 301–312.

Christophersen, E., & Sullivan, M. (1982). Increasing the protection of newborn infants in cars. *Pediatrics, 70,* 21–25.

Cliff, K., Catford, S., Dillow, I., & Swann, C. (1980). Promoting the use of seat belts. *British Medical Journal, 281,* 1477–1478.

Coppens, N. (1986). Cognitive characteristics as predictors of children's understanding of safety and prevention. *Journal of Pediatric Psychology, 11,* 189–202.

Cruikshank, R. (1952). Epidemiological methods in preventive medicine. *Proceedings of the Royal Society of Medicine, 45,* 621–628.

Dietz, P., & Baker, S. (1974). Drowning epidemiology and prevention. *American Journal of Public Health, 64,* 303–312.

Fortenberry, J., & Brown, D. (1982). Problem identification, implementation and evaluation of a pedestrian safety program. *Accident Analysis & Prevention, 14,* 315–322.

Fuller, E. (1948). Injury-prone children. *American Journal of Orthopsychiatry, 14,* 708–723.

Gallagher, S., Finison, K., Guyer, B., & Goodenough, S. (1984). The incidence of injuries among 87,000 Massachusetts children and adolescents: Results of the 1980–1981 Statewide Childhood Injury Prevention Program Surveillance System. *American Journal of Public Health, 74,* 1340–1347.

Garrettson, L., & Gallagher, S. (1985). Falls in children and youth. *Pediatric Clinics of North America, 32,* 153–162.

Gibson, J. (1961). The contribution of experimental psychology to the formulation of the problem of safety: A brief for basic research. In *Behavioral approaches to accident research.* New York: Association for the Aid of Crippled Children.

Gordon, J. (1949). The epidemiology of accidents. *American Journal of Public Health, 39,* 504–515.

Gould, M., Wunsch-Hitzig, R., & Dohrenwend, B. (1981). Estimating the prevalence of childhood psychopathology. *American Academy of Child Psychiatry, 20,* 462–476.

Graham, J. (1983). *The MMPI: A practical guide* (8th printing). New York: Oxford University Press.

Green, C. (1985). The use of psychodiagnostic questionnaires in predicting risk factors and health outcomes. In P. Karoly (Ed.), *Measurement strategies in health psychology.* New York: Wiley.

Gryfe, C., Amies, A., & Ashley, M. (1977). A longitudinal study of falls in an elderly population. I: Incidence and morbidity. *Age & Ageing, 6,* 201–210.

Gump, P. (1978). School environments. In I. Altman & J. Wohlwill (Eds.), *Children and the environment.* New York: Plenum.

Guyer, B., Talbot, A., & Pless, I. (1985). Pedestrian injuries to children and youth. *Pediatric Clinics of North America, 12,* 163–174.

Haddon, W., Jr. (1968). The changing approach to the epidemiology, prevention and amelioration of trauma: The transition to approaches etiologically rather than descriptively based. *American Journal of Public Health, 58,* 1431–1438.

Haddon, W., Jr. & Baker, S. (1981). Injury control. In D. Clark & B. MacMahon. (Eds.), *Preventive and community medicine.* Boston, MA: Little, Brown.

Harano, R., & Huber, D. (1974). *An evaluation of California's "good driver" incentive program* (Report No. 6). Scaramento: California Division of Highways.

Hillman, H., Jones, R., & Farmer, L. (1986). The acquisition and maintenance of fire emergency skills: Effects of rationale and behavioral practice. *Journal of Pediatric Psychology, 11,* 247–258.

Husband, P., & Hinton, P. (1972). Families of children with repeated accidents. *Archives of Disease in Childhood, 47,* 396–400.

Jeanneret, O., & Frutiger, P. (1980). Accidents in children: The potential contribution of the pediatrician to the field research approach. *Pediatrician, 9,* 358–367.

Jensen, G. (1959). Preventive implications of a study of 100 children treated for serious burns. *Pediatrics, 48*, 623–630.

Jones, R., Kazdin, A., & Haney, J. (1981). Social validation and training of emergency fire safety skills for potential injury prevention and life saving. *Journal of Applied Behavior Analysis, 14*, 249–260.

Kagan, J., Rosman, B., Day, D., Albert, J., & Phillips, W. (1964). Information processing in the child: Significance of analytic and reflective attitudes. *Psychological Monographs: General and Applied, 78*(578).

Keller, H. (Ed.) (1980). Behavioral assessment. *School Psychology Review, 9*, 93–98.

Keyser, D., & Sweetland, R. (Eds.) (1964). Test critiques (Vols. 1–4). Kansas City: Test Corporation of America.

Knudson-Cooper, M. (1984). The antecedents and consequences of children's burn injuries. *Advances in Developmental & Behavioral Pediatrics, 5*, 33–74.

Langley, J., McGee, R., Silva, P., & Williams, S. (1983). Child behavior and accidents. *Journal of Pediatric Psychology, 8*, 181–189.

Libber, S., & Stayton, D. (1984). Childhood burns reconsidered: The child, the family, and the burn injury. *Journal of Trauma, 24*, 245–252.

Limbourg, M., & Gerber, D. (1981). A parental training program for the road. Safety education of preschool children. *Accident Analysis & Prevention, 13*, 255–267.

Litovitz, T., & Veltri, J. (1985). The 1984 annual report of the American Association of Poison Control Centers. *American Journal of Emergency Medicine, 3*, 423–450.

McFarlane, A., & Fox, J. (1978). Child deaths from accidents and violence. *Population Trends, 12*, 22–27.

McFarland, R., & Moore, R. (1971). Childhood accidents and injuries. In N. Talbot, J. Kagen, & L. Eisenberg (Eds.), *Behavioral science in pediatric medicine*. Philadelphia: Saunders.

McGee, R., Silva, P., & Williams, S. (1984). Behaviour problems in a population of seven year old children: Prevalence, stability, and types of disorder: A research report. *Journal of Child Psychology & Psychiatry, 25*, 249–257.

McKinney, B., & Peterson, R. (1984). Review of Parenting Stress Index. In D. Keyser & R. Sweetland (Eds.), *Test critiques (Vol. 1). Kansas City: Test Corporation of America.*

McLoughlin, E., Vince, C., Lee, A., & Crawford, J. (1982). Project burn prevention: Outcome and implications. *American Journal of Public Health, 72*, 241–247.

MacAndres, C. (1965). The differentiation of male alcoholic outpatients from nonalcoholic psychiatric patients by means of the MMPI. *Quarterly Journal of Studies in Alcohol, 26*, 238–246.

Maddux, J., Roberts, M., Sledden, E., & Wright, L. (1986). Developmental issues in child health psychology, *American Psychologist, 41*, 25–34.

Manheimer, D., & Mellinger, G. (1967). Personality characteristics of the child accident repeater. *Child Development, 38*, 491–513.

Marcusson, H., & Oehmisch, W. (1977). Accident mortality in childhood in selected countries of different continents, 1950–1971. *World Health Statistics Report, 30*, 57–92.

Matarazzo, J. (1982). Behavioral health challenge to academic, scientific, and professional psychology. *American Psychologist, 37*, 1–14.

Matheny, A. (1986). Injuries among toddlers: Contributions from child, mother, and family. *Journal of Pediatric Psychology, 11*, 163–176.

Matheny, A., Jr., Brown, A., & Wilson, R. (1971). Behavioral antecedents of accidental injuries in early childhood: A study of twins. *Journal of Pediatrics, 79*, 122–124.

Matheny, A., Brown, A., & Wilson, R. (1972). Assessment of children's behavioral characteristics. *Clinical Pediatrics, 67*, 1037–1038.

Martin, H. (1970). Antecedents of burns and scalds in children. *British Journal of Medical Psychology, 43*, 39.

Mercer, C. (1979). *Children and adolescents with learning disabilities*. Columbus, OH: Merrill.

Metz, J., Allen, C., Barr, G., & Shinefield, H. (1976). A pediatric screening examination for psychosocial problems. *Pediatrics, 58*, 595–606.

Mierley, M., & Baker, S. (1983). Fatal housefires in an urban population. *Journal of the American Medical Association, 249*, 1466–1468.

National Safety Council. (1984). *Accident facts*. Chicago: National Safety Council.

Nixon, J., & Pearn, J. (1978). An investigation of socio-demographic factors surrounding childhood drowning accidents. *Social Science & Medicine, 12,* 387–390.

Noyes, R., Frye, S., Seyman, D., & Canter, A. (1978). Stressful life events and burn injuries. *Journal of Trauma, 18,* 141–144.

O'Neill, B., Williams, A., & Karpf, R. (1983). Passenger car size and driver seat belt use. *American Journal of Public Health, 73,* 588–590.

Padilla, E., Rohsenow, D., & Bergman, A. (1976). Predicting accident frequency in children. *Pediatrics, 58,* 223–226.

Pearn, J., Brown, J., Wong, R., & Bart, R. (1979). Bathtub drownings: Report of seven cases. *Pediatrics, 64,* 68–70.

Plionis, E. (1977). Family functioning and childhood accident occurrence. *American Journal of Orthopsychiatry, 47,* 250–263.

Press, E., Walker, J., & Crawford, I. (1968). An interstate drowning study. *American Journal of Public Health, 58,* 2275–2289.

Quay, H. (1977). Measuring dimensions of deviant behavior. The Behavior Problem Checklist. Journal of Abnormal Child Psychology, *5,* 277–287.

Quay, H., & Peterson, D. (1967). Manual of Behavior Problem Checklist. Champaign: Children's Research Center, University of Illinois.

Reisinger, K. (1980). Smoke detectors: Reducing deaths and injuries due to fire. *Pediatrics, 65,* 718–724.

Rivara, R. (1982). Epidemiology of childhood injuries. I. Review of current research and presentation of conceptual framework. *American Journal of Disease in Childhood, 136,* 399–405.

Rivara, F., Bergman, A., LoGerfo, J., & Weiss, N. (1982). Epidemiology of childhood injuries. II. Sex differences in injury rates. *American Journal of Disease in Childhood, 136,* 502–506.

Roberts, M., Elkins, P., Royal, G. (1984). Psychological applications to the prevention of accidents and illness. In M. Roberts & L. Peterson (Eds.), *Prevention of problems in childhood: Psychological research and applications*. New York: Wiley.

Roberts, M., Maddux, J., & Wright, L. (1984). The developmental perspective in behavioral health. In J. Matarazzo, N. Miller, S. Weiss, J. Herd, & S. Weiss (Eds.), *Behavioral health: A handbook of health enhancement and disease prevention*. New York: Wiley.

Roberts, M., & Turner, D. (1984). Preventing death and injury in childhood: A synthesis of child safety seat efforts. *Health Education Quarterly, 11,* 181–193.

Robertson, L. (1980). Crash involvement of teenaged drivers when driver education is eliminated from high school. *American Journal of Public Health, 70,* 599–603.

Robertson, L. (1983). *Injuries: Causes, control strategies, and public policy*. Lexington, MA: Lexington Books.

Rotter, J. (1966). Generalized expectancies for internal versus external control of reinforcement. *Psychological Monograph, 80,* 1–28.

Rotter, J., Liverant, S., & Crowne, D. (1961). The growth and extinction expectancies in chance controlled and skilled tests. *Journal of Psychology, 52,* 161–177.

Salvia, J., & Ysseldyke, J. (1978). *Assessment in remedial and special education*. Boston, MA: Houghton Mifflin.

Samkoff, J., & Baker, S. (1982). Recent trends in fatal poisoning by opiates in the U. S. *American Journal of Public Health, 72,* 1251–1256.

Sarason, I., Johnson, J., & Siegel, J. (1978). Assessing the impact of life changes: Development of the Life Experiences Survey. *Journal of Consulting & Clinical Psychology, 5,* 932–946.

Sibert, J. (1975). Stress in families of children who have ingested poisons. *British Medical Journal, iii,* 87–89.

Sibert, J., & Newcombe, R. (1977). Bicycle injuries in children. *British Medical Journal, i,* 613–614.

Sobel, R., & Margolis, J. (1965). Repetitive poisoning in children: A psycho-social study. *Pediatrics, 35,* 641–651.

Spyker, D. (1985). Submersion injury: Epidemiology, prevention, and management. *Pediatric Clinics of North America, 32,* 113–125.

Steele, P., & Spyker, D. (1985). Poisonings. *Pediatric Clinics of North America, 32,* 77–86.

Thomas, A., Chess, S., & Birch, H. (1968). *Temperament and behavior disorders in children*. New York: New York University Press.

Viney, L. (1971). Accident proneness: Some psychological research. *Medical Journal of Australia, 2,* 916–918.

Wadsworth, J., Burnell, I., Taylor, B., & Butler, N. (1983). Family type and accidents in preschool children. *Journal of Epidemiology & Community Health, 37,* 100–104.

Williams, A. (1982). Passive and active measures for controlling disease and injury: The role of the health psychologist. *Health Psychology, 4,* 399–409.

Williams, A., Wells, J., & Lund, A. (1983). Voluntary seat belt use among high school students. *Accident Analysis & Prevention, 16,* 161–165.

Williams, C., & Nichels, J. (1969). Internal–external control dimensions as related to accident and suicide proneness. *Journal of Consulting & Clinical Psychology, 33,* 485–494.

Williams, H., & Bowman, N. (1958). A social study of burns and scalds in children. *Medical Journal of Australia,* 599–601.

Wise, P. (1983). Differential childhood mortality in Boston. *American Journal of Disease in Childhood, 137,* 538.

Wolfe, A., & O'Day, J. (1982). Pedestrian accidents in the U.S. HSRI research review. *Highway Safety Research Institute, 12,* 1–16.

Wright, L., Flagler, S., & Litovitz, T. (1985). The Children's Repeat Poisoning Checklist. Unpublished scale.

Wright, L., Flagler, S., & Friedman, A. (1986). Demographic Screening Checklist. Unpublished scale.

Wright, L., Schaefer, A., & Solomons, G. (1979). Poisoning, accidental. In L. Wright, A. Schaefer, & G. Solomons (Eds.), *Encyclopedia of pediatric psychology*. Baltimore: University Park Press.

Ysseldyke, J. (1979). Issues in psychoeducational assessment. In C. Phye & D. Reschley (Eds), *School psychology: Perspectives and issues*. New York: Academic.

Zuckerman, B., & Duby, J. (1985). Developmental approach to injury prevention. *Pediatric Clinics of North America, 17,* 17–29.

21

Measuring and Preventing Noncompliance in Pediatric Health Care

JUDITH R. MATHEWS
EDWARD R. CHRISTOPHERSEN

INTRODUCTION

As pediatric health care becomes increasingly sophisticated, child mortality has decreased and morbidity has changed. A large portion of pediatricians' practice is now focused on prevention of illness and on behavioral aspects of chronic illness (Haggerty, 1986). The emphasis on prevention and on the availability of good pediatric care has probably resulted in children having increasing experience with medical settings, personnel, and treatments. In fact, most children will be hospitalized before they are 21 years old (Wright, Schaefer, & Solomons, 1979), and consequently may encounter potentially aversive experiences in a medical environment. Children

Preparation of this manuscript was partially supported by grants from NICHD (Grants HD 03144, HD 18435, and HD 02528) to the University of Kansas Medical Center. Judith R. Mathews submitted this manuscript as partial fulfillment of the Ph.D. requirements, in Developmental and Child Psychology at the University of Kansas.

who have long-term illnesses may require ongoing treatment at home, at the physician's office, and/or in the hospital for extended periods of their lives (Haggerty, Roghmann, & Pless, 1975). Such prolonged treatment may result in child noncompliance in order to avoid unpleasant or restrictive treatments; or it may result in poor parental adherence due to regimen complexity, physical or financial barriers, or child noncompliance. Because there are critical differences in the focus of treatment between parents' and children's noncompliance, these topics will be discussed separately. This chapter also discusses assessment in two ways: first, strategies for assessing actual noncompliance; and second, strategies for assessing predictors of noncompliance. Finally, strategies that may prevent or reduce noncompliance will be discussed.

Definition

In this chapter, *compliance** is defined as "the extent to which a person's behavior (in terms of taking medications, following diets, or executing lifestyle changes) coincides with medical or health advice" (Haynes, 1979, pp. 1–2). A *regimen* may have single or multiple components; a *procedure* is a component of a regimen that may be a one-time or a repeated event and that requires the child's physical cooperation during a medical activity implemented by medical personnel. Procedures usually occur in a medical setting and may elicit fear and/or pain responses. The vast majority of studies examining *regimen* compliance focus on the parent's behavior, including failure to follow a recommended regimen, failure to keep doctors' appointments, or errors in giving medication (Epstein & Cluss, 1982). In contrast, studies of compliance to medical *procedures* usually focus on the child's behavior.

Unfortunately, there are no established criteria distinguishing compliance from noncompliance. Most published reports consider an acceptable level of regimen compliance to range from 50 to 80 percent (Epstein & Cluss, 1982). The degree of compliance needed to ensure acceptable treatment outcome probably varies with each regimen and illness. Although one might presume that the goal is 100 percent compliance with medical procedures, little social validation of acceptable levels of compliance has been undertaken. In fact, it is likely that expectations of compliance vary according to the age of the child, the procedure, and the personnel implementing the procedure.

Incidence

Initial parental compliance rates to short-term medical regimens (such as antibiotics) have been reported to be 66 percent without intervention (Rapoff & Christophersen, 1982a), but the rate frequently decreases during the course of the medication regimen (Rapoff & Christophersen, 1982b). Understandably, both long-term regimens and multicomponent regimens yield lower compliance rates (Rapoff & Christophersen, 1982a). These estimates may be high, however, due to reactivity (i.e., parent knowledge that compliance is being measured) or to the possibility that those parents

* Because this chapter examines compliance to both medical procedures and regimens, the term *compliance* is used here for consistency of terminology. The authors acknowledge that the term *adherence* is sometimes preferred when referring to medical regimens.

willing to participate in a study may be more compliant than the general public (Ramsay, 1982).

Few studies have examined the incidence of children's compliance when they are given responsibility for their own regimens. In a study of theophylline compliance in adolescents with chronic asthma who were regulating their own regimens, Miller (1982) found that only 10 percent had serum levels in the therapeutic range. Of 27 diabetic children, Simonds (1979) found that 66 percent reported their urine test results accurately.

Children's compliance to medical procedures has often been found to decrease as invasiveness and painfulness of the procedure increase. For example, physicians reported physical resistance in less than 8 percent of their patients undergoing routine physical examinations (Chamberlin, 1975). In contrast, in a sample of 115 children undergoing bone marrow aspirations (which are presumed to be more invasive and painful than physical examinations), 34 percent required restraint because of poor cooperation (Katz, Kellerman, & Siegel, 1980). Studies of "distress" in hospitalized children have included such measures as increased pulse rate and blood pressure, sweaty palms, crying, regression, and acting-out behavior (Melamed, Robbins, & Graves, 1982). Unfortunately, noncompliance is not always analyzed separately from these other measures, and consequently it is difficult to ascertain its prevalence in hospitalized children.

ASSESSING NONCOMPLIANCE

The most common ways of assessing compliance to medical regimens (from most to least objective) are drug or tracer assays, direct observation, pill counts, treatment outcome measures, physician estimates, and patient or parent estimates (Rapoff & Christophersen, 1982a). Each method has its advantages and disadvantages. For example, the more objective measures are less likely to be biased by parent report, but are more expensive in terms of time, personnel, and laboratory costs (Rapoff & Christophersen, 1982a). Table 21.1 provides a list of the advantages and disadvantages of each method. A combination of measures may be the most useful approach (e.g., a combination of self-report and assays). Parent- or self-recording can serve a dual function: as an estimate of compliance and as a reminder of compliance. Table 21.2 gives an example of a self-monitoring form for an adolescent learning to implement his or her own regimen for atopic dermatitis. It is important to keep the form short and uncomplicated, so that it does not require much time to complete, as complicated forms may result in inaccurate or incomplete recording (Keefe & Gil, 1987). Periodic assay, observations and/or pill count measures may then be used as reliability checks. Regular checkup visits can provide the structure for doing this, as well as giving the patient ongoing feedback that may, in turn, enhance compliance (Wright, 1973).

The most common measures of noncompliance in children undergoing medical treatment procedures have been rating scales and direct observation. Parents and professionals have rated the child's level of cooperation during medical procedures on a 5- or 7-point scale from extremely compliant to extremely noncompliant (e.g., the Frankl Scale by Frankl, Shiere, & Fogels, 1962). These rating scales are global and subjective in nature but can be of value in assessing the adult's perception of

TABLE 21.1. MEASURES OF ACTUAL COMPLIANCE

Type	Advantages	Disadvantages	Feasibility
I. To Medical Regimens[a]			
Assays	1. Objective 2. Direct 3. Quantifiable	1. Pharmacokinetic variations make them difficult to interpret across individual patients 2. Measures of compliance over short periods 3. Expensive as they require lab analyses	
Observation	1. Objective 2. Superior to patient or physician estimates 3. Can be done by family members	1. Obtrusive 2. May result in parent badgering child for noncompliance	+ (if done by family members)
Pill counts	1. Easily obtained 2. Inexpensive 3. Superior to patient or physician estimates	1. Rely on patients to return medication containers 2. Overestimate compliance by 10 to 50% 3. Pills removed may not have been ingested	+
Treatment outcome	1. Identify patients who fail to improve (e.g., repeat throat cultures with strep) 2. Available and frequently used by physicians	1. Relationship to compliance inexact or unknown 2. Factors other than patient compliance affect treatment outcome	+
Physician estimates	1. Requires little time and effort 2. More accurate than patient estimates	1. Less accurate than pill counts, observation, and assays 2. Accuracy of estimates not related to physician's familiarity with patient or number of years the physician has been practicing	+
Patient estimates	1. Easily obtained 2. Accurate when patients are grossly noncompliant	1. Overestimates compliance 2. Less accurate than pill counts, assays, and physician estimates	+

TABLE 21.1. *(Continued)*

Type	Advantages	Disadvantages	Feasibility
II. To Medical Procedures[b]			
Behavioral observation	1. Objective 2. Direct 3. Quantifiable 4. Can determine patterns of interaction 4. Can determine patterns of interaction	1. Time-consuming 2. Requires operational definitions 3. Difficult to implement without independent observer	0
Rating scales Independent observer Medical personnel Parent (From most to least objective)	1. Easily obtained 2. Requires little time and effort	1. Subjective 2. May not be high agreement between observers or between rating scales and behavioral observations	+

Note: + = can be feasibly implemented by primary medical personnel; 0 = less feasible for primary medical personnel to implement.

[a]In this chapter, a medical regimen is defined as "the extent to which a person's behavior (in terms of taking medications, following diets, or executing lifestyle changes" coincides with medical or health advice" (Haynes, 1979, pp. 1–2).

[b]A medical procedure is defined as "a component of a regimen that may be a one-time or repeated event and that requires the child's physical cooperation during a medical activity implemented by medical personnel" (see text).

(*Source*: From "Improving Compliance in Pediatric Practice" by M. A. Rapoff and E. R. Christophersen, 1982, *Pediatric Clinics of North America, 29*, p. 341. Reprinted by permission.)

TABLE 21.2. EXAMPLE OF SELF-MONITORING FORM

Name: Sarah Month: May

Topic: Atopic Dermatitis Checklist

Check off each time you complete a part of your treatment:

1. Take a 15-minute sitz bath each morning.
2. Apply the cream and gauze to your legs, arms, and body. (See list on wall for the order of applying them.)
3. At noon, look at your counter and mark the number of times you scratched during the morning. Reset the counter at 0 and record again at bedtime.
4. Practice relaxation exercises before bed or when you begin itching.

Date	Bath	Cream and Gauze	Scratching		Practice Relaxation?	Comments
			A.M.	P.M.		
1						
2						
3						
4						
5						
6						
7						
8						
9						
10						
11						
12						
13						
14						
15						
16						
17						
18						

TABLE 21.2. *(Continued)*

Date	Bath	Cream and Gauze	Scratching A.M.	Scratching P.M.	Practice Relaxation?	Comments
19						
20						
21						
22						
23						
24						
25						
26						
27						
28						
29						
30						
31						

Notes:

TABLE 21.3. BEHAVIORAL ASSESSMENT OF CHILD NONCOMPLIANCE DURING MEDICAL PROCEDURES

Scale	Authors	Use	Weighted?	Number of Compliance Items / Total Number of Items	Operational Definitions
North Carolina Behavior Rating Scale (NCBRS)	Chambers, Fields, & Machen (1981)	Dentistry	No	5/8	Head movement High-hands Torso-trunk movement Leg movement Oral–physical resistance
Observation Scale of Behavioral Distress (OSBD)	Jay & Elliott (1983)	Bone marrow aspirations	Yes (1–4)	2/11	Physical resistance (4) Flail (4)

Procedure Behavioral Rating Scale (PBRS)	Katz, Kellerman, & Siegel (1980)	Bone marrow aspirations	No	5/13	Restrain Carry Flail Refusal position Cling
Behavior Profile Rating Scale (BPRS)	Melamed (1979)	Dentistry	Yes (1–5)	14/27	Clings to mother (4) Refuses to leave mother (4) Bodily carried in (5) Inappropriate mouth closing (1) Won't sit back (2) Attempts to dislodge instrument (2) Refuses to open mouth (3) Restraints used (4) Kicks (4) Stands up (4) Rolls over (4) Dislodges instruments (5) Refuses to sit in chair (5) Leaves chair (5)

the child's behavior (McMahon, 1984). While they are less objective, these global ratings have been positively correlated with direct behavioral observations, using a complex coding system (Katz et al., 1980; Melamed, 1979). They are simple to administer and are particularly useful in conjunction with direct observation.

Recently, detailed behavioral coding systems have been developed to provide a more objective analysis of the child's behavior. Most observation codes have targeted "anxious" and/or pain behaviors and consequently have included non-complaint behavior (e.g., hitting, physical resistance, refusal to open mouth) as well as less disruptive behaviors (e.g., crying, muscular rigidity, white knuckles, and verbal complaints). Table 21.3 provides a list of some commonly used behavioral scales, their operational definitions of noncompliance, and the proportion of non-compliance items relative to the overall score. Some scales have weighted the behaviors according to their severity and/or disruptiveness, thus assigning a higher score to presumably more unacceptable behaviors (e.g., the Behavior Profile Rating Scale by Melamed, 1979; the Observation Scale of Behavioral Distress by Jay, Ozolins, & Elliott, 1983). Of 11 behaviors, Jay and colleagues (1983) weighted the only two measures of physical noncompliance as highest in intensity. Others have rated all behaviors with equal weighting (e.g., the Procedure Behavioral Rating Scale by Katz et al., 1980). The behaviors are rated by independent observers in fixed intervals, and in most cases interobserver reliability is reported. Jay and Elliott (1984) found that there was little difference between recording the behavior at four phases of the procedure and recording it every 15 seconds, suggesting that the less rigorous approach may well be sufficient.

Unfortunately, noncompliance is often evaluated globally with other behaviors, which may cause confusion as to what is being measured. While measures of stress, fear, and/or pain are all important components in assessing a child's response to medical procedures, it is important to measure these components separately (Shacham & Daut, 1981). Those studies that *have* analyzed the behaviors separately (e.g., Katz et al., 1980) offer more precise implications for appropriate, individualized intervention strategies.

Assessment of actual noncompliance is important in identifying when there is a problem and in selecting potential intervention strategies for the noncompliant parent or child. Assessment of *predictors* of noncompliance may actually prevent the problem from occurring. The following section will discuss ways of identifying such predictors.

ASSESSING PREDICTORS OF NONCOMPLIANCE

It is sometimes difficult to measure noncomplaint behavior accurately due to imprecise definitions or differing criteria for acceptable levels of compliance. It is even more difficult to assess predictors of noncompliance. Clearly, factors apparently predictive of noncompliance are correlational, not necessarily causal. Nonetheless, research aimed at identifying children and parents at risk for noncompliance is an important line of investigation.

Table 21.4 provides an overview of factors thought to contribute to parental and child noncompliance. This section will review these factors and discuss strategies for assessing them individually.

TABLE 21.4. FACTORS CONTRIBUTING TO COMPLIANCE

Factors	Effect on Compliance		
	Impede	Promote	No Effect
I. Parent Compliance[a]			
A. Demographics (general)			
1. Age extremes (very young and old)	X		
2. Females	X		
3. Low socioeconomic status	X		
B. Regimen characteristics			
1. Several different medications	X		
2. Frequency of dosage (greater than four times daily)	X		
3. Side effects	X		X
4. Behavioral restrictions/life-style changes required	X		
5. Taste of oral meds (especially with younger children)	X		
6. Alternative meds for same condition			X
7. Duration of treatment	X		
C. Illness			
1. Delayed negative effects of stopping treatment	X		
2. Patients asymptomatic or in remission	X		
3. Psychiatric conditions (e.g., schizophrenia)	X		
4. Increasing symptoms	X		
5. Increased disability		X	
6. Severity of symptoms			X
D. Other			
1. Patient knowledge of illness			X
2. Continuity of care (physician familiar with patient)		X	
3. Health beliefs and perceptions	X	X	
II. Child Compliance			
A. Demographics			
Social class			X
Under 6 years old	X		
Developmental delay	X		
B. Predisposing factors			
Child's health beliefs[b]	X	X	
Child's use of multiple coping strategies		X	
Child's coping style[b]	X	X	
C. Antecedent factors			
Previous experience:			
Painless procedures		X	
Painful procedures	X		
Parent presence[b]	X		X
Peer modeling		X	
Medical personnel's behavior:			
Clear instructions		X	
Immediate reinforcement		X	
Physical affection		X	
Questioning for feeling		X	
Reassurance			X
Distraction[b]		X	X

[a]From Rapoff & Christophersen, 1982b.
[b]Data not conclusive

Parent Compliance

The focus of compliance with pediatric regimens often targets parents' behavior, since parents are usually responsible for monitoring and implementing the regimen. Factors that have been examined include demographic and predisposing variables as well as the doctor–patient relationship.

Factors. Some studies have found an association between noncompliance with medical regimens and age extremes (i.e., youthful and elderly) (Rapoff & Christophersen, 1982a); lower education and income (Shope, 1981); and single, employed mothers (Rapoff & Christophersen, 1982a). However, other studies have found no correlations between compliance and any demographic variables (Webb et al., 1984).

Some authors have suggested that compliance with a physician's recommendations can be predicted by the patient's or parents' health beliefs (i.e., whether the patient recognizes the need for medical treatment and believes that the treatment will improve his or her health). However, a clear correlation between such beliefs and compliance has rarely been established empirically (Becker et al., 1979).

An illness that has asymptomatic periods and is of longer duration has a poorer prognosis for compliance (Anderson & Kirk, 1982). Increased compliance has been associated, however, with increasing physical disability (Rapoff & Christophersen, 1982a) and previous experience with the disease (Shope, 1981). Kasl (1975) suggests that regimen characteristics are more reliable predictors of compliance than patient characteristics. Generally, the more complex and the longer the regimen, the higher the likelihood of noncompliance (Rapoff & Christophersen, 1982a). Other factors contributing to noncompliance include: (1) noxious-tasting medication (Klein & Ziering, 1983); (2) adverse side effects (Anderson & Kirk, 1982); (3) high cost of medicine; (4) increased frequency and number of medications; and (5) restrictions or interference with life-style (Haynes, 1979).

Structural and pharmaceutical barriers may also impede compliance. For example, transportation or financial problems as well as illness in the family have all been found to be predictive of poor compliance with appointment keeping (Francis, Korsch, & Morris, 1969). Increased waiting time during appointments and long lag time between referral and appointment have also been associated with decreased compliance (Haynes, 1979). Mattar, Markello, and Yaffe (1975) evaluated pharmaceutical factors contributing to noncompliance with prescribed regimens for otitis media and found that much of the surprisingly low compliance level of 5 percent could be attributed to poor or inaccurate labeling, underfilling of prescriptions, difficulty obtaining the medication through the pharmacy, and lack of standardization of teaspoon size.

Another barrier can be the parents' knowledge. Lower formal education or poor parent knowledge of the disease, medication, or regimen have been associated with noncompliance (Kasl, 1975). Lack of family support, peer or family advice discrepant from the physician's (Becker & Green, 1975), and teacher pressure (Firestone, 1982) were also found to contribute to noncompliance.

Parents' embarrassment over public manifestations of their child's illness or regimen administration can either increase or decrease compliance. In the former instance, for example, parents have been found to demonstrate higher compliance, apparently in order to avoid the embarrassment of an asthma attack in public (Radius et al., 1978). In contrast, parents are more likely to avoid administering medication in public (Bartlett, 1984).

The child's behavior can also be a major contributing factor to compliance. It has been found that parents are more likely to be noncompliant if the child resists the regimen (Firestone, 1982), particularly if the parent is single and administration of medication requires two people (Mattar et al., 1975).

Finally, higher parental compliance has been found when continuing care is from the same provider (Mattar & Yaffee, 197), when the parent considers the physician skilled, friendly, and empathic (Freemon, Negrete, Davis, & Korsch, 1971), and when physician instructions are clear and concise (Hulka, 1979).

Assessment Strategies. Many of the factors just discussed can be assessed by taking a thorough medical history. For example, Table 21.5 is a questionnaire developed by the authors and based on a compilation of individual factors that have been found to be predictive of noncompliance. While this questionnaire has not yet been validated, it offers a guideline for medical personnel of those factors thought to be predictive of medical noncompliance. Litt, Cuskey, and Rudd (1980) examined factors correlated with noncompliance to oral contraceptives in adolescents and condensed their findings into six variables that were predictive of noncompliance in 72 percent of their patients. Because several of the predictive variables were demographic and consequently unchangeable, this is a good example of how the variables can be used to identify at-risk patients, but may not indicate appropriate intervention strategies. Consequently, once such individuals can be identified, interventions designed to prevent noncompliance are a compelling focus for research.

A questionnaire such as presented in Table 21.5 can provide the physician with a focus for further investigation. A score of 3 on any individual item may indicate high risk for that particular factor. An overall cutoff score indicating that a patient is at high risk for noncompliance can only be determined once this measure is validated. The following section will discuss ways of assessing in more detail those individual factors placing the individual at risk for noncompliance.

Although not feasible for routine clinical assessment, videotaping or audiotaping clinic interviews can be useful training or research tools for assessing the interaction between the physician and patient. They may also provide cues to parental noncompliance that may have been missed during the interview.

Child Compliance

A few studies have examined child characteristics that may be predictive of noncompliance to overall regimens; these studies usually are focused on adolescents, many of whom are responsible for their own regimens. The vast majority of studies, however, examine factors associated with child compliance to specific procedures that require physical cooperation.

Factors. In being questioned about the reasons for their diabetic children's noncompliance to a prescribed regimen, parents reported the following explanations: (1) personality trait (e.g., stubbornness); (2) physical reasons (e.g., not feeling well); (3) denial (e.g., not wanting to be different from others); (4) hedonism (e.g., in-

TABLE 21.5. COMPLIANCE SCREENING INDEX

Parent Form

Child's Name: ____________ Date: ____________

Person Completing Form: ____________

Instructions: Please provide some information about yourself and your child so that we can adapt our medical recommendations to your child's individual needs. Place a check or X in the box to the right of the answer that applies best to you. Questions with an * should probably be answered after your first appointment, unless you have seen this doctor before.

	1		2		3		Comments
A. Parents 1. Age, primary caregiver	30–50		20–30 50–60		under 20 over 60		
2. Income	more than $30,000		$15–30,000		less than $15,000		
3. Financial problems	none		some		severe		
4. Highest grade of education	University		12		less than 12		
5. Marital status	married		separated		single/divorced		
6. How would you rate your marriage?	good		fair		poor		
7. Transportation problems?	none		some		severe		
8. How important is it to get medical advice when your child is ill?	very		somewhat		very little		
9. How important is it to get medical advice for your child's present illness?	very		somewhat		very little		
10. Is your child's illness embarrassing?	no		sometimes		yes		
11. How many relatives live near you?	many		a few		none		
12. Do your relatives support your decisions about your child's health?	very		neutral		not at all		

TABLE 21.5. *(Continued)*

	1		2		3		Comments
13. When your child is going to have a medical procedure, how anxious are you?	not very		somewhat		very		
*14. Do you think your doctor makes good decisions about your child's health?	yes		maybe		no		
*15. How understanding do you find your doctor?	very		somewhat		not at all		
*16. How well do you understand your child's illness?	quite well		somewhat		very little		
*17. Do you think the present recommendations will help?	yes		maybe		no		
B. Child							
18. Age	over 7		5–6		under 5		
19. Does your child have any delays in language?	no		mild		moderate–severe		
20. Does your child have any delays in motor development?	no		mild		moderate–severe		
21. Does your child have learning problems?	no		mild		moderate–severe		
22. Does your child have any other disabilities? (list)	no		mild		moderate–severe		
23. Describe your child's behavior at home	acceptable		some problems		many problems		

(Table continues on p. 534.)

TABLE 21.5. *(Continued)*

	1		2		3		Comments
24. How does your child react to medical people?	positive		neutral		negative		
25. How has your child reacted to taking medication in the past?	no problems		some problems		refused		
26. How has your child reacted to medical procedures in the past?	no problems		some problems		refused		
27. How anxious is your child before having a medical procedure?	not very		somewhat		very		
*28. How well does your child understand his or her illness?	very well		average		very little		

Other Information

A. Do you prefer to be present during medical procedures? Yes ____ No ____

B. What techniques have helped your child during medical procedures?

distraction ____
imagery____
relaxation____
watching another child ____
clenching fist ____
praise ____

C. What is your family routine?

Morning:

Afternoon:

Evening:

D. Other comments:

TABLE 21.5. *(Continued)*

Physician Form

A. Child's Name: ________________ Date: ________________

Physician's Name: ________________________

Instructions: This questionnaire is probably best used as a screening tool with new patients. However, as regimens change, it may be useful as a review of the child's and parents' status. It may be best to have the primary caregiver complete the questions with * at the end of the first appointment or between appointments. Then complete the following form yourself. Each subscore is computed by adding the items checked and dividing by the total possible number. There are some items that may not always apply; therefore, the total possible score may vary. An overall score may be derived by adding the two subtotals. Any items that are checked in the third column warrant further investigation. If your observations do not agree with the parent's report, make a note beside the question in the "Comments" column.

	1		2		3		Comments
A. Parent 1. Observed anxiety in office	not very anxious		somewhat		very anxious		
B. Child 2. Observed anxiety in office	not very anxious		somewhat		very anxious		
3. Observed compliance to parent in office	compliant		somewhat noncompliant		very noncompliant		
4. Observed compliance to medical personnel in office	compliant		somewhat noncompliant		very noncompliant		
5. Observed activity level	average activity		quite active		very active		
C. Illness Characteristics 6. Latency between illness symptoms and ending treatment	immediate		medium delay		long delay		
7. Status of illness	acute symptoms		some symptoms		asymptomatic or in remission		
8. Trend of illness	increasing symptoms		stable		decreasing symptoms		
9. Disability from illness	increasing		stable		decreasing		
10. Severity of symptoms	severe		moderate		mild		
D. Regimen Characteristics 11. Number of medications	one		2–3		more than 4		

(Table continues on p. 536.)

TABLE 21.5. (*Continued*)

	1		2		3		Comments
12. Frequency of medications	once/day		2–4 per day		over 4 per day		
13. Side effects	minimal		some side effects		severe effects		
14. Behavioral restrictions or life-style changes	minimal		some restrictions		many or severe restrictions		
15. Taste of medications	pleasant		neutral		noxious		
16. Duration of treatment	short-term		medium		long-term		

Parent Subtotal: ________

Physician Subtotal: ________

Overall Total: ________

E. Plans:

convenience); and 5) interpersonal reasons (e.g., peer pressure) (Allen, Tennen, McGrade, Affleck, & Ratzan, 1983). They found that, while children with increased responsibility for their regimens appeared to cope better, those who gave their own injections tended to have poorer diabetic control, presumably either because of inadequate knowledge or because of unpleasant aspects of the regimen. In another study with diabetic children at a summer camp, 33 percent reported falsifying their urine tests in order to gain access to increased activity or sweets or to avoid being punished (Simonds, 1979). Rapoff, Lindsley, and Christophersen (1985) asked parents of children with juvenile rheumatoid arthritis to describe the frequency and types of compliance problems they encountered. They found that children had the most negative reaction (i.e., crying, complaining, and noncompliance) to range-of-motion exercises, splint wearing, and medication (in that order). They suggest that lower compliance to exercises is due to the pain resulting from following the regimen.

Litt and colleagues (Litt & Cuskey, 1980, 1981; Litt, Cuskey, & Rosenberg, 1982) have studied compliance in adolescents, who are generally at particularly high risk for noncompliance. They found that noncompliant adolescents: (1) had social problems and poor self-esteem (Litt & Cuskey, 1980); and (2) had had the illness for a longer time, with an earlier onset and a later time of referral to a subspecialist (Litt &

Cuskey, 1981). Complaint adolescents, in contrast: (1) had had previous experience with illness in their family; (2) had family support and the expectation by their family that they would comply (Litt & Cuskey, 1980); and (3) were given responsibility for their own regimen (Litt et al., 1982). When given responsibility, however, they did better if they received supervision, particularly from someone outside the family (Litt & Cuskey, 1980). Other factors influencing compliance in adolescents parallel those of adults.

The only demographic variable consistently correlated with noncompliance to medical procedures is age. Some studies suggest that children under 6 years of age exhibit greater physical resistance for longer time periods when undergoing medical procedures than children over that age (Jay et al., 1983). Several dental studies have further divided those children under 6, and have found that by 4 or 5 years, most children are compliant (Winer, 1982). The concepts of maturation and development have been used to explain these age differences. For example, younger age is thought to be associated with greater generalization of an aversive event from one situation to another (Katz et al., 1980); poorer understanding of the procedure and instructions due to limited language development (Steward & Steward, 1981); problems with "separation anxiety" (Morris & Kratochwill, 1983); and poorer impulse control (Jay et al., 1983).

Predisposing factors thought to influence child compliance include the child's health beliefs, the child's coping style, and the child's behavior and experience with discipline at home. Steward and Steward (1981) suggest that children's conception of illness advances from concrete to abstract and that older children are better able to differentiate the functions of personnel and procedures. The organization of children's health beliefs into developmental stages has been achieved primarily by correlating self-report with various age levels, and then associating the age level with developmental theory (e.g., Bibace & Walsh, 1979). Self-report by its very nature is subjective and influenced by the language abilities of the individual child, and so is difficult to interpret. Nonetheless, it is reasonable that noncompliance could be the result of age-inappropriate instructions and explanations of illness and procedures.

Children's adjustment and subsequent compliance to medical regimens and procedures may be related to their style of coping (i.e., the use of individual cognitive strategies such as self-instruction, distraction, or information seeking) (Ross & Ross, 1984). As is the case for beliefs, direct observations of these behaviors are rarely included, and assessment is primarily self-report. Although styles of seeking or avoiding information regarding a particular procedure have only been studied in adults (Miller, 1980), Traughber and Cataldo (1983) suggest that this may be an important area of study with children. In addition, studies examining correlations between negative behavior during medical procedures and the children's reports of whether they feel that they have control over the aversive events (locus of control) have not yielded significant results (e.g., Jay et al, 1983; Rothbaum, Wolfer, & Visintainer, 1979).

Extremes such as use of punishment in fearful situations (Zabin & Melamed, 1980) or lack of structure in the home (Venham, Murray, & Gaulin-Kremer, 1979) have been associated with increased "anxiety" in children undergoing medical procedures. Firestone (1982) found that negative child behaviors were associated with noncompliance to medication for hyperactivity. It would be interesting to replicate this study with other regimens to see whether similar findings can be documented.

Events occurring prior to medical procedures can also have an impact on the child's behavior. Children's prior history can increase the likelihood of compliance or noncompliance. In addition, specific events, people, or settings can become associated with an aversive event (e.g., Shorkey & Taylor, 1973), particularly in young children, who are more likely to overgeneralize (Steward & Steward, 1981). There is a greater likelihood, as well, that a child whose noncomplaint behavior has been reinforced by the avoidance of the procedure will be noncompliant under similar circumstances in the future (Skinner, 1974). While children's avoidance behavior has not been specifically evaluated with medical procedures, use of behavior management (usually consisting of reinforcement of compliance and ignoring or time out for noncompliance) has contributed to increased compliance during various medical and dental procedures (Stokes & Kennedy, 1980; Varni, Bessman, Russo, & Cataldo, 1980).

Findings on the effect of previous experience have been contradictory. In a study examining sequential dental visits, Venham and Quatrocelli (1977) found that cooperation was directly related to the specific procedure. They concluded that, with repeated exposure over subsequent visits, children showed increased cooperation for apparently painless procedures, but decreased cooperation for injections. In contrast, the compliance of children undergoing painful bone marrow aspirations either remains stable with time (Katz et al., 1980) or improves slightly (Jay et al., 1983).

Parents can have a direct and immediate impact on their child's compliance during medical procedures by serving as models of appropriate or inappropriate behavior (Jay et al., 1983). However, a common response to parental presence—regardless of the parents' behavior—is increased negative child behavior (Gross, Stern, Levin, Dale, & Wojnilower, 1983; Shaw & Routh, 1982). Gross and colleagues (1983) suggest that most children have learned to identify their parents as a potential means of escape from aversive events. During medical procedures, however, the parents' failure to intervene may constitute an extinction contingency. A frequent initial response to extinction is increased negative behavior or aggression (Drabman & Jarvie, 1977).

Hyson, Snyder, and Andujar (1982) looked at the doctor–patient relationship in preschoolers undergoing routine checkups and concluded that children responded most positively to a physician's "warmth" (defined as close physical proximity, verbal expressions of empathy, and hugs or gifts at the end of the appointment). In another study, Weinstein, Getz, Ratener, and Domoto (1982a) reported that children showed less crying, physical resistance, screaming, whimpering, protest, and expressions of hurt and discomfort if their dentist used precise and immediate directions, positive reinforcement of specific behaviors, physical touch, and frequent queries to determine whether the child was experiencing pain. In contrast, coercion, coaxing, put-downs, and stopping treatment to manage behavior resulted in increased fear behaviors. In a subsequent study, the authors noted a circular response pattern, wherein dentists responded to children's fear behaviors with the very responses that evoked them (Weinstein, Getz, Ratener, & Domoto, 1982b). They concluded that either the dentists are not skilled in behavior management or they do not use the skills that they have learned.

Assessment. The factors just discussed can be assessed individually or globally as a part of a screening device, such as the questionnaire in Table 21.5. Identified problem areas may be dealt with by further questioning or assessment or by intervention strategies. For example, a child who is noncompliant in the office or by parent report should be assessed further to determine specific compliance problems. Parents or children who exhibit anxious behavior should be questioned further, and if the anxiety is greater than one would expect in the circumstance, standardized assessment may be warranted. Children or parents with poor understanding of the illness, procedure, or regimen can be assessed further to determine specific deficits in their knowledge. Table 21.6 discusses a number of assessment tools that have been developed to measure overall child development or behavior, child health beliefs, state or trait anxiety, self-esteem, locus of control, and the child's coping style. Most of these are self-report measures that can be completed by the parent or child while in the waiting room or at home. A few are more complex measures that require professional administration. Although some of the measures completed are not clearly correlated with noncompliance, they are included because of their prevalence in the compliance literature. If the child scores well outside the mean, a referral for further investigation or treatment may be warranted.

If a more detailed analysis of the parent–child interactions is warranted, an assessment of the child's compliance and parental behaviors, such as that presented by Forehand and McMahon (1981), might be appropriate. Another way to analyze the antecedents (i.e., events that occur prior to the behavior of concern) and consequences of compliant and noncompliant behavior is to keep an ongoing written record of the sequence of events (Barton & Ascione, 1984). Weinstein and colleagues (1982a) is an example of a detailed analysis of the interaction between children and professionals. By recording what happens before and after each occurrence of noncompliance, it may be possible to determine a pattern of behavior. For example, noncompliance may be associated with a particular person, time of day, or event. The parent or medical personnel may actually make future noncompliance more likely by inadvertently allowing the child to avoid or delay the medication or procedure, or by failing to praise compliant behavior. Such an analysis can indicate ways of changing the environment to decrease noncompliance in the future. Analyzing the antecedents can prevent the actual occurrence of noncompliance.

FURTHER ASSESSMENT OF FACTORS AFFECTING COMPLIANCE

A simple screening device such as the one presented in Table 21.5 may help a physician identify families who are at risk for noncompliance. If a family scores high on a particular item, it may be advisable to assess those factors further. Table 21.6 provides a list of standardized assessment tools that have been used to measure factors associated with noncompliance. Specifics about the measures' mode of administration, outcome measures, reliability, and validity are presented. These measures were selected for their feasibility for a physician to administer in a minimum of time. Although some of the measures listed have not been used specifically in studying medical compliance, they can be used with ease by a physician to screen for further problems. A score outside of the stated norms on any of these measures probably indicates that consideration be given to referral for treatment or more in-

TABLE 21.6. FURTHER ASSESSMENT OF FACTORS AFFECTING COMPLIANCE

Factor	Name of Test	Authors	Ages	Person Completing Test
I. Parent				
A. State-trait anxiety				
	1. State-Trait Anxiety Inventory (STAI)	Spielberger, Gorsuch, & Lushene (1980)	Grade 9 Adults	Parent
B. Family environment				
	1. Family Environment Scale (FES)	Moos, Insel, & Humphrey (1974)	Adults	Parent
C. Parenting skills				
	1. Child Development Questionnaire	Zabin & Melamed (1980)	Adult	Parent
	2. Parent Competency Inventory (PCI)	Cook & Ballenski (1983)	Parents of children under 3	Parent
	3. Parenting Stress Index (PSI)	Loyd & Abidin (1985)	Parents of children under 10	Parent
D. Health beliefs				
	1. Health Belief Questionnaire	Fincham & Wertheimer (1985)	Adult	Parent
	2. Measure of Health Beliefs	Leavitt (1979)	Adult	Parent
E. Disease/regimen knowledge				
1. Asthma	Asthma Self-Management Knowledge Questionnaire	Hindi-Alexander & Cropp (1981)	Child and adult	Child and parent
2. Diabetes	Test of Diabetes Knowledge	Johnson et al. (1982)	Child and adult	Child and parent
3. Hemophilia	1. Behavioral Assessment Inventory	Sergis-Deavenport & Varni (1983)	Adult/adolescent	Professional
II. Child				
A. Developmental level				
	1. Developmental Profile II (DPII)	Alpern, Boll, & Shearer (1980)	0–9	Parent or professional

Type of Assessment	Outcome Measure	Reliability	Validity	Comments
Self-report (40 items)	Two scores: 1. State anxiety (A-State) 2. Trait anxiety (A-Trait)	1. Test–retest (2–104 days): Trait = .70 State = .27–.54 2. Internal consistency: .80–.90	1. Construct: Item correlation with other anxiety scales 2. Experimental exposure to stressors yielded higher A-State scores, but stable A-Trait scores	
Self-report (90 items)	Two domains: 1. Relationship: Cohesion Expressiveness Conflict 2. Personal Growth: Independence Achievement orientation Intellectual/Cultural orientation Moral-religious emphasis	Test–retest (4 and 12 months): .68–.86	Compared distressed families with norms; distressed had: 1. Lower scores on: Cohesion Expressiveness Independence Intellectual/ recreational 2. Higher scores on: Conflict Control	
Self-report (14 items)	Parent management of fear behaviors in their children	Internal consistency: Significant correlations between disciplinary methods	Predictive Validity: Correlation between parent discipline and observed child anxiety (.38)	
Self-report (8–14 items)	Perceived competence Five forms: Infancy Toddlerhood Preschool School-age Adolescence	Test–retest (2 weeks): .85	Not reported	
Self-report (101 items)	Two domains of stress: 1. Child characteristics 2. Parent characteristics	1. Test-retest (3 weeks): .71–.82 2. Internal consistency: Child domain = .62–.70 Parent domain = .55–.80	Factor Analysis: Child domain: six factors accounted for 41% of variance Parent domain: seven factors accounted for 44% of variance Both domains: two factors accounted for 58% of variance	1. 20–30 minutes to complete 2. Fifth grade reading level
Self-report (129 items)	Four domains: 1. Motivations 2. Value of illness threat reduction 3. Possibility that compliant behavior will reduce illness threat 4. Modifying and enabling factors	Not reported	Results on questionnaire predicted drug defaulting in 67% of patients	Measure of drug compliance was self-report only
Self-report (125 items)	Five variables: 1. Vulnerability 2. Seriousness 1 3. Seriousness 2 4. Efficacy 5. Preventive	Not reported	Results on questionnaire predicted illness-related utilization of medical facility for three factors: 1. Vulnerability (*p*. .001) 2. Efficacy (*p*. .01) 3. Preventive (*p*. .01)	
Self-report (18 and 26 items)	Knowledge of illness Two forms: 1. Child 2. Adolescent/parent	In process of being standardized	In process of being validated; one study showed an increase score after education	
Self- or parent-report (39 and 35 items)	Two components: 1. Knowledge of illness and regimen 2. Problem solving	Internal consistency: .90 Interobserver agreement of observed competence: 88% (urine testing) and 93% (injection)	Low correlations between performance on urine testing/injections and results on knowledge/ problem-solving tests Low correlations between knowledge in eight different content areas	
Direct observation	Demonstrated ability to reach criterion performance on each of three classifications of behaviors	Interobserver: 93% (range of 77–100%)	Not standardized	Good example of task analysis; can be adapted to any other procedure to be performed by a parent or child
Structured interview (186 items)	Five subscales 1. Physical 2. Self-help 3. Social 4. Academic 5. Communication	1. Test–retest (2-day intervals): 92% were within 3 points of each other 2. Interscorer: No teachers disagreed on more than 2 items	.85 correlation between 1QE and Stanford-Binet IQ	1. 20–40 minutes for each of five areas 2. Should be used for screening only 3. Recent revison needs further standardization

TABLE 21.6. *(Continued)*

Factor	Name of Test	Authors	Ages	Person Completing Test
	2. Denver Developmental Screening Test (DDST)	Frankenburg & Dodds (1981)	2–6	Professional
B. Child behavior				
	1. Child Behavior Checklist	Achenbach & Edelbrock (1983)	4–16	Parent
	2. Diabetic Management Behavioral Inventory	Barnard (1987)	Adult	Parent
	3. Child Behavior Inventory	Robinson, Eyberg, & Ross (1980)	2–12	Parent
	4. Toddler Temperament Scale (TTS)	Carey & McDevitt (1978)	1–3	Parent
C. Depression				
	1. Child Depression Inventory (CDI)	Kovacs (1981)	7–17	Child
D. Self-esteem				
	1. Perceived Self-Competence Scale	Harter (1982)	Grades 3–9	Child
	2. Piers-Harris Children's Self-Concept Scale	Piers & Harris (1984)	Grades 4–12	Child
E. Locus of control				
	1. Children's Nowicki-Strickland	Nowicki & Strickland (1973)	Grades 3–12	Child
F. State-trait anxiety				
	1. Child Anxiety Scale (CAS)	Gillis (1980)	Grades K–5	Child
	2. Hospital Fears Rating Scale	Zabin & Melamed (1980)	4–12	Child

Type of Assessment	Outcome Measure	Reliability	Validity	Comments
Structured interview (105 items)	Four subscales 1. Gross motor 2. Fine motor/adaptive 3. Language 4. Personal-social	1. Test-retest & interexaminer: .66–.93 2. Observed behaviors had lower reliability than parent report items	.74–.97 correlation between DDST and Stanford-Binet, Revised Yale Developmental Schedule, Cattell Infant Intelligence Scale, and Bayley Scales of Infant Development	1. Widely used by physicians 2. Should be used for screening only 3. 15–20 minutes to administer 4. Small standardization sample 5. Best for years 3 and 4
Parent report (118 items)	Total Behavior Problem Score Five subscales: A. Social competence: 1. Activities 2. Social 3. School B. Behavior problems 4. Internalizing 5. Externalizing	1. Intraclass: .90 2. Test-retest (3 months): behavior problems = .84 social competence = .97	1. Construct = good 2. Misclassification for cutoffs = Non-referred: 9.8% Referred: 25.9%	1. Other forms: Teacher Direct observation Youth self-report (11–18) 2. Grade 5 reading level
Parent report (39 items)	Parents' perception of behavioral problems related to diabetes regimen Two scores: 1. Total Intensity 2. Total Behavior Problems	In process of being standardized	In process of being validated	Same format as Child Behavior Inventory
Parent report (36 items)	Two Scores of conduct problem behaviors: 1. Total intensity 2. Total behavior problems	1. Test–retest ($\bar{x}$ = 21 days): Intensity = .49 – .90 Problems = .35 – .69 2. Split-half: Intensity = .95 Problems = .94	1. 33 of items discriminated conduct problem group from normals 2. Internal: $\bar{x}$ interitem correlation: Intensity = .31 Problem = .29 3. Correlation between intensity and problems: .75	1. Easy to administer and score 2. Problem score gives parental concern
Parent report (97 items)	Nine clusters, scored from easy to difficult: 1. Activity 2. Rhythm 3. Approach/withdrawal 4. Adaptability 5. Intensity 6. Mood 7. Persistence 8. Distractibility 9. Threshold	Test–retest (1 month): .69–.89	Concurrent: a. More difficult = more optimal environment b. More difficult = higher developmental level	1. Infant form as well
Self-report (27 items)	Overall measure of childhood depression	$\bar{x}$ Test–retest: .73 (range: .42–.96)	1. Intercorrelation between scales: .21–.59	
Self-report (28 items)	Three domains: 1. Cognitive competence 2. Social competence 3. Physical competence	1. Internal consistency: .73–.86 2. Test–retest: 3 months = .70–.86 9 months = .69–.80	Factor analysis: orthogonal and oblique analyses = same factor structure; stable across sample groups	20–25 minutes to administer
Self-report (80 items)	Six cluster scores: 1. Behavior 2. Intellectual/school status 3. Physical appearance and attributes 4. Anxiety 5. Popularity 6. Happiness/satisfaction	1. Internal consistency: .93, total score .73–.81, cluster scores 2. Test–retest: $\bar{x}$ of .73 (range of .42–.96)	1. Intercorrelation between cluster scales = .21–.59 2. Moderate relationship between Piers-Harris and other measures of self-concept	
Self-report (40 items)	General measure of whether child attributes reinforcement to his or her own behavior (internal locus of control) or to some other factor (external locus of control)	1. Split-half: .63 2. Test–retest (6 weeks): .63–.71	Construct: .38–.61 correlation with Rotter	Other form: Preschool and Primary
Self-report; oral administration with tape and pictures (20 items)	Trait anxiety	1. Test–retest (immediate): .82–.92 2. Test–retest (1 week): .81 3. Internal consistency: .73	Factorial validity acceptable	15 minutes to administer
Self-report; (8 items)	State anxiety in hospital rated on a 5-point "fear thermometer"	Not standardized	Not standardized	

TABLE 21.6. *(Continued)*

Factor	Name of Test	Authors	Ages	Person Completing Test
	3. Revised Children's Manifest Anxiety Scale (RCMAS)	Reynolds & Richmond (1978)	Grades 1–12	Child
	4. State-Trait Anxiety Inventory for Children (STAIC)	Spielberger (1973)	9–12	Child
G. Health beliefs	See chapter 14 in this volume			

Note: Although some of the measures listed here were actually used in researching factors predictive of noncompliance, this table is intended only to provide the reader with available assessment tools that measure those factors. Measures were selected for their feasibility for a physician to administer with a minimum of time needed. Scores outside the norm on these measures indicate the need for referral for treatment or more in-depth assessment by a professional. Some of the information regarding specific tests was obtained from *The Ninth Mental Measurements Yearbook Vols. 1–2*, edited by J. V. Mitchell (1985).

depth assessment by a professional. Table 21.6 is divided into parent and child assessments. These will now be discussed in more detail.

Parent Factors

Because anxious parents can model inappropriate behaviors for their children, further assessment of parents reporting or exhibiting anxiety is advisable. The advantage of the State-Trait Inventory (Spielberger, Gorsuch, & Lushene, 1970) is that it has been widely used and can consistently distinguish between state and trait anxiety. The Family Environment Scale (Moos, Insel, & Humphrey, 1974) can further assess whether some of the parents' or child's anxiety can be attributed to distress in the family as a whole.

How parents manage their children's behavior generally and in relation to medical procedures can influence the child's compliance. The Parent Competency Inventory (Cook & Ballenski, 1983) and the Parenting Stress Index (Loyd & Abidin, 1985) both measure the parents' perceptions of their abilities at parenting and their home stressors. The Child Development Questionnaire (Zabin & Melamed, 1980) has been used to determine how parents report that they discipline their children if the child is exhibiting fear in medical settings.

The two measures of parent health beliefs presented in Table 21.6 (Fincham & Wertheimer, 1985; Leavitt, 1979) offer structured ways to determine whether there are potential problems in parents' perceptions of the value of treatment. Although parent education alone has not been effective in increasing compliance, lack of

Type of Assessment	Outcome Measure	Reliability	Validity	Comments
Self-report; (93 items)	Trait anxiety	1. Test–retest (9 months): .68 2. Internal consistency: .80	1. Construct: Positive correlation-with A-Trait on STAIC (no correlation with A-State) 2. Positive correlation between score and teacher report of behavior problems 3. Factor analysis: Three factors = Physiological worry; Worry and oversensitivity; Concentration anxiety	
Self-report; paper and pencil (40 items)	2 Scores: 1. State anxiety (A-State) 2. Trait anxiety (A-Trait)	1. Test–retest (2 months for A-Trait): .65–.71 2. Internal consistency: .82–.87	1. Construct: Correlation with A-Trait and: CMAS = .75; General Anxiety Scale for Children = .63 2. Discriminated between normals and emotionally disturbed 65% 3. Introduction of stressor increased A-State but not A-Trait	Narrow age range

knowledge of the illness or regimen has been associated with noncompliance. In Table 21.6, examples of measures assessing knowledge of asthma, diabetes, and hemophilia are presented. There are many other examples that are specific to individual illnesses. Interestingly, the measures of hemophilia and diabetes knowledge (Johnson et al., 1982; Sergis-Deavenport & Varni, 1983) include direct observation of the parents' regimen administration. This is considerably stronger than assessing parents' verbal or written reports of their knowledge alone.

Child Factors

It is important to determine the child's developmental level so that instructions and explanations can be adjusted accordingly. The Denver Developmental Screening Test (Frakenburg & Dodds, 1981) has the advantage of being short and easy to administer; in addition, it is already familiar to many physicians. However, it is not as valid for younger ages. The Developmental Profile II (Alpern, Boll, & Shearer, 1980) is considerably more detailed and probably provides better overall information about the child's development. Its lengthy administration, however, limits its usefulness as a screening device. Both measures can be administered by a physician without the need for training.

Assessing the child's overall behavior is important in determining whether the child is likely to listen to the parents' or physician's instructions. Both the Child Behavior Checklist (Achenbach & Edelbrock, 1983) and the Child Behavior Inventory (Robinson, Eyberg, & Ross, 1980) are well-established measures of the parents' report of their children's behavior. The Child Behavior Checklist has the advantage of measuring social behavior as well as withdrawn behavior, while the Child Behavior Inventory measures only conduct problems. The latter measure is considerably shorter, however, and offers an interesting measure of the parents' perception of whether a particular behavior is of concern to them. The Toddler Temperament Scale (Carey & McDevitt, 1978) can be used for children between 1 and 3, while the other two measures do not extend below the ages of 2 (Child Behavior Inventory) and 3 (Child Behavior Checklist). The disadvantage is that this scale measures parents' report of a construct labeled as *temperament*, which is not clearly correlated with negative child behavior.

Barnard (1987) has adapted the Child Behavior Inventory (Robinson et al., 1980) to discover parents' perceptions of their children's compliance with a diabetic regimen. This measure, which can undoubtedly be used as a model for assessment of compliance to other medical regimens, is in the process of being standardized and validated.

Measures of predisposing factors such as depression, self-esteem, locus of control, and trait anxiety can be useful in determining whether there are characteristics of a particular child that may make him or her less able to cope with the demands of a medical regimen or procedure. All of the measures listed in Table 21.6 are well standardized and have been used in studying children's reactions to medical regimens or procedures. None is directed specifically at medical regimens. Certainly in the instance of high depression, high anxiety, or low self-esteem, it would be advisable to refer for professional counseling. The implications of the outcome of a locus of control measure such as the Children's Nowicki-Strickland (Nowicki & Strickland, 1973) are less clear. It is possible that children scoring high on external locus of control should be provided with some controllability in their regimens or procedures. This is discussed in more detail in the next section.

Measures of state anxiety, such as the State-Trait Anxiety Inventory for Children (Spielberger, 1973) or the Hospital Fears Rating Scale (Zabin & Melamed, 1980), provide the clinician with important information about the impact of a procedure on a child. The former is a well-standardized measure that does not address medical regimens directly, but can be used to measure the child's anxiety in any stressful situation. In contrast the Hospital Fears Rating Scale, which is not standardized, addresses the child's fears as they apply directly to hospitalization.

Once it has been determined that a parent or child is at risk for noncompliance, there are a number of strategies that can be used to minimize compliance problems. The following section discusses anticipatory strategies that can be used once at-risk families have been identified.

TAILORING ANTECEDENTS TO ENHANCE COMPLIANCE

The context in which a behavior occurs may have a direct effect on whether a parent or child responds in a given way (Bijou & Baer, 1978). Specific environmental factors, such as physical conditions (e.g., when the medication is to be given or where the procedure is carried out), biological conditions (e.g., the child's health), or social conditions (e.g., who gives the medication or who is present during the procedure), may determine whether or how a particular response occurs. Under different conditions, the same child may respond to similar situations in an entirely different manner; for example, the smell of rubbing alcohol may evoke crying when the child is in the hospital, but not when at home. Such antecedent environmental factors have been referred to as *setting events* (Bijou & Baer, 1978).

In attempting to avoid or reduce noncompliance, one must assess how these setting events occasion both the child's and the parents' compliance, and then adjust those factors that may interfere with compliance. In addition, one can identify at-risk factors such as age or coping style and tailor treatment accordingly. Unfortunately, much of the prevention literature is anecdotal, and changing the factors merely predictive of noncompliance does not always increase compliance (Rapoff et al., 1985). This is probably due in part to the correlational nature of studies and in part to medicine's inability always to *know* that a recommended regimen will eliminate the medical problem (Epstein, 1984). This section discusses ways of tailoring regimens once at-risk families are identified.

Improving Parental Compliance

In general, short-term compliance to medical regimens can be improved greatly by providing clear, written instructions, telephone follow-ups, and standardized patient recordings of compliance (see Rapoff & Christophersen, 1982b, for examples of recording forms and concise instructions). Compliance to long-term regimens is more complex and requires life-style changes as well as the physician's ongoing feedback and reinforcement of compliance (Epstein & Cluss, 1982). Maintenance of behavioral treatment effects continues to be an area of concern in the field of psychology in general (Stokes & Baer, 1977).

Demographic Factors. Although demographics are usually unchangeable, adjustments can be made that may decrease the likelihood of parental noncompliance. For example, instructions can be adjusted to the educational level of the parents. The timing of medications can sometimes be adjusted to fit a parent's work schedule. Young, elderly, or single parents may be helped by a support group or by a referral for assistance from a public health nurse.

Predisposing Factors. Little change has been reported in compliance using single educational approaches targeting the parents' health beliefs (Clark, 1983) and knowledge regarding the disease, medication, and regimen (Casey, Rosen, Glowasky, & Ludwig, 1985). However, compliance to short-term medication regimens has been improved by using education in combination with other approaches. For example, Finney, Friman, Rapoff, and Christophersen (1985) improved compliance with medication for otitis media by using an educational handout, a self-monitoring calendar, and phone reminders.

Identification and elimination of structural and financial barriers, wherever possible, can increase compliance. This may include referring the parent to a reliable discount pharmacy, discussing the regimen with other family members, or referral to a social services agency. Finally, identification of general child behavior problems often indicates a need to provide information regarding child management or to refer the parent for assistance with child behavior problems prior to addressing problems of medical noncompliance.

Setting Events. A number of studies have shown that compliance to medical regimens can be improved by environmental changes that cue the parent to comply with the regimen. In addition to simplifying the regimen and implementing it gradually wherever possible, tailoring it to the individual's routine has been shown to improve compliance (Rapoff & Christophersen, 1982b). For example, parents are more likely to remember to administer medication if it coincides with meals, leaving for work, or brushing their teeth. In these instances, a reminder on the refrigerator, near the car keys, or by the toothpaste can serve as a cue for giving medication. In addition, the package that medication is in can improve compliance (Linkewich, Catalano, & Flack, 1974). Successful multicomponent approaches have included components such as a self-monitoring calendar (Finney et al., 1985), telephone reminders (Finney et al,, 1985), home visits (Mayo, 1981), self-recording of food intake (Stunkard, 1981), and public posting of number of exercises completed (Waggoner & LeLieuvre, 1981).

Improving Children's Compliance

Young children are at particular risk for noncompliance, presumably because of their limited language abilities. Adapting to the child's developmental level and coping style, improving overall child behavior, and arranging antecedents carefully can improve compliance.

Demographic Factors. Developmental level, which is the single greatest demographic predictor of compliance in children (Gross et al., 1983), implies changes in expectations of the child and instructions given. Because the literature is in agreement that children younger then about 6 or 7 are more likely to be noncompliant with medical procedures (Katz et al., 1980), the professional needs to anticipate this possibility and implement some preventive strategies. Since young children do not respond accurately to abstractions (Christophersen, 1986), explanations of illness or impending procedures should be short and concrete. Rehearsal or modeling with another child or doll provides a more concrete explanation than do words alone, and peer modeling has been used successfully to decrease uncooperative behavior during dental procedures (Stokes & Kennedy, 1980) and hospitalization (Melamed & Siegel, 1975). Since young children's behavior often generalizes from one procedure to all procedures, and/or from procedures to people and settings in the hospital environment (Steward & Steward, 1981), the child needs to be provided with clear distinctions between invasive and noninvasive procedures, and to associate the staff with positive consequences as well as the inevitable unpleasant ones (Traughber & Cataldo, 1983).

Older children respond more appropriately to explanations of their illness and upcoming procedures, but caution should be taken not to overwhelm children with detail beyond their language ability or attention span. In fact, Steward and Steward (1981) suggest that children may not understand the necessity of treatment and the details of their illness until they are near adolescence.

Although most factors that improve compliance in adults are similar for adolescents (Litt & Cuskey, 1980), some factors are unique to adolescents. While a few educational programs have increased regimen compliance in children (Beck et al., 1980), one study found that teaching diabetic adolescents social skills and how to resist peer pressure had more impact than disease education on improving their metabolic control (Kaplan, Chadwick, & Schimmel, 1985). Increased responsibility, but with supervision (by someone other than the family), can contribute to improved compliance in children (Litt & Cuskey, 1980); it is important, however, to ensure that the child is accurate in carrying out the regimen (Allen et al., 1983). Sallis (1985) suggests that responsibility should be given gradually, according to the child's developmental level.

Predisposing Factors. In a survey on coping with pain, administered to 994 school-age children, Ross and Ross (1984) reported that only 21 percent used any type of coping strategy. Distraction, one of the most commonly reported strategies in this study, has been found to be effective in decreasing reports of pain when combined with other approaches (Kelley, Jarvie, Middlebrook, McNeer, & Drabman, 1984). Peterson and Shigetomi (1981) found that children who were taught a combination of coping strategies (including relaxation, distraction, and comforting self-talk) in addition to viewing a filmed model were more cooperative during their hospitalization than those receiving preoperation information or any of the just-mentioned strategies alone. One complicating factor in teaching coping strategies is that children may have different styles of coping (Miller, 1980), which may influence the type of preparation most appropriate for each child. Further research is needed in order to determine whether children do in fact cope differently. At present, the professional must rely on verbal reports of the parents' and child's past experiences and preferred coping strategies.

Although there is no clear evidence for a relationship between locus of control and compliance, there are some indications that children who perceive themselves as having control of their environment may be more noncompliant than those who perceive someone else having the control (Rothbaum et al., 1979). However, if aversive events are presented without clear warnings (and thus without means of avoiding the events), a common outcome may be learned helplessness, or conditioned suppression of behavior (Maier & Seligman, 1976). Clearly, neither noncompliance nor learned helplessness is desirable. Cataldo, Jacobs, and Rogers (1982) have suggested that controllability and predictability are the two factors that can mitigate learned helplessness. Within this context, the professional may need to give the child clearly defined control. For example, control may be given to children by allowing them to choose the type of chaser after the medication, the persons who remain in the room during medical treatment, and the order in which pills are given. However, children should *not* be given control over whether or when to take medication.

As a matter of routine, assessment of the child's behavior at home as well as discipline strategies used by the parents can indicate whether behavior management training is warranted. Parents can be referred to literature on child management (e.g., Christophersen, 1982) or, in more severe cases, professional counseling may be necessary. Other behavioral approaches that have improved the child's behavior include token reinforcement of appropriate behavior (Lowe & Lutzker, 1979); token reinforcement plus rehearsal (Rapoff et al., 1985); and self-monitoring, goal setting, and behavioral contracting (Schafer, Glasgow, & McCaul, 1982). While these approaches were used in treating children and adolescents who were already behavior problems, the techniques could be used prophylactically as well.

Setting Events. In addition to making the immediate environment predictable and controllable within limits, the manner in which instructions are given may influence a child's compliance. Baron and Galizio (1983) suggest that instructions can control behavior, particularly if the child has been reinforced for compliance to instructions in the past. Instructional control can be achieved more readily if detail is kept to a minimum (Etzel & LeBlanc, 1979), particularly if the child is young (Roberts, 1984) and if eye contact precedes the instruction (Hamlet, Axelrod, & Kuerschner, 1984). Blount, Dahlquist, Baer, and Wouri (1984) taught children to accept pills by beginning with a very small object and gradually increasing the size. This is an excellent example of improving compliance by breaking down a task into small steps and teaching each step systematically.

Identification and elimination of behaviors that precede noncompliance can also help avoid behavior problems. For example, Mathews and Grantmyre (1985) increased compliance with radiation therapy by using a verbal reprimand for tears in the eyes after determining that tears preceded flailing. Frequently, medical technicians use anticipatory restraint of a limb, based on the child's age or antecedent behavior (e.g., hesitancy to enter the treatment room). However, reports of increased fear behaviors in young children who were physically restrained during medical procedures (Weinstein, 1984) indicate that this approach requires further investigation, and should be used with caution.

Little has been written about the influence of the presence of specific sensory stimuli in the physical environment prior to a child's receiving medication or a procedure. It is quite possible, however, that aversive smells or tastes may elicit a gag response that then sets the occasion for future noncompliance. Identification and elimination of such aversive stimuli may prevent further problems. In addition, adjusting meals or medication times to symptoms of the disease or side effects of treatment may prevent noncompliance. For example, because one side effect of uremia in patients with chronic renal failure is nausea and vomiting (Hoekelman, Blatman, Brunell, Friedman, & Seidel, 1978), it may be desirable to try adjusting mealtimes so that the child does not associate food with nausea. Introducing pain medication routinely rather than waiting until the child reports severe pain has been recommended prophylactically to avoid discomfort and physical complications (Schechter, 1985); in addition, it may prevent noncompliance with routine activities due to pain.

Visual stimuli have been found to influence a child's compliance. Children have been found to be less "anxious" if first interviewed in a neutral room prior to being taken into a dental surgery room (Swallow, Jones, & Morgan, 1975). Crying in a 17-month-old burned child decreased substantially when the hospital staff wore a different gown color and changed the room lighting in order to help the child discriminate between social interactions and painful procedures (Shorkey & Taylor, 1973).

Parental presence during a procedure can increase crying, but may not increase physical resistance (Gross et al., 1983). In spite of equivocal empirical evidence for the advantages and disadvantages of parental presence, parents are increasingly being encouraged to "room in" (Kellerman, 1981), to be present during medical procedures, and to participate in the child's medical care while in the hospital (Roskies, Mongeon, & Gagnon-Lefebvre, 1978). Parent participation may be useful for both the parent and child, but it is probably not appropriate for all parents or children, particularly if the parent displays high levels of anxiety. Nonetheless, further research is needed to determine the parents' influence on compliance.

Role of the Professional in Enhancing Compliance

Medical Personnel. The literature suggests that pediatricians who are warm, give positive feedback, and provide continuity of care have better success with getting patients to comply with their recommendations (Freemon et al., 1971; Mattar & Yaffe, 1974). Other approaches that the pediatrician may use to enhance compliance are: (1) explaining the regimen clearly and providing written instructions; (2) exploring the child's and parents' health beliefs and providing alternative information if the beliefs are predictive of noncompliance; (3) identifying potential barriers and collaborating with the patient in generating solutions; (4) providing a checklist for recording regimen components and discussing where to post the list; (5) determining the role of the parent and child in carrying out the regimen; (6) discussing adapting the regimen to the family's routine, and using specific environmental cues as reminders in the home; (7) discussing child management strategies that will enhance compliance, and giving management protocols where appropriate; (8) planning for follow-up; (9) when performing a medical procedure, giving clear, concise instructions to both the child and the parent; (10) introducing invasive instruments and procedures gradually whenever possible; and (11) considering procedures for reinforcing both child and parent compliance.

Changes on an Institutional Level. Because hospitals are often perceived as aversive by children, hospital administrations should explore ways to lessen the trauma of hospitalization (Cataldo, Bessman, Parker, Pearson, & Rogers, 1979). Some efforts have been made in this direction, such as showing preparatory films or giving instruction regarding hospitalization, providing playrooms and appropriately trained staff, and allowing parents to room in and in some instances accompany their children into treatment or induction rooms. Many of these efforts still need to be empirically evaluated, however. The training of professionals in child management, anticipatory guidance strategies, and patient–professional interactions is an area that clearly warrants further investigation. In addition, those variables in the physical environment that may prevent noncompliance (such as the setup of waiting rooms, placement of instruments in the treatment room, and clothing worn by the staff) need to be investigated individually in each clinical setting.

CONCLUSION

The literature reviewed in this chapter identifies a number of variables that correlate with noncompliance in health settings. Children's compliance improves with age, with consistent discipline practices at home, and with predictable variables surrounding the regimen. Identification and initial treatment of children who are general behavior problems may also help to prevent medical noncompliance.

The clinical application of the many studies reviewing factors associated with parental noncompliance is complicated. Some of these factors (e.g., demographics, clinic vs. private practice) can serve only as markers for identifying individuals at higher risk for noncompliance; others have not contributed to compliance when eliminated (e.g., limited knowledge of illness and health beliefs); still others may require substantial changes that the participants may not be willing or able to implement (e.g., better parent–doctor relationships). Furthermore, there is *not* always a direct correspondence between improved compliance and improved medical outcome (Finney et al., 1985). This last finding may have unfortunate implications. If the patient's compliant behavior does not result in improved symptoms, future compliance may become less likely.

There are two separate issues in the assessment of noncompliance: identification of high-risk parents and children; and implementation of intervention strategies for improving the likelihood of compliance once such patients are identified. The factors indicating a high risk for noncompliance may not necessarily be those factors that should be targeted for intervention. The contradictions in studies on this subject attest to the complexity and individuality of the problem. It is appealing to look for a single set of factors that can be applied universally, but it is more likely that the factors vary from person to person and even temporally for the same person.

Given this complexity, health care professionals do not have an easy task. For some patients, it is possible that the solution may be as simple as providing written handouts and monitoring sheets routinely. For others, however, the professional may need to make adaptations once the family is in the office (e.g., tailoring regimens to the parents' life-style or adapting instructions to the child's developmental level). In general, by giving clear instructions and approaching the child or parent in an individualized and caring manner, the provider can probably increase the likelihood of compliance.

Finally, there is much research needed in this area. Unfortunately, assessment strategies are difficult to study due to the complexity of factors associated with noncompliance. Nonetheless, prevention remains a compelling arena for investigation. In particular, identification and manipulation of specific physical stimuli during medical procedures, further investigation of factors contributing to child compliance with regimens, the impact of coping style on compliance, and parent instruction in child management in medical settings provide exciting areas for future research.

References

Achenbach, T. M., & Edelbrock, C. S. (1983). Behavioral problems and competencies reported to parents of normal and disturbed children aged four through sixteen. *Monographs of the Society for Research in Child Development, 46* (1, Serial No 188).

Allen, D. A., Tennen, H., McGrade, B. J., Affleck, G., & Ratzan, S. (1983). Parent and child perceptions of the management of juvenile diabetes. *Journal of Pediatric Psychology, 8,* 129–141.

Alpern, G. D., Boll, T. J., & Shearer, M. S. (1980). *Developmental profile II.* Aspen, CO: Psychological Development Publications.

Anderson, R. J., & Kirk, L. M. (1982). Methods of improving patient compliance in chronic disease states. *Archives of Internal Medicine, 142,* 1673–1675.

Barnard, M. U. (1987). *Diabetic inventory.* Manuscript submitted for publication.

Baron, A., & Galizio, M. (1983). Instructional control of human operant behavior. *Psychological Record, 33,* 495–520.

Bartlett, E. E. (1984). Effective approaches to patient education for the busy pediatrician. *Pediatrics, 74,* 19–24.

Barton, E. J., & Ascione, F. R. (1984). Direct observation. In T. H. Ollendick & M. Hersen, *Child behavioral assessment: Principles and procedures.* New York: Pergamon.

Beck, D. E., Fennell, R. S., Yost, R. L., Robinson, J. D., Geary, D., & Richards, G. A. (1980). Evaluation of an educational program on compliance with medication regimens in pediatric patients with renal transplants. *Journal of Pediatrics, 96,* 1094–1097.

Becker, M. H., & Green, L. W. (1975). A family approach to compliance with medical treatment: A selective review of the literature. *International Journal of Health Education, 19,* 173–182.

Becker, M. H., Maiman, L. A., Kirscht, J. P., Haefner, D. P., Drachman, R. H., & Taylor, D. W. (1979). Patient perceptions and compliance: Recent studies of the health belief model. In R. B. Haynes, D. W. Taylor, & D. L. Sackett (Eds.), *Compliance in health care*. Baltimore: Johns Hopkins University Press.

Bibace, R., & Walsh, M. E. (1979). Developmental stages in children's conceptions of illness. In G. C. Stone, F. Cohen, & N. E. Adler (Eds.), *Health psychology*. San Francisco: Jossey-Bass.

Bijou, S., & Baer, D. M. (1978). *Behavior analysis of child development*. Englewood Cliffs, NJ: Prentice-Hall.

Blount, R. L., Dahlquist, L. M., Baer, R. A., & Wouri, D. (1984). A brief effective method for teaching children to swallow pills. *Behavior Therapy, 15,* 381–387.

Carey, W. B., & McDevitt, S. C. (1978). Stability and change in individual temperament diagnoses from infancy to early childhood. *Journal of American Academy of Child Psychiatry, 17,* 331—337.

Casey, R., Rosen, B., Glowasky, A., & Ludwig, S. (1985). An intervention to improve follow-up of patients with otitis media. *Clinical-Pediatrics (Philadelphia), 24*(3), 149–152.

Cataldo, M. F., Bessman, D. A., Parker, L. H., Pearson, J. E. R., & Rogers, M. C. (1979). Behavioral assessment for pediatric intensive care units. *Journal of Applied Behavior Analysis, 12,* 83–97.

Cataldo, M. F., Jacobs, H. E., & Rogers, M. C. (1982). Behavioral/environmental considerations in pediatric inpatient care. In D. C. Russo & J. W. Varni (Eds.), *Behavioral pediatrics: Research and practice*. New York: Plenum.

Chamberlin, R. W. (1975). The new morbidity: Behavioral problems of preschoolers. In J. J. Haggerty, K. J. Roghmann, & I. B. Pless, *Child health and the community*. New York: Wiley.

Chambers, W. L., Fields, H. W., & Machen, J. B. (1981). Measuring selected disruptive behaviors of the 36- to 60-month-old patient: Part 1. Development and assessment of a rating scale. *Pediatric Dentistry, 3,* 251–256.

Christophersen, E. R. (1982). *Little people: Guidelines for common sense child rearing*. Shawnee Mission, KS: Overland.

Christophersen, E. R. (1986). Anticipatory guidance on discipline. *Pediatric Clinics of North America, 33,* 789–798.

Clark, N. M. (1983). Response: The application of theory in childhood asthma self-help programs. *Journal of Allergy & Clinical Immunology, 72,* 578–580.

Cook, A. S., & Ballenski, C. B. (1983). The Parent Competency Inventory. Unpublished manuscript, Fort Collins. CO.

Drabman, R. S., & Jarvie, G. (1977). Counseling parents of children with behavior problems: The use of extinction and time-out techniques. *Pediatrics, 59,* 78–85.

Epstein, L. (1984). The direct effects of compliance on health outcome. *Health Psychology, 3,* 385–393.

Epstein, L. H., & Cluss, P. A. (1982). A behavioral medicine perspective on adherence to long-term medical regimens. *Journal of Consulting & Clinical Psychology, 50,* 950–971.

Etzel, B. C., & LeBlanc, J. M. (1979). The simplest treatment alternative: The law of parsimony applied to choosing appropriate instructional control and errorless-learning procedures for the difficult-to-teach child. *Journal of Autism & Developmental Disorders, 9,* 361–382.

Fincham, J. E., & Wertheimer, A. I. (1985). Using the health belief model to predict initial drug therapy defaulting. *Social Science & Medicine, 20,* 101–105.

Finney, J. W., Friman, P. C., Rapoff, M. A., & Christophersen, E. R. (1985). Improving compliance with antibiotic regimens for otitis media. *American Journal of Diseases of Children, 139,* 89–95.

Firestone, P. (1982). Factors associated with children's adherence to stimulant medication. *American Journal of Orthopsychiatry, 52,* 447–457.

Forehand, R. L., & McMahon, R. J. (1981). *Helping the noncompliant child: A clinician's guide to parent training*. New York: Guilford.

Francis, V., Korsch, B. M., & Morris, M. J. (1969). Gaps in doctor–patient communication: Patients' response to medical advice. *New England Journal of Medicine, 280*, 535–540.

Frankenburg, K., & Dodds, J. B. (1981). Denver Developmental Screening Test. Denver: LADOCA.

Frankl, S. N., Shiere, F. R., & Fogels, H. R. (1962). Should the parent remain with the child in the dental operatory? *Journal of Dentistry in Childhood, 29*, 150–163.

Freemon, B., Negrete, V. F., Davis, M., & Korsch, B. M. (1971). Gaps in doctor–patient communication: Doctor–patient interaction analysis. *Pediatric Research, 5*, 298–311.

Gillis, J. S. (1980). Child Anxiety Scale. Champaign, IL: Institute for Personality and Ability Testing.

Gross, A. M., Stern, R. M., Levin, R. B., Dale, J., & Wojnilower, D. A. (1983). The effect of mother–child separation on the behavior of children experiencing a diagnostic medical procedure. *Journal of Consulting & Clinical Psychology, 51*, 783–785.

Haggerty, R. J. (1986). The changing nature of pediatrics. In N. A. Krasnegor, J. D. Arasteh, & M. F. Cataldo (Eds.), *Child health behavior: A behavioral pediatrics perspective*. New York: Wiley.

Haggerty, R. J., Roghmann, K. J., & Pless, I. B. (1975). *Child health and the community*. New York: Wiley.

Hamlet, C. C., Axelrod, S., & Kuerschner, S. (1984). Eye contact as an antecedent to compliant behavior. *Journal of Applied Behavior Analysis, 17*, 553–557.

Harter, S. (1982). The Perceived Competence Scale for Children. *Child Development, 53*, 87–97.

Haynes, R. B. (1979). Determinants of compliance: The disease and the mechanics of treatment. In R. B. Haynes, D. W. Taylor, & D. L. Sackett (Eds.), *Compliance in health care*. Baltimore: Johns Hopkins University Press.

Hindi-Alexander, M., & Cropp, G. J. A. (1981). Community and family programs for children with asthma. *Annals of Allergy, 46*, 143–148.

Hoekelman, R. A., Blatman, S., Brunell, P. A., Friedman, S. B., & Seidel, H. M. (1978). *Principles of pediatrics: Health care of the young*. New York: McGraw-Hill.

Hulka, B. S. (1979). Patient–clinician interactions and compliance. In R. B. Haynes, D. W. Taylor, & D. L. Sackett (Eds.), *Compliance in health care*. Baltimore: Johns Hopkins University Press.

Hyson, M. C., Snyder, S. S., & Andujar, E. M. (1982). Helping children cope with checkups: How good is the "good" patient? *Children's Health Care, 10*, 139–144.

Jay, S. M., & Elliott, C. (1984). Behavioral observation scales measuring children's distress. The effects of increased methodological rigor. *Journal of Consulting & Clinical Psychology, 52*, 1106–1107.

Jay, S. M., Ozolins, M., Elliott, C. H. (1983). Assessment of children's distress during painful medical procedures. *Health Psychology, 2*, 133–147.

Johnson, S. B., Pollak, T., Silverstein, J. H., Rosenbloom, A. L., Spillar, R., McCallum, M., & Harkavy, J. (1982). Cognitive and behavioral knowledge about insulin-dependent diabetes among children and parents. *Pediatrics, 69*, 708–713.

Kaplan, R. M., Chadwick, M. W., & Schimmel, L. E. (1985). Social learning intervention to promote metabolic control in type 1 diabetes mellitus: Pilot experiment results. *Diabetes Care, 8*(2), 152–155.

Kasl, S. V. (1975). Issues in patient adherence to health care regimens. *Journal of Human Stress, 1*, 5–15.

Katz, E. R., Kellerman, J., & Siegel, S. E. (1980). Behavioral distress in children with cancer undergoing medical procedures: Developmental considerations. *Journal of Consulting & Clinical Psychology, 48*, 356–365.

Keefe, F., & Gil, K. M. (1987, March). *Pain management training techniques*. Workshop presented at the meeting of the Society for Behavioral Medicine, Washington, DC.

Kellerman, J. (1981). *Helping the fearful child*. Chicago: Contemporary Books.

Kelley, M. L., Jarvie, G. J., Middlebrook, J. L., McNeer, M. F., & Drabman, R. S. (1984). Decreasing burned children's pain behavior: Impacting the trauma of hydrotherapy. *Journal of Applied Behavior Analysis, 17*, 147–158.

Klein, G. L., & Ziering, R. W. (1983). Improving drug administration in young children with asthma and allergic rhinitis. *Immunology & Allergy Practice, 5*, 49–53.

Kovacs, M. (1981). Rating scales to assess depression in school-aged children. *Acta Paedopsychiatrica, 46*, 305–315.

Leavitt, F. (1979). The health belief model and utilization of ambulatory care services. *Social Science & Medicine, 13A*, 105–112.

Linkewich, J. A., Catalano, R., & Flack, H. L. (1974). The effect of packaging on instruction on outpatient compliance with medication regimens. *Drug Intelligence & Clinical Pharmacy, 8*, 10–15.

Litt, I. F., & Cuskey, W. R. (1980). Compliance with medical regimens during adolescence. *Pediatric Clinics of North America, 27*, 3–15.

Litt, I. F., & Cuskey, W. R. (1981). Compliance with salicylate therapy in adolescents with juvenile rheumatoid arthritis. *American Journal of Disabled Child, 135*, 434–436.

Litt, I. F., Cuskey, W. R., & Rosenberg, A. (1982). Role of self-esteem and autonomy in determining medication compliance among adolescents with juvenile rheumatoid arthritis. *Pediatrics, 69*, 15–17.

Litt, I. F., Cuskey, W. R., & Rudd, S. (1980). Identifying adolescents at risk for noncompliance with contraceptive therapy. *Journal of Pediatrics, 96*, 742–745.

Lowe, K., & Lutzker, J. R. (1979). Increasing compliance to a medical regimen with a juvenile diabetic. *Association for Advancement of Behavior Therapy, 10*, 57–64.

Loyd, B. H., & Abidin, R. R. (1985). Revision of the Parenting Stress Index. *Journal of Pediatric Psychology, 10*, 169–177.

Maier, S. F., & Seligman, M. E. P. (1976). Learned helplessness: Theory and evidence. *Journal of Experimental Psychology, 105*, 3–46.

Mathews, J. R., & Grantmyre, J. D. (1985, November). *Increasing compliance to radiation therapy in a two-year-old child*. Paper presented at the meeting of the Association for the Advancement of Behavior Therapy, Houston.

Mattar, M. E., Markello, J., & Yaffe, S. J. (1975). Pharmaceutic factors affecting pediatric compliance. *Pediatrics, 55*, 101–107.

Mattar, M. E., & Yaffe, S. J. (1974). Compliance of pediatric patients with therapeutic regimens. *Postgraduate Medicine, 56*, 181–188.

Mayo, N. E. (1981). The effect of a home visit on parental compliance with a home program. *Physical Therapy, 61*, 27–32.

McMahon, R. J. (1984). Behavioral checklists and rating scales. In T. H. Ollendick & M. Hersen (Eds.), *Child behavioral assessment: Principles and procedures*. New York: Pergamon.

Melamed, B. G. (1979). Behavioral approaches to fear in dental settings. In M. Hersen, R. M. Eisler, & P. M. Miller (Eds.), *Progress in behavior modification* (Vol. 7). New York: Academic Press.

Melamed, B. G., Robbins, R. L., & Graves, S. (1982). Preparation for surgery and medical procedures. In D. C. Russo & J. W. Varni (Eds.), *Behavioral pediatrics: Research and practice*. New York: Plenum.

Melamed, B. G., & Siegel, L. J. (1975). Reduction of anxiety in children facing hospitalization and surgery by use of filmed modeling. *Journal of Consulting & Clinical Psychology, 43*, 511–521.

Miller, K. A. (1982). Theophylline compliance in adolescent patients with chronic asthma. *Society for Adolescent Medicine, 3*, 177–179.

Miller, S. M. (1980). When is a little information a dangerous thing? Coping with stressful events by monitoring vs. blunting. In S. Levine & H. Ursin (Eds.), *Coping and health*. New York: Plenum.

Mitchell, J. V. (Ed.) (1985). *The ninth mental measurements yearbook* (Vols. 1–2). Lincoln, NE: University of Nebraska Press.

Moos, R. H., Insel, P. M., & Humphrey, B. (1974). *Family work and group environment scales manual*. Palo Alto: Consulting Psychologists Press.

Morris, R. J., & Kratochwill, T. R. (1983). *Treating children's fears and phobias: A behavioral approach*. New York: Pergamon.

Nowicki, S., & Strickland, B. R. (1973). A locus of control scale for children. *Journal of Consulting & Clinical Psychology, 40*, 148–154.

Peterson, L., & Shigetomi, C. (1981). The use of coping techniques to minimize anxiety in hospitalized children. *Behavior Therapy, 12*, 1–14.

Piers, E. V., & Harris, D. B. (1984). *Piers–Harris Children's Self-Concept Scale (The Way I Feel about Myself)*. Los Angeles: Western Psychological Services.

Radius, S. M., Becker, M. H., Rosenstock, I. M., Drachman, R. H., Schuberth, D. C., & Teets, K. C. (1978). Factors influencing mothers' compliance with a medication regimen for asthmatic children. *Journal of Asthma Research, 15*, 133–149.

Ramsay, J. A. (1982). Participants in noncompliance research: Compliant or noncompliant? *Medical Care, 20,* 615–622.

Rapoff, M. A., & Christophersen, E. R. (1982a). Improving compliance in pediatric practice. In E. R. Christophersen (Ed.), *The Pediatric Clinics of North America, 29*(2). Philadelphia: Saunders.

Rapoff, M. A., & Christophersen, E. R. (1982b). Compliance of pediatric patients with medical regimens: A review and evaluation. In R. B. Stuart (Ed.), *Adherence, compliance and generalization in behavioral medicine.* New York: Brunner/Mazel.

Rapoff, M. A., Lindsley, C. B., & Christophersen, E. R. (1984). Improving compliance with medical regimens: Case study with juvenile rheumatoid arthritis. *Archives of Physical Medicine & Rehabilitation, 65,* 267–269.

Rapoff, M. A., Lindsley, C. B., & Christophersen, E. R. (1985). Parent perceptions of problems experienced by their children in complying with treatments for juvenile rheumatoid arthritis. *Archives of Physical Medicine & Rehabilitation. 66,* 427–429.

Reynolds, C. R., & Richmond, B. O. (1978). "What I think and feel": A revised measure of children's manifest anxiety. *Journal of Abnormal Child Psychology, 6,* 271–280.

Roberts, M. W. (1984). An attempt to reduce time out resistance in young children. *Behavior Therapy, 15,* 210–216.

Robinson, E. A., Eyberg, S. M., & Ross, A. W. (1980). The standardization of an inventory of child conduct problem behaviors. *Journal of Clinical Child Psychology, Spring,* 22–29.

Roskies, E., Mongeon, M., & Gagnon-Lefebvre, B. (1978). Increasing maternal participation in the hospitalization of young children. *Medical Care, 16,* 765–777.

Ross, D. M., & Ross, S. A. (1984). Childhood pain: The school-aged child's viewpoint. *Pain, 20,* 179–191.

Rothbaum, F., Wolfer, J., & Visintainer, M. (1979). Coping behavior and locus of control. *Journal of Personality, 47,* 118–135.

Sallis, J. F. (1985). Improving adherence to pediatric therapeutic regimens. *Pediatric Nursing, 11,* 118–120, 148.

Schafer, L. C., Glasgow, R. E., & McCaul, K. D. (1982). Increasing the adherence of diabetic adolescents. *Journal of Behavioral Medicine, 5,* 353–362.

Schechter, N. L. (1985). Pain and pain control in children. *Current Problems in Pediatrics, 15,* 3–67.

Sergis-Deavenport, E., & Varni, J. W. (1983). Behavioral assessment and management of adherence to factor replacement therapy in hemophilia. *Journal of Pediatric Psychology, 8,* 367–377.

Shacham, S., & Daut, R. (1981). Anxiety and pain: What does the scale measure? *Journal of Consulting and Clinical Psychology, 49,* 468–469.

Shaw, E. G., & Routh, D. K. (1982). Effect of mother presence on children's reaction to aversive procedures. *Journal of Pediatric Psychology, 7,* 33–42.

Shope, J. T. (1981). Medication compliance. *Pediatric Clinics of North America, 28,* 5–21.

Shorkey, C. T., & Taylor, J. E. (1973). Management of maladaptive behavior of a severely burned child. *Child Welfare, 52,* 543–547.

Simonds, J. F. (1979). Emotions and compliance in diabetic children. *Psychosomatics, 20,* 544–551.

Skinner, B. F. (1974). *About behaviorism.* New York: Vintage.

Spielberger, C. D. (1973). *State-Trait Anxiety Inventory for Children.* Palo Alto, CA: Consulting Psychological Press.

Spielberger, C. D., Gorsuch, R., & Lushene, R. (1970). *State-Trait Anxiety Inventory Manual.* Palo Alto, CA: Consulting Psychological Press.

Steward, M. S., & Steward, D. S. (1981). Children's conceptions of medical procedures. In R. Bibace & M. E. Walsh (Eds.), *Children's conceptions of health, illness, and bodily functions.* San Francisco: Jossey-Bass.

Stokes, T. F., & Baer, D. M. (1977). An implicit technology of generalization. *Journal of Applied Behavior Analysis, 10,* 349–367.

Stokes, T. F., & Kennedy, S. H. (1980). Reducing child uncooperative behavior during dental treatment through modeling and reinforcement. *Journal of Applied Behavior Analysis, 13,* 41–49.

Stunkard, A. J. (1981). Adherence to medical treatment: Overview and lessons from behavioral weight control. *Journal of Psychosomatic Research, 25,* 187–197.

Swallow, J. N., Jones, J. M., & Morgan, M. F. (1975, July–August). The effect of environment on a child's reaction to dentistry. *Journal of Dentistry for Children,* 42–44.

Traughber, B., & Cataldo, M. F. (1983). Biobehavioral effects of pediatric hospitalization. In P. J. McGrath & P. Firestone (Eds.), *Pediatric and adolescent medicine: Issues in treatment.* New York: Springer.

Varni, J. W., Bessman, C. A., Russo, D. C., & Cataldo, M. F. (1980). Behavioral management of chronic pain in children: Case study. *Archives of Physical Medicine and Rehabilitation, 61,* 375–379.

Venham, L. L., Murray, P., & Gaulin-Kremer (1979). Personality factors affecting the preschool child's response to dental stress. *Journal of Dental Research, 58,* 2046–2051.

Venham, L., & Quatrocelli, S. (1977). The young child's response to repeated dental procedures. *Journal of Dental Research, 56,* 734–738.

Waggoner, C. D., & LeLieuvre, R. B. (1981). A method to increase compliance to exercise regimens in rheumaoid arthritis patients. *Journal of Behavioral Medicine, 4,* 191–201.

Webb, K. L., Dobson, A. J., O'Connell, D. L., Tupling, H. E., Harris, G. W., Moxon, J. A., Sulway, M. J., & Leeder, S. R. (1984). Dietary compliance among insulin-dependent diabetics. *Journal of Chronic Disease, 37,* 633–643.

Weinstein, P. (1984). Influence of dentist variables on patient behavior: Managing child behavior in the operatory. In J. D. Matarazzo, S. M. Weiss, J. A. Herd, N. E. Miller, & S. M. Weiss (Eds.), *Behavioral health: A handbook of health enhancement and disease prevention.* New York: Wiley.

Weinstein, P., Getz, T., Ratener, P., & Domoto, P. (1982a). The effect of dentists' behaviors on fear-related behaviors in children. *Journal of the American Dental Association, 104,* 32–38.

Weinstein, P., Getz, T., Ratener, P., & Domoto, P. (1982b). Dentists' responses to fear- and nonfear-related behaviors in children. *Journal of the American Dental Association, 104,* 38–40.

Winer, G. A. (1982). A review and analysis of children's fearful behavior in dental settings. *Child Development, 53,* 1111–1133.

Wright, L. (1973). Handling the encopretic child. *Professional Psychology, 4,* 137–144.

Wright, L., Schaefer, A. B., & Solomons, G. (1979). *Encyclopedia of pediatric psychology.* Baltimore: University Park Press.

Zabin, M., & Melamed, B. G. (1980). The relationship between parental discipline and children's ability to cope with stress. *Journal of Behavioral Assessment, 2,* 17–38.

22

Assessing Risk for Addictive Behaviors in Adolescence

LAURIE CHASSIN
CLARK C. PRESSON
STEVEN J. SHERMAN
JOHN McGREW

This chapter examines procedures for identifying adolescents who are at high risk to initiate addictive behaviors. The assessment of risk for addictive behaviors has important practical consequences provided it can facilitate development of primary preventive interventions directed at an adolescent population. In the field of addictive behaviors (e.g., alcoholism, cigarette smoking, hard drug use) the outcomes of treatment interventions for addicted individuls have been disappointing in the sense of producing short-term success but high relapse rates (National Institute on Drug Abuse, 1984). Because of the disappointing outcome of treatment, the interventive focus has turned to primary prevention as a potentially more effective way to combat substance abuse. Some evidence of this potential has already been documented, at least in the field of cigarette smoking (see Flay, 1985, for a review), although it has not been possible consistently to isolate effective components of

Preparation of this chapter was supported in part by NIH grant HD 13449.

prevention, and many outcome studies are limited by methodological shortcomings. In any case, given the prominent role of primary prevention as a way of combating substance abuse, the question of assessing risk for addictive behaviors becomes particularly important.

In this chapter we focus on our ability to assess risk in the preadolescent and early adolescent years. These are particularly important developmental periods because onset of substance use behavior occurs during these years (NIDA, 1984). Accordingly, these are the age groups at which preventive interventions have been directed. However, it is important to remember that risk assessment for addictive behaviors may be achieved with different degrees of success or be characterized by attention to different high-risk factors at different points in the life cycle.

We focus on the norm-violating subset of addictive behaviors, which involve the use of substances that are either illegal (e.g., hard drugs) or legal for adult use but not for adolescent use (e.g., alcohol). Thus we exclude the eating disorders (obesity, anorexia, bulimia), although it can be argued that they are forms of "addictive" behaviors. Even though eating disorders and substance use behavior may share some conceptual similarities (in the sense that they involve misregulations in self-control), the two types of addictive behaviors take quite different forms in adolescents. Unlike the eating disorders, adolescent substance use is associated with other forms of norm-violating, delinquent behavior (Johnston, O'Malley, & Eveland; 1978). Eating disorders (particularly anorexia) more often appear in conventional, even perfectionistic adolescents who strive to conform to adult expectations (Minuchin, Rosman, & Baker, 1978).

Although the substance use behaviors considered in this chapter are closely associated with more general forms of delinquent and antisocial behaviors, we confine ourselves to the assessment of risk for substance use and abuse. Antisocial behavior and delinquency are considered only to the extent that they are themselves risk factors in predicting subsequent substance abuse (Johnston et al., 1978). There exists a quite large and distinct literature on the prediction of delinquent behavior (see Loeber & Dishion, 1983, for a review), which is beyond the scope of this chapter.

The chapter is structured into four different sections. First, we consider some of the basic conceptual questions that arise in assessing risk for addictive behaviors. Before we can assess risk, we must have a conceptual model of addictive behaviors and a clear definition of the criterion behavior that we are trying to predict. Second, we review the empirical evidence concerning adolescent risk for addictive behaviors. This evidence is derived mainly from large-scale longitudinal studies that have attempted prospectively to predict the initiation of different substance use behaviors. Third, we consider the success of these risk factors, combined into a multivariate assessment instrument, at identifying adolescents at risk for the adoption of an addictive behavior—cigarette smoking. We provide an empirical example of risk assessment from our own longitudinal research, and we consider different ways of evaluating the adequacy of risk assessment. Finally, given the level of success of risk measures in accurately identifying adolescents at high and low risk for substance use, we discuss the uses to which such information can be put. Although there are both practical and ethical concerns with using risk assessment to target individuals for preventive intervention, we suggest several other important ways in which risk assessment can be used to aid primary prevention programs.

BASIC QUESTIONS: ASSESSING RISK FOR WHAT?

Common Syndrome versus Individual Addictive Behaviors

A key issue in the assessment of risk for addictive behaviors is whether these behaviors are best conceived as separately and independently determined or whether it is more useful to conceive of behaviors such as cigarette smoking, marijuana use, alcohol use, hard drug use, etc. as constituting a single "syndrome." To the extent that the addictive behaviors are separate and are the outcomes of different antecedent conditions, different risk assessment tools would have to be developed for each behavior. If, on the other hand, the behaviors represent alternative outcomes of similar antecedent conditions and if they serve similar psychological and social functions, a single risk assessment instrument for addictive behaviors would be feasible. In the strongest sense of the term, a syndrome should consist of behaviors that are linked by common causal factors. Given the correlational nature of the existing empirical data bases, a strong case for common causes underlying individual addictive behaviors cannot be made. However, aside from the issue of common cause, there is much supporting evidence for the co-occurrence and co-variation of addictive behaviors.

Perhaps the clearest supportive data are provided by the Jessors and their colleagues (Donovan & Jessor, 1985; Jessor & Jessor, 1977), who identify a syndrome of adolescent "problem behavior" including cigarette smoking, problem drinking, drug use, and precocious sexual activity. These alternative behaviors are viewed as achieving the same basic goal—premature transition to adult behaviors in violation of age norms. As such, the behaviors should co-occur in the same individuals and should be able to substitute for one another. The Jessors and their colleagues have been able to demonstrate that several conditions for a common syndrome have been met. In several different cohorts these behaviors have been shown to co-occur, to correlate negatively with indices of conventional behaviors, and to have common psychosocial predictors (Donovan & Jessor, 1985; Jessor & Jessor, 1977). On this basis, a consideration of risk for "general problem behavior" rather than for individual substance use behaviors seems warranted.

Common Syndrome versus Sequentially Linked Behaviors

One potential problem with the syndrome notion is that it may obscure the sequential nature of an adolescent's engagement in different problem behaviors. Kandel (1975; Kandel & Margulies, 1978) argues that some of the similarity in the determinants of different problem behaviors may be spurious. According to Kandel, adolescents progress through a series of distinct stages of problem behaviors—specifically from beer or wine to cigarettes or hard liquor, to marijuana, and finally to other illicit drugs. What appear to be common determinants of these different behaviors may actually reflect predictors of an adolescent's involvement at an earlier stage of problem behavior. Kandel's data suggest that an assessment of risk for problem behavior must consider the adolescent's current stage of problem behavior. Involvement with an early stage of problem behavior (e.g., beer drinking) is itself a risk for further involvement (e.g., hard drug use). This approach assumes not that the different addictive behaviors constitute a syndrome, but rather that they represent earlier and later stages in a sequence of nonnormative behaviors. Thus for Kandel any assessment of risk for addictive behaviors would involve measuring the specific addictive behaviors in which the adolescent has already engaged. A most important predictor of future stages in the substance use chain would be involvement with a substance at an earlier stage.

Whether the criterion addictive behaviors merely co-occur, form a conceptually unified syndrome, or represent a clear and necessary sequencing of steps is an empirical question. It is, however, a question of significant importance for prevention programs, dictating both the kinds of screening and the kinds of interventions that must be undertaken. If behaviors are simply co-occurring, then both screening and intervention should be narrowly targeted to specific addictive behaviors. If these behaviors form a sequence of steps, then screening and intervention should focus on the early stages of the progression. However, if these behaviors form a conceptually unified syndrome, then broadly targeted screening and intervention aimed at preventing problem behavior are indicated.

Risk for Use versus Risk for Abuse

Another issue that must be considered in defining the domain of risk assessment is the individual's level of involvement with any one particular addictive behavior. Any substance use behavior can range in involvement from occasional experimentation to a pattern of dependent use involving multiple negative consequences for the individual's home, school, and peer functioning. Given the very high frequency of some substance use behaviors in adolescence (e.g., use of alcohol), it is not clear that simply engaging in substance use per se should be considered a problem behavior. For clinical purposes, the criterion behavior that is most appropriate for defining risk is most likely to be substance *abuse* rather than substance *use*.

In terms of assessing risk, the distinction between normal adolescent experimentation and problematic substance abuse raises several possibilities. First, determinants of substance abuse may be quite different from determinants of "normal" experimental use. For example, it has been suggested (Carman, 1979; Chassin, Tetzloff, & Hershey, 1985) that social and environmental factors may raise risk for adolescent experimentation although other factors (such as anxiety reduction, mood management) may raise risk for substance abuse. Thus there may in fact be different risk factors for substance use and substance abuse.

Second, rather than different risk factors for use and abuse, it is possible that there are a given number of risk factors, and that what is critical in distinguishing use from abuse is simply the *number* of these risk factors that are present for a particular individual (Bry, McKeon, & Pandina, 1982). Bry and colleagues suggest that adolescent substance use involvement is a general coping strategy rather than a response to particular types of stressors. In their data, the degree of adolescent substance use involvement increased with the number of risk factors. In addition to simply counting the *number* of risk factors, one might wish to consider the *degree* of any risk factor.

Third, it is possible that what is important for risk assessment is an understanding of the determinants of initial substance use. An addictive model suggests that, regardless of factors that raise risk for initial use, later-stage behaviors become controlled by the physiological and addictive properties of the substance itself (cf.

Lettieri, Sayers, & Pearson, 1980). According to an addictive model, risk screening for prevention should concentrate on the determinants of initial use. Within an addictive model, the factors that determine initial onset would be most useful for intervention purposes.

Thus the distinction between use and abuse raises several alternative conceptual models to guide preventive screening and intervention. Risk for use and abuse may be characterized either by different *types* of risk factors or simply by *number* of risk factors. Alternatively, risk for use and abuse may be identical for practical purposes if the transition between use and abuse is determined merely by repeated exposures to the substance and by its addictive properties. Further, the utility of these different models may vary for different substances. In general, however, risk assessment research that is geared toward preventive intervention should allow for the possibility that substance use and abuse are qualitatively as well as quantitatively distinct phenomena.

The discussion to this point has emphasized fundamental conceptual questions about what assessment of risk entails. We now turn to more empirical issues concerned with identification of specific kinds of factors that have been demonstrated to be important in the assessment of risk for adolescent addictive behaviors.

FACTORS THAT PLACE ADOLESCENTS AT RISK FOR ADDICTIVE BEHAVIOR

Factors that place adolescents at risk for addictive behavior can best be identified from longitudinal research that prospectively predicts the *initiation* of these behaviors. Such longitudinal studies allow us to identify the types of adolescents at high risk for problem behavior. Several large-scale longitudinal studies have been conducted, and the risk factors described here are derived primarily from the work of the Jessors (Jessor & Jessor, 1977, 1984), Kellam and his colleagues (Kellam, Brown, & Fleming, 1982; Kellam, Brown, Rubin, & Ensminger, 1983), and Kandel and her colleagues (Kandel, 1978, 1984; Kandel, Kessler, & Margulies, 1978), and from our own work (Chassin, Presson, Sherman, Corty, et al., 1984). Risk factors consist of both intrapersonal and interpersonal variables. In addition, risk factors can be divided into those that have been widely replicated and whose status is clearly documented and those where there has been less consistent empirical support.

Demographic Predictors

In a recent review of the epidemiological literature, Miller (1981) has suggested that the predictive power of demographic factors in adolescent substance use has declined dramatically over the last decade, and that there are now few consistent demographic differences in substance use. Although males have traditionally reported greater use, these sex differences have been decreasing (Wechsler & McFadden, 1976). In addition, although both socioeconomic and ethnic differences in substance use have been found, the pattern of differences has shown only small and inconsistent effects of socioeconomic status and ethnicity (Kandel, 1980). The most consistent demographic correlate of substance use is age, with increasing use at older age levels (Kandel, 1980).

In general, demographic risk factors are useful for prevention in terms of allocating resources toward demographic groups in which high rates of substance use are found. However, in terms of guiding the content of prevention programs, the important question often requires identifying the high-risk individuals *within* a particular demographic category (e.g., identifying high-risk middle school students within a particular community). To accomplish this goal, other sorts of risk factors, particularly potentially *modifiable* risk factors (e.g., personality characteristics, attitudes and beliefs, interpersonal influences), become more important than demographic factors.

Widely Replicated Intrapersonal Risk Factors

The most widely agreed-upon high-risk factors are those that describe substance use behavior as part of a rebellious and nonconforming life-style (see, e.g., Cox, Lun, & Loper, 1983). A clear and widely replicated set of findings is that the typical adolescent at high risk for addictive behavior is characterized by:

Rebellion and nonconformity (e.g., Brook, Lukoff, & Whiteman, 1977; Chassin et al., 1984; Smith & Fogg, 1978)

Aggression and antisocial behavior (e.g., Ensminger, Brown, & Kellam, 1982; Loney, 1984)

Extroversion (sociability, impulsivity, sensation seeking) (e.g., Brook, Whiteman, Brook, & Gordon, 1981; Segal, 1975; Smith, 1970)

Attitudinal tolerance for norm-violating behavior (e.g., Chassin, Presson, Sherman, Corty et al., 1984, Jessor & Jessor, 1977)

Poor educational achievement, low educational aspirations (e.g., Johnston, O'Malley, & Eveland, 1978)

Adolescents with these personality characteristics are likely to be at risk for addictive behaviors for several reasons. These are adolescents who may use substances to express alienation from conventional adult values. They are also likely to be part of a social network that encourages substance use. Moreover, the impulsivity of these adolescents makes them unlikely to consider carefully the long-term consequences of their acts, including the addictive and health consequences involved in substance use. Finally, of course, it is possible that this set of personality characteristics describes a particular genotype at risk for addictive behaviors.

Other Intrapersonal Risk Factors

Another group of personality risk factors that have been less widely replicated describe substance abuse and norm-violating behaviors as a way of coping with or managing negative affect and threats to a fragile sense of self-esteem. In this view, an adolescent at high risk for addictive behaviors would be characterized by:

Low self-esteem (Kaplan, 1975, 1980)

Depression, anxiety (Kandel et al., 1978; Pandina & Scheule, 1978; Paton & Kandel, 1978)

Self-handicapping tendencies (Berglas & Jones, 1978)

Because self-handicapping is a recently developed and less well known concept than the other factors, some discussion of this risk factor is warranted. *Self-handicapping* refers to attempts to protect fragile self-esteem from failure experiences. When individuals are faced with future poor performances in areas where they have moderately high but uncertain self-images, they may adopt external impediments to performance. Although such impediments will make failure more likely, they also will allow potential failures to be justified without diminishing self-esteem. For example, a student who gets drunk the night before an important examination can explain a poor performance as a result of drinking rather than as a result of a lack of ability. Substance use, in fact, has been identified as a possible self-handicapping strategy (Berglas & Jones, 1978). Self-handicapping is an especially interesting risk factor because it allows an understanding of substance abuse by segments of the adolescent population that are not otherwise rebellious or nonconventional. Unfortunately, because the construct is so new, strong empirical support is still lacking.

In general, empirical support for the notion of adolescent substance use as a way of managing negative affect is somewhat inconsistent. In part this may be due to methodological shortcomings of the studies themselves (see Chassin, 1984, for a review). However, negative affect and low self-esteem may play a more important role in later stages of heavy substance use involvement than in predicting risk for initiation. Studies that seek to differentiate users and nonusers of a substance often fail to find differences in self-esteem or in negative affect. However, these factors differentiate users from abusers (see Chassin, 1984).

Attitudes and Beliefs as Risk Factors

To this point, the risk factors described have been personality characteristics or enduring mood states. Previous literature suggests that our ability to predict behavior from personality characteristics alone is limited (Mischel, 1968; Sherman & Fazio, 1983). The combination of personality characteristics and attitudes and beliefs may allow for better prediction.

Studies of adolescent substance use suggest that adolescents at risk to initiate substance use behavior have more positive attitudes toward the behavior and more positive beliefs about the consequences of its use. For example, longitudinal research has applied the Ajzen and Fishbein (1980) *theory of reasoned action* to predict substance use behavior from adolescents' attitudes toward the act of use and from their normative beliefs about what others in their social world would want them to do (Chassin, Presson, Sherman, Corty et al., 1984; Schlegel & DiTecco, 1978).

Research in the area of attitude–behavior relations suggests that attitudes are not always good predictors of subsequent behavior. However, attitudes that are measured at the same level of specificity as the subsequent behavior and attitudes that are based on direct experience with the attitude object are much better predictors of behavior (Fazio & Zanna, 1981; Fishbein & Ajzen, 1974).

Behavioral Intentions as a Risk Factor

One way to assess the likelihood of subsequent behavior is to ask people their future intentions with respect to that behavior. This would appear to be a simple and straightforward method. In fact, previous research indicates that behavioral intentions are sometimes excellent predictors of behavior (see Ajzen & Fishbein,

1980, for a review). However, there are reasons that make this a less than perfect approach. In the first place, in order that intentions be good predictors of behavior, these intentions must be measured at a point in time close to the target behavior. For preventive interventions, this is not ideal. In addition, individuals must have control over the target behaviors in order for intentions to predict behavior very well. Many adolescents may not plan or intend to engage in substance use, but may do so because of strong situational external pressures that they feel they cannot resist.

Moreover, behavioral intentions simply reflect people's predictions of what they will do in the future. Research has indicated that predictions are quite poor in areas involving behaviors that have a social desirability component (Sherman, 1980). In addition, once these "mispredictions" are made, they tend to have an influence on subsequent behavior. Thus measures of behavioral intentions are reactive, and may actually alter the likelihood of the future behavior.

Behaviors as Risk Factors

As previously discussed, stage models of substance use suggest that early forms of substance use behaviors are particularly important risk factors for predicting later stages in the progression (Kandel et al., 1978). Moreover, other forms of norm-violating behaviors, particularly aggressive and antisocial behaviors, are important predictors of substance use (Loney, 1984).

INTERPERSONAL RISK FACTORS

There is widespread agreement that the adolescent at high risk for addictive behavior is characterized by social environments including:

Peer and parent models for addictive behavior (Huba, Wingard, & Bentler, 1979; Kandel, 1978; Krosnick & Judd, 1982; Smart & Fejer, 1972)

Peer and parent attitudes that tolerate addictive behavior (e.g., Akers, Krohn, Lanza-Kaduce, & Radosevich, 1979)

Alienation from parents (e.g., Dembo, Farron, Des Jarleis, Burgos, & Schmeidler, 1981; Ensminger et al., 1982; Hirschi, 1969)

Parent disciplinary practices including lack of monitoring and ineffective discipline (cf. Loeber & Dishion, 1983)

Most of the research on parent and peer influence is based on social learning theory (Bandura, 1969; Bandura & Walters, 1963), which would suggest that substance behaviors are acquired both by vicarious conditioning and by the social reinforcement provided by significant others in the social network. These factors refer to parent and peer behavior and attitudes specific to substance use. However, other more general aspects of parent and peer relations (e.g., perceived distance or parent discipline practices) may also be important. As discussed in Chapter 23 of this volume, particular parent–child interactions raise risk for general antisocial behavior that is highly correlated with substance abuse.

AN EMPIRICAL EXAMPLE OF RISK ASSESSMENT FOR ADOLESCENT CIGARETTE SMOKING

Given that longitudinal studies have been conducted to identify the prospective predictors of substance use behaviors, and given that these studies converge in identifying a large number of factors that place adolescents at high risk, is it possible to use these factors effectively to assess risk with a multivariate battery? Before such a battery can be used to screen individuals for preventive intervention, it is obviously important to examine the degree of accuracy with which such an assessment could identify individuals at risk to initiate addictive behavior. In order to discuss the utility of assessing substance use risk, we present an empirical example from our own longitudinal investigations of adolescent cigarette smoking. We will examine the accuracy of prediction and discuss ways in which a multivariate risk measure might be used.

Subjects

Subjects were all consenting sixth through twelfth graders from a midwestern county school system who were present in school on the days of testing. Demographic figures reveal a community that is predominantly White (96 percent). The influence of a large university community is reflected in the educational status of parents, with 38 percent holding a bachelor's degree or higher.

Procedure

Using a cohort-sequential design, questionnaires were group administered in classrooms by a member of the research team unconnected with the school system. The data reported here are from two administrations of the questionnaire performed over a 1-year interval. The questionnaire included four general kinds of predictor variables: personality characteristics (e.g., relative unconventionality, rebelliousness, and deviance proneness); attitudes and beliefs about cigarette smoking; the distal perceived environment (e.g., perceptions of the quality of relationships with peers and parents); and the proximal perceived environment (e.g., the smoking behavior and attitudes of peers and parents). A more detailed description of the questionnaire can be found in Chassin and colleagues (1981). Cigarette-smoking status was assessed by a single self-report item (validated with a bogus pipeline procedure; see Evans, Hansen, & Mittelmark, 1977). For prospectively predicting smoking transitions, the subjects of interest here are those who at Time 1 of measurement were either Never Smokers or Triers (had smoked one or two cigarettes, just to try, but had not smoked in the past month).

Results

To examine the accuracy of prediction, discriminant function analyses were performed comparing initial Never Smokers who did and did not go on to smoke over the 1-year period. Parallel analyses compared initial Triers who did and did not go on to become regular smokers. Separate discriminant functions were done for middle school (grades six through eight) and high school subsamples. Each subject was classified by the discriminant function (on the basis of scores on predictor variables) as predicted either to make or not to make a transition in smoking status. Table 22.1 compares the predicted transitions to actual transitions separately for initial Never Smokers and initial Triers in middle school and in high school. The percentage correctly classified for each group ranged from 80.6 to 96.7.

The question of assessing the adequacy of risk assessment is not straightforward. Given the hit rates achieved by our instrument, several tests of its adequacy are possible. One possibility is to test the improvement in prediction relative to a random 50–50 classification into those who will and will not make a transition (the success rate of which would, of course, be 50 percent). Clearly, prediction using our assessment instrument does significantly better than this classification (chi-square comparisons, p's $< .001$). However, this would be a weak test of improvement when the criterion behavior (transition) occurs far less frequently than 50 percent of the time.

When the base rate of the criterion behavior is very low (as in the present case), one can obviously attain a large percentage of correct classification by simply predicting that no one will change status. For example, only 14 percent of middle school Never Smokers make the transition. By predicting that no one will become a smoker, correct classification would be achieved 86 percent of the time. However, this procedure has no utility for preventive screening and intervention, because no one would be predicted to be at risk.

A more appropriate and extremely stringent comparison looks at the number of successful and unsuccessful predictions compared to the level of success that would be achieved simply by considering the base rate of actual transition and the base rate of predicted transition. This produces a two-cell chi-square (number of successes and number of failures) in which the observed and expected frequencies can be compared. This chi-square compares the efficacy of the predicted classification against a random selection given the base rate of actual and predicted transitions. In our data, the chi-squares were 26.8, 26.9, 26.5, and 25.8 (all p's $< .001$). Thus in each case prediction based on our assessment instrument was a significant improvement over the minimum level expected by chance.

Just as the base rate of actual transition and the base rate of predicted transition set the empirical limits for minimal success, we can estimate the maximum prediction possible from these base rates (see Loeber & Dishion, 1983, for a detailed discussion). Loeber and Dishion (1983) suggest that both the minimum and maximum levels of prediction be calculated and used to specify the range of possible prediction. They then propose an index that represents the improvement over chance achieved by the assessment instrument as a percentage of this range (designated as the *relative improvement over chance*). In our data, the relative improvement over chance ranged from 67 to 87.5 percent. Thus, although the question of assessing the efficacy of prediction is not at all straightforward, our data demonstrate both a statistically significant and relatively highly efficient gain over chance using a variety of indices. By all of the indices, it is clear that the instrument was able to identify the adolescents at risk to make transitions in smoking status.

However, even when successful prediction has been demonstrated over a variety of indices, the utility of the instrument in screening adolescents for risk for addictive behaviors has not been established. Rather, an evaluation of the instrument's utility depends on the uses to which the obtained information can be put.

TABLE 22.1. ACCURACY OF RISK ASSESSMENT FOR SMOKING TRANSITIONS FOR INITIAL NEVER SMOKERS AND TRIERS IN MIDDLE SCHOOL AND HIGH SCHOOL

A. *Subpopulation:* Initial *Never Smokers* in year 1—middle school

		Predicted status: Predict no transition	Predicted status: Predict transition		
Actual status in year 2	No transition	(Valid negatives) 508	(False positives) 12	520	Base rate of actual transition: 14.0%
	Made transition to increased smoking	(False negatives) 55	(Valid positives) 30	85	
		563	42	$N = 605$	
		Base rate of predicted transition = 6.9%			

Canonical $R = .5015$

Correctly classified = 88.9%

Predictive efficiency (relative increase over chance) = 66.7%

B. *Subpopulation*: Initial *Never Smokers* in year 1—high school

		Predicted status: Predict no transition	Predicted status: Predict transition		
Actual status in year 2	No transition	(Valid negatives) 208	(False positives) 14	222	Base rate of actual transition: 22.9%
	Made transition to increased smoking	(False negatives) 22	(Valid positives) 44	66	
		230	58	$N = 288$	
		Base rate of predicted transition = 20.1%			

Canonical $R = .6244$

Correctly classified = 80.6%

Predictive efficiency (RIOC) = 68.9%

TABLE 22.1. *(Continued)*

C. *Subpopulation*: Initial *Triers* in year 1—middle school

Actual status in year 2	Predicted status: Predict no transition	Predicted status: Predict transition	Total	
No transition	(Valid negatives) 176	(False positives) 4	180	Base rate of actual transition: 10.0%
Made transition to increased smoking	(False negatives) 4	(Valid positives) 16	20	
	180	20	$N = 200$	
	Base rate of predicted transition = 10.0%			

Canonical $R = .668$

Correctly classified = 96.0%

Predictive efficiency (RIOC) = 75.0%

D. *Subpopulation*: Initial *Triers* in year 1—high school

Actual status in year 2	Predicted status: Predict no transition	Predicted status: Predict transition	Total	
No transition	(Valid negatives) 243	(False positives) 3	246	Base rate of actual transition: 11.2%
Made transition to increased smoking	(False negatives) 7	(Valid positives) 24	31	
	250	27	$N = 277$	
	Base rate of predicted transition = 9.7%			

Canonical $R = .675$

Correctly classified = 96.4%

Predictive efficiency (RIOC) = 87.5%

GROUP VERSUS INDIVIDUAL LEVELS OF RISK ASSESSMENT

Risk assessment can serve two main purposes. First, at a group level, knowledge of risk factors can be used to build theories of the acquisition of problem behaviors. An understanding of the acquisition process can then be used to guide the development of intervention programs (Chassin, Presson, & Sherman, 1985). Second, at the individual level, risk assessment can be used to target particular individuals as high-risk cases and to select those individuals for intervention efforts. We consider here whether risk assessment for addictive behaviors can effectively and ethically be used at the individual level.

In some sense, screening individuals and identifying them as high-risk individuals might, in itself, be an effective form of primary prevention. If an individual recognizes that he or she has particular vulnerability to substance use, that person may arrange his or her life-style to avoid exposure to the substance. For example, individuals identified at particular risk for heart attacks may take special care with their diet and exercise so as to avoid the risk of heart disease. Similarly, individuals who feel that they have particular risk for alcoholism may strictly abstain from using alcohol. Thus there can be positive preventive effects of simply informing individuals of their risk status.

Unfortunately, however, identifying particular individuals as high-risk cases has potentially negative effects as well. The major obstacle to an individual-level use of risk assessment has to do with both practical and ethical concerns that are brought about by errors of prediction and misidentification. These errors are particularly critical when intervention decisions are made about specific individuals as a result of their risk designation. For example, labeling effects can be created when a person is mistakenly designated a high-risk individual. That is, individuals labeled as potential candidates for addictive behaviors may react negatively to such labeling. They may feel weak or deviant. This can have effects on self-concept. In addition, self-fulfilling prophecies can result, and a negative cycle can be set in motion. The label itself may create its own reality because of changes in the behavior of the labeled individual or because of the reactions of others to the label. Any time that the individual is made aware of his or her own risk status, or significant others in the person's life are made aware of that status, the risk of labeling effects and self-fulfilling prophecies occurs. This situation could arise in the context of a research study where high-risk individuals are merely followed rather than targeted for intervention. However, it is more often a problem when risk assessment is used to select particular individuals for preventive intervention.

If errors are made in risk designation, then individuals who are actually at low risk may be subjected to unnecessary intervention. In some cases this may mean no more than an unnecessary expenditure of intervention resources. However, any intervention can have negative as well as positive effects. For example, there have been occasional reports of drug education programs that have led to increases in drug use (Stuart, 1974). Thus all intervention carries some risk of doing harm. Generally (for individuals who are suffering from some disorder or individuals who are at high risk for disorder), the chance of treatment gains is thought to offset the risk of negative effects. However, for individuals who are actually at low risk for substance abuse but are mislabeled and given unnecessary intervention, there is no potential gain to balance the risk of harm. Because of the risk of labeling effects and the risk of harm from intervention, an individual-level application of risk assessment requires an extremely high degree of accuracy in pinpointing high-risk adolescents.

As we have seen, evaluating the degree of accuracy of risk assessment is not a simple matter. Hit rates alone can provide misleading information because it is necessary to interpret the hit rates within the context of base-rate information. As the base rate decreases, the ability of prediction to improve upon simple base rate information decreases (Meehl & Rosen, 1955). Because substance abuse is a low-base-rate behavior, considerable care must be taken in interpreting the results of risk assessment.

Moreover, when evaluating rates of hits and misses, any inaccuracy must be decomposed into two kinds of errors—false positives and false negatives. False positives occur when individuals are mistakenly predicted to initiate the addictive behaviors. These individuals would then be subject to unnecessary intervention. False negatives occur when high-risk individuals are mistakenly thought to be at low risk for addictive behavior. In this case, intervention would fail to reach part of the important audience.

An example of the importance of false negatives and false positives can be seen by examining our prediction for the middle school initial Never Smokers (see Table 22.1). For this subpopulation, intervention with the high-risk group would be inefficient because the predicted high-risk group includes only 35.3 percent of the true high-risk group. Using the same assessment device, we can adopt a different selection ratio (by changing the cutoff score). With changes in the selection ratio, we were able to use our same assessment measure to identify 80.0 percent of the high-risk group, which considerably reduces the number of false negatives. However, by this new criterion, 21.3 percent of low-risk subjects ($N = 111$) were mistakenly predicted to begin to smoke. This represents an increase in false positives. The trade-off between false positives and false negatives in this population might then mean that 111 adolescents get subjected to unnecessary intervention. It is important to remember that our prediction was better than chance at forecasting a low-base-rate behavior (using a stringent test) and that it achieved a relative increase over chance of considerable magnitude. Even with this extent of success, the number of false positives and negatives may still be so high that for practical and ethical reasons the instrument cannot be used to screen individuals for intervention.

Even if research were to demonstrate acceptably low levels of false positives and false negatives, there are several concerns that remain in taking instruments developed for research purposes and applying them as screening devices to target individuals for preventive interventions. Methodologically, there is a question of whether the large-scale longitudinal studies have validated their risk factors against an accurate assessment of substance use behavior. Most studies are forced to rely on self-report measures that are obviously limited when the target behavior is illegal or nonnormative. Self-reports of these types of behaviors are subject to social desirability biases. Adolescents are likely to be afraid of the consequences of admitting to such behaviors. In some cases, investigators have attempted to solve this problem by using more objective measures such as bioassays to detect the presence of metabolites of substances such an nicotine. Unfortunately, however, these bioassays have been limited as measures of adolescent use of substances. For example, with cigarette smoking, these assays often fail to detect the low levels of use that are characteristic of adolescent populations. In short, caution is required in applying risk measures developed from the existing longitudinal studies because of their reliance on self-report measures of the criterion behavior. A more accurate measure of the criterion behavior might reveal a different degree of predictability or a different set of risk factors.

When moving from instruments developed for research purposes to the level of individual risk assessment, additional concerns arise from the question of generalizability. First, the degree of predictive power or the type of risk factors identified may vary considerably in different populations. For example, in our data in trying to predict the initial onset of smoking, the same instrument did a better job of minimizing false negatives among high school than among middle school students. The same variables that prove useful in large-scale longitudinal research studies might fail if applied to individual-level risk assessment with a different type of population.

The generalizability of findings from large-scale longitudinal investigations to individual-level risk assessment is also limited by sampling and attrition biases within the longitudinal research. Most of the large-scale longitudinal studies cited in this chapter have attempted to study representative samples of the adolescent population by selecting public school students as subjects. Unfortunately, this sample is likely to exclude the most high-risk subjects—school dropouts, truants, or students in nontraditional educational settings. This problem of sample selection is compounded in longitudinal studies with repeated measurements over time. Attrition in these studies is rarely random. Rather, the adolescents at highest risk for substance abuse behavior are the ones who are most likely to be lost to follow-up. Thus the prospective prediction of the criterion behavior may be performed using a population that is not the most representative for individual-level risk assessment.

Finally, the success of the research instruments (such as the one from our study) does not necessarily provide a practical measure for individual use. These measures are typically lengthy and time-consuming to administer. For example, our questionnaire required an hour to complete. In addition, the number of instruments available for inclusion in a general risk assessment battery for substance abuse behavior is quite large. One potential solution would be to compile a measure by selecting a smaller subset of variables that have been proven useful in different studies. However, such an instrument is unlikely to achieve the accuracy of the original questionnaires. Changing the multivariate context can change the level of prediction achieved by a single variable.

Thus we have identified several important issues that suggest caution in moving from research-group-level uses of a risk assessment to clinical prediction of risk at the individual level in order to target adolescents for intervention. The overall success of the research instruments must be carefully examined in terms of false positives and false negatives. Even with acceptably low levels of false positives and false negatives, it may be unwise to generalize from the school-based research populations to the clinical target audiences (especially given subject attrition in the longitudinal studies). The research findings may also be limited by inaccurate assessment of the criterion variable. These potential losses in accuracy in applying risk measures from research to clinical practice become particularly serious because of the ethical concerns inherent in targeting specific individuals for preventive intervention.

THE SOCIOCULTURAL CONTEXT OF RISK ASSESSMENT

A final concern in moving from group level to individual levels of risk assessment is the need to consider the larger cultural and historical context in which risk assessment is conducted. Data bases are necessarily limited by the particular time and culture in which they have been generated. The degree of predictability, the types of predictor variables, and the very social meaning of the behavior itself can change with time and culture. For these reasons, any risk assessment must consider variables that go beyond the individual level of analysis and must also consider the social and cultural context of the assessment.

The meaning of any act (including addictive behaviors) is of course determined by the sociocultural and historical context in which that act is embedded. The very same behavior can be interpreted and evaluated in quite different ways by a society at different stages of that society's historical development. In this regard, one possible interpretation of norm-violating behavior is that the level of such behavior by individuals within a society is fairly constant. However, specific behaviors that are judged as violations of norms may change dramatically over time. Thus premarital sex or cigarette smoking may be regarded as quite deviant at one point in history and as quite normative or acceptable at another time. Addictive behaviors may then increase or decrease partly because of their social meaning.

Interestingly, this view implies that the increases and decreases in addictive behaviors across historical periods may differ dramatically among different subgroups of society. As a behavior (e.g., smoking) becomes more acceptable, it may be adopted more by those in the society who are norm followers and who are not deviance prone. On the other hand, when a behavior becomes labeled as more norm violating, its adoption is likely by a very different segment of the population, the deviance-prone individuals. Taking into account the social meaning (especially the degree of nonnormativeness) of any behavior can help us understand the apparent faddish nature of certain addictive behavior patterns.

An example can be drawn from patterns of tobacco use in this country over the last 80 years. At the beginning of this century, smokeless forms of tobacco were the most prevalent uses. The shift to cigarettes as the primary form of tobacco use was caused in part by a change in the perceived meaning and accessibility of smoking and chewing tobacco. Chewing came to be seen as a greater health risk than smoking due to the risk of spreading tuberculosis bacilli through spitting in public (Christen, Swanson, Glover, & Henderson, 1982). Ironically, at the present time, we may be seeing the reversal of this pattern. In the past decade, as awareness of the pervasive and severe health risks of smoking has grown, there has again been a shift in the perceptions of the relative health risks of chewing versus smoking. There has also been a rise in the prevalence of smokeless tobacco use (Gritz, Ksir, & Mccarthy, 1985).

The example of tobacco use behavior illustrates the importance of considering risk for any individual substance use behavior in a larger social context. Societally relevant behaviors are judged very differently depending on the context in which they appear (Parducci, 1968; Sherman, Ahlm, Berman, & Lynn, 1978). Social judgment effects of assimilation and contrast are well documented for evaluations of a variety of stimuli (Anderson, 1975; Pepitone & DiNubile, 1976; Sherif & Hovland, 1961). We can analyze the adoption of addictive behaviors in the light of these social judgment processes.

One of the deterrents to substance use is likely to be the degree of negativity attached by the individual and by the larger society to the possible outcomes of such use. How negatively will an individual evaluate the possibility of cancer following cigarette smoking or the possibility of addiction or loss of job due to drug use? This will depend in part on the context of other possible negative outcomes with which one is confronted. As extremely negative and threatening events become salient and/or prevalent, the judgment of less threatening outcomes (such as addiction or the possibility of heart disease in the distant future) becomes much less negative because of contrast effects. In recent years extremely negative salient and vivid problems such as nuclear war, AIDS, and international terrorism have become highly publicized. In the context of these problems, some kinds of substance use may appear far less negative in terms of their potential consequences.

CONCLUSION

We have illustrated that large-scale longitudinal research projects have achieved successful prospective prediction of adolescents' initiation of addictive behaviors. These studies have thus identified individuals *at risk* for substance use. However, we have also argued that there is considerable reason for caution in attempting to apply these risk assessment measures as screening devices to select individual adolescents for preventive intervention. There are both practical and ethical concerns that limit the utility of these research instruments as screening devices for intervention. Given these cautions, what then is the utility of risk assessment for substance use?

We suggest that there are three important ways in which risk assessment can be used. First, risk assessment can contribute to knowledge and theory building in studying substance use. One of the goals of the longitudinal studies has been to gain an understanding of the psychological processes and mechanisms underlying the acquisition of substance use behavior. That is, the studies were not simply descriptive in nature, but rather represented attempts to test and develop theories of substance use. The studies have achieved a substantial degree of success in this regard, and a number of complex theories and models have emerged in recent years (Huba & Bentler, 1982; Jessor & Jessor, 1977; Kandel et al., 1978).

Second, the identification of a high-risk group is advantageous for research that attempts an even more detailed analysis of the substance use acquisition process. Researchers who wish to examine the onset of substance use will find the process less costly and more efficient if they can oversample from the high-risk group. This ensures that they will have sufficient numbers of onset incidents to allow for a microanalysis of the onset process.

Third, once a theory of acquisition has been developed (in part on the basis of risk assessment procedures) this understanding of acquisition can be used to develop individual intervention programs. Intervention that is based on an understanding of acquisition processes is more likely to be effective. As we have argued elsewhere (Chassin, Presson, & Sherman, 1985), intervention that is based on an understanding of the acquisition process can combat the specific causes of target behavior, allow a better prediction of the implications of intervention, and facilitate the evaluation of intervention efforts. Research using risk assessment can contribute to substance use prevention efforts by building the data base on which preventive interventions draw.

As described earlier, we have argued that using risk assessment to select specific individuals for intervention has both practical and ethical problems. However, even without selecting high-risk individuals, a knowledge of the high-risk group and the high-risk factors can be important for preventive intervention. In the field of substance use prevention, most intervention programs are in fact conducted with a general (unselected) population of public school students. When the prevention audience is unselected, knowledge of risk factors can be used to guide the content of the program. Preventive messages can be constructed to combat the specific risk factors that have been identified. Moreover, the messages can be geared to influence the high-risk individuals within the unselected audience. For example, if adolescents at high risk to initiate substance use are relatively nonconventional and "deviance prone," then using traditional school leaders to deliver preventive messages may not be maximally effective. Preventive messages could be made more effective by considering the values and aspirations of deviance-prone adolescents. Thus the utility of risk assessment for preventive intervention does not necessarily depend on selecting specific *individuals* for intervention. Rather, risk assessment can be used to select specific *factors* to be combated in intervention programs.

We hope it is clear that throughout this chapter we have not advocated a position that is either strictly in favor of or against the concept or practice of risk assessment for addictive behaviors. Rather, we have tried to identify and clarify the limitations of risk assessment and the concerns that are necessary to address. Most important, we have tried to spell out the appropriate uses to which risk assessment could be put and the benefits that are achievable from these appropriate uses.

References

Ajzen, I., & Fishbein, M. (1980). *Understanding attitudes and predicting social behavior*. Englewood Cliffs, NJ: Prentice-Hall.

Akers, R. L., Krohn, M. D., Lanza-Kaduce, L., & Radosevich, M. (1979). Social learning and deviant behavior: A specific test of a general theory. *American Sociological Review, 44*, 635–655.

Anderson, N. H. (1975). On the role of context effects in psychophysical judgment. *Psychological Review, 82*, 462–482.

Bandura, A. (1969). *Principles of behavior modification*. New York: Holt, Rinehart & Winston.

Bandura, A., & Walters, R. H. (1963). *Social learning and personality development*. New York: Holt, Rinehart & Winston.

Berglas, S., & Jones, E. E. (1978). Drug choice as a self-handicapping strategy in response to noncontingent success. *Journal of Personality & Social Psychology, 36*, 405–417.

Brook, J., Lukoff, I., & Whiteman, M. (1977). Peer, family, and personality domains as related to adolescents' drug behavior. *Psychological Reports, 41*, 1095–1102.

Brook, J., Whiteman, M., Brook, D., & Gordon, A. (1981). Paternal determinants of male adolescent marijuana use. *Developmental Psychology, 17*, 841–847.

Bry, B., McKeon, P., & Pandina, R. (1982). Extent of drug use as a function of number of risk factors. *Journal of Abnormal Psychology, 91*, 273–279.

Carman, R. S. (1979). Motivations for drug use and problematic outcomes among rural junior high school students. *Addictive Behaviors, 4*, 91–93.

Chassin, L. (1984). Adolescent substance use and abuse. In P. Karoly & J. Steffen (Eds.), *Adolescent behavior disorders: Foundations and contemporary concerns*. Lexington, MA: Heath.

Chassin, L., Presson, C. C., & Sherman, S. J. (1984). Cigarette smoking and adolescent psychosocial development. *Basic & Applied Social Psychology, 5*, 295–315.

Chassin, L., Presson, C. C., & Sherman, S. J. (1985). Stepping backward in order to step forward: An acquisition-oriented approach to primary prevention. *Journal of Consulting & Clinical Psychology, 53*, 612–622.

Chassin, L., Presson, C. C., Sherman, S. J., Bensenberg, M., Corty, E., & Olshavsky, R. W.. (1981). Predicting adolescents' intentions to smoke cigarettes. *Journal of Health & Social Behavior, 22*, 445–455.

Chassin, L., Presson, C. C., Sherman, S. J., Corty, E., & Olshavsky, R. W. (1984). Predicting the onset of cigarette smoking in adolescents: A longitudinal study. *Journal of Applied Social Psychology, 14*, 224–243.

Chassin, L., Tetzloff, C., & Hershey, M. (1985). Self-image and social-image factors in adolescent alcohol use. *Journal of Studies on Alcohol, 46*, 39–47.

Christen, A. G., Swanson, B. Z., Glover, E. D., & Henderson, A. H. (1982). *Journal of the American Dental Association, 105*, 821–829.

Cox, W. M., Lun, K.-S., & Loper, R. G. (1983). Identifying prealcoholic personality characteristics. In W. M. Cox (Ed.), *Identifying and measuring alcoholic personality characteristics*. San Francisco: Jossey-Bass.

Dembo, R., Farrow, D., Des Jarlais, D., Burgos, W., & Schmeidler, J. (1981). Examining a causal model of early drug involvement among inner-city junior high school youths. *Human Relations, 34*, 169–193.

Donovan, J., & Jessor, R. L. (1985). Structure of problem behavior in adolescence and young adulthood. *Journal of Consulting & Clinical Psychology, 53*, 890–904.

Ensminger, M., Brown, C. H., & Kellam, S. (1982). Sex differences in antecedents of substance use among adolescents. *Journal of Social Issues, 38*, 25–42.

Evans, R., Hansen, W., & Mittelmark, M. (1977). Increasing the validity of self-reports of behavior in a smoking in children investigation. *Journal of Applied Psychology, 62*, 521–523.

Fazio, R. H., & Zanna, M. P. (1981). Direct experience and attitude-behavior consistency. In L. Berkowitz (Ed.), *Advances in experimental social psychology* (Vol. 14). New York: Academic.

Fishbein, M., & Ajzen, I. (1974). Attitudes toward objects as predictors of single and multiple behavioral criteria. *Psychological Review, 81*, 59–74.

Flay, B. R. (1985). Psychosocial approaches to smoking prevention: A review of findings. *Health Psychology, 4*, 449–489.

Gritz, E. R., Ksir, C., & McCarthy, W. J. (1985). Smokeless tobacco use in the United States: Present and future trends. *Annals of Behavioral Medicine, 7*, 24–27.

Hirschi, J. (1969). *Causes of delinquency*. Berkeley: University of California Press.

Huba, G., & Bentler, P. (1982). A developmental theory of drug use: Derivation and assessment of a causal modeling approach. In P. B. Baltes & O. G. Brim (Eds.), *Life-span development and behavior* (Vol. 4), New York: Academic Press.

Huba, G., Wingard, J., & Bentler, P. (1979). Beginning adolescent drug use and peer and adult interactional patterns. *Journal of Consulting & Clinical Psychology, 47*, 265–276.

Jessor, R., & Jessor, S. L. (1977). *Problem behavior and psychosocial development: A longitudinal study of youth*. New York: Academic.

Johnston, L., O'Malley, P., & Eveland, L. (1978). Drugs and delinquency: A search for causal connections. In D. B. Kandel (Ed.), *Longitudinal research on drug use: Empirical findings and methodological issues*. New York: Wiley.

Kandel, D. B. (1975). Stages in adolescent involvement in drug use. *Science, 190*, 912–914.

Kandel, D. B. (1978). *Longitudinal research on drug use: Empirical findings and methodological issues*. New York: Wiley.

Kandel, D. B. (1980). Drug and drinking behavior among youth. *Annual Review of Sociology, 6,* 235–285.

Kandel, D. B. (1984). Family and peer processes in adolescent drug use. In S. Mednick, M. Harway, & K. Finello (Eds.), *Handbook of longitudinal research* (Vol. 2). NIDA research monograph 48. Washington, DC: US Government Printing Office.

Kandel, D. B., Kessler, R., & Margulies, R. (1978). Antecedents of adolescent initiation into stages of drug use: A developmental analysis. In D. B. Kandel (Ed.), *Longitudinal research on drug use: Empirical findings and methodological issues*. New York: Wiley.

Kaplan, H. B. (1975). *Self-attitudes and deviant behavior*. Pacific Palisades, CA: Goodyear.

Kaplan, H. B. (1980). *Deviant behavior in defense of self*. New York: Academic.

Kellam, S., Brown, C. H., & Fleming, J. (1982). Social adaptation to first grade and teenage drug, alcohol, and cigarette use. *Journal of School Health, 52,* 301–306.

Kellam, S. G., Brown, C. H., Rubin, B. R., & Ensminger, M. E. (1983). Paths leading to teenage psychiatric symptoms and substance use: Developmental epidemiological studies in Woodlawn. In S. B. Guze, F. J. Earls, & J. E. Barett (Eds.), *Childhood psychopathology and development*. New York: Raven.

Krosnick, J., & Judd, C. (1982). Transitions in social influence at adolescence: Who induces cigarette smoking? *Developmental Psychology, 18,* 359–368.

Lettieri, D. J., Sayers, M., & Pearson, H. W. (Eds.). (1980). *Theories on drug abuse: Selected contemporary perspectives*. Rockville MD: National Institute on Drug Abuse.

Loeber, R., & Dishion, T. (1983). Early predictors of male delinquency: A review. *Psychological Bulletin, 94,* 68–99.

Loney, J. (1980). The Iowa theory of substance abuse among hyperactive adolescents. In D. J. Lettieri, M. Sayers, & H. W. Pearson (Eds.), *Theories on drug abuse: Selected contemporary perspectives*. Rockville MD: National Institute on Drug Abuse.

Meehl, P. E., & Rosen, A. (1955). Antecedent probability and the efficiency of psychometric signs, patterns, or cutting scores. *Psychological Bulletin, 52,* 194–216.

Minuchin, S., Rosman, B., & Baker, L. (1978). *Psychosomatic families: Anorexia nervosa in context*. Cambridge, MA: Harvard University Press.

Mischel, W. (1968). *Personality and assessment*. New York: Wiley.

Pandina, R. J., & Scheule, J. (1978). Psychosocial correlates of substance use. In R. J. Pandina (Ed.), *Coping with adolescent substance use*. New Brunswick, NJ: Rutgers Center on Alcohol Studies.

Parducci, A. (1968). The relativism of abolute judgments. *Scientific American, 219,* 84–90.

Paton, S., & Kandel, D. B. (1978). Psychological factors and adolescent illicit drug use: Ethnicity and sex differences. *Adolescence, 13,* 187–200.

Pepitone, A., & DiNubile, M. (1976). Contrast effects in judgments of crime severity and the punishment of criminal violators. *Journal of Personality & Social Psychology, 33,* 448–459.

Schlegel, R. P., & DiTecco, D. (1978). *Mediational adequacy of the Fishbein model under conditions of varying behavioral complexity*. Unpublished manuscript, University of Waterloo, Ontario, Canada.

Segal, B. (1975). Personality factors related to drug and alcohol use. In D. J. Lettiary (Ed.), *Predicting adolescent drug use: A review of issues, methods, and correlates*. Rockville, MD: National Institute on Drug Abuse.

Sherif, M., & Hovland, C. I. (1961). *Social judgment: Assimilation and contrast effects in communication and attitude change*. New Haven, CT: Yale University Press.

Sherman, S. J. (1980). On the self-erasing nature of errors of prediction. *Journal of Personality & Social Psychology, 39,* 211–221.

Sherman, S. J., Ahlm, K., Berman, L., & Lynn, S. (1978). Contrast effects and their relationship to subsequent behavior. *Journal of Experimental Social Psychology, 14,* 340–350.

Sherman, S. J., & Fazio, R. H. (1983). Parallels between attitudes and traits as predictors of behavior. *Journal of Personality, 51,* 308–345.

Smart, R. G., & Fejer, D. (1972). Drug use among adolescents and thir parents: Closing the generation gap in mood modification. *Journal of Abnormal Psychology, 79,* 153–160.

Smith, G. M. (1970). Personality and smoking: A review of the empirical literature. In W. A. Hunt (Ed.), *Learning mechanisms in smoking*. Chicago: Aldine.

Smith, G., & Fogg, C. (1978). Psychological predictors of early use, late use, and nonuse of marijuana among teenage students. In D. B. Kandel (Ed.), *Longitudinal research on drug use: Empirical findings and methodological issues*. New York: Wiley.

Stuart, R. B. (1974). Teaching facts about drugs: Pushing or preventing? *American Journal of Drug & Alcohol Abuse, 4,* 55–64.

Wechsler, H., & McFadden, M. (1976). Sex differences in adolescent alcohol and drug use: A disappearing phenomenon. *Journal of Studies on Alcohol, 37,* 1291–1301.

23

Assessing Aggressive and Violent Parent–Child Interaction

JAMES SNYDER
JEANETTA RAINS
JAMES POPEJOY

OVERVIEW AND DEFINITION

There is a tendency to think of aggressive and violent parent–child interactions in terms of a typology. These interactions occur in some families, but not in others. For example, parents are classified as abusive if their children show evidence of "non-accidental, physical injury (or injuries) that are the result of acts (or omissions) on the part of the parents . . . that violate community standards concerning the treatment of children" (Parke & Collmer, 1975, p. 510). Parents whose children do not show such evidence are not considered abusive. This "either–or" typology is utilitarian in several respects. It identifies those parents whose behavior toward their children is sufficiently dangerous that it requires immediate intervention. It fulfills the legal obligation of helping agents to report abusive behavior. It delineates a group of violence-prone parents needed effectively to research the cause of violence and to develop and assess intervention strategies for such families.

Alternately, parent–child interaction can be construed along a qualitative continuum ranging topographically from positive social exchange to extreme violence, with neutral and milder forms of verbal and physical aggression falling between the extremes (Zigler, 1980). The qualitative aspects of parent–child interaction observed in a specific family can be expressed as a range on this continuum. A second, quantitative dimension can be added that describes the rate with which those various qualitative behaviors are performed by family members. The qualitative range and frequency distributions descriptive of interaction in aggressive and normative families are shown in Figure 23.1 (calculated from Reid, 1978). Situational variables affect where, within this range, parent–child interaction will fall at any moment in time. The qualitative range and the frequency distribution may slowly shift as a result of intra- and extrafamilial variables that occur over long periods of time.

The use of a continuum model of child-directed parent behavior does not preclude the selection of a cutoff point to define extreme, abusive families, but offers several conceptual advantages over the typology model. First, it suggests that parental aggression toward children is a dynamic process. Within short periods of time, there are identifiable variables that influence where, within a qualitative range, a parent's child-directed behavior will fall. Over longer periods of time, there are identifiable developmental variables that influence the breadth of the qualitative range and the frequency distribution of behaviors used by parents to relate to their children. Thus aggression toward children is not easily explained by a static, parent trait causal model (Wolfe, 1985). Second, the interaction patterns of aggressive and abusive families are not dramatically different, on the whole, from those of non-distressed families. Their qualitative range is somewhat broader, and the distribution

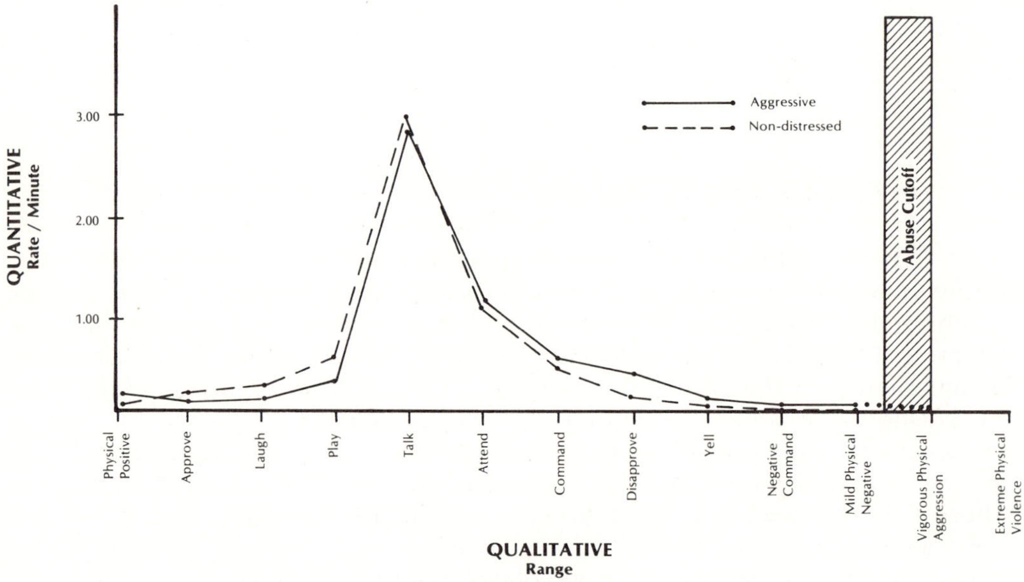

FIGURE 23.1. The continuum model of social exchange.

of behaviors within that range indicates the use of slightly more aversive and slightly fewer positive interactions; however, the majority (85 to 95 percent) of the interactions in aggressive and abusive families fall in the positive and neutral portion of the continuum. Third, the development of aggressive and abusive family interaction is not discontinuous from that of normative interaction. Expansion of the qualitative range toward the abusive pole may often be preceded by, or be contiguous with, an increase in the frequency of milder forms of verbal and physical aggression. Those variables that situationally elicit and maintain aversive parent–child interaction may also play a role in the expansion of the range toward physical violence. Parents who frequently direct mild and moderately intense aggression toward their children may be at risk for more extreme, abusive behavior. Fourth, whereas extreme forms of physical aggression are, by definition, dangerous to the child, less extreme *but frequent* parental aggression is also associated with negative child development outcomes. High-frequency parental aggression is predictive of negative developmental sequelae such as aggression, criminality, impaired social and work skills, and other forms of psychopathology (Patterson, 1982; Patterson, Reid & Dishon, 1987; Snyder & Patterson, 1986). Aggressive as well as abusive treatment of children is an important target of clinical assessment and intervention.

This chapter has two goals. The first is to develop a conceptualization of aggressive and abusive parent–child interactions. This conceptualization provides the framework needed to define variables that are relevant to the systematic assessment of aggressive and abusive family interaction. A major facet of this conceptualization is a discussion of those factors that lead to progressive increases in the frequency and severity of aggressive interactions. Using this framework, the second goal is to discuss specific assessment issues and to review tools relevant to the measurement of aggressive and abusive parent–child interaction.

A SOCIAL INTERACTIONAL APPROACH TO AGGRESSIVE AND ABUSIVE PARENT–CHILD INTERACTION

Aggressive and abusive treatment of children by parents can be understood by identifying antecedents that precipitate and consequences that maintain such behavior. Two classes of variables contribute to family violence: microsocial and macrosocial. Microsocial variables are those that operate in the immediate parent–child interactional context. Microsocial variables include the overt behavior observed during the interaction and the feelings, thoughts, and images experienced by the parties during that interaction. Macrosocial variables are observable events occurring distal to the interaction that influence the affective, cognitive, and behavioral repertoire family members bring to microsocial interaction. At both the microsocial and the macrosocial level, parents and children contribute to aggressive and abusive interaction; the influence is bidirectional (Bell, 1981). Let us first consider microsocial variables.

Microsocial Variables: Aversive Parent–Child Interaction

Mild forms of aversive parent–child interaction can be observed in all families. Children often engage in behaviors aversive to parents. Infants cry and fuss, toddlers hit and have temper tantrums, school-age children whine and fight. These behaviors may occur because the child is wet, hungry, or tired. They may also result from parental limit setting, commands, and inattention, or from sibling teasing and hitting. The average child emits three to four aversive acts per hour. Consequently, the typical parent is confronted with literally thousands of aversive child behaviors during a child's development.

Nearly all parents occasionally respond to these misbehaviors with commands, cajoling, and disapproval. Even harsh parental responses are relatively frequent; parents in nondistressed families spank their children on an average of once every 10 to 15 days. It is in these garden-variety discipline situations that more extreme forms of parental aggression most frequently occur (Herrenkohl, Herrenkohl, & Egolf, 1983). Given that aversive parent–child interaction is frequent and ubiquitous, why do parental responses to discipline situations sometimes escalate to harsh and abusive intensities in some situations in some families?

Research points to three related microsocial processes that contribute to this escalation: (1) high-frequency aversive parent–child interaction; (2) distorted parental perceptions along with unrealistic parental expectations of the child's behavior; and (3) parental physiological and emotional arousal during discipline situations. Let us consider each of these in more detail.

Harsh and abusive treatment of children tends to occur in those families characterized by high-frequency aversive parent–child interaction. Children in those families engage in more aversive and problematic behaviors than children from nondistressed families (Reid, 1978, 1983; Reid, Taplin, & Lorber, 1981; Snyder, 1977). They present their parents with frequent discipline situations. Their parents, in turn, are unable to ignore even relatively innocuous child misbehavior, but rather tend to scold, threaten, command, and hit (Patterson, 1982). In terms of absolute frequency or in terms of the proportion of total interaction, they direct more aversive behavior toward their children than parents in nondistressed families (Burgess & Conger, 1978; Bousha & Twentyman, 1984; Lahey, Conger, Atkeson, & Treiber, 1984; Lorber, Felton, & Reid, 1984; Snyder, 1977). Their primary response to child misbehavior is to punish and/or to coerce the child to stop misbehaving.

Coercive responses to child misbehavior are not effective in reducing the frequency of that misbehavior. High-rate punishment often results in a paradoxical increase in the rate of child misbehavior. The child tends to respond to parental punishment with continued misbehavior. This coercion–countercoercion process is a result of the high-frequency use of punishment by the parents. As children are frequently exposed to low-intensity punishment, they acclimate to punishment at that intensity. Increasingly severe punishment is required to control the child's behavior (Azrin, 1958; Azrin, Holz, & Hake, 1963). As commands and disapproval lose their power, the parent resorts to threats and hitting. However, it is simply not possible to use such high-intensity punishers consistently each time children misbehave, especially if that misbehavior is very frequent. As the parent uses punishment inconsistently and intermittently, the child is more likely to misbehave persistently, even in the face of punishment (Deur & Parke, 1970). The child, as well as the parent, learns that if he or she persists in an aversive interchange, the other person will give in at least some of the time. Thus persistent aversive behavior is negatively (and often positively) reinforced on an intermittent schedule. Unwittingly, parents who use frequent punishment are supporting their children's misbehavior. As the frequency of aversive interaction increases, there is an increased chance that violent parental behavior will (inadvertently) occur; the more fights, the more likely it is that someone will be hurt.

With increased frequency of aversive parent–child interaction, the duration of episodes of aversive interaction also increases (Patterson, 1982; Reid, 1983). Each person has learned that if he or she persists, the other person will give in. There is also a tendency for the intensity of aversive behavior to increase as an aversive interchange persists. Each party "ups the ante" in an attempt to out-coerce the other. Most harsh and abusive parent actions occur toward the end of long (30- to 45-second) aversive interchanges. Because of the physical superiority of the parent, the child is usually the victim. Violence toward children is the end result of an interactional process in which family members reciprocally cue and reinforce each other's coercive means of control. Situationally, violence is most likely to occur when the parent is unable quickly to terminate an aversive interchange with the child.

What constitutes child misbehavior is in the eye of the beholder. Parental misperception of child behavior often plays an important role in the frequency–intensity escalation process. Punitive and abusive parents may have a low tolerance threshold for child misbehavior (Lahey et al., 1984). They perceive normal and relatively innocuous misbehavior as noxious. They are more annoyed than nondistressed parents by crying infants, whining toddlers, and demanding school-age children, and they overestimate the frequency and severity of their children's misbehavior (Frodi & Lamb, 1980; Holleran, Littman, Freund, & Schmaling, 1982; Schmaling & Patterson, 1984). Because of a lack of knowledge about normal development, abusive and punitive parents often have unrealistic expectations about their children's capabilities (Mash, Johnson, & Kovitz, 1983). These parents tend to make negative child-internal and -stable attributions about their children's misbehavior (Larrance & Twentyman, 1983). These distorted perceptions and expectations facilitate the escalation process. A parent who engages in this distorted tracking is more likely to initiate aversive interchanges (i.e., to respond aversively to misperceived innocuous child behavior), to reciprocate aversive child behavior (i.e., to be unable to ignore innocuous aversive and irritating behavior), and to respond with an intensity disproportionate to the child's misbehavior (i.e., to explode).

Highly aggressive, abusive parents report more anger during discipline situations (Reid, 1983), report more frustration at their own inability to deal effectively with their children's misbehavior (Rosenberg & Reppucci, 1983), and are more physiologically aroused when exposed to noxious and nonnoxious child behaviors (Frodi & Lamb, 1980; Wolfe, Fairbank, Kelly, & Bradlyn, 1983) than their nondistressed counterparts. Affective and physiological arousal is thought to potentiate the intensity of aversive responses to provoking situations (Berkowitz, 1983). The parents' anger, frustration, and physiological arousal may "fuel" a response that is explosive and out of proportion to the child's irritating or problematic behavior. Consequently, harsh and abusive parental responses to child misbehavior may be the result of such arousal, or the result of an interaction between this arousal and the escalation process that occurs in long-duration aversive parent–child interactions.

In summary, the probability and frequency of harsh and abusive parental treatment of children are a function of several related parent–child interactional processes. High-rate child misbehavior coupled with ineffective parental disciplinary skills, especially those involving the frequent and inconsistent use of punishment, lead to a developmental progression characterized by aversive parent–child interchanges of increased frequency, duration, and intensity. Thus the range of aversiveness slowly shifts up the continuum over time. Situationally, harsh and abusive treatment is most likely to occur when the child misbehaves, the parent perceives such misbehavior as intentional, the parent does not have an effective nonviolent means of dealing with the misbehavior, and the parent experiences frustration and anger.

Microsocial Variables: Positive Parent–Child Interactions

Parents and children in aggressive and abusive families engage in less positive interaction (and often less total interaction) than their counterparts in nondistressed families (Bousha & Twentyman, 1984; Burgess & Conger, 1978). They provide less tactile and auditory stimulation to infants (Dietrick, Starr, & Kaplan, 1980), engage in less interactional play (Bousha & Twentyman, 1984; Snyder, 1977), and less frequently demonstrate affection (Bousha & Twentyman, 1984; Lahey et al., 1984). Abusive and aggressive parents appear to lack the motivation, time, or skills to engage their children positively.

This lack of positive interaction may both contribute to and result from frequent aversive interaction. Parents are the primary socialization agents of children during infancy and preschool years (Sigel, McGillicuddy-DiLisi, & Johnson, 1980; Patterson, 1982). Even by the fifth grade, children only spend an average of 1 hour of nonschool time outside the home (Stouthamer-Loeber, Patterson, & Loeber, 1983). In the relative absence of positive family interaction, a child may have few opportunities to learn developmentally appropriate self-care, social, and work skills. This lack of skills may lead to frequent child misbehavior with which aggressive and abusive parents have difficulty. Whereas children who are treated harshly by their parents may display difficulties of constitutional origin (prematurity, physical and mental handicaps, hyperactivity), many of their difficulties may result from poor positive parenting practices (Kelly, 1983).

Frequent aversive parent–child interaction may also contribute to a reduction in positive interchanges. Because the parent–child interaction is primarily organized around aversive interchange, each party has a negative stimulus value for the other. Children treated in a harsh or abusive manner tend to avoid their parents and other caretakers. They are affectively withdrawn and respond to social overtures with aggression (George & Main, 1979; Snyder & Brown, 1983). In a complementary fashion, aggressive and abusive parents perceive their children as less skilled and more problematic than they really are (Mash et al., 1983). Because these children are, or are perceived to be, so aversive, their parents avoid interaction with them (Patterson, Reid, & Dishon, 1987). The tension and lack of affection and joy are apparent to persons who observe these families (Reid, 1985).

Microsocial Variables: A Summary

High-rate aversive and low-rate positive interaction play a central and reciprocal role in the development of aggressive and abusive treatment of children. Both parents and children contribute to this process. Aggressive and abusive parents appear to lack the requisite skills to socialize their children. They spend little time teaching skilled behavior, and they lack effective means to deal with discipline situations. This results in high-frequency aversive child behavior. The parents and children reciprocate these aversive interchanges because their aversive responses are occasionally reinforced. This leads to increasingly long aversive interchanges that tend to escalate in intensity to harsh and abusive levels. The negative stimulus value of each family member for the other leads to continued avoidance and minimally positive interaction, further exacerbating children's skills deficits and problematic behavior.

Macrosocial Variables

Parent–child interaction does not occur in a vacuum. Macrosocial or contextual variables from both within and outside the family influence that interaction by altering the mood, perceptual set, and behavior that the parent and child bring to the interaction. Macrosocial conditions that increase the use of aversive behavior and decrease the use of positive behavior contribute to the harsh and abusive treatment of children. This section will review macrosocial variables found to be related to child maltreatment and will analyze the mechanisms by which those variables affect microsocial parent–child interaction.

Socioeconomic Disadvantage and Insularity. Many researchers have reported an association between socioeconomic disadvantage and violence toward children. A higher incidence of parental aggression toward children is found in families with low income, chronic unemployment, poor-quality housing, inadequate parental education, and a lack of social supports (Gaines, Sandgrund, Green, & Power, 1978; Garbarino, 1976; Garbarino & Sherman, 1980; Rutter, 1978; Snyder & Patterson, 1986; Wahler & Dumas, 1983). Such disadvantage is neither a necessary nor a sufficient condition for violence toward the child. Harsh and abusive treatment occurs in only a minority of disadvantaged families (Smith & Hanson, 1974; Smith, Hanson, & Noble, 1974) and has been observed in middle- and upper-class families (Steele & Pollock, 1968).

The impact of socioeconomic disadvantage on violence toward children may be moderated by at least two factors: the degree to which parents perceive disadvantage as aversive or debilitating; and the availability of positive social contacts. Those parents who perceive disadvantage as personally painful and overwhelming are more likely to interact with their children in an aggressive fashion (Conger, Burgess, & Barrett, 1979; Mash et al., 1983; Rosenberg & Reppucci, 1983). Insularity, or the lack of positive, supportive social contacts, is also associated with an increased risk of child maltreatment. Parents (particularly mothers) who have a limited social network (Salzinger, Kaplan, & Artemyeff, 1983) or who have few positive relative to unpleasant contacts with family, friends, and helping agents (Wahler, 1980; Wahler, Leske, & Rogers, 1979) are more likely to engage in frequent and intense aversive interactions with their children.

There are several specific mechanisms by which economic disadvantage and social insularity may influence parent–child interaction. High levels of stress (e.g., socioeconomic disadvantage) and low levels of coping resources (e.g., insularity) are associated with parental irritability, depression, and somatic complaints. Somatic and affective distress disrupts existing parenting skills or interferes with the development of such skills (Conger et al., 1979; Lahey et al., 1984; Patterson, 1982; Wolfe, 1985). Parental distress is associated with reduced positive and increased aversive parent–child interaction (Hops & Biglan, 1985; Lahey et al., 1984). The daily frequency of aversive parent–child interaction covaries with daily parent reports of irritability and depression (Patterson, 1982; Snyder & Patterson, 1984; Wahler & Dumas, 1983). High-level parental distress is also associated with increased misperception of child behavior (Lorber, Felton, & Reid, 1982; Wahler & Dumas, 1981). Such contextual alterations provide "fuel" for the escalation process both situationally and longitudinally.

The lack of supportive social relationships also reduces the parents' opportunity to learn good parenting skills and to get feedback about their current styles of interaction (Kelly, 1983). Children in disadvantaged and insular families are frequently exposed to persons who model deviant behavior and are infrequently exposed to persons who model skilled behavior. The impact of such modeling experiences on the child's behavioral repertoire may also contribute to aggressive parent–child interaction (Bronfenbrenner, 1979).

Family Structure and Conflict. In addition to conditions external to the family, stressors emanating from within the family may lead to violence toward children. Harsh and abusive parent–child interaction has been associated with discord and violence in the marital relationship (Emery, 1982; Porter & O'Leary, 1982; Snyder & Patterson, 1986; Strauss, Gelles, & Steinmetz, 1980). Child maltreatment appears to be one facet of a generally coercive and violent style of family relating (Burgess & Conger, 1978; Lahey et al., 1984; Lorber, Felton, & Reid, 1984; Reid et al., 1981). Child maltreatment is also more frequent in single-parent households (Elmer, 1977; Gil, 1970; Smith et al., 1974; Wahler, 1980; Wahler and Dumas, 1983) and in families with many children (Gil, 1970; Light, 1973; Wahler, 1980).

Marital conflict and divorce often disrupt effective parenting skills. Parents who are in conflict are less consistent and effective in dealing with child misbehavior. They make fewer demands for self-sufficient, skilled child behavior and less consistently track and encourage such behavior (Hetherington, Cox, & Cox, 1979, 1980; Lutzker, 1980). The disruption of parenting skills consequent to conflict and divorce results in more frequent child misbehavior and in reduced child competence (Porter & O'Leary, 1980; Wolfe, Jaffe, Wilson, & Zak, 1985). Increased child misbehavior and lack of competence, in turn, result in more frequent discipline situations, further taxing already inadequate or disrupted parenting skills. The consequence is more frequent aversive parent–child interaction, which, over time, escalates in intensity. The lack of a supportive partner and the innumerable demands made by a large family may also affect the quality of parenting. In both situations, there simply may be less time adequately to monitor and consequate child misbehavior and to elicit and encourage skilled behavior.

Characteristics of the Child. Children who are the target of parental aggression are often seen as difficult to manage. They are frequently reported to be hyperactive, irritable, and colicky, and to have physical and intellectual handicaps or delays (Elmer & Gregg, 1967; Helfer, 1973; McCrae, Furgeson, & Lederman, 1973; Smith & Hanson, 1974). The high-rate misbehavior and lack of skills posed by such children are a challenge even to parents who have excellent skills, and may be particularly conducive to the frequent use of excessive punishment by unskilled, depressed, insular parents. However, the direction of causality has not been established in these studies. It is equally plausible that punitive and aggressive parenting contributes to developmental lags and to various child misbehaviors.

HARSH AND ABUSIVE PARENT–CHILD INTERACTION: A SUMMARY

By definition, harsh and abusive treatment of children by parents is an unfolding, interactional event. Since all children misbehave and the parents' role is to socialize their children, the opportunity (potential) for abusive treatment occurs in all families. Two basic parenting skills are needed effectively to discourage child misbehavior. First, parents need to track misbehavior. Tracking consists of accurately defining what behaviors are problematic and systematically noting their occurrence. Second, when such problematic behavior occurs, parents need to respond consistently in a manner that discourages the misbehavior. Parents who are overreactive to frequent but relatively innocuous aversive child behaviors and who use verbal and physical punishment to respond to child misbehavior are at risk for aggression toward their children. The failure to engage in adequate tracking and discipline often leads to a *coercion–countercoercion process* characterized by an increasing frequency and intensity of aversive parent–child interaction, situationally and longitudinally, until it reaches harsh and abusive dimensions. Both the child and the parent contribute to this process. Simultaneously, there is a lack of positive parent–child interaction as a result of parental skill deficits and of affective and behavioral withdrawal consequent to frequent aversive interchange. This provides the child with fewer opportunities to acquire and perform age-appropriate skills and competencies. The resulting child deficits further frustrate parents and contribute to the aversive interchange. The escalation may also be enhanced by the affective and physiological arousal experienced by the parents during interaction with their children. Such arousal may lead to explosive responses to discipline situations.

Variables distal to the immediate interaction may also play a role in parental aggression toward children. Stressors such as socioeconomic disadvantage, insularity, marital conflict, single parenting, and large families may preclude effective learning of parenting skills or may disrupt their use. The influence of stressors on aggression toward children is further mediated by the parent–child interactional process. Stress often enhances parental irritability and depression. This affective distress is associated with increases in aversive and decreases in positive parent–child interaction, eliciting or further contributing to the microsocial escalation process. A summary of the relationship of these variables is shown in Figure 23.2.

The determinants of maltreatment of children do not appear to be homogeneous across families. The lack of parenting skills, a difficult child, marital conflict or divorce, insularity, and socioeconomic disadvantage are not uniformly descriptive of all families in which aggression toward children occurs. The exact contribution of each of these factors may also depend on the point in the longitudinal escalation process at which the family is observed and assessed. A flexible assessment approach is required in order to identify the idiosyncratic combination of variables contributing to harsh and violent parent–child interaction at any given point in time.

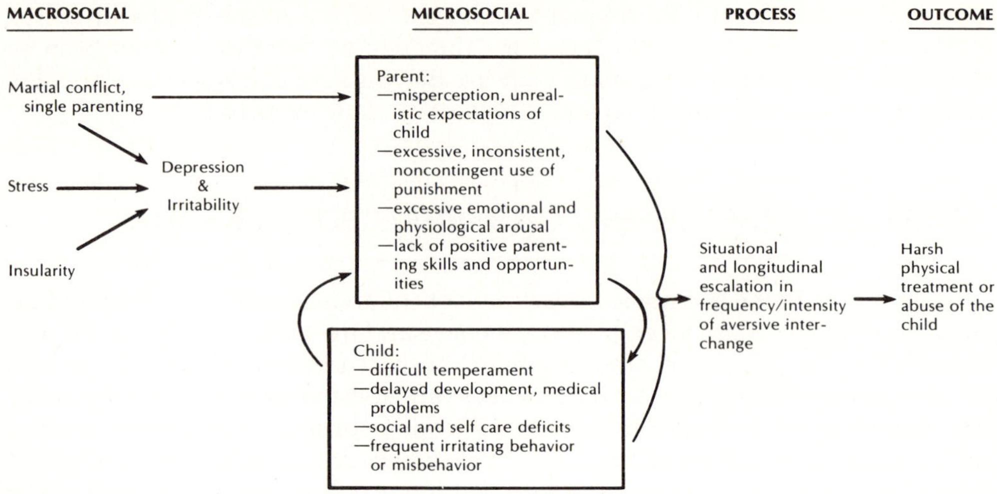

FIGURE 23.2. The contribution of macrosocial and microsocial variables to aggressive and violent parent–child interaction.

ASSESSMENT OF HARSH AND ABUSIVE PARENT–CHILD INTERACTION

Overview

Assessment of aggressive parent–child interaction has four goals. First, it is necessary to specify variables contributing to aggressive parent–child interaction in order to design and implement an effective behavior change program. Second, assessment involves the selection and measurement of target behaviors used to estimate treatment outcome; systematic evaluation of treatment outcome is particularly critical in order to ensure that aggressive interaction does not continue to escalate and that violence does not recur. Third, assessment must focus on prediction of violent parent–child interactions in view of both ethical and legal responsibilities to protect the client and to report abuse. The prediction of violent behavior is particularly difficult (Monahan, 1981). Fourth, the relational tone of the clinician–client relationship is established during assessment. Because of the special circumstances that operate in working with aggressive and abusive families, adequate assessment requires that clinicians foster family members' openness, cooperation, and involvement in the overall assessment process. In the absence of a strong collaborative relationship between the clinician and the family, the fulfillment of other assessment goals will be extremely difficult.

Special Circumstances in Assessment

Clinicians often cannot directly observe harsh and abusive parent–child interactions. These interactions are low-base-rate events that most frequently occur in the privacy of the home. The clinician has to rely on the *report* of the parents, a report that may be strongly biased in view of the illegal and socially undesirable nature of violence toward children. While this bias may be reduced by establishing a collaborative relationship with family members, it is also important to obtain converging information using other behavioral targets and assessment methods. One strategy is to observe high-base-rate behaviors occurring in family interaction that are assumed to be related to the low-base-rate but more violent behaviors of interest. The frequency and duration of parent–child exchanges involving verbal and mild physical aggression appear to be reliable correlates of more violent interactions. These exchanges are important targets in their own right because of their role in the escalation of aggression in family interaction.

Aggressive and abusive parents who do not voluntarily seek help are difficult to engage in the assessment and therapeutic process. They may deny the existence of any problem and may see the clinician as another "outsider" who is intruding into their private affairs and who is blaming and critical. This leads to resistance to assessment and treatment procedures characterized by a lack of candor, noncompliance to assessment and treatment tasks, missing sessions, and outright anger and hostility. The relationships and responsibilities of the client, the clinician, and the legal or child-protective agencies must be clarified, and special efforts must be made to develop a working client–clinician relationship.

Whereas the selection of information-gathering procedures must meet multiple assessment goals, be consistent with the multiple determinants of aggressive and abusive parent–child interaction, and adjust for the inherent bias in parent self-report, it is important to consider the degree to which various procedures are seen as intrusive, threatening, and mysterious by parents. Given the parents' ability to subvert the assessment process and to distort information, assessment procedures should be selected that are collaborative in tone, that are directly relevant to helping the parents deal with their troublesome children, and that bear an obvious (to the parents) relationship to treatment. It is generally better to select procedures that focus on problematic parent–child interactions than on parental "character flaws."

Assessment of aggressive and abusive parent–child interaction requires multiple methods and data sources. Such a multiple method–multiple source approach provides a convergence of information appropriate to the covert nature and seriousness of the problem, and is necessitated by the multiple goals of assessment. However, selection of assessment procedures must be tempered by realistic time constraints and expense to the clinician and clients, and by the urgency of the problem. Consequently, a number of assessment procedures and devices will herein be discussed. This discussion will move from the most general and least expensive to the most specific and time-consuming strategies. This sequence does not necessarily reflect their utility in assessing child maltreatment. Ultimately, the clinician must select the procedures to be used, balancing time and expense with the need to fulfill the various assessment goals.

Interviewing

On initial contact with parents in aggressive and abusive families, it is important to create an atmosphere in which the parents and the clinician can work together to produce beneficial change. The parents need to feel that the clinician is sensitive to their problems and wishes to address those problems, rather than to blame and berate them for their actions. This can be accomplished, in part, by framing the initial interview in terms of the daily problems the parents have in dealing with their children, in contrast to focusing on specific punitive and abusive incidents. An attempt is made to "join" the parents in their feelings of frustration and lack of control. The focus is on problems in the style of interaction rather than whether punitive parental actions occurred, were too harsh, or were warranted. The goal is to create a problem-solving orientation relevant to the parents' perspective.

While punitive and abusive episodes are deemphasized, the clinician also needs to make clear that such actions are not condoned. This can be established by communicating to the parents that the content of assessment and treatment is protected by legal and ethical standards of confidentiality, and that this confidentiality *will be broken* as prescribed by law. Such prescriptions should be presented in a matter-of-fact manner, and should include those conditions under which confidentiality would be broken (i.e., the clinician's awareness of plans or actions by the client that would endanger the client or others, including child abuse).

In developing a collaborative set, it is useful to discuss the specific ways in which assessment and therapy will help the family. The focus is on providing the parents with skills in dealing with difficult disciplinary situations, irritating child behaviors, and intra- and extrafamilial stressors. It may also be useful to discuss how assessment and treatment may be beneficial to the parents in relationship to legal and child-protective agencies. For example, as the parents find alternate and additional means to respond to their children's misbehavior, and as they are actively involved in assessment and treatment, these agencies may monitor the family less intensively. As the parents are making progress in intervention, the clinician may serve as an advocate for the parents in relation to these agencies.

A collaborative set may also be enhanced by describing the assessment procedures and their rationale to the parents. The objective of assessment is to help the family change, and not to blame or to obtain a confession for past mistakes. The focus is on reducing the rate and intensity of aversive parent–child interactions and on promoting positive interaction rather than on a preoccupation with the dangerous but infrequent occurrence of abuse and harsh punishment. The goal is to abort the situational and longitudinal escalation process by teaching parents effective child management skills.

In addition to establishing rapport and trust, the interview is an inexpensive, flexible means of gathering information concerning factors that contribute to aggressive parent–child interaction. In an interview, the parents can communicate their perception of problematic and positive interactions with their children, and of distal, macrosocial variables (such as family structure, marital relationship, socioeconomic disadvantage, social supports, and mood states) that contribute to the problematic parent–child interaction. The information to be obtained can be construed in a stimulus–organism–response–contingency–consequence (S–O–R–K–C) format as shown in Table 23.1.

The interview and concomitant informal observations provide a broad overview of the variables potentially relevant to child maltreatment in a particular family. Those variables that appear to contribute importantly to aggressive parent–child interactions can then be pursued more systematically via interviewing and other assessment procedures. Data obtained from interviews are tentative, because they are subject to intentional and nonintentional biases. Family members may withhold or distort information in order to present themselves in a positive light. Even when this is not the case, information obtained in an interview represents the generalized

TABLE 23.1. INTERVIEW QUESTIONS RELEVANT TO AN S-O-R-K-C FUNCTIONAL ANALYSIS

	Target	Relevant Questions
Stimulus	Problematic child behaviors	What types of (mis)behaviors lead to discipline confrontations?
	Temporal, situational, and setting effects	When do discipline situations occur? Are there problems at bedtime, dinnertime, etc.? Does it involve fighting with sibs? Do these confrontations occur outside of the home? Do they occur following a marital dispute?
Organism	Parental psychopathology	Is the parent psychotic? Does the parent intentionally seek to harm the child? Are violent episodes associated with drug use or intoxication?
	Parental knowledge and expectations of child development and behavior	Does the parent have realistic expectations about the child's behavior given the child's age? Does the parent make negative internal and stable attributions about the child?
	Parental depression	Is the parent depressed? How severely? Does this affect the quality of parent–child interaction?
	Parental anger and irritability	Is the parent generally irritable? Does the parent experience significant anger and arousal during discipline situations? Does the parent have difficulty controlling anger?
	Child physical and behavioral problems	Does the child display frequent behavioral problems? What type? Is the child physically handicapped or developmentally delayed? What is the child's temperament?
	Child skills and competence	Does the child carry out age-appropriate self-care skills? How does the child relate to peers and siblings? How does the child perform and behave in school?
Response	Parent child-management skills	What tactics are used by the parents to discipline the child? Is aggressive treatment the result of poor child-management skills? Does the parent have the needed skills?
	Parental interaction skills	Is the parent able to interact effectively in everyday situations (talking, giving attention, playing games, teaching)? How frequently do such interactions occur?
	Child response to discipline	How does the child respond to the disciplinary tactics used by the parents?

(*Table continues on p. 592.*)

TABLE 23.1. (*Continued*)

	Target	Relevant Questions
	Child interaction skills	Does the child initiate interaction with the parents? Is the child responsive to parental overtures? Is the child "difficult" or minimally responsive?
Contingency and Consequence	Utility of (harsh or abusive) discipline	Does parental discipline stop aversive child behavior, at least for a short time? What is the reaction of the spouse and siblings to such discipline?
	Utility of positive social interaction	How do the spouse, child, and siblings respond to positive social attention to the child?

perception of family members concerning the macrosocial and microsocial functioning of the family; as such, it is subject to selective memory, and to preconceived explanations and rationales that may be more a function of the members' attitudes, attention, and values than of what is actually occurring. While these perceptions are important assessment data in their own right, the sole use of data subject to such biases is problematic in meeting assessment goals. The direction and magnitude of these biases are difficult to estimate in the absence of data gathered using more objective assessment procedures.

Data relevant to identifying the determinants of child maltreatment, predicting its future occurrence, and evaluating treatment outcome must involve the use of systematic assessment procedures in addition to interviewing. Such procedures add to the cost of assessment, but are critical to meeting the goals of assessment. These procedures include structured self-report inventories and standardized tests, self-monitoring or participant observation, and direct observation.

Self-Report Inventories and Standardized Tests

Self-report inventories and standardized tests are relatively inexpensive means of systematically gathering information relevant to aggressive parent–child interaction. They provide quantitative information concerning family members' (most often parents') responses to a standard set of stimuli. The psychometric properties of these devices have been established and the family members' responses can be compared to those of normative or known problematic samples. Although these characteristics offer relative advantages over interview data, the data from tests and inventories are based on family members' self-report and are consequently subject to intentional or nonintentional biases. This does not obviate the usefulness of such data; however, such data should not be treated as unbiased simply because they were collected by using standardized stimuli.

Standardized tests and inventories relevant to child maltreatment focus primarily on organismic variables and on intra- and extrafamilial macrosocial stimuli that contribute to aggressive parent–child interaction. These devices do *not* produce data directly reflective of that interaction. Data from self-report tests and inventories are generally based on global assessments of experiences or global observations averaged across settings and time. They are not very sensitive to the temporal and situational variation in affect, cognition, and behavior. An exhaustive list of such measures for each variable is not attempted; rather, a sample of measures will be presented that have been commonly used with aggressive families and that have adequate psychometric characteristics and normative data.

Parental Affect. As indicated earlier, parental irritability and depression negatively influence the quality of parent–child interaction; affectively distressed parents engage in less positive interaction and in more aversive interaction with their children and their partners than their nondistressed counterparts (Biglan et al., 1985; Lahey et al., 1984). Negative parental affect is also associated with a negative perceptual bias toward the child's behavior (Griest, Forehand, Wells, & McMahon, 1980).

As indicated in Table 23.2, several measures of parental depression and irritability are available. The MMPI is a good screening device for general psychopathology as well as hostility and depression. The Beck Depression Inventory provides a "trait" measure of depression whereas the Depression Adjective Checklist provides a "state" measure of depression that may be useful in measuring covariation between depressive affect and interactional variables. In a similar manner, the Buss-Durkee Hostility Inventory and the Novaco Anger Inventory provide stable measures of anger and hostility while the Multiple Affect Adjective Checklist can be used to assess fluctuations in irritability and depression over time. These affect measures are not specific to family interaction, but focus on the general affect of the parent.

Parental Stress and Insularity. High levels of stress, particularly in the absence of adequate coping skills and social supports, also disrupt effective family management skills. It is possible to estimate gross stress levels from general socioeconomic and family structural data obtained in the interview. These data can be used to calculate a disadvantage index by summing, on a 0 (nondisadvantaged) or 1 (disadvantaged) basis, a number of indicators: changes in residence during the past year, marital separation or divorce, the use of community services, family income, parent unemployment, parent education, large family size, source of referral, and areas of residence (for details see Rutter, 1971; Dumas & Wahler, 1983).

A more refined and specific estimate of stress and insularity can be obtained using self-report inventories. Table 23.2 provides a list of several useful inventories. Parental stress can be measured by focusing on major life changes (Life Experiences Inventory) or on more frequent daily irritants and demands (Hassles and Uplifts Scales). Though currently lacking sufficient psychometric study, scales are also available to assess stress specific to family life involving both younger (Early Parenting Dimensions of Stress) and older (Family Crisis List) children. Stress can also be measured via parental self-reports of physical symptoms and emotional distress (Cornell Medical Index, General Health Questionnaire). Stress measures can be complemented by inventories that ask parents to report the extent and quality of social support networks (Social Support Questionnaire, Perceived Social Support). Mood, stress, social support, physical symptoms, and emotional distress are mod-

TABLE 23.2. SELF-REPORT INVENTORIES AND TESTS

Domain	Test or Inventory	Variables	Reference
Parental affect	MMPI	General psychopathology, depression, hostility, impulsivity	
	Beck Depression Inventory	Depression	Beck, 1973
	Depression Adjective Checklist	Depression	Levitt & Lubin, 1973
	Buss-Durkee Hostility Inventory	Anger	Buss & Durkee, 1957
	Anger Inventory	Anger	Novaco, 1975
	Multiple Affect Adjective Checklist	Anger, depression	Zuckerman & Lubin, 1965
Parental stress–social support	Life Experiences Inventory	Major stress	Sarason, Johnson, & Siegal, 1978
	Hassles and Uplifts Scales	Daily demands and irritants	Kanner, Coyne, Schaefer, & Lazarus, 1981
	Stress of Early Parenting	Familial stress	Weinberg & Richardson, 1981
	Family Crisis List	Familial stress	Patterson, 1982
	Cornell Medical Index	Somatic and emotional distress	Cornell University Medical College, 1949
	General Health Questionnaire	Somatic and emotional distress	Goldberg & Hillier, 1979
	Social Support Questionnaire	Number and quality of relationships	Sarason, Levine, Basham, & Sarason, 1983
	Perceived Social Support	Social supports from family and friends	Procidano & Heller, 1983
Child problems and competencies	Eyberg Child Behavior Inventory	Child conduct problems	Eyberg & Ross, 1978
	Child Behavior Checklist	Child behavior problems and competencies	Achenbach & Edelbrock, 1982
	Infant Temperament Questionnaire	Temperament (ages 1 to 3)	Carey & McDevitt, 1978
	Behavior Style Questionnaire	Temperament (ages 3 to 7)	McDevitt & Carey, 1978
	Michigan Screening Profile of Parenting	Knowledge and expectations of child age-appropriate behavior	Helfer, Hoffmeister & Schneider, 1978
Marital relationship	Dyadic Adjustment Scale	Marital satisfaction and conflict	Spanier, 1976
	Marital Adjustment Scale	Marital satisfaction	Locke & Wallace, 1959
	Conflict Tactics Scale	Marital aggression	Straus, 1979

erately correlated. While the exact nature of their relationship is open to debate (Lazarus & Folkman, 1984), assessment of some of these variables is warranted if interview data suggest they are contributing to problematic parent–child interaction.

Child Problems and Competencies. Children who are the targets of parental maltreatment are often described as "difficult" or "problematic." Several parent-report inventories are useful in assessing the behavioral characteristics of younger (Infant Temperament Questionnaire) and older (Eyberg Child Behavior Inventory,Child Behavior Checklist, Behavioral Style Questionnaire) children (see Table 23.2). Results from these inventories reflect parental *perceptions* of their children's behavior. Aggressive and abusive parents often overestimate their children's problematic behavior and often underestimate skilled behavior because of unrealistic expectations or a lack of a normative judgment base (Mash et al., 1983; Reid, Baldwin, Patterson, & Dishon, 1985). The degree to which parents have unrealistic expectations of or inaccurate knowledge about their children can be assessed via the Michigan Screening Profile of Parenting. More objective information concerning the children's capabilities and behaviors can be assessed via age-appropriate developmental scales (McCarthy Scales of Children's Ability—McCarthy, 1972; Bayley Scales of Infant Development—Bayley, 1969), by seeking information from other informants (e.g., teachers), and by direct observation of the child. While it is not clear that the behavioral characteristics of the child are causally related to maltreatment, the existence of problems and current capabilities of the child will influence the nature of the intervention and the measures used to assess treatment outcome.

Marital Relationship. The quality of the marital relationship and the nature of marital interaction influence parent–child interaction. Marital conflict and violence are associated with reduced positive and increased aversive parent interaction with children. The Dyadic Adjustment Scale and the Marital Adjustment Scale (see Table 23.2) provide reliable and valid indices of general marital satisfaction. If physical violence is suspected, the Conflict Tactics Scale may serve as a useful adjunct to the general satisfaction inventories. The reader is referred to Weiss and Margolin (1977) for a more thorough discussion of marital assessment.

OBSERVATIONAL ASSESSMENT

Data obtained from interviews, self-report inventories, and standardized tests (1) focus primarily on organismic and macrosocial setting variables, (2) are often based on the perception of family members and consequently subject to bias and distortion, (3) provide global estimates of family members' thinking, mood, experience, and behavior over time and across settings, and (4) primarily address noninteractive characteristics of specific family members, of the family as a whole, and of the community–family interface. Such data are valuable in assessing child maltreatment, yet, sole reliance on such data is insufficient.

Interview and self-report data must be complemented by information obtained from observational procedures. *Observational* assessment refers to data collected (1) by an agent using preset, concrete, and finite categories to summarize individuals' behavior, (2) over a specified time period in a specified setting, (3) minimizing the use of the agent's memory and judgment, (4) which are subject to reliability and accuracy checks (Reid et al., 1985). Observational procedures provide the means to assess concrete parent and child behaviors occurring in the natural setting. In addition to accessing the actual frequency and topography of the behaviors that family members direct to one another, it is possible to delineate the functional relationships between one member's behavior and that of other family members. Antecedents and consequences for aversive child behavior and aggressive parental responses can be specified. A similar functional analysis can be implemented for positive parent–child interaction. In this way, problematic child behaviors and parenting skill deficits can be measured in a direct fashion. Observational data are not subject to the same sort of biases operating in interviewing and self-report data. Observational methods are ideally suited to the situational, interactive process that elicits and maintains aggressive and abusive treatment of children.

In addition to its critical role in identifying the determinants of maltreatment, direct observation provides quantitative measurement of positive and aversive parent–child interaction, independent of parent report, needed for assessing treatment outcome. Family members are reactive to observation, but the resultant bias is different from that operating in self-reports. While actual abusive episodes may not be observed because of reactivity, family members cannot or do not suppress less noxious aggressive behaviors. In fact, abusive parents have been known to hit and spank their children even though they knew they were being observed because of their abusive history (Reid, 1985). In any case, more frequent but less severe aggressive interactions are important in their own right; these interactions frequently serve as situational antecedents for highly punitive and abusive episodes, and are the engines that drive the longitudinal escalation process.

Predicting child maltreatment is a very difficult task. The traditional approach to prediction utilizes organismic trait variables that only weakly predict violence (Monahan, 1981). Although untested, data derived from the observation of family interaction may serve as better predictors of child maltreatment. The frequency with which family members initiate aversive interaction, the likelihood that they reciprocate aversive interaction, the duration of chains of aversive interaction, and the intensity of the aversive interchange have been postulated to be accurate indices of how far along a family is in the escalation process (Patterson, 1985).

Two types of observational procedures are available: participant observation, or self-monitoring, and observation by independent agents.

Participant Observation

In participant observation, a family member is trained systematically to observe, record, and report his or her own and other family members' behavior as it occurs in the home or in other natural settings. The behaviors to be observed are concretely specified, and the family member is trained accurately to discriminate and track the target behaviors. The data can be collected by daily phone calls or by mail. This observational method is very economical. Only a few hours of participant observer training are needed, and the resultant data are easily summarized. Such data have acceptable accuracy and temporal stability (Chamberlain, 1980) and good concurrent validity when compared to independent observations (Reid, 1982) or against other objective indices of behavior (Loeber, Dishon, & Patterson, 1984). It is an especially useful method for collecting data concerning covert, low-base-rate events not amenable to direct observation. It is flexible and can be individualized to reflect the specific characteristics and concerns of a particular family.

This method would seem to be highly intrusive, reactive, and subject to conscious distortion. However, these threats can be minimized by introducing the observation in a manner congruent with a collaborative set, and may even be used to enhance that set. For example, it is possible to target for observation those child behaviors that the parents find particularly frustrating or troublesome. Requesting parents to record their responses to these behaviors as they occur in the home setting is congruent with the goal of providing the parents with more effective ways of dealing with problematic child behavior (Reid et al., 1985). Care should be taken not to present this method in a fashion that arouses parent resistance ("I want to know what's going on in your home"). It is better presented as a straightforward and logical means of collecting information relevant to helping the parents improve their child management skills ("Let's see how often your child misbehaves and what kind of actions you currently use to deal with that misbehavior"). It desensitizes parents to providing information about what is occurring in the home and consequently facilitates a veridical report when the clinician is suspicious of harsh or abusive child treatment.

To convey the flexibility, relevance, and utility of participant observation procedures, an example of potential target behaviors is shown in Table 23.3. The

TABLE 23.3. EXAMPLES OF TARGET BEHAVIORS FOR PARTICIPANT OBSERVATION

		Affective–Subjective Judgments	
Child Behaviors	Parental Response*	Anger	Response Severity
Dawdling in the AM	______	1 2 3 4 5	1 2 3 4 5
Talking back	______	1 2 3 4 5	1 2 3 4 5
Lying	______	1 2 3 4 5	1 2 3 4 5
Hit sibling	______	1 2 3 4 5	1 2 3 4 5
Whining	______	1 2 3 4 5	1 2 3 4 5
Complied	______		
Played nicely	______		
Was helpful	______		
Did chores	______		
Was affectionate	______		

* Choose from yell, threaten, spank, ignore, set in corner, take away TV, command (for negative behavior), and from praise, compliment, physical affection, ignore (for positive behavior)

Contacts with others:

Person	#	Time	Pleasant	Neutral	Unpleasant
Friend	____	__ min.	____	____	____
Relative	____	__ min.	____	____	____
Co-worker	____	__ min.	____	____	____
Agency–doctor	____	__ min.	____	____	____
Stranger	____	__ min.	____	____	____
Other ______	____	__ min.	____	____	____

targets of observation may focus on parent and child behaviors, on feelings of the participant specific to an interaction, on positive as well as aversive behavior, and on daily reports of macrosocial and organismic variables.

The data obtained from participant observation are less global than those obtained from the interview or from self-report inventories. The data are descriptive of specific, objectively defined behaviors and experiences occurring within a relatively brief time period in a specified setting. Although these characteristics minimize nonintentional bias, they are still based on parental report. If there is reason to suspect the willingness or ability of the observing family member to provide veridical data, independent observation is indicated.

Independent Observation

In independent observation, the moment-by-moment interaction of family members is observed and coded by agents other than family members. There are several advantages to independent observation: (1) The information is not mediated through the norms and unique experience of a family member; using objectively defined categories, the observer records the specific overt behaviors displayed by family members during interaction. (2) The data are precise, quantitative, and interactive; they can be compared to normative data and allow a description of the exact linkages between child and parent behaviors that influence the rate and topography (form and duration) of aversive and positive interactions. (3) The procedure is highly flexible; target behaviors to be observed can be selected according to their relevance to a particular family and its problems. (4) The behavior can be observed in the natural setting in which the problem exists. Independent observation, then, provides direct access to actual microsocial family interactional processes that situationally and longitudinally promote harsh and abusive treatment of children.

These advantages are balanced by some disadvantages. Independent observation is relatively expensive. Observers must be thoroughly trained, and 3 to 6 hours of observation is required to achieve stable estimates of family members' behavior. There is travel time and cost for the observers, and summarizing the data is a difficult and time-consuming process. On the average, an observational session costs $30 to $40 per hour (a total of $180 to $240 for 6 hours of observation) (Reid et al., 1985). Whereas this cost may appear prohibitive, it is often comparable to that of a comprehensive personality assessment. The cost can be reduced if observations are made in a standardized clinic setting rather than in the home.

Another problem is reactivity, or variation from usual family interaction due to being observed. The family may engage in "impression management," either to look good or to look bad. Of course, this impression management is not unique to independent observation. The research on observation of aggressive families suggests that they have difficulty "faking good" (Johnson & Lobitz, 1974; Lobitz & Johnson, 1975). The habitual manner in which these families interact appears to provide constraints against gross distortion of typical interaction. Some distortion probably occurs, but the elements of the basic process are clearly observable (Reid et al., 1985). For example, abusive mothers are observed to hit and threaten their children more than nonabusive mothers even when they are aware of being observed because of their abusive behavior (Reid et al., 1981). The members of highly aggressive families are observed to hit and threaten at twice the rate of nonproblem family members (Reid, 1978).

Independent Observation in Standardized Settings. Compared to home observation, observation of family interaction in a clinic or lab setting is a convenient and economical procedure. It is possible to minimize home–laboratory differences by simulating a home setting (e.g., a family room) such that the immediate stimulus field is similar to that in the natural environment (Parke, 1979). Observational data collected in structured settings have been shown to differentiate abusive and aggressive from nonproblem families, and the functional effect of the behavior of one family member's behavior on that of others is comparable to that obtained from observations in the home (Dietrich et al., 1980; Hops & Biglan, 1985; Snyder, 1977).

Observation in standardized settings can be implemented under structured or unstructured conditions. In structured conditions, the family is instructed to engage in certain activities like child-directed play, parent-directed play, pick-up time, and playing a specific game (e.g., Robinson & Eyberg, 1981). Observational data collected in standardized settings can be used to define the antecedents and consequences associated with child maltreatment and as treatment outcome measures. To date, the utility of such data to predict the occurrence or recurrence of harsh and abusive parent–child interaction has not been assessed.

Independent Observations in Natural Settings. Although expensive, inconvenient, and intrusive, the observation of family interaction in home and other natural settings provides the richest, most face-valid information about microsocial family process. The data are obtained in the setting in which the problem occurs and thus provide an ecologically valid estimate of each family members' behavior and the functional effect of that behavior on family interaction. It is a very sensitive tool for identifying factors that elicit child maltreatment and for assessing the efficacy of intervention (Patterson & Reid, 1984). Though largely untested, observational data may be accurate predictors of parental aggression toward children (Patterson, 1985).

Observation of family interaction in the home requires a number of decisions by the clinician. Usually, some constraints are placed on the family in order to maximize the collection of relevant interactive data. All family members must be present during the observation, they must remain in one or two adjacent rooms, they cannot watch TV, no outgoing phone calls are allowed, and incoming calls are limited (Reid, 1978; Wahler, House, & Stambaugh, 1976). The clinician must also decide when to sample the family interaction. Observations are frequently made around evening meal time; everyone is typically home and this is often a chaotic time for the family. However, very little is known about variations in family interaction depending on the time of day and the predominant activity around which interaction is organized. It would seem reasonable to sample during times indicated by the parents as particularly problematic; this is likely to vary according to the family and the age of the child. The frequency and total duration of observations must also be specified; beyond the data indicating that a 3- to 6-hour total duration is necessary for stable estimates of behavior, there are few empirical guidelines. Observation produces a large amount of data that must be summarized in order to be useful. Summary indices can range from frequency counts and simple behavior probabilities to conditional probabilities and complex sequential analyses. This is a time-consuming task. Hartman (1982) and Cairns (1979) discuss these issues in detail.

Observational Coding Systems. Many coding systems are currently available for observing family interaction in structured and natural settings. These systems vary in terms of simplicity, specificity, and bandwidth. While it is possible to develop a coding system (see Cairns, 1979, for suggestions), this is a tedious and difficult task. It is much easier to select from existing coding systems that have demonstrated reliability and validity. Several coding systems relevant to the observation of aggressive family interactions are described in Table 23.4. In the table, the coding systems are rank-ordered in approximate ease of training, use, and analysis. All of the coding systems except the Social Interaction Scoring System and the Family Process Code can be implemented via paper and pencil recording. Generally, the richness of the data is inversely related to the ease and simplicity of the coding system. For clinical use, the simpler systems are recommended because of their economy. They provide sufficiently specific data to meet assessment goals. For intensive research study, complex codes are recommended because they make possible fine-grained analyses needed thoroughly to understand the family processes that may promote and maintain aggressive interaction. In any case, a careful study of the available alternatives is warranted before selecting a coding system.

TABLE 23.4. FAMILY INTERACTION OBSERVATION CODING SYSTEMS

Code Name	Time Base	Categories	Reference
Response Class Matrix	Interval	7 parent and 6 child behaviors	Mash, Terdal, & Anderson, 1973
Behavioral Coding System	Interval	Binary decision of child appropriate–inappropriate behavior; 8 parent and 2 child behaviors	Forehand & McMahon, 1981
Dyadic Parent–Child Interaction Coding System	Interval	19 or 22 parent and child behaviors	Robinson & Eyberg, 1981
Family Interaction Coding System	Interval	29 parent and child behaviors	Reid, 1978
Ecological Assessment of Child Behavior Problems	Interval	19 child and 5 parent–sibling behaviors	Wahler, House, & Stambaugh, 1976
Social Interaction Scoring System	Continuous	Multidimensional rating of interaction on type, content, and affect	Conger, 1982
Family Process Code	Continuous	25 parent and child behaviors, 5 affect codes	Dishon, Gardner, Patterson, Reid, Spyrou, & Thidobeaux, 1984

Observer impressions are a useful and inexpensive supplement to independent observation. Observers are asked to make systematic judgments by rating their impressions of family characteristics and behaviors using a Likert scale. These global ratings are independent of parent report, and are selected in terms of relevance to the particular family and to specific assessment and intervention goals. Weinrott, Reid, Bauske, and Brummett (1981) provide an example of such an instrument and have demonstrated its potential validity, reliability, and clinical utility.

Observational Assessment: A Summary

Observational procedures are a critical part of the assessment of harsh and abusive parent–child interaction. They address multiple assessment goals. They are necessitated by the potential for intentional and nonintentional distortion of parent self-report data and by the interactive nature of child maltreatment. For clinicians who have limited time and resources, participant observation and/or observation in structured settings are highly recommended as complements to parent report data. Independent observation in the home is ideal because of its ecological validity, but quite demanding in terms of time and money.

INTEGRATING ASSESSMENT AND TREATMENT

The selection of assessment procedures discussed in this chapter is tied closely to treatment goals. These goals are: a reduction in the rate of aversive family interaction; an increase in the rate of positive family interaction; decreased use of physical punishment; increased use of effective nonphysical forms of discipline; a quick and effective resolution of discipline confrontations; a reduction in parental anger and arousal during such confrontations; and the development of accurate perceptions and expectations for age-appropriate child behavior. Distal, macrosocial problems such as stress, depression, irritability, marital discord, and insularity may also be targeted for intervention as indicated.

The use of assessment procedures closely tied to treatment goals facilitates the involvement of family members in the therapeutic process. The communication of assessment data to the family is problem oriented. It focuses on providing parents with assistance in learning and using alternate strategies to deal with frustrating and anger-provoking child behaviors, and with conflictual and stressful marital and community relationships. It maximizes parent motivation and collaboration prerequisite to successful treatment. Without such conditions, parent training programs and other forms of intervention are met with resistance, early termination, and dropout (Chamberlain, Patterson, Reid, Kavanaugh, & Forgatch, 1984; Conger & Lahey, 1982; McMahon, Forehand, Griest, & Wells, 1981; Wolfe, Aragona, Kaufman, & Sandler, 1980).

SUMMARY

This chapter has provided an overview of the conceptualization and assessment of aggressive and abusive parent–child interaction. Parental aggression toward children has multifaceted and heterogeneous causes occurring at both microsocial and macrosocial levels. Such aggression is largely a function of behavior exchanged by family members during interaction and of familial and community contextual variables.

Any multidimensional problem requires a multidimensional, flexible approach to assessment. Therefore, a wide variety of assessment procedures have been presented, including interviewing, self-report, and participant and independent observation. It is not expected that clinicians will use all of these procedures. The goal has been to offer clinicians a variety of procedures in order to help them select those that are most relevant to a particular family and to a specific clinical setting.

Issues that are particularly characteristic and problematic in the assessment of parental maltreatment of children were emphasized. Assessment of aggressive families is not solely a technological problem. There are numerous legal, ethical, and relational issues critical to valid and clinically relevant assessment. Parents in such families are often coerced into treatment. Even when not coerced, the clinical problem for which they are seeking assistance is socially disapproved. Consequently, parents' perceptions of the problem and their willingness or ability to provide veridical data challenge the assessment process. These difficulties are compounded by the infrequent and private nature of the problematic behavior. Adequate assessment requires establishing trust, openness, and collaboration of family members. Establishing such conditions requires skills and strategies not easily operationalized and communicated. It entails such clinician behaviors as joining the client, reframing the problem, knowing when to confront, support, question, and teach, as well as qualities like sensitivity, empathy, and tenacity (Alexander & Parsons, 1982; Haley, 1973; Kolko & Milan, 1983; Patterson, 1984).

The status of the assessment of aggressive and abusive families has improved dramatically over the last 5 years. Reasonably good procedures and devices are now available to meet most assessment goals. Nonetheless, a glaring deficiency is the lack of reliable and valid procedures to assess parental perceptions and expectations of children. An improved methodology for prediction must be developed and tested, perhaps using a combination of parent-report, objective, and observational measures. The development of such a methodology will necessarily involve a clearer understanding of the developmental processes occurring in the family that promote an escalation in aggression and violence.

References

Achenbach, T., & Edelbrock, C. S. (1982). *Manual for the Child Behavior Checklist and Child Behavior Profile*, Burlington: University of Vermont.

Alexander, J. F., & Parsons, B. V. (1982). *Functional family therapy*, Monterey, CA: Brooks/Cole.

Azrin, N. H. (1958). Some effects of noise on human behavior. *Journal of the Experimental Analysis of Behavior, 1*, 183–200.

Azrin, N. H., Holz, W. C., & Hake, D. F. (1963). Fixed ratio punishment. *Journal of the Experimental Analysis of Behavior, 6*, 141–148.

Bayley, N. (1969). *Bayley Scales of Infant Development*. New York: Psychological Corporation.

Beck, A. T. (1973). *Diagnosis and management of depression*. New York: Atheneum.

Bell, R. Q. (1981). Introduction to symposium on parent, child, and reciprocal infuences: New experimental approaches. *Journal of Abnormal Child Psychology, 9*, 299–301.

Berkowitz, L. (1983). Aversively stimulated aggression: Some parallels and differences in research with animals and humans. *American Psychologist, 38*, 1135–1144.

Biglan, A., Hops, H., Sherman, L., Friedman, L., Arthur, J., & Osteen, V. (1985). Problem solving interaction of depressed women and their husbands. *Behavior Therapy, 16,* 431–451.

Bousha, D. M., & Twentyman, C. T. (1984). Mother–child interaction style in abuse, neglect and control groups: Natural observation in the home. *Journal of Abnormal Psychology, 93,* 106–114.

Bronfenbrenner, U. (1979). *The ecology of human development*. Cambridge, MA: Harvard University Press.

Burgess, R. L., & Conger, R. (1978). Family interactions in abusive, neglectful, and normal families. *Child Development, 49,* 1163–1173.

Buss, A. H., & Durkee, A. (1957). An inventory for assessing different kinds of hostility. *Journal of Consulting Psychology, 21,* 343–349.

Cairns, R. D. (1979). *The analysis of social interaction: Methods, issues and illustrations*. Hillsdale, NJ: Erlbaum.

Carey, W., & McDevitt, S. (1978). Revision of the Infant Temperament Questionnaire. *Pediatrics, 61,* 735–739.

Chamberlain, P. (1980). *Standardization of a parent report measure*. Unpublished doctoral dissertation, University of Oregon.

Chamberlain, P., Patterson, G. R., Reid, J. B., Kavanaugh, K., & Forgatch, M. S. (1984). Observation of client resistance. *Behavior Therapy, 15,* 144–155.

Conger, R. D. (1982). *Social Interaction Scoring System: Observer training manual*. Unpublished manuscript, University of Illinois.

Conger, R. D., Burgess, R., & Barrett, C. (1979). Child abuse related to life changes and perceptions of illness: Some preliminary findings. *Family Coordinator, 28,* 73–78.

Conger, R. D., & Lahey, B. B. (1982). Behavioral intervention for child abuse. *Behavior Therapist, 5,* 49–53.

Cornell University Medical College (1949). *Cornell Medical Index*. New York: Author.

Deur, J. L., & Parke, R. D. (1970). The effects of inconsistent punishment on aggression in children. *Developmental Psychology, 2,* 403–411.

Dietrich, K. N., Starr, R. H., & Kaplan, M. G. (1980). Maternal stimulation and care of abused infants. In T. M. Field, S. Goldberg, D. Stern, & A. M. Sostik (Eds.), *High-risk infants and children: Adult and peer interactions*. New York: Academic.

Dishon, T., Gardner, K., Patterson, G., Reid, J., Spyrou, S., & Thibodeaux, S. (1984). *The family process code: A multidimensional system for observing family interaction*. Unpublished manuscript, Oregon Social Learning Center, Eugene.

Dumas, J., & Wahler, R. G. (1983). Predictions of treatment outcome in parent training: Mother insularity and socioeconomic disadvantage. *Behavioral Assessment, 5,* 301–313.

Elmer, E. (1977). *Fragile families, troubled children*. Pittsburgh: University of Pittsburgh Press.

Elmer, E., & Gregg, G. S. (1967). Developmental characteristics of abused children. *Pediatrics, 40,* 596–602.

Emery, R. (1982). Interparental conflict and the children of discord and divorce. *Psychological Bulletin, 92,* 310–330.

Eyberg, S., & Ross, A. (1978). Assessment of child behavior problems: The validation of a new inventory. *Journal of Clinical Child Psychology, 7,* 113–116.

Forehand, R. L., & McMahon, R. J. (1981). *Helping the noncompliant child: A clinician's guide to parent training*. New York: Guilford.

Frodi, A. M., & Lamb, M. E. (1980). Child abusers' responses to infant smiles and cries. *Child Development, 51,* 238–241.

Gaines, R., Sandgrund, A., Green, A. H., & Power, E. (1978). Etiological factors in child maltreatment: A multivariate study of abusing, neglecting and normal mothers. *Journal of Abnormal Psychology, 87,* 531–540.

Garbarino, J. (1976). A preliminary study of some ecological correlates of child abuse: The impact of socioeconomic stress on mothers. *Child Development, 47,* 178–185.

Garbarino, J., & Sherman, D. (1980). High risk neighborhoods and high risk families: The human ecology of child maltreatment. *Child Development, 51,* 188–198.

George, C., & Main, M. (1979). Social interaction of young abused children: Approach, avoidance and aggression. *Child Development, 50*, 306–318.

Gil, D. G. (1970). *Violence against children: Physical child abuse in the United States*. Cambridge, MA: Harvard University Press.

Goldberg, D. P., & Hillier, V. F. (1979). A scaled version of the General Health Questionnaire. *Psychological Medicine, 9*, 139–145.

Griest, D. C., Forehand, R., Wells, K. C., & McMahon, R. J. (1980). An examination of differences between nonclinic and behavior-problem clinic referred children and their mothers. *Journal of Abnormal Psychology, 89*, 497–500.

Haley, J. (1973). *Uncommon therapy: The psychiatric techniques of Milton H. Erickson M.D.* New York: Norton.

Hartman, D. P. (1982). *Using observers to study behavior*. San Francisco: Jossey-Bass.

Helfer, R. E. (1973). The etiology of child abuse. *Pediatrics, 51*, 777.

Helfer, R. E., Hoffmeister, J. K., & Schneider, C. (1978). *A manual for use of the Michigan Screening Profile of Parenting*. Boulder, CO: Test Analysis and Development Corporation.

Herrenkohl, R. C., Herrenkohl, E. C., & Egolf, B. P. (1983). Circumstances surrounding the occurrence of child maltreatment. *Journal of Consulting & Clinical Psychology, 51*, 424–431.

Hetherington, E. M., Cox, M., & Cox, R. (1979). Family interaction and the social, emotional and cognitive development of children following divorce. In V. Vaugh & T. Brazelton (Eds.), *The family: Setting priorities*. New York: Science and Medicine.

Hetherington, E. M., Cox, M., & Cox, R. (1981). Effects of divorce on parents and children. In M. Lamb (Ed.), *Nontraditional families*. Hillsdale, NJ: Erlbaum.

Holleran, P. A., Littman, D. C., Freund, R. D., & Schmaling, K. B. (1982). A signal detection approach to social perception: Identification of negative and positive behaviors by parents of normal and problem children. *Journal of Abnormal Child Psychology, 10*, 547–557.

Hops, H., & Biglan, T. (1985). *Family interactions of depressed women*. Paper presented at the annual meeting of the Association of Behavior Therapy, Houston.

Johnson, S. M., & Lobitz, G. A. (1974). Parental manipulation of child behavior in home observations. *Journal of Applied Behavior Analysis, 7*, 23–31.

Kanner, A. D., Coyne, J. C., Schaefer, C., & Lazarus, R. S. (1981). Comparison of two modes of stress measurement: Daily Hassles and Uplifts versus Major Life Events. *Journal of Behavioral Medicine, 4*, 1–39.

Kelly, J. A. (1983). *Treating child abusive families: Intervention based on skills training principles*. New York: Plenum.

Kolko, D. J., & Milan, M. A. (1983). Reframing and paradoxical instructions to overcome "resistance" in the treatment of delinquent youths: A multiple baseline analysis. *Journal of Consulting & Clinical Psychology, 51*, 655–660.

Lahey, B. B., Conger, R. D., Atkeson, B. M., & Treiber, T. A. (1984). Parenting behavior and emotional status of physically abusive mothers. *Journal of Consulting & Clinical Psychology, 52*, 1062–1071.

Larrance, D. T., & Twentyman, C. T. (1983). Maternal attributions and child abuse. *Journal of Abnormal Psychology, 92*, 449–457.

Lazarus, R. S., & Folkman, S. (1984). *Stress, appraisal and coping*. New York: Springer.

Levitt, E. E., & Lubin, B. (1975). *Depression: Concepts, controversies and some new facts*. New York: Springer.

Light, R. J. (1973). Abused and neglected children in America: A study of alternative policies. *Harvard Educational Review, 43*, 556–598.

Locke, H. J., & Wallace, K. M. (1959). Short marital adjustment and predictive tests: Their reliability and validity. *Journal of Marriage & Family Living, 13*, 251–255.

Lobitz, W. C., & Johnson, S. M. (1975). Parental manipulation of the behavior of normal and deviant children. *Child Development, 46*, 719–726.

Loeber, R., Dishon, T. J., & Patterson, G. R. (1984). Multiple gating: A multistage assessment procedure for identifying youth at risk for delinquency. *Journal of Research in Crime & Delinquency, 21*, 7–32.

Lorber, R., Felton, D., & Reid, J. B. (1982). *The relationship between parental tracking and labelling of child aggressive behavior and abusive behavior of mothers toward their children*. Unpublished manuscript, Oregon Social Learning Center, Eugene.

Lorber, R., Felton, D. K., & Reid, J. B. (1984). A social learning approach to the reduction of coercive processes in child abusive families: A molecular analysis. *Advances in Behavior Research & Therapy, 6,* 29–45.

Lutzker, J. R. (1980). Deviant family system. In B. B. Lahey & A. E. Kazdin (Eds.), *Advances in clinical child psychology* (Vol. 3). New York: Plenum.

Mash, E. J., Johnson, C., & Kovitz, K. (1983). A comparison of mother–child interaction of physically abused and nonabused children during play and task situations. *Journal of Clinical Child Psychology, 12,* 337–346.

Mash, E. J., Terdal, L., & Anderson, K. (1973). The response-class matrix: A procedure for recording parent–child interactions. *Journal of Consulting & Clinical Psychology, 40,* 163–164.

McCarthy, D. (1972). *McCarthy Scales of Children's Abilities.* New York: Psychological Corporation.

McCrae, K. N., Furgeson, C. A., & Lederman, R. S. (1973). The battered child syndrome. *Canadian Medical Association Journal, 108,* 859–866.

McDevitt, S., & Carey, W. (1978). The measurement of temperament in 3 to 7 year old children. *Journal of Child Psychology & Psychiatry, 19,* 245–253.

McMahon, R. J., Forehand, R., Griest, D. C., & Wells, K. C. (1981). Who drops out of therapy during parent behavioral training? *Behavioral Counseling Quarterly, 1,* 79–85.

Monahan, J. (1981). *Predicting violent behavior.* London: Sage.

Novaco, R. W. (1975). *Anger control: The development and evaluation of an experimental treatment.* Lexington, MA: Lexington.

Parke, R. D. (1979). Interactional design. In R. B. Cairns (Ed.), *The analysis of social interaction: Methods, issues and illustrations.* Hillsdale, NJ: Erlbaum.

Parke, R. D., & Collmer, C. W. (1975). Child abuse: An interdisciplinary analysis. In E. M. Hetherington (Ed.), *Review of child development research* (Vol. 5). Chicago: University of Chicago Press.

Patterson, G. R. (1982). *Coercive family process.* Eugene, OR: Castilia.

Patterson, G. R. (1985). *Family Process: Loops, levels and linkage.* Paper presented to the SCRD Study Group on "Interacting Systems in Human Development," Cornell University, Ithaca, NY.

Patterson, G. R. (1984). Beyond technology: The next stage in the development of an empirical base for parent training. In L. L. Abate (Ed.), *Handbook of family psychology and psychotherapy.* Homewood, IL: Dow, Jones, Irwin.

Patterson, G. R., & Reid, J. B. (1984). Social interactional processes within the family: The study of moment by moment transactions in which social development is embedded. *Journal of Applied Developmental Psychology, 5,* 237–262.

Patterson, G. R., Reid, J. B., & Dishon, T. J. (1987). *A social learning approach: A model for child antisocial behavior.* Eugene, OR: Castilia.

Porter, B., & O'Leary, K. D. (1980). Marital discord and child behavior problems. *Journal of Abnormal Child Psychology, 80,* 287–295.

Procidano, M. E., & Heller, K. (1983). Measures of perceived social support from friends and family: Three validation studies. *American Journal of Community Psychology, 11,* 127–139.

Reid, J. B. (1978). *A social learning approach to family intervention: Vol. 2. Observation in home settings.* Eugene, OR: Castilia.

Reid, J. B. (1982). Social interactional patterns in families of abused and nonabused children. In C. Zahn-Waxler, M. Cummings, & M. Radke-Yarrow (Eds.), *Social and biological origins of altruism and aggression.* New York: Cambridge.

Reid, J. B. (1983). *Child Abuse: Developmental factors and treatment.* NIMH Final Report.

Reid, J. (1985). Behavioral approaches to intervention and assessment of abuse. In P. Bornstein & A. E. Kazdin (Eds.), *Handbook of clinical behavior therapy with children.* Homewood, IL: Dorsey.

Reid, J. B., Baldwin, D. V., Patterson, G. R., & Dishon, T. J. (1985). *Some problems relating to the assessment of childhood disorders: A role for observational data.* Unpublished manuscript, Oregon Social Learning Center, Eugene.

Reid, J. B., Taplin, P. S., & Lorber, R. (1981). A social interactional approach to the treatment of abusive families. In R. Stuart (Ed.), *Violent behavior: Social learning approaches to prediction, management and treatment.* New York: Brunner/Mazel.

Robinson, E. A., & Eyberg, S. (1981). The dyadic parent–child interaction coding systems: Standardization and validation. *Journal of Consulting & Clinical Psychology, 49*, 245–250.

Rosenberg, M. S., & Reppucci, N. D. (1983). Abusive mothers: Perceptions of their own children's behavior. *Journal of Consulting & Clinical Psychology, 51*, 647–682.

Rutter, M. (1971). Parent–child separation: Psychological effects on children. *Journal of Child Psychology & Psychiatry, 12*, 233–260.

Rutter, M. (1978). Family, area and school influences in the genesis of conduct disorders. In A. Hersov, M. Berger, & D. Schaffer (Eds.), *Aggression and antisocial behavior in childhood and adolescence*. Oxford: Pergamon.

Sarason, I. G., Johnson, J. H., & Siegal, J. M. (1978). Assessing the impact of life changes: Development of the Life Experiences Survey. *Journal of Consulting & Clinical Psychology, 46*, 932–946.

Sarason, I. G., Levine, H. M., Basham, R. B., & Sarason, B. R. (1983). Assessing social support: The social support questionaire. *Journal of Personality & Social Psychology, 43*, 127–139.

Salzinger, S., Kaplan, S., & Artemyeff, C. (1983). Mothers' personal social networks and child maltreatment. *Journal of Abnormal Psychology, 92*, 68–76.

Schmaling, K., & Patterson, G. R. (1984). *Maternal clarifications of deviant and prosocial child behavior and reactions to the child in the home*. Unpublished manuscript, Oregon Social Learning Center, Eugene.

Sigel, I. E., McGillicudy-DiLisi, A. V., & Johnson, J. E. (1980). *Parental distancing beliefs and children's representational competence within the family context*. Research Report. Princeton, NJ: Educational Testing Service.

Smith, S. M., & Hanson, R. (1974). Battered children: a medical and psychological study. *British Medical Journal, 3*, 666–670.

Smith, S. M., Hanson, R., & Noble, S. (1974). Social aspects of the battered baby syndrome. *British Journal of Psychiatry, 125*, 568–582.

Snyder, J. J. (1977). A reinforcement analysis of interaction in problem and non-problem families. *Journal of Abnormal Psychology, 86*, 528–535.

Snyder, J., & Brown, K. (1983). Oppositional behavior and noncompliance in preschool children: Environmental correlates and skills deficits. *Behavioral Assessment, 5*, 333–348.

Snyder, J. J., & Patterson, G. R. (1986). Family interaction and delinquent behavior. In H. C. Quay (Ed.), *Handbook of juvenile delinquency*. New York: Wiley.

Spanier, G. B. (1976). Measuring dyadic adjustment: New scales for assessing the quality of marriage and similar dyads. *Journal of Marriage & Family Living, 38*, 15–28.

Starr, R. H. (1982). A research-based approach to the prediction of child abuse. In R. Starr (Ed.), *Child abuse prediction: Policy implications*. Cambridge, MA.: Ballinger.

Steele, B. F., & Pollock, C. B. (1969). A psychiatric study of parents who abuse infants and small children. In R. E. Helfer & C. H. Kempe (Eds.), *The battered child*. Chicago: University of Chicago Press.

Stouthamer-Lorber, M., Patterson, G. R., & Lorber, R. (1983). *Parental monitoring and antisocial behavior in boys*. Unpublished manuscript. Oregon Social Learning Center, Eugene.

Straus, M. A. (1979). Measuring intrafamily conflict and violence: The Conflict Tactics (CT) scale. *Journal of Marriage & the Family, 41*, 75–88.

Straus, M. A., Gelles, R. J., & Steinmetz, S. K. (1980). *Behind closed doors: Violence in the American family*. Garden City, NY: Anchor.

Wahler, R. G. (1980). The insular mother: Her problems in parent–child treatment. *Journal of Applied Behavior Analysis, 13*, 207–219.

Wahler, R. G., & Dumas, J. E. (1983). Predictors of treatment outcome in parent training: Mother insularity and socioeconomic disadvantage. *Behavioral Assessment, 5*, 301–314.

Wahler, R. G., House, A. E., & Stambaugh, E. E. (1976). *Ecological assessment of child behavior problems: A clinical package for home, school, and institutional settings*. New York: Pergamon.

Wahler, R. G. Leske, G., & Rogers, E. S. (1979) The insular family: A deviance support system for oppositional children. In L. A. Hamerlynck (Ed.), *Behavioral systems for the developmentally disabled: I. School and family environments*. New York: Brunner/Mazel.

Weinberg, S. C., & Richardson, M. S. (1981). Dimensions of stress in early parenting. *Journal of Consulting & Clinical Psychology, 49,* 686–693.

Weinrott, M. R., Reid, J. B., Bauske, B. W., & Brummett, B. (1981). Supplementing naturalistic observations with observer impressions. *Behavioral Assessment, 3,* 151–160.

Weiss, R. L., & Margolin, G. (1977). Assessment of marital conflict. In A. Ciminero, K. Calhoun, & H. Adams (Eds.), *Handbook of behavioral assessment*. New York: Wiley.

Wolfe, D. A. (1985). Abusive parents: An empirical review. *Psychological Bulletin, 97,* 462–482.

Wolfe, D. A., Aragona, J., Kaufman, K., & Sandler, J. (1980). The importance of adjudication in the treatment of child abusers: Some preliminary findings. *Child Abuse & Neglect, 4,* 127–135.

Wolfe, D. A., Fairbank, J., Kelly, J. A., & Bradlyn, A. S. (1983). Child abusive parents' physiological responses to stressful and nonstressful behavior in children. *Behavioral Assessment, 5,* 363–371.

Wolfe, D., Jaffe, P., Wilson, S. K., & Zak, L. (1985). Children of battered women: The relation of child behavior to family violence and maternal stress. *Journal of Consulting & Clinical Psychology, 53,* 657–665.

Zigler, E. (1980). Controlling child abuse: Do we have the knowledge and/or the will? In G. Gerbner, C. J. Ross, & E. Zigler (Eds.), *Child abuse: An agenda for action*. New York: Oxford University Press.

Zuckerman, M., & Lubin, B. (1965). *Manual for the Multiple Affect Adjective Checklist*. San Diego, CA: Educational and Industrial Testing Service.

APPENDICES

DIRECTIONS AND ISSUES IN TRAINING

APPENDIX 1

Training the Child Health Psychologist

MICHAEL C. ROBERTS
DEBRA FANURIK
PAULINE D. ELKINS

The specialty of pediatric psychology developed as practitioners found they could not meet the challenge of critical problems in childhood within the frameworks of traditional pediatrics and traditional clinical child psychology. As noted in several surveys, the types of problems presenting in pediatric practices involve a significant number of psychological, developmental, behavioral, educational, and child management issues (McClelland, Staples, Weisberg, & Berger, 1973). As depicted in the other chapters in this book, child and developmental issues abound in health care. Problems commonly presented in pediatric health care settings include many psychological–medical concomitants of physical illness, handicap, or medical procedures (e.g., sequelae to burns, spina bifida, adjustment to diabetes, anxiety about hospitalization and surgery). Additionally, there are many medical–psychological disorders for which effective psychological assessment and interventions are available (e.g., encopresis, failure to thrive, abdominal pain).

We will use the terms *pediatric psychology* and *child health psychology* interchangeably in this chapter because we find the differences to be fairly negligible. The term *pediatric psychology* has more historical usage. It is flexible and broad enough to accommodate a wide diversity of practices even outside the traditional pediatric setting. Thus we adopt the definition articulated by Roberts, Maddux, and Wright (1984):

> Pediatric psychology as a field of research and practice has been concerned with a wide variety of topics in the relationship between the psychological and physical well-being of children, including behavioral and emotional concomitants of disease and illness, the role of psychology in pediatric medicine, and the promotion of health and prevention of illness among healthy children. (pp. 56–57)

Also, for purposes of this discussion we will use *predoctoral training* to designate university-based training (coursework, practica) leading to a doctorate in psychology prior to the internship. The term *internship* will be used to indicate clinical predoctoral training taken upon completion of coursework. The internship training experience is typically a year-long formalized program in a medical center, school system, mental health center, or child guidance clinic. The term *postdoctoral training* will be reserved for formalizing training after receipt of the doctoral degree including postdoctoral fellowships and internships, respecialization, and continuing education. Of course, most psychologists undergo a considerable amount of postdoctoral learning "on the job" in whatever position is taken. The formal programmatic nature of postdoctoral training will be stressed in our discussion here.

There are several aspects to this work in child health psychology that relate to training. In the brief period of work in this area (less than 20 years), a number of conceptualizations have developed for the roles and functions of pediatric psychologists (Roberts, Maddux, Wurtele, & Wright, 1982). These functional roles of the area should give rise to a set of definitional criteria for training. However, no guidelines have been established for training in child health psychology. Because there were no formalized sequences of training in this developing specialty, psychologists frequently received on-the-job training ("self-training") in pediatric settings after taking positions that often required considerable adaptation (Ottinger & Roberts, 1980).

Surveys of the members of the Society of Pediatric Psychology, the primary organizational home for child health psychologists, indicate a diversity of backgrounds of current professionals in the field (La Greca, 1985; Stabler & Mesibov, 1984). In many ways, this diversity has served the area well by bringing into it a wealth of approaches and ideas. Thus it is common to find in literature and practice the perspectives of not only clinical psychologists, but also developmental, social, experimental, school, and counseling psychologists. The diversity also may produce some lack of consensus over what constitutes "proper" training.

Increasingly, however, as the field has grown, more pediatric psychologists have called for a delineation of basic training necessary for competent practice. Such an outline of training would not preclude involvement of many other specializations within psychology, but could provide a conceptualization for trainers to educate future workers in the field. As noted by Roberts, Erickson, and Tuma (1985), a lack of training criteria poses professional, ethical, and social responsibility problems. This situation of no training standards could lead to potentially harmful or needless interventions and eventual disenfranchisement of the field.

There have been national training conferences in the two specialties particularly relevant to pediatric psychology: health psychology (Stone, 1983) and clinical child psychology (Tuma, 1985). The Health Psychology Training Conference did not address children's health issues to any significant degree (Maddux, Roberts, Sledden, & Wright, 1986; Maddux, Roberts, & Wright, 1986), and recommendations for training any type of health psychologists were imprecise. At the Conference on Training Clinical Child Psychologists held at Hilton Head, South Carolina, in May 1985, a series of recommendations were adopted that bear directly on the training of child health psychologists, whether or not one conceptualizes the field as requiring a clinical background. For example, the conference endorsed the scientist–professional model of clinical training and emphasized the role of developmental bases of behavior.

Many of the training recommendations adopted by the Clinical Child Psychology Conference derived from the set prepared by the Training Task Force of the Division of Child, Youth, and Family Services of the American Psychological Association (Division 37; see Roberts et al., 1985). These Division 37 recommendations are clearly the most relevant set of training criteria for application to child health psychology. As noted by Roberts and colleagues (1985), the basics of psychological work with children were delineated in these training guidelines, but other interested groups were encouraged to add any uniquely relevant qualifications and training for specialty training. The Clinical Child Psychology Conference did this for "clinical child psychology" by endorsing in principle the Division 37 recommendations among other resolutions (Tuma, 1985). Additionally, the more generic training recommendations of Division 37 were approved as guiding principles with no additions or modifications by the Executive Board of the Society of Pediatric Psychology (Society of Pediatric Psychology, 1984). However, no group or publication, to our knowledge, has provided a conceptualization of training specifically for pediatric or child health psychology.

In this chapter we will attempt to outline the basic and specialty components we assert are necessary for training competent child health psychologists or pediatric psychologists based on an adaptation of the Division 37 recommendations. We will provide a justification of each recommended experience and note particular relevance to pediatric psychology. Finally, particular concern will be given to the various levels at which training can and should occur (predoctoral, internship, and postdoctoral). Throughout this chapter, reflecting a similar stance taken by Roberts and colleagues (1985), no presumption is made that all child health psychologists must proceed through the type of training sequence followed in clinical training programs accredited by the American Psychological Association (Committee on Accreditation, 1980). We are affiliated with such a program, and some biases may be evident in this chapter. However, it is not our intent to imply that there is a single route to competence as a child health psychologist (Koocher, 1983). There are many competent professionals researching and working in the field who come through different sequences.

We do assume that certain fundamentals of psychology have been acquired by the trainee while mastering the essentials of specialization. A principle of the APA accreditation criteria for doctoral programs in professional psychology states that one is a psychologist first and a specialist second (Committee on Accreditation, 1980). Fundamental psychology requires a firm grounding in individual differences and biological, cognitive—affective, and social bases of behavior as well as scientific and professional ethics and standards. Furthermore, fundamental psychology requires knowledge of research design and methodology, statistics, psychological measurement, and history and systems of psychology. With these as a basis, under the APA criteria, professional courses and experiences are added, such as psychodiagnostics and assessment, intervention procedures, consultation, program evaluation, and research training for the professional psychologist. Then, in addition to these basic and specialized training components, further specialization can occur for clinical child psychology and pediatric psychology.

As noted by Tuma and Grabert (1983), there have been two positions about whether pediatric psychology is a subspecialty of clinical child psychology or a specialty in its own right. These positions have implications for how training should be handled. If pediatric psychology is a subspecialty, then greater emphasis would be placed on the predoctoral, university-level training of the basics of clinical psychology and clinical child psychology. Specialization in pediatric psychology would come at the internship or postdoctoral levels. If pediatric psychology is a specialty in its own right, then intensive training specifically in child health psychology could be made at the predoctoral level with additional work at the internship and postdoctoral levels. Of course, there are additional considerations of how pediatric psychology relates to the larger domain of health psychology. Without debating the merits of any of these positions, we would argue that there are basics of psychology and specialty courses that can be articulated as very relevant to psychological practice in the area of children's health. The generic nature of the training recommendations from the Division 37 deliberations has the advantage of being applicable to *all* psychology work with children, youth, and families. Thus it is a relatively easy task to apply the training recommendations to child health psychology.

A number of surveys have been taken to determine the training backgrounds of various groups and to ascertain what professionals involved in training think are necessary courses and experiences. These surveys are useful for developing ideas on requisite coursework and applied clinical work for child health psychology. For example, in a survey of internship programs in pediatric psychology, Tuma and Grabert (1983) found that a majority of directors endorsed predoctoral (preinternship) coursework and experiences in intellectual assessment, developmental, personality assessment, psychotherapy, child psychology, projective testing, psychopathology, personality, and abnormal psychology. Of course, these are basic courses obtained typically in APA-accredited predoctoral clinical programs regardless of any further specialty. Tuma and Grabert (1983) also found internships for pediatric psychology offered training that consisted of basic clinical seminars and supervised clinical work such as psychodiagnostics and treatment, with a few additional seminars in adolescent medicine, behavioral medicine, and neuropsychology. These trainers of pediatric psychologists defined specialty practice as applying traditional clinical child psychology techniques to health-related problems, while additionally requiring further specialized skills and techniques. The reliance of child health psychology on clinical child psychology is evident. Indeed, Tuma and Grabert (1983) suggest that pediatric psychology is clinical child psychology's entry into the health psychology domain.

In a comparison of pediatric psychologists and health psychologists, Stabler and Mesibov (1984) surveyed the members of the Society of Pediatric Psychology and the APA Division of Health Psychology (38). They found that the majority of both groups had graduate training in clinical psychology. (This finding for pediatric psychology is similar to one obtained earlier by Routh, 1977.) The remaining pediatric psychologists tended to have backgrounds in developmental, educational, and school psychology, whereas the remaining health psychologists had training in social or experimental psychology. Another noteworthy finding of this survey is that pediatric psychologists function mostly as therapists, diagnosticians, consultants, and teachers, while less time is spent in research and administration.

The Training Committee of the Society of Pediatric Psychology (SPP) recently conducted a survey of members to determine their training backgrounds and attitudes toward coverage of specific content areas in training (La Greca, 1985). Preliminary analyses indicate results paralleling previous surveys, in that clinical and clinical child psychology formed the major field of study for the majority of SPP members with school, developmental, counseling, and experimental psychology comprising much smaller percentages. The respondents endorsed the importance of the following content areas in coursework: child development, child psychopathology, child intellectual assessment, child assessment (overview), child personality or emotional assessment, child psychotherapy (overview), behavior therapy, infancy, developmental disabilities, child or adolescent medical disorders, child achievement testing, behavioral assessment, adolescence, legal or ethical issues, family assessment, and family therapy. Similar content areas were rated important for applied work with the addition of training in consultation or liaison. These pediatric psychologists generally endorsed clinical child training with a developmental psychology emphasis as the most satisfactory model for predoctoral training. However, those surveyed responded that the major thrust of specialized training should be at the internship and postdoctoral levels.

These surveys indicate that the majority of current child health psychologists received their training as clinical psychologists for their doctorate. Despite one's training background or personal opinions about requisite skills to be a child health psychologist, perhaps more than anything the training in this specialty should be shaped by what roles and functions are actually assumed by the pediatric psychologist. The types of cases seen define the area more than any other definitional criteria. Roberts (1986) has compiled the referral problems reported by three different types of pediatric psychology services (Kanoy & Schroeder, 1985; Ottinger & Roberts, 1980; Walker, 1979). A fairly consistent pattern of practice emerges, with negative behaviors, school-related problems, and personality problems comprising a high percentage of referrals to pediatric psychology. These data indicate that a large proportion of current practice in child health psychology reflects more traditional clinical child psychology issues. This compilation of actual functioning notably speaks to the need for training in clinical and clinical child psychology before further specialization in pediatric or child health psychology. Also well represented in this compilation of referral problems were issues more typically considered pediatric psychology, such as physical complaints, adjustment to disease, developmental delays, toileting, and infant management problems. Ability to provide competent service for these problems requires more specialized training.

Since child health psychologists provide a variety of services and fulfill a multitude of roles, training should be geared toward the common basic requirements at the predoctoral level with more specialized work obtained at internship and postdoctoral levels as the psychologist forms a clearer idea of his or her future roles. The recommendations for training child health psychologists outlined here are based firmly in training for psychologists to work with children, youth, and families. We believe that the child health psychologist first must be a psychologist with a background in providing competent services to and for children. Specialization to provide child health psychological services comes after or is intertwined with mastery of generic clinical child psychology. This specialization can occur at the predoctoral level and, most certainly, should also occur at the internship and postdoctoral levels.

Our orientation derives from several factors. First, we believe that there are certain basics of psychology necessary for professional practice that must be present before specialization should occur. Second, when considering the types of clinical cases seen in pediatric psychology practices, the necessity becomes evident that child health psychologists should be able to work with more generalized problems of childhood as well as with the specialized problems presenting in children's health care settings. Finally, we view child health psychology as a specialized professional area occurring at the overlap of clinical child psychology and health psychology. While pediatric psychology should be recognized as a specialty in its own right, there seem to be many more aspects of clinical child psychology that relate to practice and research in this area than there are from health psychology per se.

The topics listed here form an ideal training program for child health psychology. To our knowledge, there are a few programs actually providing the bulk of these topics. However, there are several programs that provide some, but not all, topics listed (Roberts, 1985). Roberts and colleagues (1985) provide examples of how three training programs provide the basics of psychology to work with children, youth, and families through university-based programs of clinical, school, and applied developmental psychology. The increased specialization required of child health psychologists will automatically narrow the number of available training places. This list of topics may be helpful to faculty in designing a program for child health psychology, as well as for students considering a program for possible matriculation.

BASIC COMPETENCE

A critical consideration for defining the training standards for child health psychologists as well as for describing, in essence, who can work in this area, must be the Ethical Standards of the American Psychological Association, the Principle 2 of Competence: "Psychologists recognize the boundaries of their competence."(American Psychological Association, 1981, p. 2). For those psychologists choosing to practice professionally in the area of child health psychology, the Standards for Providers of Psychological Services also apply: "Psychologists shall limit their practice to their demonstrated areas of professional competence" (Standard 1.6: American Psychological Association, 1977). The recommendations outlined here attempt to define training experiences and coursework useful in becoming a competent pediatric psychologist. However, these are not necessarily sufficient to guarantee such competence. We do endorse the concept that competence in psychological work with children, youth, and families in health care settings is directly linked to training for that competence (Roberts et al., 1985; Wohlford, 1978).

Goals of Training Child Health Psychologists

1. Training should provide, at a minimum, those entry-level skills for providing professional psychological services to children, in general, and for children's

health, in particular. Child health psychology specialists should be competent to assess children's psychological problems, understand their etiologies, and intervene and prevent on behalf of children and their significant adults in different settings. Thus training should provide exposure to and experience with a broad range of child populations, disorders, and settings.

2. Pediatric psychology training should include more specialized coursework and experiences related to practice in health care settings and with child health issues.
3. Training should provide the scientific basis for applications in professional psychology and should include specialized research contributing to an understanding of human development. Training should include the evaluation of therapeutic interventions with children and families. Particular research expertise should include health issues in both mental and physical domains, and their interaction.
4. The training of child health psychologists requires concerted efforts at all three levels: predoctoral, internship, and postdoctoral. Topics for training should be articulated across levels with particular emphases included at each. There are several adequate ways to achieve quality training for competent professionals in this field. These suggested topics and coverage delineate what is needed within whatever form the training program may have.

TOPICS OF TRAINING

In this section, we outline topic areas that may be covered in various ways in order to accomplish the goals of training child health psychologists. This outline of specialty topics is not a listing of courses, but is an indication of what is desirable for training the child health psychologist to be a competent provider of psychological services. Most of the basic and specialized topics can be covered at the predoctoral level without overburdening the students. Additional specialty emphasis and experiences in clinical applications then can be gained through internship programs and postdoctoral work oriented to pediatric psychology.

Basic Topics

Life span developmental psychology with emphasis on child development
Psychopathology (child and adult)
Mental retardation and developmental disabilities
Child psychotherapy and behavior change
Parent, family, and school intervention techniques
Research methods in child psychology

Ethics and legal issues related to children and families

Specialty Topics

Health psychology (life cycle)
Assessment in child health psychology

Interventions in child health psychology
Clinical practica in child health psychology

Each of these topics is elaborated in the next section with a brief description of coverage and a rationale for inclusion in training programs for child health psychologists.

Topics and Coverage

Life Span Developmental Psychology with Emphasis on Child Development. Knowledge of normal development and behavior is essential for understanding abnormal development and behavior. Professional psychological practice in child health psychology requires a basic understanding of the developmental process and its impact on the child as well as the eventual adult (Maddux, Roberts, Sledden, & Wright, 1986; Roberts, Maddux, & Wright, 1984). Consequently, developmental milestones and transitions should be taught. Topical coverage should include social, physical, personality, cognitive, perceptual, language, and emotional development across the life span. Developmental psychology should be acquired with a life span perspective covering the periods of prenatal, neonatal, infant, toddler, nursery school, middle childhood, adolescent, young adulthood, middle adulthood, and late adulthood.

Psychopathology (Child and Adult). Abnormal development should be examined with a particular emphasis on childhood. Different theoretical viewpoints on deviant behavior need to be presented. A basis for understanding the etiology of disorders, conducting assessment, and developing a clinical diagnosis should be obtained for the range of emotional, behavioral, cognitive, and learning disorders across the life span. Training should include exposure to physical disorders that have psychological concomitants as well as those of a primary psychological nature.

Mental Retardation and Developmental Disabilities. Coverage should include etiology, assessment and diagnosis, intervention, and prevention of mental retardation and other developmental disabilities. Students should receive exposure to significant research, applied experiences with developmentally delayed children and their families, and consultation regarding programming for these clients. Since developmentally disabled children and their families represent a large proportion of clientele in many pediatric settings, specialty training ought to be oriented to meeting their special needs.

Child Psychotherapy and Behavior Change. This topic covers various theoretical approaches to treating children and families including, for example, behavioral, cognitive, educational, play, and traditional therapies. Examination should be made of the empirical bases of these therapeutic approaches. Additionally, instruction should be provided in strategies for determining the applicability of specific interventions, prognosis, and therapeutic outcome.

Parent, Family, and School Intervention. The child lives in the context of other systems; recognition of these should be made. Coursework and practica should cover the basics of therapeutic interventions with parents and other family members in addition to school teachers, counselors, and principals when indicated. Training should cover the determination of when interventions are indicated to be most appropriate.

Research Methods in Child Psychology and Specialties. Basic research methodology in psychology should be covered in addition to more specific research techniques developed for child and family psychology. Instruction might include coverage of cross-sectional and longitudinal research, group versus individual subjects designs, behavior analysis, observational research, treatment outcome, and laboratory and naturalistic experimentation.

Ethics and Legal Issues Related to Children, Youth, and Families. Attention should be given to the rights of children related to psychologists' activities in different settings (e.g., medical care, courts, mental health care, schools). Students should become alert to protecting children's rights in such issues as informed consent or assent for medical and psychological treatment or for research participation, substituted judgment, child custody, confidentiality, testing, and school placement.

Health Psychology (Life Cycle). Development and change occur across the life span with significant implications for health attitudes and behavior. Life cycle health psychology reflects an orientation to development and meeting the health needs of children while they are children and to help later when they are adults. Additionally, attention is directed to the changing health status as adults develop. The developmental perspective for child health psychology, indeed, for all health psychology, aids in deciding: (1) when during a life span preventive and remediative interventions are most needed and for what problems; (2) when services would be most effective and acceptable for recipients; and (3) what types of services would be most effective for what age child and adult (Roberts, Elkins, & Royal, 1984). Training should be devoted to this developmental orientation with attention to the various health concerns in the life cycle.

Assessment in Child Health Psychology. Competent assessment and diagnosis of children's problems require special training experiences. Didactic coursework and clinical experience should cover general assessment of children such as for intelligence and achievement, personality, learning disabilities, and general behavioral problems. Additionally, more advanced and specialized instruments are needed in the diagnosis of child health problems and related conditions as covered in other chapters in this book. Assessment training should be available for special populations of physically handicapped children, disadvantaged and minority children, speech- and hearing-impaired children, developmentally delayed children, and neuropsychologically impaired children. Students need to be trained in how to decide which assessment instruments are most appropriate for which disorders and how to use information gained from such assessments in formulating the treatment plans. While actual experience with all assessment modalities available may be impossible, basic approaches to assessment should be provided with information about the uses and availability of various instruments. The assessment measures discussed in the present text are indicative of the specialized instruments and approaches necessary for child health psychology in such topics as family assessment, health beliefs, and medical compliance. It would be useful also to provide training in procedures for designing and evaluating new instruments to help meet the often immediate needs for special assessment when confronted with unique problems for which present techniques may be inadequate.

Interventions in Child Health Psychology. There are specific disorders in child health psychology with empirically based interventions (e.g., diabetes, asthma, migraine headaches, enuresis, encopresis). Didactic instruction is necessary prior to intensive applications in clinical practice. An orientation to early intervention, prevention, and health promotion is essential for the child health psychologist. Prevention covers both prevention of psychological disorders and prevention of physical problems. These efforts should include improving health behaviors for the well-being of children while they are children and for improvement of health in the later adult life. Prevention and promotion are the keys to competent, economical, and high-quality health care for children. This orientation should emphasize the concepts of behavioral health.

Clinical Practica in Child Health Psychology. Applied clinical experiences are necessary to complement didactic coursework covered in the other topics. Students must obtain basic clinical experiences with children and adults in other practica prior to working with specialized populations and problems. The special needs of many clients and families presenting in pediatric settings require advanced trainees who have mastered the fundamentals of psychotherapeutic work. The specialized clinical practica would provide extra experiences with a variety of child and family problems and demographic characteristics. For training in the basic aspects of clinical child psychology, these advanced practica could be conducted in a variety of settings (e.g., schools, residential treatment centers and psychiatric inpatient units, community mental health centers, psychological clinics, and child guidance or child study centers). However, for the child health psychology trainee, such advanced practica might also take place in pediatric or medical settings such as general hospital units or departments (e.g., general pediatrics wards, outpatient adolescent medicine), special treatment units with inpatient and/or outpatient services (e.g., pediatric burn ward, endocrinology treatment, dialysis, or oncology), and pediatricians' clinic or office practices. Exposure to alternative models of intervention and professionals of other disciplines (e.g., pediatrics, social work, psychiatry) should be available. We acknowledge that it would be impossible for a predoctoral student (or an intern) to obtain experience with all possible settings and health issues. Time and availability of resources pose legitimate constraints. These limits on training should pose few problems for later practice in child health psychology since there is considerable overlap in psychological approaches to assessment and treatment across disorders and settings.

Internship

Thus far, we have focused primarily on the predoctoral aspects of training child health psychologists, although most of the topics outlined do require coverage at all levels. The intensive predoctoral internship is a necessary component for training the psychologist to be competent in providing psychological services. The nature and quality of training at the internship level have not been well articulated for child health psychology or for any specialty outside of the APA Accreditation Criteria (Committee on Accreditation, 1980). The Division 37 recommendations for training psychologists to work with children, youth, and families (Roberts et al., 1985) merely noted that a child-oriented internship should be completed with rotations to different child and family settings for maximal exposure and training. It is further suggested that no less than two-thirds time of an internship should be devoted to child-related work. These points were endorsed by the Conference on Training Clinical Child Psychologists with a few additional provisions (Tuma, 1985). The final recommendations adopted by the Conference included the following statement:

> Internship programs in clinical child psychology should be broad based with regard to populations serviced, theoretical orientation, and experiences provided. In addition to the need for experiences with adults, the clinical child psychology intern should receive experiences with children from as broad an age range as possible with experiences with infants through adolescents being the goal.
>
> Diversity in gender, SES background, ethnic origin, and presenting problem of clients served is a desired goal. An understanding of the nature of the problem presented by the child must take into account the developmental level of the child. (Tuma, 1985, p. 5).

Additionally, the Conference recommended that:

> Internship training in clinical child psychology should include didactic and supervised training in at least assessment, intervention strategies, case management and consultation skills. In addition, training and experience in prevention is highly desirable. The nature of didactic training and supervised experiences in each of these areas should be as broad based and varied as possible. Case management conferences should be utilized to integrate assessment, treatment, and consultation, with ethical considerations and an increased awareness of [the need for] evaluating the success of our chosen interventions also being considered. (Tuma, 1985, p. 5)

Building on these recommendations for clinical child psychology, additional criteria need to be elaborated for the child health psychologist's training. Indeed, La Greca's (1985) survey of SPP members determined that the greatest endorsement of pediatric psychology training came for internship level training. Internships in health care settings are perhaps in the best position to provide intensive, focused training in child health psychology. Interns in these settings can be exposed to a greater variety of pediatric health cases and general pediatric issues. Internship faculty are not required to teach all the basic knowledge and skills necessarily taught at the predoctoral level. Furthermore, the larger pool of faculty mentors can often provide more exposure to child health psychologists as clinicians, researchers, and teachers.

Internship programs with an emphasis on child health psychology typically note the wide variety of training experiences and caseloads. These include pain management, noncompliance with medical regimens, reactions to disfigurement and physical disabilities as a result of illness or injury, preparation for hospitalization or outpatient medical procedures, substance abuse, attempted suicide, eating disorders, child abuse, coping with life-threatening illness, and counseling parents of premature and seriously ill infants. These problems are most frequently encountered in hospitals or associated outpatient specialty clinics. However, many internship programs also note training opportunities in primary child health care settings where psychological problems are often observed by physicians or reported by parents in the course of medical treatment. School and learning problems, developmental disabilities, psychosomatic symptoms, behavior problems due to poor child management skills, hyperactivity, enuresis, and encopresis are commonly presented in these settings (e.g., Kanoy & Schroeder, 1985; Walker, 1979). Additionally, the primary care setting gives the intern experience in helping parents anticipate and cope with issues of normal psychosocial development in their children (e.g., temper tantrums, toilet training, getting ready for kindergarten, sex education). The types of health care settings and presenting problems noted above require a wide variety of assessment techniques and instruments that have been the subject matter of earlier chapters in this book. While at their internship, students will be called upon to determine the level of intellectual, emotional, behavioral, and social functioning in children and their families. In addition to refining the basic assessment skills acquired through earlier predoctoral experience, the intern in a health care setting will have more opportunities for infant assessment and neuropsychological assessment. Somewhat surprisingly, a survey of pediatric internship programs by Tuma and Grabert (1983) revealed that learning disabilities were the most frequently seen disorder among pediatric patients. Therefore, assessment skills in this area are clearly indicated as part of a comprehensive training program.

Postdoctoral Training

Additional specialized experiences are available for training in child health psychology. Many current professionals received their training in postdoctoral experiences with special work in particular areas within pediatric psychology. In addition, La Greca's (1985) survey of SPP members found that a large percentage of respondents viewed postdoctoral training as "essential" to provide child health care services. Postdoctoral experiences often permit more focused training in the area than is allowed in most predoctoral graduate programs or internship programs that have the mandate to provide basic and therefore more general training. We combine in this category three types of training: postdoctoral fellowships and internships, respecialization training, and continuing education.

Postdoctoral Fellowships and Internships. Since the field of child health psychology has not established its own recommendations regarding postdoctoral training, we borrow some from the 1983 National Working Conference on Education and Training in Health Psychology. There was general agreement among the conference working groups that postdoctoral training in health psychology should occur through a 2-year postdoctoral residency that follows both "mentor" and "didactic" training models. Although a background in health psychology prior to the postdoctoral training was considered preferable, this was not considered a requirement for entrance into a formal postdoctoral program in health psychology. Also recommended was that such postdoctoral programs be accredited by APA's Education and Training Board.

In Tuma's (1984) *Directory of Internship Programs in Child Clinical and Pediatric Psychology*, there are 21 postdoctoral internships and fellowships in pediatric psychology. This number reflects an increase in programs over the past several years. Postdoctoral programs in pediatric psychology are typically found within medical centers in departments of pediatrics or developmental centers. They usually require a 1- to 2-year commitment and are often autonomous from, but cooperative with, psychiatry (Faust, Ulissi, & Thurber, 1980; Tuma, 1982b). In their review of available postdoctoral programs, Faust and colleagues (1980) determined that approximately 25 percent of the trainees' time is typically spent in didactic training and formal supervision. The greater part of the remaining time is allotted to providing direct services to children, followed by teaching, consultation to hospital personnel and community agencies, and unfunded research. Tuma (1982b) has noted that the conduct of research is more feasible in a postdoctoral program because of the longer time commitment. As one example of this type of training, Faust and colleagues (1980) described a postdoctoral fellowship in pediatric psychology.

Formal postdoctoral training programs in pediatric psychology should provide the opportunity for advanced training for those doctoral psychologists not previously trained in a child health area in addition to those wishing further to develop expertise in the specialty of pediatric psychology. Regardless of the students' previous levels of training in pediatric psychology, postdoctoral work in this area should build on the basic clinical skills developed during the predoctoral internship. The student lacking in pediatric psychology training does need to have a background similar to the content outlined earlier, however it is obtained. Obtaining these clinical skills prior to entering the postdoctoral program for nonclinical psychologists constitutes respecialization. A second-year option for postdoctoral work for some fellows or residents may be taken depending on individual interests and training opportunities.

Respecialization. Respecialization, or the lateral change of specialty within psychology (Stricker, 1983), can provide the opportunity for the psychologist who has been previously trained in a nonclinical field to enter the field of child health psychology (if one conceives it as a clinical specialty). According to APA policy (Conger, 1976), respecialization should take place through a formal program, including both coursework and internship. Therefore, professionals desiring to change to clinical careers proceed through a truncated graduate program in clinical psychology (recognizing previous doctoral work) and then complete a clinical internship. A recent survey identified 43 graduate programs offering respecialization training in clinical psychology (Stricker, Hull, & Woodring, 1984). Several of these programs have been described (e.g., Page, 1983; Silber, 1983). Respecialization programs typically involve 2 years of clinical coursework, followed by the internship. The nonclinical psychologist who seeks to be a provider of health services to children might most appropriately follow these formal respecialization procedures. Some expertise might also be most useful in clinical child psychology. After completing the clinical coursework, the student can proceed to complete a postdoctoral internship or fellowship in pediatric psychology. The APA Committee on Accreditation (1984) has stated that, while it is not inappropriate for an APA-accredited clinical internship program to offer training to those without a clinical background (e.g., the developmental psychologist), this training does not constitute professional respecialization.

Continuing Education in Child Health Psychology. The Conference on Training Clinical Child Psychologists noted a critical need for child psychologists continually to be aware of the current state of knowledge. The conference recommended that continuing education should be an "ethical responsibility of all clinical child psychologists" (Tuma, 1985, p. 5). It was further noted that such education should be continually renewed in the areas of assessment, intervention, consultation, and prevention. Given the rapidly changing specialty of pediatric psychology, continuing education needs are perhaps even greater for the specialist.

The American Psychological Association provides overview and approval of continuing education offerings. Continuing education credits are required for maintaining licensure in some states. As a result, a number of groups (both professional and private, profit making) have begun to provide training of this type. Several professional organizations provide opportunities for earning continuing education credits with a significant number of their programs directly related to concerns of child health psychology. The APA Division of Clinical Psychology (12) sponsors Postdoctoral institutes every year for several days prior to the APA Convention. Recent topics included child behavioral assessment, child sexual abuse, and neuropsychology. The Division of Health Psychology (38) also sponsors continuing education workshops at the APA convention, with recent ones on pediatric health psychology, anorexia and bulimia in adolescence, and patient compliance with health recommendations. The Society of Behavioral Medicine holds an annual conference with basic and advanced workshops on such topics as anorexia nervosa, pain management, medical noncompliance, and childhood injury prevention. Similarly, the Association for the Care of Children's Health holds an annual conference with relevant continuing education programming on children's health issues (e.g., pediatric oncology, chronic illness in childhood, psychosocial programming in hospitals). The Society of Pediatric Psychology has developed a mechanism for proposing specialty programs at the various regional conventions in order to provide greater access to child health psychology for interested professionals. The Society also has program time on substantive issues at the APA annual convention with recent topics on prevention and promotion, sequelae to pediatric conditions, assessment in pediatric psychology, and family involvement in health issues.

THE PROGRAM AT THE UNIVERSITY OF ALABAMA*

The clinical child psychology training concentration at the University of Alabama (Tuscaloosa) exemplifies one of the many programs across the country that provide the components of training clinical child psychology with additional work in child health psychology following the format outlined in this chapter. In presenting a

*This section is based on the grant application to the National Institute of Mental Health for training in child mental health awarded to the University of Alabama, which was prepared by Carl B. Clements, Clinical Training Director, and Michael C. Roberts, Coordinator of Clinical Child Psychology.

description of the Alabama program, we do not want to imply that it is the only one conducting training relevant to the specialty. Indeed, there are several programs with excellent reputations for producing quality professionals and researchers. For example, we are aware of quality predoctoral training in clinical child psychology with an overlay in pediatric psychology at Purdue University, the University of Miami, and the University of Florida, among others. We should also note that the Alabama program does not purport to train child health psychologists per se; the training is in clinical psychology with a concentration of study in clinical child psychology and additional opportunities for work in pediatric psychology through practica and research activities. This format is consistent with the recommended training components outlined earlier and endorsed in principle by a variety of concerned organizations. We describe the details of this program to illustrate concretely how the rather abstract recommendations can be put into practice.

The basic goal of training in the Alabama clinical program is to develop scientist–practitioners who can apply research and intervention skills to the understanding, prevention, and treatment of human behavioral and physical problems. The basic doctoral program in psychology for the department emphasizes the importance of core knowledge in the social, cognitive, developmental, and biological aspects of behavior as well as the methodological foundations necessary to scientific advancement. Clinical psychology students take an additional sequence of courses designed to prepare them with the knowledge and skills for further understanding, assessing, and intervening in broad areas of behavioral problems. The clinical core includes: psychological assessment (two semesters), principles of psychotherapy, modification of behavior, psychopathology, and supervised practica in psychotherapy and intervention (two semesters). A portion of each of these core courses is devoted to child and family issues.

Beyond these core curricula (general and clinical), specialty students take coursework and practica in the clinical psychology concentration. A variety of employment experiences also expands the background in child-related psychology. Coursework, basic practica, specialty practica, and research requirements are usually completed in a 4-year period. Clinical students then receive internship training in which they solidify and refine their clinical skills particularly with children and families.

The specialty program relies on several faculty directly involved in publishing and serving in clinical child psychology with additional expertise in child health psychology areas. Additional expertise is provided by adjunct professors in pediatrics, psychiatry, family medicine, pharmacology, neuropsychology, and community mental health. The clinical training program heavily utilizes the department's Psychological Clinic, a fully functioning mental health agency. The clinic provides psychological assessment, referral, treatment planning, and direct intervention for a variety of clinical populations. All predoctoral clinical students receive most of their first 2 years of training in the clinic. All students, regardless of specialty, take the basic two-semester practicum. Sixty-eight percent of the assessment and intervention cases in this clinic involve children and/or families. Students additionally interact with a staff social worker, a consulting psychiatrist, local school teachers, juvenile court officers, and physicians. The clinic also serves as the contact point for a variety of community agencies and programs that have become a part of the clinical training resources.

Didactic Components of Specialty Training

Added to the general and clinical doctoral core curricula noted earlier, the clinical child specialty curriculum includes:

Child development, psychopathology, and treatment (two semesters)
Professional issues seminar in clinical child psychology
Mental retardation and developmental disabilities
Advanced clinical child practica (two semesters)

Within these courses, a considerable amount of attention is devoted to specialized work in child health psychology topics. Numerous other experiences (e.g., work stipend experiences and volunteered professional work) and courses (e.g., neuropsychology, psychopharmacology) augment these basic and specialized training components.

Child Development, Psychopathology, and Treatment. The didactic foundation of the specialty program consists of a two-semester course sequence. The first of the two semesters is designed to familiarize the student with an overview to the normal development of children, to behavior problems arising in childhood, and to the psychological treatment approaches for childhood psychopathology and physical syndromes. The last two topics include psychopathology in children in terms of etiology, diagnosis, and treatment from empirical, theoretical, and practical standpoints. The second semester of this course focuses on specific psychological and physical syndromes, their distinguishing characteristics, and research-supported treatment interventions. A range of clinical problems are covered including childhood emotional, behavioral, learning, physical, and cognitive disorders. Instructional modules of reading, lectures, and discussions include developmental psychopathology, prevention of psychological disorders, childhood psychosis and autism, psychological causalities and intervention in psychosomatic disorders, childhood depression, conduct disorders, learning and language disabilities, and residential, educational, and community treatment.

A required literature review paper of current important topics in child mental health is written by the student over the two semesters. Topics recently covered include conceptions of death, adolescent sexual behavior, children's perceptions of handicapped peers, and childbirth. There are five basic textbooks for this two-semester course (Walker & Roberts, 1983; Mash & Terdal, 1981; Quay & Werry, 1979; Ripple, Biehler, & Jaquish, 1982; Ross, 1981). Additional readings are selected from a list of books and journals in the pediatric psychology area (e.g., *Journal of Pediatric Psychology, Journal of Clinical Child Psychology, Pediatrics*).

Professional Issues Seminar. A seminar is offered on a continuing basis and is team-taught by faculty in the specialty. Students take the seminar for one credit each semester and are required to have a total of four credits. However, specialty students usually choose to participate whether registered or not for the course. The continuing and evolving nature of the seminar allows for a wide range of topics to be covered over a student's tenure in the program. The course format includes faculty lectures, journal and research reviews, student presentations, case conceptualizations, guest lectures, observations at various settings, and a class project each term. Topics covered in the past have included: psychological adjustment to chronic disease, special assessment techniques, family violence, public policy issues, ethics of research and treatment, learning disabilities, and autism. Guest lecturers have included social workers, a lawyer, child advocates, a speech therapist, a school psychologist, and a psychologist based at a community health center.

Students have made participatory observations at an infant stimulation program for motorically impaired or delayed infants (cerebral palsy, spina bifida, seizures, hydrocephalus, and premature infants) and a special summer program for autistic children.

Mental Retardation and Developmental Disabilities. This course provides an overview of the field of mental retardation and related disorders. It covers topics of definition and classification, diagnosis, causes, speech and language problems, care and education, research, and legal aspects. One section also deals with associated and complicating conditions of physical defects, epilepsy, cerebral palsy, autism, learning disabilities, and other psychological disorders. Enrolled students are assigned an apprenticeship with a staff psychologist at the state school for mentally retarded clients during which they conduct evaluations and participate in treatment planning of residents. The basic text is *Mental Retardation in School and Society* (Macmillan, 1982) with additional readings assigned on selected topics.

Advanced Clinical Child Practica. These advanced practica are required of upper-level students (typically fourth year) at the Capstone Medical Center (the principal training site of the university's medical school residency program in family medicine). Under the supervision of a medical center staff psychologist and department faculty, the students function through the outpatient clinics in psychiatry and pediatrics. They provide consultation with center staff and medical students for psychological problems arising in the medical clinics. Other clients are referred to the psychiatry clinic for assessment and treatment of psychological disorders and psychological concomitants to medical problems. Three psychiatrists with adjunct appointments in the psychology department and three pediatric faculty in the medical school provide consultation and referrals. The learning objectives of this practicum are for the student to:

1. Become familiar with the psychological problems present in a primary medical population and the interventions that have been demonstrated to be effective in these cases
2. Learn to conduct diagnostic interviews and psychometric assessments in response to referrals by medical personnel in order to determine the nature of psychological processes presented in a case and the effective treatment
3. Learn to initiate, upon referral, effective treatment interventions in the areas of behavior therapy, psychotherapy, parent training, and family therapy
4. Learn to initiate referrals to other community agencies where treatment might be more effectively delivered

5. Learn to evaluate the effectiveness of treatment interventions and modify the delivery of treatment in accordance with this evaluation
6. Learn to communicate the results of assessment and treatment to referring medical personnel in a brief understandable report, along with recommendations for future action on their part
7. Learn effectively to communicate issues, techniques, and underlying principles in clinical psychology to medical personnel through formal didactic teaching and informal case-related interactions
8. Become familiar with various service delivery settings for children, youth, and families including, for example, pediatric practices, a hospital pediatric ward, special education programs, day-care centers, and a speech and hearing center

Resource texts are also used in these specialized practica (e.g., Magrab, 1984; Roberts & Peterson, 1984; Tuma, 1982a; Varni, 1983; Wright, Schaefer, & Solomons, 1979).

Additional Learning and Employment Experiences

Using stipends from a National Institute of Mental Health training grant in child mental health, funded students in clinical child psychology obtain additional experiences in several settings. These activities include clinical work in the Adolescent Medicine Unit of Children's Hospital of Alabama (in Birmingham), a group home for delinquent boys, Parents Anonymous and a parent training program sponsored by the Family Counseling Center, the outpatient clinics of the medical center, and the local comprehensive mental health center. Clinical duties in these settings vary, but typically extend the basic experiences of assessment and therapy received in the department's clinic.

Other learning opportunities are through paid positions and volunteer work with two child programs related to the department. Brewer-Porch Children's Center is a residential center for emotionally disordered children administered in conjunction with the department. Third-year students assume funded positions as unit psychologists under the direction of two staff psychologists and working with educational specialists and social workers. Experiences include treatment planning, assessment, and individual therapy. The Early Childhood Education Day Care Center, also administered through the department, provides day-care experiences for disadvantaged preschoolers based on behavioral teaching techniques. Students have been involved in both experiential and research aspects of this program.

In an outside funded position, students also work on an adolescent unit of Bryce Hospital, a self-contained residential facility for the most severely and chronically disordered or psychotic adolescents in the state. Psychology trainees provide treatment planning and therapy under the supervision of staff psychologists who have adjunct professorships with the department.

Specialty Internships

After completing the doctoral curriculum, students go on to pediatric or clinical child psychology oriented internships, typically at medical centers. Recent settings have included the University of Oklahoma Health Sciences Center, University of Mississippi Medical Center, Oregon Health Sciences Center, and Children's Memorial Hospital of Chicago.

Specialty Research Activities

A master's thesis project on a child-related research problem is required of all clinical child students. These projects research various aspects of child health. In their third or fourth year, students develop an extensive literature review and conceptualization for a dissertation research topic. The preliminary examination includes an evaluation of a written document and an oral defense. Students then conduct, analyze, and write up the research, which is frequently on pediatric psychology topics. Recent theses and dissertations have been on topics of reducing stress due to medical procedures, preventing fetal alcohol syndrome, improving children's perceptions of physical and psychological disorders, effects of caffeine and sugar consumption on normal children, prevention of sexual abuse, and increasing children's use of car safety devices.

While in the specialty program, students collaborate with faculty on research projects resulting in publications and convention presentations. Recent articles have been on pediatric psychology topics such as prevention of injury and promotion of health in childhood, alleviating children's fears of medical settings, events, and personnel, improving children's attitudes toward chronically ill peers, family reactions to home apnea monitoring, and failure to thrive.

OPPORTUNITIES FOR TRAINING IN CHILD HEALTH PSYCHOLOGY

What should a student do who wants to go into child health psychology? We propose that students carefully consider the predoctoral programs providing clinical child specialty training and those providing other relevant training such as applied developmental psychology and counseling psychology. The training models and some programs are described by Roberts (1982) and a list of university programs is presented in Mannarino and Fischer (1982). The latest edition of the *Graduate Study in Psychology* manual (American Psychological Association, 1985) also should be reviewed. Based on these lists, the prospective student can write for application materials, which should be carefully examined for program goals and training content with respect to psychologists working with children, youth, and families (or more narrowly, for clinical child psychology). The student can rely on the topic descriptions noted in this chapter and the guiding principles of training psychologists to work with children, youth, and families (Roberts et al., 1985; Tuma, 1985). A comparison of programs' listed offerings with these suggested topics will help in selecting appropriate graduate programs. The prospective student should not necessarily rely on a program's accurate self-labeling as providing specialty training (Roberts, 1985). The research and professional contributions of the faculty listed for the various university programs can be obtained by consulting *Psychological Abstracts* to see what types of relevant work are being produced in a department. Examination of articles published in the *Journal of Pediatric Psychology*, *Health Psychology*, *Children's Health Care*, and other related journals can help identify institutional affiliations that might be conducive to specialty interests and training in child health psychology. Similarly, the editorial boards of these journals may indicate a strong professional identity with this area. In addition, the student can ask training directors to list where recent students from their program went for clinical internships. If their interns went to medical centers with significant availability of training in child work, then the preparatory work at the predoctoral level is more likely to be a useful background for child health psychology.

There are some lists available in which several programs are cited for training in pediatric psychology based on different criteria. None of these lists are definitive; they are only suggestive for the student to look further at the course offerings and faculty involvement. Routh (1985) listed the university origins of doctorates for members of the Society of Pediatric Psychology and found the top 10 were Purdue University, University of Iowa, University of Michigan, New York University, Boston University, Case Western Reserve University, University of Pittsburgh, George Peabody College, and Temple University. In another analysis, as evidence of where pediatric psychology research was being done, Routh (1980) listed the top 11 university affiliations of authors of articles cited by articles in the *Journal of Pediatric Psychology* and found University of Iowa, Columbia University, University of Michigan, Stanford University, Yale University, University of Illinois, University of Washington, University of Chicago, Harvard, University of Minnesota, and University of Pennsylvania. Of course, these lists will change over time, reflecting growth and development in the field, so prospective students are encouraged to examine more recent years of the relevant journals. These resources should be considered starting points with additional follow-up by the applicant to check out the content of training. There are published descriptions of predoctoral programs in clinical child psychology with some work in pediatric psychology (Purdue University—Ottinger & Roberts, 1980; Case Western Reserve University—Drotar, 1975; University of Alabama—Roberts, 1982; University of Washington—Perry, 1978).

Several internships have developed reputations for training pediatric psychologists. These include (but are not restricted to) University of Oklahoma Health Sciences Center, the University of North Carolina Medical School, Children's Hospital Medical Center in Boston, Children's Hospital of Chicago, and the University of Maryland, among others (Roberts, Quevillon, & Wright, 1979; Roberts et al., 1982). Again, we note that reputations wax and wane over time with changing faculty, interests, and resources. The prospective pediatric psychologist will find it necessary to check out the actual content of specialty training at the internship level. These lists are also problematic because there are likely several other programs with which we are not as familiar. With regard to postdoctoral training, Faust and colleagues (1980) listed the relevant considerations of programs as well as the various training sites offering postdoctoral training and fellowships.

June Tuma compiles a regularly updated *Directory of Internship Programs in Clinical Child and Pediatric Psychology* (latest edition: 1985–1986). This directory is a compendium of information about internship and postdoctoral programs including a listing of prerequisites, type and amount of specialty training, stipend, supervision, client characteristics, and caseload. The directory is the single most useful source in identifying internship programs for child health psychology. (The latest edition can be obtained for $8.00 from June Tuma, Department of Psychology, Louisiana State University, Baton Rouge, LA 70803.)

References

American Psychological Association (1985). *Graduate study in psychology*. Washington, DC: Author.

American Psychological Association (1977). *Standards for providers of psychological services*. Washington, DC: Author.

American Psychological Association (1981). *Ethical principles of psychologists*. Washington, DC: Author.

Committee on Accreditation, American Psychological Association (1980). *Accreditation Handbook*. Washington, DC: Author.

Committee on Accreditation, American Psychological Association (December 1984). Applied training for developmental psychologists. *Capsule: Newsletter from the APA Committee on Accreditation and the Staff of the Accreditation Office*.

Conger, J. J. (1976). Proceedings of the American Psychological Association, Incorporated, for the year 1975: Minutes of the annual meeting of the Council of Representatives, *American Psychologist, 31*, 406–434.

Drotar, D. (1975). Clinical psychology training in the pediatric hospital. *Journal of Clinical Child Psychology, 4*, 46–49.

Faust, D. S., Ulissi, S. M., & Thurber, S. (1980). Postdoctoral training opportunities in pediatric psychology: A review. *Journal of Pediatric Psychology, 5*, 277–286.

Kanoy, K. W., & Schroeder, C. S. (1985). Suggestions to parents about common behavior problems in a pediatric primary care office: Five years of follow-up. *Journal of Pediatric Psychology, 10*, 15–30.

Koocher, G. P. (1983, August). Competence in serving children: Credentials protectionism and public policy. Paper presented at annual convention of the American Psychological Association, Anaheim.

La Greca, A. M. (1985). Training survey results. *Newsletter of the Society of Pediatric Psychology, 9*(3), 19–21.

Maddux, J. E., Roberts, M. C., Sledden, E. A., & Wright, L. (1986). Developmental issues in child health psychology. *American Psychologist, 41*, 25–34.

Maddux, J. E., Roberts, M. C., & Wright, L. (1986). Health psychology for children: A step-child/stepping stone. *Journal of Clinical Psychology, 42*, 383–386.

Magrab, P. (Ed.). (1984). *Psychological and behavioral assessment in pediatric psychology*. New York: Plenum.

Mannarino, A. P., & Fischer, C. (1982). Survey of graduate training in clinical child psychology. *Journal of Clinical Child Psychology, 12*, 22–26.

Mash, E. J., & Terdal, L. G. (Eds.). (1981). *Behavioral assessment of childhood disorders*. New York: Guilford.

McClelland, C. Q., Staples, W. P., Weisberg, I., & Berger, M. E. (1973). The practitioners' role in behavioral pediatrics. *Pediatrics, 82*, 325–331.

Ottinger, D. R., & Roberts, M. C. (1980). A university-based predoctoral program in pediatric psychology. *Professional Psychology, 11*(5), 707–713.

Page, H. A. (1983). Review of a clinical post-doctoral training program. *The Clinical Psychologist, 36*, 65–66.

Perry, M. A. (1978). Development of a clinical child psychology training program. *Professional Psychology, 9*, 677–684.

Quay, H. C., & Werry, J. S. (Eds.). (1979). *Psychopathological disorders of childhood*. New York: Wiley.

Ripple, R. E., Biehler, R. F., & Jaquish, G. A. (1982). *Human development*. Boston: Houghton-Mifflin.

Roberts, M. C. (1986). *Pediatric psychology: Psychological intervention strategies for pediatric problems*. New York: Pergamon.

Roberts, M. C. (1985). The *places rated almanac* and training in clinical child psychology. *Journal of Clinical Child Psychology, 14*, 285–288.

Roberts, M. C. (1982). Clinical child programs: What and where are they? *Journal of Clinical Child Psychology, 11*, 13–21.

Roberts, M. C., Elkins, P. D., & Royal, G. P. (1984). Psychological applications to the prevention of accidents and illness. In M. C. Roberts & L. Peterson (Eds.), *Prevention of problems in childhood: Psychological research and applications*. New York: Wiley.

Roberts, M. C., Erickson, M. T., & Tuma, J. M. (1985). Addressing the needs: Guidelines for training psychologists to work with children, youth, and families. *Journal of Clinical Child Psychology, 14,* 70–79.

Roberts, M. C., Maddux, J. E., & Wright, L. (1984). The developmental perspective in behavioral health. In J. D. Matarazzo, N. E. Miller, S. M. Weiss, J. A. Herd, & S. M. Weiss (Eds.), *Behavioral health: A handbook of health enhancement and disease prevention.* New York: Wiley.

Roberts, M. C., Maddux, J., Wurtele, S. K., & Wright, L. (1982). Pediatric psychology: Health care clinical psychology for children. In T. Millon, C. J. Green, & R. B. Meagher (Eds.), *Handbook of clinical health psychology.* New York: Plenum.

Roberts, M. C., & Peterson, L. (Eds.). (1984). *Prevention of problems in childhood: Psychological research and applications.* New York: Wiley.

Roberts, M. C., Quevillon, R. P., & Wright, L. (1979). Pediatric psychology: A developmental report and survey of the literature. *Child & Youth Services, 2,* 1–9.

Ross, A. O. (1981). *Child behavior therapy.* New York: Wiley.

Routh, D. K. (1977). What is a clinical child psychologist? *Clinical Psychologist, 30,* 23–25.

Routh, D. K. (1980). Research training in pediatric psychology. *Journal of Pediatric Psychology, 5,* 287–293.

Routh, D. K. (1985, August). Training of pediatric psychologists: Discussion. Presented at the annual convention of the American Psychological Association, Los Angeles.

Silber, D. E. (1983). The emergence of a post-doctoral retraining program in clinical psychology. *Clinical Psychologist, 36,* 63–65.

Society of Pediatric Psychology. (1984). Minutes of the Executive Board mid-winter meeting, February 2-3, 1984. *Journal of Pediatric Psychology, 9,* 525–528.

Stabler, B., & Mesibov, G. B. (1984). Role functions of pediatric and health psychologists in health care settings. *Professional Psychology, 15,* 142–151.

Stone, G. C. (1983). *Proceedings of the National Working Conference on Education and Training in Health Psychology.* Special Issue of *Health Psychology,* 2(5).

Stricker, G. (1983). Respecialization in clinical psychology: The Adelphi model. *Clinical Psychologist, 36,* 62–63.

Stricker, G., Hull, J. W., & Woodring, J. (1984). Respecialization in clinical psychology. *Professional Psychology, 15,* 210–217.

Tuma, J. M. (Ed.). (1982a). *Handbook for the practice of pediatric psychology.* New York: Wiley.

Tuma, J. M. (1982b). Training in pediatric psychology. In J. M. Tuma (Ed.), *Handbook for the practice of pediatric psychology.* New York: Wiley.

Tuma, J. M. (Ed.). (1984). *Directory of Internship programs in clinical child and pediatric psychology: 1984-1985* (4th ed.). Baton Rouge, LA: Author.

Tuma, J. M. (1985). Recommendations: National Conference on Training Clinical Child Psychologists. Presented at annual convention of the American Psychological Association, Los Angeles.

Tuma, J. M., & Grabert, J. (1983). Internship and postdoctoral training in pediatric and clinical child psychology: A survey. *Journal of Pediatric Psychology, 8,* 245–260.

Varni, J. W. (1983). *Clinical behavioral pediatrics.* New York: Pergamon.

Walker, C. E. (1979). Behavioral intervention in a pediatric setting. In J. R. MacNamara (Ed.), *Behavioral approaches to medicine: Applications and analysis.* New York: Plenum.

Walker, C. E., & Roberts, M. C. (Eds.). (1983). *Handbook of clinical child psychology.* New York: Wiley.

Wohlford, P. (1978). A challenge to clinical psychology: Better training to serve children. *Journal of Clinical Child Psychology, 11,* 27–34.

Wright, L., Schaefer, A. B., & Solomons, G. (1979). *Encyclopedia of pediatric psychology.* Baltimore: University Park Press.

APPENDIX 2

Needs and Directions in Pediatric Medical Education

DANIEL L. COURY

The previous chapters of this handbook have discussed the various levels, specialized foci, and orientations of different perspectives of biopsychosocial assessment. What has yet to be described is how we are going to train health professionals, particularly pediatricians, in the use of these tools in their everyday practice. This chapter will discuss the current status of behavioral science training in pediatric programs in the United States and the needs for this training in pediatrics as perceived by different factions. We will then discuss the current obstacles preventing training in behavioral pediatrics from being more widely instituted, and possible directions for circumventing these obstacles.

A HISTORICAL PERSPECTIVE ON BEHAVIORAL PEDIATRICS

The term *behavioral pediatrics* has become popular in recent years despite the lack of a clear definition. It has been defined as "an area within pediatrics which focuses on the psychological, social and learning problems of children and adolescents" (Friedman, 1975, p. 515). This definition was later expanded to "the branch of medicine that treats the behavioral or psycho-social aspects of pediatric practice, teaching and research" (Friedman & Sarles, 1980, p. 219). The Task Force on Pediatric

Education in 1978 defined biosocial problems as "those health problems which are socially induced or complicated by social and environmental factors." A committee of the Society for Behavioral Pediatrics, which has been given the assignment of developing a definition of behavioral pediatrics, has yet to report on their progress with this task. Lastly, Levine, Carey, Crocker, and Gross (1983), in the preface to their text, *Developmental–Behavioral Pediatrics*, made the point that many children with disabilities or handicapping conditions develop "behavioral" concerns, while those with "psychosocial problems" commonly harbor underlying developmental problems. They went on to conclude that "the interplay makes it unjust to classify as exclusively behavioral or developmental such conditions as attention deficit, bedwetting, colic, teenage pregnancy, and mental retardation." The result of this thinking was that they titled their book *Developmental–Behavioral Pediatrics*.

For the purposes of this chapter, the terms *biosocial pediatrics, biopsychosocial pediatrics, psychosocial pediatrics*, and *behavioral pediatrics* will be used interchangeably.

Training in the area of biosocial pediatrics first received attention from the American Board of Pediatrics in 1951 in a statement on training requirements in growth and development. The board of examiners discovered that pediatric residents had no difficulty memorizing the facts related to motor skills development and psychological development, but had very little understanding of the clinical application of this knowledge in the treatment of patients. With the development of new vaccines and antibiotics for the treatment and prevention of infectious diseases, it is easy to see why many departments paid little attention to these recommendations in their training programs. Those programs that made attempts to teach the clinical relevance of these facts often did so through liaisons between their pediatric departments and departments of child psychiatry. Although the significance of this may have been missed by department heads, pediatric practitioners were finding that it was an important gap in their education.

The rationale behind forming liaisons with departments of child psychiatry is fairly clear. Most child development teaching at that time was based on the Gesell scales. The more behavioral aspects of the child's growth became the province of the child psychiatrist, who would be consulted whenever a child's behavioral activities did not fit the norm. Through the theoretical constructs of Freud and others, child psychiatry attempted to explain why the child developed these behavior patterns, and through psychotherapy worked on changing these into more normal behavior patterns. The result of these liaisons with departments of pediatrics was that pediatricians became aware of the severity of some childhood problems. However, these problems were so serious that they required the skills of a child psychiatrist for treatment. Many pediatricians thus felt unable to manage these problems, and learned only to refer to a child psychiatrist when they encountered such patients. Other pediatricians who wished to manage such problems in their practices found themselves left with no choice other than to pursue formal training through divisions of child psychiatry for a period of 1 or 2 years. The education received in such programs was aimed toward a career in child psychiatry, rather than being focused on the practice of pediatrics. This was perhaps in part due to the fact that child psychiatry evolved out of departments of adult psychiatry rather than having pediatrics as its foundation. As a result the psychiatric orientation of the management of childhood behavioral problems comes from a perspective of deviancy, while the practicing pediatrician is oriented more toward normalcy and the variations of normal.

The utilization of departments of child psychiatry to provide training in the behavioral aspects of pediatrics in many ways helped perpetuate the gap between this area and that of organic diseases. Behavioral pediatric problems were identified more with the child psychiatrist than with the pediatrician, and the lack of sufficient qualified teaching faculty in the department of pediatrics helped to maintain this identification.

Liaisons with divisions of pediatric psychology were the next attempt at providing training in behavioral issues. Pediatric psychology focuses on the mental health needs of children and is often based in a pediatric inpatient service or other pediatric health setting. By moving psychology into the pediatric arena, rather than having the pediatrician visit the psychologist's home turf, headway was made into convincing pediatricians of the usefulness of this knowledge of behavioral medicine in their daily practice. The success with programs of this type is variable, but it does manage to avoid some of the problems of child psychiatry liaisons. Awareness of the heavy workload of pediatricians in training and an ability to adapt to their schedules are an important part of helping such arrangements work effectively.

CURRENT STATUS OF BEHAVIORAL SCIENCE TRAINING IN PEDIATRIC PROGRAMS

As it became clearer that behavioral issues needed to be identified as pediatric responsibilities, pediatric departments began to make a more concerted effort to incorporate relevant training into the curriculum. The impetus behind such a move varied. In some institutions the primary motive was an attempt to comply with the recommendations of the Task Force on Pediatric Education, which will be discussed later. Some departments felt that this was an important part of the training and simply emphasized it for that reason. Still other departments were encouraged through the availability of monies from either private foundations or federal agencies. The Department of Health and Human Services offered funding for primary care residency grants that were based in internal medicine and family practice as well as pediatrics. Training in psychosocial and behavioral aspects of medical care was an important requirement for approval of such grant proposals, necessitating appropriate changes in the curriculum for all residents in order to receive funding for a few. The William T. Grant Foundation began funding behavioral pediatric programs in 1976. Although their emphasis was on incorporation of behavioral pediatrics in residency training, they had not required any specific format for this teaching. As a result, each of the 11 behavioral pediatric programs funded by the Grant Foundation has varied in its approach toward this training. Settings utilized have included outpatient clinics, intensive care units, inpatient wards, schools, and day-care centers. The format for teaching the residents varied from block rotations to continuity of care experiences through continuity clinics.

Friedman, Phillips, and Parrish (1983) have reported heavy utilization of the continuity clinic experience in a number of programs. They noted that the continuity clinic can be a very effective method of teaching behavioral pediatrics if it is perceived as a strong program in its individual institution. The advantages of utilizing continuity clinics for the teaching of behavioral pediatrics are several. First, the emphasis in such clinics tends to be on well child care. In this way, the role of the pediatrician is emphasized as the health care provider who should be involved with prevention or treatment of common behavioral disorders. Utilization of practitioners as preceptors in these clinics further enhances this model. Many ambulatory pediatric faculty members have limited patient practices and as a result many have limited experience with managing behavioral problems. The emphasis among many ambulatory faculty is on acute care in an outpatient setting. By utilizing competent community practitioners as teachers in continuity clinics, pediatricians in training learn the importance of a working knowledge in behavioral issues. For those situations requiring additional help, liaisons as previously described with departments of pediatric psychology have been very helpful. By utilizing such liaisons in continuity clinic settings, the pediatrician in training is able not only to encounter a patient with a behavioral problem (as he or she would in a block rotation) but also to follow the management and resolution of this problem over a period of time in the continuity clinic. One disadvantage of emphasizing biosocial pediatrics in the continuity clinic setting is the fact that some trainees will perceive this to be an outpatient issue and fail to recognize the relevance to care of inpatients.

In July 1977 the Department of Pediatrics at the University of Maryland instituted a structured 2-year behavioral pediatric residency program. This program was mandatory for all house staff training in their facility. The structure, implementation, and evaluation of this program has been discussed in several articles (Felice & Friedman, 1982; Friedman et al., 1983; Phillips, Friedman, Smith, & Felice, 1983). This program consisted of 4 months of formal training: the first 2 months occurring in the PL-1 year, and the second 2 months in the PL-2 year. The program was under the supervision of a full-time behavioral pediatrician in the department of pediatrics, and was emphasized to house staff candidates during their interviews with the program. Specific goals of the first 2 months of the PL-1 year were to teach basic skills and fundamental concepts in psychosocial issues and to influence pediatric house officers early in their training (so as to develop a positive attitude towards biosocial pediatrics). Topics identified as pertinent for pediatric interns included interviewing skills, knowledge of child development and common behavioral problems including hyperactivity, obesity, and enuresis; reaction of children and families to hospitalization; and grief and dying. Instruction was carried out not only by behavioral pediatricians and child psychiatrists but also by child life workers, social workers, psychologists, and nurses. Special efforts were made to have pediatric subspecialists involved as well. Subjects such as effects of hospitalization or death and dying were discussed by those specialists commonly encountering these problems, such as nephrologists and hematologists. In this way, emphasis was placed on behavioral aspects of pediatrics appearing not only in the outpatient setting but also in the inpatient setting. This also allowed the identification of numerous faculty members as role models, rather than relying on only the behavioral pediatrician or child psychologist.

The format for teaching was weighted heavily on didactic sessions during the first 4 weeks of the rotation. The last 4 weeks of the rotation saw increased patient responsibility, with a decrease in the number of didactic sessions. The didactic sessions totaled approximately 100 hours of direct contact between faculty and the pediatric residents on the rotation. Patients encountered during the rotation were then assigned to the resident for continuity of care through the resident's own continuity clinic. An individual behavioral pediatric supervisor was assigned to each resident for the rest of the year in order to assist and direct the resident in management of the patient.

The formal objectives for the second-year rotation were to expand the resident's clinical experience in behavioral problems; engage the resident as a member of a multidisciplinary team in the assessment of behavioral problems; and increase the awareness of the resident of the nonhospital management of these problems in schools and community agencies. Patient care took up approximately 75 percent of the teaching time during this rotation, with the remainder being didactic material. Clinical experiences during that second-year rotation focused on out-of-hospital visits to schools and day-care centers. Didactic seminars focused on learning problems, including mental retardation, special education, and chronically ill children in schools; family dynamics and family problems, including adoption, delinquency, and divorce; and pediatric intervention, such as family counseling and behavior modification.

The Task Force on Education in Developmental Pediatrics produced and field-tested a curriculum in developmental pediatrics in 1982 (Bennett, Guralnick, Richardson, & Heiser, 1984). This curriculum, often referred to as the Nisonger curriculum or the Ohio State curriculum, was field-tested in eight pediatric centers across the country, reflecting the different clinical facilities that are available at various institutions. The curriculum identified several specific topics such as mental retardation, motor disabilities, autism, learning disorders, and family issues, with which pediatric residents should be familiar.

The format of the curriculum utilized clear goals and objectives for each topic area. For example, one of the goals under "critical aspects of development and screening" was for the resident to describe common patterns of normal development and typical variations in those patterns. More detailed objectives under this goal were to describe a child's developmental status in the speech and language, cognitive, socioemotional, fine motor, gross motor, visual, and hearing areas. Content outlines for the topic area were then developed so as to display clearly the knowledge the resident was expected to acquire. Suggested clinical experiences were then described. Appropriate clinical experiences and an appropriate amount of time allotted to this training were two issues clearly addressed by the task force in developing this curriculum. They noted that some programs may only have 3 weeks allotted for such a rotation while others may allot two months. For this reason, they felt that the content of the curriculum was very important to outline. The structure or implementation was not as important as the end result of conveying the total content to the resident. Similarly, in regards to appropriate clinical experiences they noted that it was not necessary to have a specific clinic such as a cerebral palsy clinic, but that there was a need for a predictable mechanism by which residents could evaluate children with cerebral palsy or other handicapping conditions.

It was hoped that the Ohio State curriculum would be widely adaptable for the teaching of developmental pediatrics. Although not strictly behaviorally oriented, the subject matter does overlap with what others have called behavioral pediatrics and represents another format for incorporating behavioral pediatric training in residency programs.

THE NEED FOR BEHAVIORAL SCIENCE TRAINING IN PEDIATRICS

The greatly improved health of children in this country accompanying the decline of infectious diseases brought about by mass immunization practices has resulted in a changing of the traditional role of the pediatrician. While 50 years ago pediatric practitioners were predominantly concerned with battling life-threatening illnesses, over the past two decades they have become more concerned with the total well-being of the child, including social, behavioral, and developmental aspects. This trend has been described as the "new morbidity" and has been proposed as the new thrust and focus for pediatrics. A recent study of pediatric practitioners in the Rochester, New York, area has documented that pediatricians are indeed addressing more problems in behavior and development in their practices than in years past (Roghmann, Hoekelman, & McInerny, 1984). In addition, the general movement medicine has made away from exclusive consideration of disease and biological processes to a broader perspective has encouraged pediatricians to incorporate the growing knowledge of psychological, social, cultural, and environmental issues into their practice. Pediatricians are now reviewing the relationship between emotion and physical disease and beginning to address this and other issues in a more systematic fashion.

Changes in the population typically seen in a pediatric practice also have served to emphasize the importance of understanding behavioral and developmental issues. For example, children with chronic illnesses are constituting an increasingly large percentage of the patients in a pediatrician's practice. Improved technologies, new antibiotics, and various other medical treatments are allowing children with these diseases to live on into adulthood. Their physical illnesses impair their emotional and behavioral development in a manner not previously appreciated. Chronic illness has biological, behavioral, and social manifestations, and even the effects of stable biological conditions manifested in the behavioral and social aspects of a child's life will change over time. To treat this expanding segment of the patient population most effectively, pediatricians must be knowledgeable about behavioral and developmental issues and skilled in treating disturbances manifested in behavioral or developmental terms. To acquire this knowledge, pediatricians need training experience with children having behavioral and developmental problems. Increases in the prevalence of other disorders typically seen by the pediatrician, such as emotional and behavioral problems, have also served to focus attention on the pediatrician's need for knowledge and skills in behavioral and developmental pediatrics. Furthermore, these children often receive their care from a wide variety of health professionals within diverse settings. The pediatrician is thus in a unique position to serve as the coordinator of the child's care; however, in order to do so effectively he or she must have knowledge of other available resources and services. Of particular importance is a working knowledge of the interdisciplinary process as it relates to the health care of the child.

Physician Assessment of Needs in Pediatric Training

This chapter has thus far discussed the attempts of several training programs to provide training in behavioral–developmental pediatrics. Their motivating forces differ according to the decade in which they were initiated, accessibility to funds from granting agencies, and the program's perceived importance on the part of department chairmen. The future needs of pediatricians as envisioned by the American Board of Pediatrics in 1951 were becoming clearer by the late 1960s. Pediatric practices were beginning to change, and medical educators began a stronger emphasis on the behavioral sciences in medical training in order to meet these changing needs. Thus two intertwined forces became more apparent: professional needs as assessed by medical educators, and needs of the consumer receiving health care. Together these forces have impacted on medical education and promoted behavioral science education.

In 1969, the newly created National Center for Health Services Research and Development funded a 30-month study of the role of behavioral sciences in medical education. Due to the center's focus upon the delivery of health services, particular attention was aimed at the interplay between health services delivery, the behavioral sciences, and ongoing or potential curriculum changes within medical schools. During this same time, in early 1970, the National Board of Medical Examiners voted to establish an ad hoc committee to explore the possibility of establishing a new test committee covering the field of behavioral sciences. The early work of this ad hoc committee led to eventual formal recognition as one of the basic science test committees, along with anatomy, pathology, biochemistry, and others. The behavioral science portion of the national board examination was first formally given in June of 1972.

Coinciding with these two developments was a third major event. The National Institute of Child Health and Human Development sponsored a series of conferences known as the Allenberry Conferences. These dealt with the roles of psychology, sociology, and anthropology in medical school curricula. The persons involved in the presentation of these conferences established what later became known as the Association for Behavioral Sciences in Medical Education (ABSAME). This organization has remained active in promoting and developing behavioral science curricula in medical schools across the country. ABSAME also sponsored the publication of the summary report of the project funded by the National Center for Health Services Research and Development. This report, "Teaching Behavioral Science in Schools of Medicine," has been widely disseminated among medical educators in the United States.

The next major assessment of the needs of pediatric education came in the 1978 report of the Task Force on Pediatric Education. This interorganizational task force, with representatives from the American Academy of Pediatrics, Society for Adolescent Medicine, Ambulatory Pediatric Association, and Association of Medical School Pediatric Department Chairmen, among others, met monthly over a 2-year period. The members of the task force reviewed previously published materials and embarked on new research as well. In assessing the health needs of children and the educational needs of pediatricians who will serve them, they identified several core issues that posed problems. First, they identified biosocial and developmental problems as widespread and serious issues, and felt that all pediatricians should have the skill to cope with them. Secondly, they noted that the care provided to children with chronic handicapping conditions was inadequate, and recommended that residency programs emphasize this aspect more clearly. Thirdly, they also noted that the health needs of adolescents were being inadequately met and recommended improving health care and research in this area. Finally, they expressed an awareness of the fact that most pediatric practice is based in the office, while most pediatric education is centered in the hospital. They lamented the emphasis given to hospital care while recognizing that revenues generated from this care are the primary source of funding for pediatric programs. They called for a reevaluation and revision of reimbursement formulas to encourage pediatricians to treat biosocial and developmental problems. Many of the issues they identified are still issues today; the underlying problems continue to obstruct pediatric departments in their efforts to change pediatric education. The task force itself noted that it had no power to enforce its recommendations but hoped that they would be implemented as much as possible in various pediatric centers.

A study by Dworkin, Shonkoff, Leviton, and Levine (1979) added further credence to the concerns of the leaders in medical education. In this study, 97 randomly selected board-certified pediatricians in New England were surveyed to examine their attitudes toward their residency training and their current knowledge of developmental pediatrics. Their responses were overwhelmingly critical of the child development aspects of their training programs. Seventy-nine percent of the pediatricians rated their training in child development as inadequate and 47 percent rated the training received in medical school as having no value. Only 30 percent of the physicians viewed their residency experience as highly valuable. This lack of training had a significant effect on their practice of medicine, since 60 to 70 percent reported at least monthly interactions with the school nurse, a social worker, and a learning disabilities specialist. Forty to fifty percent acknowledged a similar frequency of communication with an audiologist, guidance counselor, classroom teacher, speech pathologist, and psychologist. Almost half of the physicians felt that this interdisciplinary communication was a highly valuable ongoing source of knowledge. The overwhelming majority felt that their accumulated clinical experience was highly valuable, but they just as strongly stated that they did not regard it as an adequate substitute for formal training. The Ambulatory Pediatric Association has also been actively involved in the introduction of appropriate behavioral developmental topics into undergraduate and graduate education in pediatrics. Through the "Standards for Graduate Medical Education in Pediatric Ambulatory Care" (1978) and the 1984 "Educational Guidelines for Training in General/Ambulatory Pediatrics" it has attempted first to set appropriate standards for training and then to delineate more clearly those topics that should be addressed at both levels of training. The "Guidelines" were organized around the three content areas of well child care, emergency pediatrics, and organ systems. The health care approach stressed in this document emphasizes physical, psychosocial, and cognitive development, as well as cultural and ethical issues.

The guidelines systematically present the knowledge areas the trainee is expected to acquire. For example, one objective under the section "anticipatory guidance" is for the trainee to "discuss contraception and venereal disease prevention with adolescent patients." The age group targeted in this instance is the adolescent, and the clinical experience is expected to occur in a health care setting that treats adolescent patients. Potential learning experiences for this objective would be both patient contact and didactic presentation from a faculty person to the trainee. Suggested methods of evaluation for this objective consist of observation of the student actually discussing this topic with a patient. Other objectives may have other targeted age groups, potential learning experiences, and suggested methods of evaluation.

The APA guidelines, like the report of the 1978 Task Force on Pediatric Education, are intended to serve as broad outlines for the content of undergraduate and residency training in general and ambulatory pediatrics. There is no accrediting agency that requires their complete or even partial utilization. They allow great latitude within their guidelines and make no attempt to be national standards of pediatric training. Nonetheless, their utilization, along with certain requirements of the Residency Review Committee for pediatrics, help ensure that pediatric training programs in this country do meet certain minimal standards.

Although the recommendations of the Task Force on Pediatric Education have had some influence on residency training, it has not been as widespread or strong as some would like. Weinberger and Oski (1984) surveyed pediatric residencies in an attempt to monitor the effect of the report and to assess the changes it effected on residency training programs. By requesting data from programs regarding training during the years 1980–1983 and training in the same program a decade earlier, they hoped to determine the impact of the report of the task force. A significant change was the number of programs requiring their residents to participate in continuity of care experiences, increasing by fifty percent during that period. There were also advances made in the availability of electives in the "new morbidity," but few programs required their residents to participate. Experiences in adolescent medicine and handicapping conditions were the same before and after the 1978 report. The authors noted that their survey failed to demonstrate any uniformity in residency training experiences in the area of the new morbidity. Considering the wide latitude allowed by the accreditation board for training programs, and the lack of power for the task force to enforce the recommendations, this is not totally unexpected. However, their conclusion that the traditional structuring of the content area had not changed dramatically since the report was published was disappointing.

A similar survey by Zebal and Friedman (1984) had comparable results. In assessing the status of behavioral pediatric residency training, they found that 49 percent of programs had a "formal" behavioral training program, with 38 percent offering some training and 13 percent offering no training. The types of training experiences offered, categorized as continuous training or block rotations, were fairly evenly split (52 and 48 percent respectively). It was noted that continuous training experiences were much more likely to be mandatory ($p < .01$) than block rotations, and mandatory experiences were offered significantly more frequently ($p < .01$) than electives. The nature of the training offered (whether it was formal, some, or none) did not differ according to whether the program was university affiliated, in a children's hospital, military hospital, or other setting.

Included in that survey were the 11 programs in behavioral pediatrics training funded by the W.T. Grant Foundation that were described by Friedman and colleagues (1983). Guidelines issued by the foundation for emphasizing behavioral pediatrics training included:

1. The formal inclusion of behavioral pediatric training experiences in the residency curriculum
2. The distribution of these experiences in all 3 years of pediatric residency training
3. The requirement that these be mandatory experiences for all residents in the program

There was no mandate from the funding agency requiring that each program follow an identical curriculum. As a result, each program was unique in content and implementation. Three of the programs mandated a continuous training experience through ongoing behavioral pediatrics teaching in a continuity clinic setting, while the other 8 programs developed block rotations that were primarily taken during PL-1 and PL-2 years (Friedman et al., 1983). Those programs instituting block rotations justified their choice by describing behavioral pediatrics as the equivalent of any other core area of pediatrics, with the resident requiring freedom from other major responsibilities in order to learn the material adequately. Those programs utilizing the continuity clinic approach were successful by seeing to it that the continuity clinic had a level of importance equal to that of other major rotations in the residency program.

The effectiveness of these programs has been described in several articles. Phillips and colleagues (1983) described the impact upon first-year residents of the Maryland program funded by the W.T. Grant Foundation. The residents were assessed for both knowledge and attitude regarding behavioral pediatrics. The residents' self-reported competence increased significantly over the course of the rotation. They noted an increase not only in the behavioral entities emphasized during the rotation, but in those not emphasized as well. The clearest effects of the training program were found for the residents' self-reported competence in diagnosis and management of behavioral entities, their perceived ability to advise and counsel parents and patients, and their knowledge of available resources for the management of children with behavioral problems.

Trent, Hock, and Yancy (1982) reported a similar evaluation of the W.T. Grant funded program at Duke University. They found that the residents entered the training program with positive attitudes about the relevance of behavior and development concepts to pediatric practice, and that they maintained these attitudes through their training. They also showed increasingly higher self-ratings on issues of competence as they progressed through the program.

Finally, Phillips, Friedman, and Zebal (1985) compared knowledge of both behavioral and organic aspects of pediatrics among residents taking the in-training exam of the American Board of Pediatrics. Her group broke down the residency programs into those funded by the W.T. Grant Foundation to institute training in behavioral pediatrics, those not funded by the foundation but providing mandatory training in this area, those that did not require behavioral training, and all others. They found a small to moderate positive correlation between the scores on the in-training exam and scores on behavioral questions. This correlation was highest for the "other" group and significantly lower for the funded programs, indicating that behavioral knowledge was more independent of knowledge of organic problems for the funded residents than it was for other residents. Funded and control (no required training) residents were significantly different in the PL-3 year, a difference out of proportion to the difference noted when these residents entered their training programs. Although residents entering the funded programs began with greater knowledge of behavioral pediatrics, they maintained a higher level of knowledge than residents in programs not emphasizing this training.

The effectiveness of a more structured curriculum focusing on developmental pediatrics has been demonstrated by Bennett and colleagues (1984). They evaluated the curriculum developed by the Task Force on Developmental Pediatrics in 1979, which was subsequently implemented in 11 pediatric programs. On a 7-point subjective scale the mean rating of the curriculum's usefulness was 6.0 and the residents' perceived competence in the skills of developmental pediatrics was 5.2. The mean percentage of this competence that the residents attributed to this structured curriculum–based rotation was 56.6. Although not compared with alternative forms of training in developmental pediatrics, the curriculum appears to be effective, and may reduce the wide variation in competencies in this area of resident training.

Child Health Needs Affecting Training

Despite strong recommendations from those bodies governing pediatric education, and the availability and effectiveness of model programs in behavioral–developmental pediatrics, there are indications that pediatricians are still not being adequately trained to provide this aspect of care in their practices. Deisher and colleagues (1965) reported that one out of four mothers was most concerned with her child's development, and one out of five with her child's behavior. A decade and a half later these concerns have changed very little. Reim and Adams (1980), in assessing mothers' concerns, found that half were worried about their child's behavior and one-fourth expressed concerns about their child's social skills or ability to pay attention. Hickson, Altemeier, and O'Connor (1983) interviewed 207 mothers seeking child care in private pediatric offices. They reported that only 30 percent of the mothers listed their child's physical health as their major concern. The remaining 70 percent described problems falling into the categories of psychosocial concerns. These included personalities and social development, mental development, adjustment to divorce and other life changes, discipline, mother–child interaction time, and adolescent transition. Yet only 28 percent of these mothers had discussed these concerns with their pediatrician. Reported reasons for not communicating with their physician on these subjects included a perception that their pediatrician could not help them, or that he or she lacked any ability or interest in helping them. One of the characteristics that correlated significantly with communication of psychosocial concerns was the physician's self-perceived ability and interest in handling these problems.

Another viewpoint on the role the pediatrician should take in evaluating and managing behavioral and psychosocial needs of the patient comes from a survey by Roghmann and colleagues (1984). This study described the changing pattern of pediatric practice in Rochester, New York, between the late 1960s and the later 1970s, and showed that the pediatric population had shrunk 21 percent from 1970 to 1980. It also noted a 24 percent decrease in the number of emergency room visits to the hospitals in the community, a reduction in the number of pediatric inpatient beds in the community, and a decrease in the pediatric bed occupancy rate from 70.9 percent in 1970 to 54.9 percent in 1981. During this same decade, the number of full-time-equivalent practicing pediatricians increased slightly. As a result, the number of patients seen and the number of telephone consultations weekly both decreased. Well child and preventive care visits accounted for approximately 40 percent of all visits to the pediatrician's office. The authors concluded that the decreased patient population and decreased acute care required by these children will allow pediatricians to spend more time on preventive, developmental, and psychosocial needs of these patients. It is clear that pediatricians will find themselves providing such care in the future not only because of the benefits to the patient but for economic reasons as well. Expertise in managing children's behavioral problems will likely be a marketing tactic in an effort to attract patients by offering expanded services.

NEW DIRECTIONS IN PEDIATRIC TRAINING

Guidelines of Accrediting Organizations

The scope and content of any pediatric training program are influenced by a great number of factors. Guidelines for pediatric training from the American Board of Pediatrics, and the need to be certified by this organization, help provide a minimal level of training in the spectrum of pediatric medicine. Certification by the American Board of Pediatrics requires training in an accredited pediatric training program. For a program to be accredited it must meet the general requirements for all residency training programs described by the Accreditation Council for Graduate Medical Education (ACGME) as well as the special requirements for training programs in pediatrics. These special requirements are approved by the residency review committee, its sponsoring organizations (the American Board of Pediatrics, the AMA Council on Medical Education, and the American Academy of Pediatrics), and the ACGME. The ACGME itself is composed of representatives of the five national associations interested in medical education. These are the American Board of Medical Specialties, the American Hospital Association, the American Medical Association, the Association of American Medical Colleges, and the Council of Medical Specialties Societies. Additional representatives include a resident in training, and federal and public representatives.

The general requirements for training programs delineate responsibilities of the institutions involved in the program, their organization, the eligibility and selection of residents for the program, and the appropriate evaluation of the residents in the program. The special requirements for residency training in pediatrics give more specifics regarding the structure of the curriculum. In the special requirements for 1986–1987 there is discussion of a minimum of 6 months of experience in primary care or ambulatory pediatrics. Less specific is the note that there must also be evidence of structured educational experiences in adolescent medicine, child development, psychology, and the care of the handicapped child. Other specifics mentioned include minimum and maximum numbers of months in certain specialty areas. The framework outlined by the residency review committee thus provides a well-rounded pediatric education by setting forth minimum and maximum amounts of training in specific areas. The specific content for those areas, however, is not always as clearly identified.

Additional guidelines and recommendations from the Task Force on Pediatric Education and the Ambulatory Pediatric Association give additional direction, again with the intent of meeting a minimal standard. This flexibility allows emphasis on specific topics to come from the person or persons developing the training program. A department chairman or director of residency training provides major influence on training in this way. Further direction of the proposed curriculum is then influenced by available faculty to teach the content; and their interests and skills in their respective specialties modify the content further. After the establishment of a written curriculum or an outline of content, judgments are made regarding the amount of time necessary to attain adequate knowledge in areas designated. Trainee assignment to various clinical areas is again dependent on factors that may be in conflict with the training process itself. Learning experiences in a certain content area may be limited by lack of patients, lack of faculty trained in the area, or lack of clinical facilities at the institution suitable for training in this area.

Altered Reimbursement Plans

There is also an influence from the number of patients in other health care delivery areas that may demand a greater allocation of trainees in order to provide appropriate patient care.

This has become a major problem during the last two decades. The leaders of pediatrics in America foresaw a change in the practice of pediatrics more than 30 years ago, and they have repeated attempts to develop appropriate training programs for the pediatricians of the latter half of this century. The attempts to broaden the pediatric training focus to include the new morbidity repeatedly run into the conflict of providing immediate care to the "newer morbidity." The newer morbidity encompasses those patients and conditions that have arisen from the great technological breakthroughs in medicine in the past 25 years. Before pediatricians can care for the new morbidity problems of a 2-year-old former premature, they must provide patient care and service to the newer morbidity problems of the sick premature in the hospital. Advances in pharmacologic and technologic management of cardiorespiratory problems have helped physicians to save many lives. Management of critically ill patients is very time and labor intensive, with a very high professional-to-patient ratio. Emergency rooms, neonatal intensive care units, and critical care units for older children can place a high demand on trainee allocation, especially in large tertiary care centers. The service demand for more residents in these newer morbidity areas results in decreased available time for training in the new morbidity.

The newer morbidity influences pediatric training in other ways as well. These time and treatment intensive areas generate high revenues that are a primary source of funding for residency and fellowship programs. Reimbursement for typical new morbidity treatments such as well child visits and anticipatory guidance is negligible if not nonexistent. Such financial considerations are often deciding factors in determining the role of behavioral pediatrics in a pediatric training program. Zebal and Friedman (1984), in their survey of behavioral pediatric training in residency programs, found that inadequate funding was the most frequently cited barrier to the expansion of behavioral pediatric training. Those programs that have the most success with behavioral pediatric training have received extensive outside funding.

A major advance in pediatric behavioral science training, then, would be a change in reimbursement policies of third-party payers that would encourage more practice in this area. Reimbursement at a level equal to that for acute care visits in outpatient facilities would greatly enhance the ability of programs to expand this area of training. Health maintenance organizations and other prepaid health care delivery systems could be of some benefit in this area. Because of their emphasis on promoting the wellness of the patient, strategies that would influence the development or management of psychosocial and behavioral problems can be implemented as part of well child care. Several such strategies have been developed, and many have been shown to be useful (Christophersen, Finney, & Friman, 1986).

With proven effectiveness and strong support for these activities by the American Academy of Pediatrics, third-party reimbursement for such preventive measures should be provided in a manner akin to that for routine dental checkups.

Structured Behavioral Training

The method in which behavioral training is delivered may vary between high-intensity block rotation and low-intensity continuous or longitudinal experiences; but, in either case, it is clear that a systematic process is needed. Previous studies by Phillips and colleagues (1985) and Bennett and colleagues (1984) have shown the effectiveness of systematic curricula in the teaching of behavioral and developmental pediatrics. Of special interest was the study by Phillips and colleagues in which they found not only that knowledge of behavioral pediatrics was unrelated to knowledge of more organic aspects of medicine, but also that training in this area did not limit the residents' acquisition of organic knowledge as shown by scores on the in-training examination given by the American Board of Pediatrics.

Systematic curricula can be implemented in more than one way. Block rotations, during which time the resident's major obligation is to learn behavioral developmental pediatrics, have some advantages. The resident is primarily devoted to experiences in child development and behavior, with ward duties generally being limited to night call. Behavioral pediatric training being delivered as a block rotation also gives it the status equal to that of other specialty areas. Lastly, evaluation of the trainee is simplified and the effectiveness of the rotation can be documented with few confounding variables. A disadvantage is the possibility that the resident will not carry these skills and knowledge into management of patients in other patient care areas.

Continuity clinics are a frequently used format for teaching behavioral pediatric issues. The concept fits well with the continuity of care delivered in a primary care setting. However, the implementation of such a plan is very highly dependent on strong support from the department, especially the department chairman. Friedman and colleagues (1983), in their review of the 11 programs funded by the W.T. Grant Foundation, noted that only 2 of the 11 programs gave the continuity clinic program equal importance with other major rotations. In those 2 programs, the chairman and the faculty had made it clear that ward and other responsibilities were to wait when the resident was scheduled to be in the continuity clinic. In one program, the department chairman would personally call those residents who were late or absent from the continuity clinic. Such emphasis, when present, can make a longitudinal experience such as the continuity clinic as effective as a block rotation. The additional use of a systematic curriculum for presenting select psychosocial issues can further enhance teaching in this setting. However, it must be emphasized that the low priority often given to continuity clinic programs can seriously undermine the effectiveness of this teaching approach.

Training of New Faculty

The lack of appropriately trained faculty described by Zebal and Friedman (1984) is a problem that is being addressed in various ways. The Department of Health and Human Services' Bureau of Maternal and Child Health is presently funding behavioral pediatric fellowship programs in a few select centers. Their emphasis is on the development of future academicians in the area of behavioral pediatrics, with a long-range goal of reducing the deficit of appropriately trained faculty. Other programs have found other methods for funding fellowship training in behavioral pediatrics. As a result, the Ambulatory Pediatric Association in their 1985 Fellowship Survey noted the only program area that increased in size from 1984 to 1985 was developmental behavioral pediatrics. Their survey showed an increase from 10 to 25 programs over that period, with an increase in fellows in training from 27 to 50.

Even the establishment of fellowship training programs will not meet the needs of pediatric residents unless these future academicians have a similar knowledge base from which to teach the essentials of behavioral pediatrics. Fellowship training, like residency training, tends to follow an apprenticeship model, with the result being a fellow who may have great expertise in one area but lack seemingly basic skills in another. In a survey of existing fellowship curricula in behavioral pediatrics, Coury, Mulick, and Haines (1986) reported that 16 of 60 programs responding to a questionnaire stated that they had no formal curriculum. Fourteen of the 60 programs reported that they designed the fellowship program around each fellow's individual interests and needs. The remaining 30 programs described a wide range of materials that they considered to be their curriculum. These curricula ranged from suggested reading lists to mandatory clinical experiences and rotations. Less than 15 percent of the programs described objectives and goals to be attained by the fellow during the training. Friedman (1985) has mentioned a need for "quality control" in behavioral pediatrics, and the use of structured curricula can address such a concern.

The Department of Pediatrics at Ohio State University, with funding from a grant through the federal Bureau of Maternal and Child Health, has developed a core curriculum in behavioral pediatrics at a fellowship level (Coury et al., 1986). Designed to train future academicians in the field, the curriculum addresses not only factual knowledge of behavioral and developmental issues, but other areas in which academicians must be knowledgeable. These include health legislation and policy planning, psychosocial aspects of chronic conditions, and the development of research and teaching skills. This curriculum is presently being used in the fellowship program in behavioral developmental pediatrics at Ohio State University, and plans for utilization in other centers are under way. Like the guidelines for ambulatory pediatric training of the Ambulatory Pediatric Association, and the recommendations of the Task Force on Pediatric Education, the curriculum is meant to provide a minimal standard of training in behavioral developmental pediatrics with great latitude for each fellow's scholarly pursuit of personal areas of interest.

Implementation of Curricula

The implementation of behavioral pediatric training curricula at both fellowship and residency levels requires more than a core faculty devoted to the field. It is imperative that the entire departmental faculty support the program, and that they emphasize behavioral issues in the management of patients in each specialty area.

Felice and Friedman (1982) described the involvement of the faculty in the development and implementation of a behavioral pediatric program at a residency level. Multiple day-long retreats were held for the purpose of discussing the program. Faculty fears, opinions, criticisms, and ideas were discussed and clarified. In the implementation of the program, faculty from throughout the department of pediatrics were utilized to cover the topics. A pediatric hematologist discussed death and dying; a pediatric nephrologist led the discussion on chronic illness and its effects on the family. Efficient implementation of a program is required if it is to be accepted and respected by pediatric trainees. Optimal implementation has multiple benefits. It improves the skills of the entire faculty; promotes subspecialists as role models, thus emphasizing that behavioral pediatrics is part of every patient contact; and promotes more thoroughness in patient care, in accordance with the recommendations of pediatric governing bodies and the interests of consumers.

Another proposed method for providing more behavioral pediatric training to those physicians who will be providing primary care is the possibility of pediatric training splitting into two tracks after the second postgraduate year. At that time, the pediatric resident would choose between a third year focusing on primary care and behavioral issues, or one geared toward subspecialty training and an academic career. Those trainees opting for the primary care route then have greater emphasis on ambulatory and psychosocial issues for their third year of training, while those selecting the subspecialty path would emphasize hospital care and research. Although this model may seem to put the major emphasis on behavioral issues in the training of those physicians planning on a career in practice, it perpetuates the division between organic and psychosocial factors in the practice of medicine. Subspecialists would be more highly focused on specific organ systems and conditions, and even less oriented toward the behavioral developmental concomitants of illness. In addition, it has been recommended (Friedman et al., 1983) that experiences in behavioral pediatrics should begin early in training at a time when attitudes regarding patient care are being formed. Institution of a two-track system would not completely resolve the current problem; the emphasis on behavioral pediatrics should come during the first 2 years of training, not the third.

An additional obstacle to behavioral pediatric training in residency programs has been the lack of meaningful research productivity. Department chairmen strongly emphasize research activity and publication of scientific articles as criteria for academic success; those faculty members who are highly productive in their field tend to garner more respect among their departmental colleagues. Respect and support for behavioral pediatric programs must not only come from department chairman and faculty, but must be earned and justified through solid research, just as any other section of a pediatric department earns respect. It is clear that more research will be done in the area in the near future. The W.T. Grant Foundation, which in the past has been a great supporter of behavioral pediatric training, has recently placed its emphasis in support of behavioral pediatric research. The Robert Wood Johnson Foundation has also focused on psychosocial issues, with funding for programs that improve the functional status of patients with chronic conditions among its interests. Future funding from federal sources is unclear in light of recent governmental cuts in appropriations, but in the long run should increase. The sound research being conducted by behavioral pediatricians in a few centers will hopefully continue and spread through other centers through the development and training of future academicians.

SUMMARY

The practice of pediatrics has changed remarkably over the last three decades. Near elimination of several once common childhood illnesses and a reduction in the severity and frequency of acute illnesses due to modern health care practices have changed the focus of the pediatrician's health care interventions. Once fatal diseases are now chronic conditions, and modern technology has saved many lives but posed new problems. The model for pediatric training must adapt to these changes in order to prepare pediatricians adequately for the delivery of contemporary primary care. Appropriately designed curricula to meet the needs of future pediatricians must take behavioral sciences into account, but not to the exclusion of the advances in other basic science areas. Training must move from the old model of the physician with encyclopedic knowledge to the new model of the physician as problem solver, with a sound fund of knowledge, awareness of the multiple factors influencing patient wellness and illness, and ability to access appropriate information or consultation as the need arises. The apprenticeship model of postgraduate training is evolving into a more standardized format, and should continue to head in this direction. The ultimate goal is not for each pediatrician to be a cloned product of such training, but for a continually rising baseline of competence in both behavioral and organic aspects of medicine.

Structured, systematic curricula for training pediatricians in behavioral and psychosocial issues have been shown to be effective. The major obstacle at this point is finding the time in their training to expose them to these issues, and securing appropriately trained faculty to present these subjects. The possibility of carving out a block rotation rests in the hands of individual pediatric departments and their chairmen, and is unlikely ever to become mandatory due to more pressing patient care demands in critical care areas. Increased and mandatory involvement in resident continuity of care clinics is more feasible and likely to occur. Such involvement can be mandated through the guidelines of the residency review committee for pediatrics.

An influx of appropriately trained faculty is on the horizon. The Department of Health and Human Services' Bureau of Maternal and Child Health has recently funded several new fellowship programs with the expressed purpose of training future academicians in the field of behavioral pediatrics. In the interim, appropriate role models can be found in many pediatric communities by including practitioners as potential teachers. Ancillary services such as pediatric psychology, social service, and special education can also augment the skills of these practitioners and serve as models of interdisciplinary care for physicians in training. Pediatric residents will better appreciate the importance of these issues when they see a respected local practitioner addressing them in an exemplary fashion through a continuity clinic setting. Such programs would have the additional benefit of serving as models for pediatricians in practice, and the potential of continuing medical education through these programs exists. In this way the training needs of present and future pediatricians can be met, and attention to psychosocial issues can become a more routine part of medical practice.

References

Bennett, F. C., Guralnick, M. J., Richardson, H. B., & Heiser, K. E. (1984). Teaching developmental pediatrics to pediatric residents: Effectiveness of a structured curriculum. *Pediatrics, 74,* 514–522.

Christophersen, E. R., Finney, J. W., & Friman, P. C. (Eds.) (1986). Prevention in primary care. *Pediatric Clinics of North America, 33* (4).

Coury, D. L., Mulick, J. A., & Haines, G. K. (1986). *Current status of fellowship curricula in developmental–behavioral pediatrics.* Unpublished data, Ohio State University.

Coury, D. L., Mulick, J. A., Eaton, A. P., Heron, T. E., Bruce, N. M., & Showers, J. (1986, May). *Structure and implementation of a fellowship curriculum in developmental–behavioral pediatrics.* Workshop presented at the annual meeting of the Ambulatory Pediatric Association.

Deisher, R. W., Engel, W. L., Spielholz, R., and Standfast, S. J. (1965). Mothers' opinions of their pediatric care. *Pediatrics, 35,* 82.

Dworkin, P. H., Shonkoff, J. P., Leviton, A., & Levine, M. D. (1979). Training in developmental pediatrics. *American Journal of Diseases of Children, 133,* 709–712.

Felice, M. E., & Friedman, S. B. (1982). Teaching behavioral pediatrics to pediatric residents: The state of the art and description of a program. *Journal of Developmental & Behavioral Pediatrics, 3,* 225–231.

Friedman, S. B. (1985). Behavioral pediatrics: Interaction with other disciplines. *Journal of Behavioral Pediatrics, 6,* 202–208.

Friedman, S. B. (1975). Foreword on Symposium on Behavioral Pediatrics. *Pediatric Clinics of North America, 11,* 515–516.

Friedman, S. B., Phillips, S., & Parrish, J. M. (1983). Current status of behavioral pediatric training for general pediatric residents: A study of eleven funded programs. *Pediatrics, 71,* 904–908.

Friedman, S. B., & Sarles, R. M. (1980). Introduction to issues in behavioral pediatrics. *Pediatric Annals, 9,* 219.

Hickson, G. B., Altemeier, W. A., & O'Connor, S. (1983). Concerns of mothers seeking care in private pediatric offices: Opportunities for expanding services. *Pediatrics, 72,* 619–624.

Phillips, S., Friedman, S. B., Smith, J., & Felice, M. E. (1983). Evaluation of a residency training program in behavioral pediatrics. *Pediatrics, 71,* 406–412.

Phillips, S., Friedman, S. B., & Zebal, B. H. (1985). Residents' knowledge of behavioral pediatrics. *Journal of Developmental & Behavioral Pediatrics, 6,* 268–272.

Riem, K. F., & Adams, R. E. (1980). Assessment of mothers' concerns about infants, toddlers and preschoolers. *Infant Mental Health Journal, 1,* 56.

Roghmann, K. J., Hoekelman, R. A., & McInerny, T. K. (1984). The changing pattern of primary pediatric care: Update for one community. *Pediatrics, 73,* 363–374.

The Task Force on Pediatric Education. (1978). *The future of pediatric education.* Evanston, IL: American Academy of Pediatrics.

Trent, P. J., Hock, R. A., & Yancy, W. S. (1982). Evaluation of behavioral and development training for pediatric residents. *Journal of Medical Education, 57,* 113–118.

Weinberger, H. L., & Oski, F. A. (1984). A survey of pediatric resident training programs 5 years after the task force report. *Pediatrics, 74,* 523–526.

Zebal, B. H., & Friedman, S. B. (1984). A nationwide survey of behavioral pediatric residency training. *Journal of Developmental & Behavioral Pediatrics, 5,* 331–335.

Author Index

Subject Index